CLINICAL INTENSIVE CARE

Clinical Intensive Care

KEN HILLMAN
The Liverpool Health Service,
Sydney

GILLIAN BISHOP
The Liverpool Health Service,
Sydney

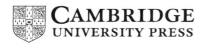

CAMBRIDGE
UNIVERSITY PRESS

Published by the Press Syndicate of the University of Cambridge
The Pitt Building, Trumpington Street, Cambridge CB2 1RP
40 West 20th Street, New York, NY 10011-4211, USA
10 Stamford Road, Oakleigh, Melbourne 3166, Australia

First published 1996

Printed in the United States of America

Library of Congress Cataloging-in-Publication Data

Hillman, Ken.
Clinical intensive care / Ken Hillman, Gillian Bishop.
p.   cm.
Includes index.
ISBN 0-521-47812-X (pbk.)
1. Critical care medicine – Handbooks, manuals, etc.   I. Bishop,
Gillian.   II. Title.
[DNLM: 1. Intensive Care – methods – handbooks.   WX 39 H654c   1995]
RC86.8.H54   1995
616′.028–dc20
DNLM/DLC
for Library of Congress   94-45762

A catalog record for this book is available from the British Library.

ISBN 0-521-47812-X paperback

CONTENTS

v

PREFACE

The book is intended for junior members of a medical staff who rotate through intensive care units (ICUs), as well as for other physicians who are involved in managing patients in an ICU, but not as their primary specialty. It may also prove useful to any member of the paramedical or nursing profession who is involved in acute medical care. The book initially arose from the need to give resident medical staff rotating through our own ICU a crash course in intensive care medicine. At present, this subject is not universally taught to undergraduates, and too often their exposure to it at the post-graduate level turns out to be a matter of learning by experience.

Intensive care medicine is an exciting and rapidly developing specialty. There are two major problems inherent in writing a book about it at this time. Firstly, it may be out of date before it is published, and secondly, it may not capture the flavour of intensive care medicine. Just as convening a committee of specialists, each representing a different organ system, may not necessarily be the best way to approach the multiorgan problems of the critically ill, a book on the specialty of intensive care medicine that only summarizes the conventional wisdom from other specialties may not be the best book on intensive care medicine. It is a new specialty, drawing on the knowledge of other specialties, but also having expertise unique to itself. The specialty has its own journals and meetings as well as nursing and medical specialists. We have tried to make this book reflect the uniqueness of intensive care medicine. We have also incorporated as much recent knowledge as possible, in order to prevent premature ageing.

The core of the book concentrates on areas common to all critically ill patients, rather than on specific diseases. These chapters are to be found mainly in the first part of the book. It is essential to understand the basic pathophysiological principles common to all seriously ill patients before concentrating on individual disease entities. Thus, the chapters on routine care of the seriously ill, fluids, nutrition, cardiovascular failure, respiratory failure, infection, resuscitation, sedation, ventilation, monitoring, and intracranial disasters are relevant to all seriously ill patients, no matter what the cause of the disease process. These chapters represent the core knowledge of intensive care medicine. We have devoted the remaining chapters to specific problems and diseases: haematology, gastroenterology, nephrology, endocrinology, the respiratory system, cardiovascular pathology, poisoning, and neurology. Discussion in these chapters is limited to its relevance in the setting of the seriously ill. The reader is continually referred from these specific chapters to core chapters. Finally, no matter what size a book about intensive care is, it cannot afford to dismiss economic and ethical issues. These are covered in one of the earlier chapters. Readers are encouraged to familiarize themselves with the core chapters and to refer to chapters on individual diseases as necessary. At the end of each chapter we have included a list of articles and books for further reading.

Many chapters also have problem-oriented guidelines to aid the reader, for there are numerous problems encountered by junior medical staff that are common to different diseases, but are not often specifically addressed. Examples include the sections on fighting the ventilator, interpreting non-specific opacities on the chest radiograph, dealing with a confused patient and dealing with the sudden onset of hypoxia. We have tried to identify the most important topics so as to assist the resident when confronted with these practical problems in the ICU. These guidelines are scattered throughout the book in relevant chapters, and for easy access, a list is provided at the beginning of the book.

Because of the rapidly developing nature of intensive care medicine, we have drawn on recent publications and integrated their findings into 'accepted practice'. Accepted practice is, of course, a variable and mobile concept. One of dilemmas is to distinguish between initial enthusiasm and a growing weight of opinion. For example, we believe that there is a trend away from invasive monitoring to non-invasive monitoring, and we have put what we consider appropriate emphasis on that development. Similarly, we sense a tendency to select a ventilatory strategy relevant to a given patient, rather than simply employing controlled mandatory ventilation. Time and more research will demonstrate whether or not this is correct. In combining the latest information with the accepted practice, we have tempered the final guidelines with what we have found to work in the clinical situation. We make no apology for the clinical flavour of the book.

As much as one might wish to avoid controversy in a text-book, that could be achieved only by reverting to bland and vague suggestions such as 'support the patient', 'give fluids', and 'give oxygen'. We have tried, wherever possible, to give precise and meaningful 'bottom-line messages'. In doing so, we run the risk of giving advice that is not accepted by everyone. We have taken that risk, rather than resorting to vague and safe alternatives, secure in the knowledge that the individual specialists who supervise junior medical staff encourage appropriate modifications in patient management within the unit's own protocols.

Finally, we would like to gratefully acknowledge the inspiration and pleasure we have experienced while working with all our junior medical colleagues and nursing staff in intensive care over the years.

ACKNOWLEDGEMENTS

Books such as this come about only as a result of inspiration and input from many sources. The list of people who contributed to this work is long. First and foremost is Sue Williams, the secretary to our department, who not only typed many drafts but also corrected them and contributed valuable advice. Additional assistance in preparing the manuscript was provided by Jacquelene Barnes. We are indebted to Richard Barling at Cambridge University Press for his patience, inspiration, and support.

Our colleagues generously contributed a great deal of their time to review many of the chapters. Special thanks to Mike Buist, whose wisdom and knowledge are greatly appreciated, especially in regard to the cardiovascular chapters. Thanks also to Ian Gosbell, at Liverpool Hospital's microbiological department, for adding a much needed dimension to the sections on infection. Stephen Deane brought clarity and new perceptions to our approach to acute limb conditions. We borrowed or modified many gems from Howard Roby, our specialist colleague in the intensive care unit. Others to whom we are indebted include Stephen Streat, at Auckland Hospital in New Zealand, for his contributions to the chapters on trauma and nutrition, and Marcus Cremonese, for his excellent illustrations.

The inspiration for this book came from many nursing and junior medical colleagues with whom we have been privileged to work over the years. They infused life and meaning into the messages contained in this book and kept us honest.

1
ORGANIZATION OF AN INTENSIVE CARE UNIT

THE SPECIALTY OF INTENSIVE CARE MEDICINE

It is generally agreed that the specialty of intensive care medicine began in Copenhagen in the early 1950s. During the poliomyelitis epidemic at that time, patients were treated by tracheostomy and prolonged manual ventilation. As a result of those measures, the mortality rate was reduced from 87% to an impressive 40%.

Although there are now many types of intensive care units (ICUs), such as medical, paediatric, respiratory, surgical, neurosurgical, cardiothoracic surgery, and trauma, they all perform the same basic function: caring for the seriously ill. Caring for a group of these patients in a single space makes economic and medical sense. Our expertise in intensive care has increased enormously since the early 1950s, and there are now specialized medical and nursing staff devoted solely to intensive care medicine.

Specialists working with the seriously ill must be familiar with complicated technology, physiology, and pharmacology, as well as conventional medicine. However, it is even more important to become familiar with the unique requirements of critically ill patients – to develop expertise in their individual patterns of illness. These patients often do not conform to the conventional artificial divisions of medicine: 'Surgical' patients can develop 'medical' diseases. 'Medical' patients may develop 'surgical' diseases. The body must be looked at as a whole, rather than as a series of independent organs. This requires that we break away from the tendency toward increasing medical specialization based on individual organs. Rather than a 'super-specialty', intensive care medicine is a very broad general specialty, based on the body as an integral system, rather than an organ-based super-specialty.

Advice from all of the single-organ specialists must often be sought. The intensive care specialist must balance all such expert opinions and fit them into an overall strategy. What is good for one organ may be detrimental to others, as well as to the patient's overall condition. One cannot take a committee approach to the seriously ill. One doctor must take ultimate responsibility and make the final decision, and that doctor must have appropriate training in intensive care medicine and not be an absentee landlord. It matters little from what background intensivists come – anaesthetics, medicine, or surgery – as long as they have highly developed clinical skills. Such skills can be gained only by spending time with seriously ill patients. The problem of territorial control by the various specialties (which physician controls which patients) was an early feature of this specialty, but that attitude is gradually being replaced by practice based on what is best for the patient.

Intensive care medicine arose from the need for physicians with skills in acute medicine. In a referral ICU, it is too much to expect a nurse from a general ward or a doctor who works only in another specialty to be able to cope with all of the problems unique to the critically ill. Both doctors and nurses in ICUs require specialized training, specialized books and journals for reference, and specialized meetings to share their knowledge and experience. Above all, they need to be working regularly with the seriously ill. This does not mean that they should not seek advice from colleagues in other specialties, when needed, just as is done in all branches of medicine. However, a permanent clinical and administrative medical and nursing presence is essential for the best clinical practice.

INTENSIVE CARE PERSONNEL

The permanent senior medical and nursing staff must provide continuity of care and ensure that standards are maintained within an ICU. They are responsible for the orientation, education, and training of new staff. Junior medical staff usually rotate through the ICU for varying periods, and that can lead to inconsistency in the care of patients unless standardization is ensured through protocols, supervision, and educational programmes.

Maintaining a constant high standard of intensive care is the greatest challenge for an ICU. The nursing staff are the mainstay in achieving that goal. They are responsible for most of the minute-to-minute monitoring and treatment. In addition to conventional nursing responsibilities, much of the clinical decision making can be decentralized to a skilled nursing staff. This requires investment in teaching, in-service programmes, and audits directed at the bedside nurse. Examples of the expanded nursing role include the following:

WEANING The weaning process (e.g., adjusting ventilatory rates and pressures) can be carried out by the nursing staff using laboratory data and bedside monitoring.

DRUGS Inotropes, vasodilators, sedatives, analgesics, insulin, and many other drugs can be given by continuous intravenous infusion. Adjustments of infusion rates can be decided by nursing staff, based on clinical and laboratory data.

FLUIDS Transient oliguria and hypotension are common in intensive care patients. Most patients will respond to a fluid challenge. This can be done by nursing staff, with recourse to medical staff if the fluid challenge fails.

OTHER ASPECTS OF WARD FUNCTION The nursing staff should be integrated into all aspects of administration of the ICU, in addition to taking care of the patients and dealing with their friends and relatives. Other additions to the intensive-care staff may include physiotherapists, ward clerks, social workers, and ward attendants. They are all essential for an efficiently run team. Although it is difficult to measure the effect on patient outcome of a well-organized team with high morale and a sense of job satisfaction, most experienced intensivists value this aspect of their unit highly and invest time and energy in achieving it.

WARD ROUNDS AND CONTINUITY

There should be at least one comprehensive ward round each day. The half-life for major decisions regarding seriously ill patients is approximately 24 hours, whereas for patients in general wards it is approximately 3–4 days. The medical staff, nursing staff, and others involved in a patient's management should formulate a strategy for the next 24 hours. This is a framework around which fine tuning can occur, depending on changes in the patient's condition and the findings on laboratory tests. Like other strategies, it must be flexible enough to allow changes according to the patient's condition. Rather than using a system that features a provisional diagnosis and final diagnosis, one must take a problem-oriented approach to seriously ill patients (see p. 11).

Despite the drama involved in the ups and downs of the critically ill, there are many predictable patterns. Apart from the initial resuscitation period, these patients usually become 'stably unstable' rather than 'unstably unstable' – a new equilibrium is reached, and the patient usually remains at that plateau for some time.

Apart from the on-site personnel, a senior member of the medical staff should be on call or on duty 24 hours per day for clinical or administrative consultation.

BOUNDARIES OF INTENSIVE CARE MEDICINE

Acute-care hospitals are becoming increasingly expensive. There is considerable pressure on clinicians to reduce the time that patients must spend in the hospital. For example, many surgical patients undergo day-only surgery, and many of those who do not are assigned to early discharge programs in order to achieve more efficient and less expensive forms of treatment. Physicians who manage medical patients are subject to the same pressures. The aged, the dying, and the chronically ill are being managed in more efficient, less acute, and probably more appropriate environments. Many investigations are being carried out on an outpatient basis, and medical procedures often are performed on a day-only basis. Acute-care hospitals are increasingly becoming limited to the role of caring for acutely ill patients with reversible illnesses. This means that the role of the intensive care specialist is becoming more important. ICUs are now being asked to care for groups of patients at different levels of illness. A seriously ill patient on assisted ventilation requires a 1:1 nurse:patient ratio, whereas a patient who has had, for example, a thoracic epidural insertion for abdominal and thoracic injuries and is being given continuous positive airway pressure (CPAP) may require a 1:2 ratio, and a non-intubated post-operative patient with uncomplicated vascular disease may need only a 1:3 ratio. Nevertheless, the skills required for managing the most seriously ill patients are similar to the skills necessary during immediate post-operative care for patients with complicated conditions. Increasingly we expect to see a blurring of the general-ward role and the intensive care role.

Despite the fact that we strive for excellence in caring for seriously ill patients in the ICU, an important factor in a patient's outcome is what happened immediately before that patient was admitted to the ICU. The importance of the initial resuscitation period for a patient who has suffered severe trauma has been appreciated for many years. The concept of the 'golden hour' derives from the finding that the outcome is largely determined by how rapidly the patient's airway is restored to patency and the cardiorespiratory status is stabilized. Many hospitals now have rapid-response teams skilled in airway management and rapid resuscitation. It would seem to make sense to define similar criteria for other medical and surgical conditions. If the factors that lead to life-threatening deterioration or even cardiorespiratory arrest could be identified, then a rapid-response team consisting of the most skilled and senior clinicians could be dispatched to rapidly assess and resuscitate such patients. The era in which the most junior and most inexperienced doctors have been caring for the most seriously ill patients in general wards and in emergency departments is passing. A 24-hour system for providing resuscitation and review by more experienced, senior personnel before patients deteriorate or go into cardiorespiratory arrest will ultimately make the efforts of the intensive care staff more successful and more rewarding.

RELATIVES AND FRIENDS

The condition of a patient should be explained in an honest and forthright manner to relatives and friends. There is no place for false hope and avoidance of difficult explanations – even if it means admitting that many aspects of the patient's disease process are as yet unknown. Much of the practice of intensive care medicine is titrational (eg trying an inotrope or antibiotic and looking for a response, without necessarily understanding all aspects of the interactions involved), and this should be explained honestly to the relatives.

It helps to have a special information pamphlet for the patient's friends and relatives that will explain certain matters:

- relevant aspects of the hospital's functioning
- visiting policy at the ICU

- the invasive lines and machines that may be encountered, with an explanation of their functions in lay terms; labelled photographs of the various pieces of equipment and lines, with a short description of each, can be displayed in the waiting room

An explanation of the possible time course of the patient's illness must be given. Many relatives wish to maintain an all-night vigil during the early part of a critical illness, when the patient conceivably could remain stable for days or weeks. It is important to inform relatives of such possibilities so that they can arrange their schedules regarding sleep, work, and other responsibilities. Relatives and friends should be told to prepare themselves for a marathon, rather than a 100-m dash. It is important to provide ongoing support and counselling for relatives and friends, either by the medical and nursing staff or by more specialized personnel.

QUALITY ASSURANCE

Quality assurance (QA), auditing, and peer review are all concepts that generally have to do with monitoring and attempting to improve current practice. The idea behind most efforts in this area is that practitioners can demonstrate to themselves and to others the quality and quantity of work they are doing.

The principles of QA and total quality management (TQM) readily lend themselves to managing an ICU. QA is not simply a matter of conducting an audit; it encompasses the principles of how an organization should be run – in our case an ICU. The Japanese have run their industries on a similar basis for decades. They call the concept *kaizen,* or 'the continuous search for improvement' in oneself and in the system. In order to accomplish this effectively, we need to shed much of our previous conditioning and training. Decision making and autonomy must be decentralized to the bedside. The ability to make decisions comes through education. Making changes is difficult, and many who have been trained in a different way will feel uncomfortable. We need, ultimately, to reach the point at which we begin to feel comfortable with many of the unpredictable aspects of our practice, until eventually we can thrive on the non-routine. Managers must learn to authorize others to solve their problems, and managers themselves must learn to find ways of saying yes, rather than finding fault and being obstructionist. The staff need to be encouraged to be autonomous and to speak out when the system is not working. We need to eliminate senseless rules, and we need to carefully examine everything we do and always ask why. Rules should be replaced by guidelines and priorities. A collective rhythm must be created whereby quality can be coaxed out of the available resources, which often are inadequate. The key to an organization's success is to master the art of orchestrating collective thinking. The common good should always be put above one's own. This system will not be the place for large egos that are easily bruised.

The principles of this new style of management include the following:

• The quality of patient care can be improved by removing the causes of problems in the system.

• Problems can be solved only after they have been identified.

• The person who is doing the job probably is the one most knowledgeable about that job.

• People want to be involved in running the unit and doing their jobs well.

• People should be authorized and encouraged to bypass managers and solve problems themselves.

• Fear and defensive attitudes are easily instilled; it is much more difficult to get people to commit to an adventurous new vision. Supervisors and managers must be specialists who will support their people when problems arise. Authority must come from within.

• A structured problem-solving process, with all of the relevant players being involved, will produce better solutions than an unstructured process.

• There will be a lot of resistance to implementation of this new style, both within the unit and, more importantly, outside the unit, during the period of transition. This must be resolved along the way, and, if necessary, a little pocket of excellence must be developed.

The philosophy of QA must be deployed to permeate all aspects of the running of the ICU and must be extended to all areas with which the ICU interacts. For example, the outcome for a patient who has suffered major trauma will depend as much on the system in place for initial management as on the treatment given in the ICU. All parts of the larger system must communicate in terms of QA if treatment is to be improved (Figure 1.1).

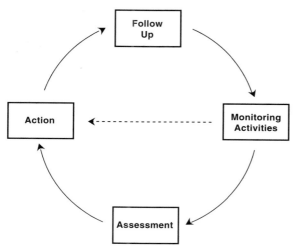

FIGURE 1.1   The quality-assurance cycle.

Examples of QA programmes in intensive care are as follows:

- mortality review (exclude if death is expected)
- review of patients' and relatives' complaints
- review of readmissions rate to the ICU
- review of prolonged length of stay (eg more than 30 days)
- review of fire and safety practices
- problem-identification workshops using flow charts
- review of nursing practices in order to eliminate outmoded practices (eg the way in which observations are recorded and action is taken)
- publication of newsletters
- critical-incident monitoring for unexpected events

Honest peer review of QA cannot be imposed. If the programme is to work properly, it must have the cooperation and commitment of all staff. This should lead to a system in which power is shared to produce the outcomes agreed on, rather than focusing only on the process.

TROUBLESHOOTING

ASSESSING A SERIOUSLY ILL PATIENT OVER THE TELEPHONE

The ICU often receives calls from other areas within the hospital or from other hospitals seeking advice or requesting a transfer to the ICU. The following are some guidelines on how to handle such requests:

ALWAYS BE HELPFUL, NEVER BE PATRONIZING. The ICU and its staff have equipment, skills, and expertise that should be shared in a positive fashion.

Patient

Assess the severity of the problem.
Identify the major problem, and take a quick history of the illness.
Determine the level of consciousness.
Determine the state of the airway (eg intubated or not).
Assess the breathing (eg respiratory rate, oxygenation).
Assess the circulation (eg blood pressure, heart rate, and rhythm, and urine output).
Record the relevant past history.
Determine the current treatment and the lines and monitors being used.

Manpower and equipment
Your advice on treatment will depend on the status of the person to whom you are speaking, that is, regarding seniority and experience. It is important not to assume that the conferring person or institution will have skills the same as your own (eg for intubation, central-line insertion), nor should you overestimate the availability of equipment in the referring hospital (eg sophisticated ventilators).

Support
The person whom you are advising usually will have less equipment and expertise than are available in your ICU. Your advice should be aimed at stabilizing the patient in the simplest and most responsible fashion, followed by support for the conferee's decision either to continue the current management or to transfer the patient to the ICU.

It is often helpful to monitor progress and provide encouragement by repeat telephone calls.

If the patient is transferred to your ICU, it is important to provide feedback to the referring institution regarding the patient's progress.

2

ROUTINE CARE OF THE SERIOUSLY ILL

- The practice of good intensive care medicine is about the methodical application of basic routines.
- ABC – Always maintain a good airway, ensure adequate oxygenation, and rapidly correct hypovolaemia.
- In a critically ill patient, one will miss more by not performing a thorough clinical examination than by under-monitoring and under-investigating.

HOW TO APPROACH A PATIENT IN INTENSIVE CARE

When the specialty of intensive care was being defined, many of the problems were new to us. As the problems had not been documented in conventional text-books, they had to be learnt at the bedside. Our specialty owes a lot to those first-generation intensivists. It was soon learnt that complex single- and multiple-organ failure (MOF) often occurred in certain patterns. There are also certain features that seriously ill patients have in common. These patterns have been taken into account as part of the routine care of seriously ill patients, making the more unpredictable aspects of complex illness easier to recognize and manage. It is these common and routine aspects that are described in this chapter.

Seriously ill patients often present with complex sets of problems that make a conventional approach difficult. For example, the conventional approach of differential diagnosis, provisional diagnosis, investigations, and final diagnosis is often irrelevant in seriously ill patients with multiple problems. Moreover, this approach inhibits the practice of good intensive care medicine. Not only is it rare that there will be only a single diagnosis, but in attempting to make the patient fit into our current bank of knowledge, there is the danger that the patient's unique problems will be ignored. The patient's problems are what the staff should address. Nursing and medical staff work more closely together in intensive care than in ordinary wards. As they both have to deal with the same problems, they should be documented together. For example, pressure areas and hypotension are common problems, perhaps even related, and should not be considered as separate medical and nursing problems – they are the patient's problems.

THE WARD ROUND

In order not to get lost in the morass of information available about each individual patient, there has to be some structure in your approach to them. The following is one way of doing this. Team management is crucial in intensive care, and this problem-oriented approach ensures that all team members will focus on a patient's problems.

1. History   Critically ill patients are often treated before a definitive diagnosis is made and a history taken. Ambulance officers, patient's relatives, and the local doctor can all give valuable information after the patient has been stabilized.

2. Hand-over   The problems encountered by the previous shift will help to establish a picture of the patient's current status.

3. Physical examination   Physical examination is discussed later (see p. 13).

4. Review of investigations, monitoring, and correct medications   Biochemistry, haematology, arterial blood gases, monitoring, chest x-ray, CT scan, and so forth.

5. List of problems and strategy   Bring together all the information about history, examination, and previous problems, and then list the current problems. The problems may be related (eg HYPOTENSION, OLIGURIA, FEBRILE) and have a common cause (eg SEPTICAEMIA). The problems need not be elaborated on, and the plan, if obvious, need not be stated in all cases, unless there is some specific investigation or treatment (eg HYPOTENSION need not be followed in the plan by 'FIND CAUSE' or 'CORRECT' if it is related to an obvious cause, such as septicaemia, and is treated with a unit protocol). The problem sheet is meant to focus the team's thoughts on overall management strategy. It is more useful than writing reams of continua-

TABLE 2.1   A MNEMONIC TO ASSIST IN THE TASKS OF JUNIOR MEDICAL STAFF

A. AIRWAY	Is it well strapped? Is it well positioned? Is it time for a tracheostomy? Remember to exclude cervical spine damage in trauma patients.
B. BREATHING	Check the ventilator settings AND the respiratory observation chart. Examine the respiratory system, and check blood gases.
C. CIRCULATION	Check haemodynamic monitoring and 12-lead ECG. Conduct a cardiovascular examination, especially peripheral perfusion.
D. DRUGS	Check regular chart, p.r.n. chart, stat chart, and any infusions: Are all the drugs necessary? Are there any missing? Do you need blood levels checked?
E. ENTERAL	Is the patient being fed, either by IVN or enteral nutrition? If not, why not?
F. FLUIDS	Review quantity and content of all input and output – some output may need analysis (eg urine or abdominal drain for electrolytes and protein).
G. GIT	Examine abdomen.
H. HAEMATOLOGY	Check all blood results (eg biochemistry, serology, white-cell count).
I. INVESTIGATIONS	
J. JVP	Jugular venous pressure and CVP are unreliable guides to fluid status.
K. KELVIN	Check temperature and temperature chart.
L. LINES	Review the lines (insertion site, date inserted), and ask yourself, Are they necessary? (NG tube, indwelling catheter, epidural, etc)
M. MICROBIOLOGY	Check results, and ensure that antibiotics are appropriate. Should they be discontinued?
N. NEUROLOGICAL	Examine the neurological system in each patient (at least GCS in all patients).
O. OLD NOTES	Determine the patient's pre-morbid history (current and previous admissions).
P. PAIN RELIEF	Is it charted (including sedation, if necessary)?
Q. QUERY	Have other specialists involved in the case been informed?

(continued)

R. RELATIVES	Determine further history. Have they been informed of the latest changes?
S. SKIN	Examine the skin, especially pressure areas, for signs of systemic disease (including mouth, teeth, ears, and sinuses).
T. TRAUMA	Ensure that a thorough secondary survey is complete in trauma patients (eg limbs, back, perineum, eyes, ears, etc.).
U. YOU	YOU must communicate with the specialist.
V. VICTUAL	Be sure you get appropriate breaks and meals.
W. WHERE TO	Have an overall plan for patient management.
X. X-RAY	Check the chest x-ray.
Y. WHY	Why is the patient here? (Ask yourself each day if you are heading in the right direction.)
Z. Zzzz	Sleep when you can.

tion notes and could even replace them if filed appropriately in the patient's notes. Fine tuning is needed within this overall management plan, and further problems may emerge before the next major ward round. These will need to be addressed during the course of the day. Table 2.1 outlines a quick way of reviewing patients.

6. Relatives and friends   Information given to relatives needs to be consistent. All team members should agree on the 'party line'.

PHYSICAL ASSESSMENT

It is important to thoroughly examine a 'stable' critically ill patient at least once a day. Conventional examination techniques may have to be modified, as these patients often are unconscious, usually with a plethora of monitoring equipment, invasive lines, and drains attached. A sound picture can be built up only after a thorough examination of the patient, in combination with knowledge of the patient's history, monitoring trends, and concurrent therapy. There is a definite art to examining the seriously ill. Like all other forms of physical assessment in medicine, a set routine guarantees that little is missed. Table 2.2 provides an outline.

TABLE 2.2 DAILY ROUTINE EXAMINATION OF PATIENTS IN INTENSIVE CARE

---

1. Address the patient by name, and explain what you intend to do.
2. Rapidly assess the airway, breathing, circulation, level of consciousness, and gross abnormalities.
3. Expose the patient's whole body, placing the patient supine if possible.
4. **Airway and head**

   Check natural airway, artificial airway (cuff, type of tube and securing method, cuff pressure, diameter).

   Inspect scalp, sinuses, mouth, ears, NG tube, cervical nodes, eyes (especially pupils and corneal abrasions).

   Check for neck stiffness.
5. **Neurological system**

   Check GCS trends and current level of consciousness, and inquire of nursing staff about GCS and limb movement.

   Assess sedation in the light of need, as well as liver and renal functions.

   Exclude seizures.

   If necessary, check brain-stem reflexes.

   Obtain gross information using focal neurological signs, and then, if necessary, make a more detailed examination.
6. **Respiratory system**

   Inspect chest movement, respiratory rate and effort.

   Check interaction of patient with ventilator, and observe F_{IO_2}, peak inspiratory pressure, PEEP levels, ventilator mode, tidal and minute volumes, and respiratory swings with spontaneous respiration.

   Assess gas exchange (colour, oximetry, arterial blood gases).

   Auscultate the chest, especially posterior and lateral bases.

   Check ICC for bubbling and fluid.

   Correlate findings with chest x-ray.

   Ask nursing staff about the patient's ability to cough and the type of secretions.
7. **Circulatory system**

   Inspect precordium.

   Observe neck veins.

   Assess peripheral pulses and rhythm.

   Exclude peripheral oedema.

   Assess peripheral perfusion.

(continued)

Auscultate the precordium.

Check the trends in blood pressure, pulse rate, urine output, and other, more complex measurements, such as cardiac output, $\dot{V}o_2$, and Do_2.

8. Gastro-intestinal tract

Observe the abdomen for distension, wounds, and drains.

Study the underlying surgery and recent imaging (eg CT scan or ultrasound).

Palpate for tenderness, tenseness, and masses.

Listen for bowel sounds.

Inquire about NG aspirate, efficacy of enteral feeding, and bowel interactions.

9. Limbs

Inspect for rashes, oedema, and wounds.

Remove dressings, where possible, and inspect wounds.

Study the underlying fractures, traction, surgery, and relevant radiological appearances.

GENERAL

Address the patient by name, even if the patient is unconscious, and explain what you are going to do.

The initial routine inspection includes rapid assessment of the airway, breathing, circulation, level of consciousness, and gross abnormalities. More is missed by not looking than by not knowing, and there is a lot to be seen in the seriously ill.

Lift the sheet off the patient, and expose as much of the body as possible. Start the general examination from the top, and work down. Turn the patient into the lateral position, and inspect the back of the trunk and legs. Inspect the skin for features such as jaundice, rashes, and bruising. Observe early pressure areas, especially around the heels, and feel for dependent oedema.

Inspect the eyes, looking carefully for corneal ulceration, as a result of drying. Inspect the mouth, nose, and teeth. Inspect all invasive-equipment sites, such as surgical drains, intercostal catheters (ICCs), intravenous and intra-arterial lines, and endotracheal tubes (ETTs). Remove all dressings, and inspect wounds. Look for abnormal bleeding into wounds or bleeding from puncture sites. It is important to know exactly where surgical drains have been placed and

TABLE 2.3 SIGNS PECULIAR TO THE CRITICALLY ILL

Bounding in the neck and precordium often indicates sepsis.

An indentation ring in the skin, left after listening for bowel sounds with a stethoscope, indicates extensive peripheral oedema.

The silhouette of the head seen over the mediastinum on an upright chest x-ray is a poor prognostic sign and is usually followed by intubation within the next 24 hours.

Attempts to breathe against the ventilator, despite what appears to be an adequate minute volume, often are due to severe metabolic acidosis.

Rapid deterioration in cardiorespiratory signs can indicate a pneumothorax.

for what purpose and to inspect the drainage fluid for amount and appearance. Ensure that the lines and drains are secure and working efficiently. Ask yourself if they are really needed, and consider removal if there is doubt. During the examination, ensure that the patient is not lying on equipment, such as intravenous lines and catheters, as they can cause pressure areas. The type of monitoring, the fluids used, the rate and content of the infusion pumps, the ventilatory settings, and the support equipment will give you a good idea of the patient's problems and their severity.

Some signs peculiar to the critically ill are listed in Table 2.3.

NEUROLOGICAL ASSESSMENT

The most important features of a neurological examination in the intensive care unit (ICU) are the level of consciousness, brain-stem function, and lateralizing signs in the limbs. The patient's level of consciousness is usually monitored by the Glasgow coma scale (GCS) (see p. 25). Look at the GCS trends. Further information can be gained from the nursing staff. Assess the level of consciousness in light of the amount of sedation. Sedation may take days to wear off, especially in the presence of hepatic and renal insufficiency. A consistent painful stimulus is recommended to test the level of response. Vigorous stimulation of the outer aspects of the eyebrow can cause nerve palsies, and rubbing of the sternum with one's knuckles can cause unsightly bruising. The nailbed or nipple may offer more suitable areas to elicit a reaction to a painful stimulus. The presence of seizures should be noted. Neck stiffness, fever, and photophobia suggest meningeal irritation due to the presence of blood or infection.

Reflexes, such as pupil size and reaction to light, gag reflex, corneal reflex, and respiration pattern, will give an indication of brain-stem function.

Information on focal neurological deficits can be grossly elicited by inquiring about movement of the limbs from the nursing staff, and if there is any doubt, limb reflexes and tone can be elicited. A nerve stimulator may be useful in determining residual paralysis, especially after prolonged use of muscle relaxants.

RESPIRATORY SYSTEM

Always assess the adequacy of the airway, even if the patient has an ETT or tracheostomy tube in place. It may be kinked or blocked. Note the diameter of the ETT, as narrow tubes can be the greatest contributors to the work of breathing. Ask the nursing staff about the nature and amount of tracheal secretions. Check the way the airway has been secured, check cuff pressures, and inquire about the appropriateness of the cuff for long-term use. Monitoring of ventilator variables and gas exchange will also provide valuable information about respiratory function (see Chapter 20). Assess oxygenation, in terms of colour, pulse oximetry, and fractional concentration of inspired oxygen (FIO_2). Note the breathing rate, the tidal volume, the respiratory effort, and, if ventilated, the positive end-expiratory pressure (PEEP), the peak inspiratory pressure, and the breathing mode. Look for asymmetry of chest movement and position of the mediastinum, as judged by the trachea and apex beat. Observe how the patient is interacting with the ventilator.

Auscultation remains important in the ICU. Intrapulmonary shadows on a chest x-ray can be difficult to interpret, but bronchial breath sounds will indicate that pneumonia is more likely than adult respiratory distress syndrome (ARDS) or pulmonary oedema. Decreased air entry, indicating collapse, and rhonchi, indicating the degree of bronchospasm, are important aspects in examining the respiratory system in the critically ill. Check for chest drains and flail segments. Look for bubbling from the ICC, as well as the amount and type of drainage. The best single means of assessing respiratory status is an upright chest x-ray. Other considerations in interpreting chest x-rays in the seriously ill are discussed later (see Chapter 18). Examine the trend of arterial blood gases.

CARDIOVASCULAR SYSTEM

There is often 'information overload' concerning cardiorespiratory variables in the ICU. Amongst all these hard data it is important not to overlook simple vital signs such as arterial blood pressure, pulse rate and rhythm, urine output, and peripheral perfusion. Current values should be seen in light of previous trends. Information may also be available for cardiac output, peripheral resistance, oxygen delivery and consumption, and other estimates of cardiac function derived from echocardiography. Despite the cardiovascular measurements available, careful physical examination of the patient is important. Assess peripheral pulses, and auscultate the precordium for added sounds, murmurs, and bruits. Examine the patient for peripheral oedema.

There are signs peculiar to the seriously ill. For example, a bounding precordium in the neck is usually seen with systemic sepsis and is due to the hyperdynamic cardiovascular status accompanying that state. This is obvious from the end of the bed. Many signs in the seriously ill can be modified by the disease process or by drugs (eg urine output in the presence of diuretics or renal failure). Patients with sepsis will often have tachycardia and low blood pressure, even with normal filling pressures. Peripheral temperature is a good empirical guide to adequate circulating volume, but it is difficult to interpret in the presence of sepsis and a fever.

GASTRO-INTESTINAL TRACT

It is important to carefully examine the gastro-intestinal tract (GIT) at least once each day. Carefully inspect the face, for signs of sinusitis, and the nose and mouth, especially in the presence of artificial airways and tubes, as they can make thorough inspection difficult. Examine the ears, and feel for cervical nodes.

The abdomen should be observed for distension, wounds, and drains. Palpate for tenderness, tenseness, and abnormal masses. Listen for bowel sounds, and inquire about bowel actions and absorption of oral feeds. The presence of bowel sounds means that air and fluid are present, but their absence does not mean a non-functioning GIT. It is important to be familiar with all abdominal drains – where they originate and what they are draining. A clear diagram of any abdominal surgery displayed in the notes at the patient's bedside can clarify the complexities of the abdominal surgery. Carefully observe the perineum for signs of swelling, inflammation, and discharge.

RENAL AND FLUIDS

Note the adequacy of the intravascular volume, as reflected by pulse rate, blood pressure, peripheral perfusion, urine output, pulmonary artery wedge pressure (PAWP), central venous pressure (CVP), and so forth.

Note the state of hydration (eg skin turgor, dry tongue).

Assess the fluid-balance chart, noting any major losses and the sources of those losses (eg nasogastric losses, drains).

Review the ward urinalysis.

Check electrolytes (sodium, potassium, calcium, phosphate, and magnesium) at least once each day.

Check urea, creatinine, and urine outputs as markers of renal function.

The urinary catheter must be inserted using strictly aseptic technique, with urine drainage collected in a closed sterile system. There is a good argument for using Silastic catheters in seriously ill patients, as they are associated with fewer long-term complications. The catheter should be taped to the patient's skin to prevent trauma caused by traction. For a male patient who will have a catheter in place for more than several days, it should be taped just below the umbilicus, with gentle traction pulling the penis superiorly to prevent urethral damage.

LIMBS

Attention to a patient's limbs is sometimes overlooked in the ICU. They should be carefully inspected for rashes, oedema, and adequacy of perfusion. Hands, feet, and nails should also be inspected. Dressings should be taken down and inspected where applicable. The details of underlying fractures should be known, and close communication with orthopaedic surgeons is essential. Fractures are often associated with wounds. It is important that plaster be regularly removed so that the wounds can be inspected. Orthopaedic surgeons should be encouraged to pin or plate fractures, as traction makes nursing and patient care very difficult.

HAEMATOLOGY

Check for obvious oozing or bleeding. Note the results of coagulation tests (see p. 716) and platelet counts. Check the haemoglobin and blood count. Assess anticoagulation therapy, if appropriate.

THROMBOEMBOLISM

There are many risk factors associated with the formation of venous thromboemboli in the critically ill – immobility, decreased blood flow secondary to intermittent positive-pressure ventilation (IPPV), surgery, or trauma, and low-flow states. Despite the reported high risk for venous thromboembolism, there does not appear to be an associated high incidence of local clinical manifestations, nor of pulmonary emboli.

Prophylaxis
• frequent turning
• passive mobilization
• graded compression stockings
• low-dosage subcutaneous heparin
• pneumatic full-length leg compression

PATIENT POSITIONING

Unless sitting up is contraindicated, patients in intensive care should be sat up to an angle of at least 30°. Pressure measurements can be taken in this position as long as the transducers are correctly placed. Upright patients usually have better oxygenation and decreased work of breathing. Moreover, lower intracranial pressure (ICP) usually can be achieved in patients who are sitting upright.

As for the head-down position, apart from specific purposes, such as the insertion of central venous lines, a patient should not be placed with the head down, not even as a temporary measure for hypotension. Posture-related hypotension should be corrected by intravascular fluids, not by placing the patient head-down.

In a patient with a unilateral lung abnormality, hypoxia can be exacerbated when the patient is positioned with the affected lung down; this position should be avoided if the hypoxia is severe. For the same reason, when assessing serial blood gases or performing pulse oximetry, the position of the patient at the time should be noted.

Stable, critically ill patients should be turned regularly, usually every 2 hours. This helps with oxygenation and may prevent pressure sores.

ROUTINE MONITORING, OBSERVATIONS, AND INVESTIGATIONS

Patients should have their vital signs, such as pulse rate, arterial blood pressure, respiratory rate, and urine output, measured regularly. Continuous electrocardiogram (ECG) monitoring and oximetry are usually necessary in all seriously ill patients. Other measurements, such as CVP, PAWP, and cardiac output, may also be necessary. Oxygenation and ventilation should be monitored by regularly measuring the inspired oxygen fraction, respiratory rate, and blood gases. If a patient is artificially ventilated, tidal volumes, inspiratory pressures, and respiratory frequency may also require monitoring. For more details on cardiorespiratory monitoring, see Chapter 21.

The patient's level of consciousness should be charted according to a consistent scale, such as the GCS.

Central temperature, rather than oral or skin temperature, should be measured either rectally or by probe in the oesophagus, bladder, or stomach.

There is a trend toward the use of continuous noninvasive monitoring, such as blood pressure, capnography, tonometry, and pulse oximetry (see p. 490).

As part of quality assurance, the staff at the ICU should continually be asking questions: WHY IS THIS PARAMETER BEING MEASURED? DOES IT NEED RECORDING? It may be more productive to invest time and resources in educating the primary health giver (ie the nurse at the bedside) to act on information, rather than simply recording it. A beautiful chart, with every possible variable meticulously recorded, may not necessarily reflect a high standard of patient care. Early action, rather than simply recording abnormal observations, is preferable.

Theoretically, computers should offer more sophisticated documentation and information on trends for all intensive care measurements; charts may not be necessary in the future. However, the computers that are currently available are expensive and often duplicate what is recorded in charts, encouraging information overload. The more modern monitoring devices usually feature printouts and graphic displays of trends. These may replace handwritten charts, if records are thought still to be necessary.

ROUTINE INVESTIGATIONS

There are certain routine tests that should be performed in all seriously ill patients. Many hospitals now have auto-analysers, which makes selective tests impractical. The following are guidelines to the minimum routine tests for the seriously ill:

Four-hourly determinations

Blood-sugar levels should be measured in all seriously ill and unconscious patients at least 4-hourly and sometimes hourly.

Twice daily determinations

• arterial blood gases
• potassium

Daily determinations

• urea and creatinine
• haemoglobin
• white-cell count
• platelets
• phosphate

• magnesium
• calcium
• chest x-ray
• 12-lead ECG

Twice weekly determinations

- so-called liver function tests (ie serum bilirubin, alkaline phosphatase and aminotransferase activities, and serum albumin)
- prothrombin time (PT)
- partial thromboplastin (PTT)

Radiology

The stethoscope is useful for detecting chest abnormalities, but daily chest x-rays are essential. Patients should always have upright chest x-rays, with every attempt made to standardize exposures, making comparisons easier. Large viewing boxes with room for representative and consecutive films should be available. Ideally, a radiologist with experience in interpreting these films, together with the intensive care team, should look at all the day's films. The interpretation of chest x-rays is discussed in more detail later (see Chapter 18).

Microbiology

Microbiology is an important area for investigation in the seriously ill. Unlike the situation in biochemistry, the findings are never clearcut; they must be interpreted, and daily consultation with a microbiologist with clinical experience is an advantage. Specific tests and routine surveillance must be carefully tracked. Antibiotic treatment should be reviewed daily and not continued nor commenced unnecessarily (see p. 204).

INTRAVASCULAR LINES

This book does not cover the anatomic and procedural aspects of cannulation. There are, however, several important points relating to intravascular lines:

Peripheral lines

- Use large-bore lines (>18 gauge) in ICU patients.
- Remove all resuscitation lines (eg those inserted in the emergency

department within the first 24 hours), as they may have been placed in less than strictly aseptic conditions.

• Peripheral lines should all be changed after 48 hours, as the infection rate increases exponentially.

• Drugs with powerful α-agonist action should not be transfused through peripheral lines, except in an emergency.

Central lines

• Beware of covered patients during central-line insertion – the head-down position is dangerous in the seriously ill. Staff can focus their attention on pressure waveforms and technical difficulties during intravascular cannulation, rather than monitoring the patient. Someone must be assigned to watch and monitor the patient. Frequent blood-gas determinations or pulse oximetry may be needed because of the potential for hypoxia in the head-down position.

• Pulmonary artery catheters ideally should be removed between 48 and 72 hours.

• Multilumen central venous lines should be placed early if the patient has MOF, requiring multidrug support. They allow CVP measurements to be performed without interruption of essential drugs, and they minimize the danger of flushing highly concentrated and potentially dangerous solutions directly into the heart chambers.

• Catheters should be inspected at least daily and removed if there are any signs of inflammation. There is no evidence to suggest that routine changing of central venous catheters reduces the incidence of infection. Central lines can be resited at the existing catheter site if it is neither red nor inflamed.

• Femoral lines do not have a higher incidence of infection than other central lines.

Arterial lines

Keep the arterial-line site in view at all times. Disconnection can lead to catastrophic haemorrhage.

• Arterial lines have a low incidence of complications, and their insertion can be justified for multiple sampling of blood gases alone.

• However, as little as 2 ml of air inadvertently flushed through an arterial line can retrogradely cause cerebral air embolism.

General points

1. Some points to remember when dressing intravascular lines:
- strict aseptic technique
- no topical antibiotics
- local application of povidone iodine
- secure with a suture if necessary

2. Blood cultures should be taken from lines only when they are first inserted. The connections soon become colonized and may give misleading results.

3. Note the amount of fluid used in the flushing of lines every 24 hours. Often it can amount to at least 500 ml, and that should be included in the patient's fluid-balance chart.

INTUBATION AND TRACHEAL CARE

Intubation is necessary in many seriously ill patients to

- secure an adequate airway
- facilitate removal of secretions
- facilitate ventilation and oxygenation

General complications of ETT and tracheostomies include

- malposition
- dislodgement
- disconnection
- obstruction
- infection
- local trauma to larynx and trachea that can result in long-term damage
- interference with normal humidification and warming of inspired gases

INTUBATION

BE PROPERLY PREPARED, with the necessary equipment.

Pre-oxygenate for 5 minutes with 100% oxygen.

Seriously ill patients need someone who can intubate expertly and rapidly. It is not the time for teaching. In fact, it is preferable to have a second experienced doctor on hand at the time of intubation, to monitor and, if necessary, to help resuscitate the patient.

There is often a dilemma concerning which artificial airway should be used – nasotracheal tube (NTT), orotracheal tube (OTT), or tracheostomy. Each ICU will develop its own policy based on some of the following considerations.

NASOTRACHEAL TUBE

Advantages

• easier to secure than an OTT.

• does not move within the trachea as easily as an OTT.

• does not require a constricting bandage around the neck, which possibly could interrupt venous drainage.

• allows easier access to the mouth for routine care.

• precludes occlusion, due to the patient biting on the tube.

Disadvantages

• An NTT can cause trauma to the nose.

• An NTT is technically more difficult to insert than an OTT.

• An NTT can cause nasal cartilage necrosis.

• An NTT necessitates a narrower-lumen tube, which, because of its high resistance, will make spontaneous breathing more difficult.

• The fragile cuffs on the tubes sometimes develop leaks, as a result of trauma as the tube is being passed through the nose.

• Occlusion of sinuses can occur, with stasis, and infection can occur. THIS CAN BE AN IMPORTANT OCCULT SOURCE OF SEPSIS (see p. 203).

• An NTT should not be used when there is a suspicion that the base of the skull is fractured.

OROTRACHEAL TUBE

Advantages

• A larger-lumen tube can be passed through the mouth than through the nose, facilitating spontaneous breathing by decreasing the work of breathing.

• Insertion of an OTT is a quicker and easier technical procedure than inserting an NTT. This may be particularly important when rapid intubation is necessary.

• An OTT makes it easier to pass a suction catheter.

Disadvantages

• An OTT is more difficult to secure than an NTT.

• The bandage around the neck can impede venous drainage (important if there is an elevated ICP) and cut into the corners of the mouth.

• Because of difficulty in securing it, there is more movement of the OTT within the trachea.

• It is difficult to conduct mouth care in the presence of an OTT.

• There can be chronic laryngeal dysfunction and tracheal stenosis at the cuff site.

• Patients can cause occlusion by biting on the tube.

TRACHEOSTOMY

An OTT or NTT usually can be left in place for 7–21 days before tracheostomy is considered. Even then, some units delay tracheostomy. A tracheostomy tube simply bypasses a part of the OTT or NTT. The tracheal tube and cuff remain in the trachea, and that is the source of most morbidity and mortality. However, laryngeal dysfunction and even vocal-cord paralysis can occur with an OTT or NTT. The decision to perform a tracheostomy after 7–10 days is largely dictated by unit policy and whether or not prolonged airway access will be required. If a prolonged period of intubation is anticipated, some units now perform tracheostomy within the first few days.

Tracheostomy should be performed by an experienced surgeon or intensivist. The best procedure is to use the smallest incision, with the greatest preservation of cartilage, between the first and second cartilage rings. Experience with percutaneous tracheostomy is increasing. It is a simple procedure that can be performed in the ICU by members of the intensive care staff. Percutaneous tracheostomies have been shown in comparative trials to have half the complication rates of conventional surgical tracheostomies.

Advantages

• There is better patient tolerance than for an OTT or NTT.
• The tube is easier to secure and enhances patient mobility.
• There is not trauma to mouth, nose, and larynx. Oral toilet is easier.
• It is easier to introduce suction catheters.
• A larger-diameter tube is possible, decreasing dead space, resistance and the work of breathing during spontaneous breathing.

Disadvantages

• An operation is involved, with small, but documented, rates of mortality and morbidity.
• The wound almost always becomes superficially infected.
• There can be difficulty in reinserting the tracheostomy tube if it becomes dislodged, especially in the first few days after operation.
• There can be tracheal stenosis at the cuff site and erosion into adjacent structures.

MINITRACHEOSTOMY

Minitracheostomy tubes are available in pre-packaged kit form. They can be inserted using local anaesthetic and cricothyroid cartilage puncture in the ICU. Minitracheostomy tubes can also be inserted through a tracheostomy stoma after the tracheostomy tube has been removed, in order to facilitate suction.

Indications

The main indication is to facilitate suction of secretions, typically in patients with chronic lung disease and patients with copious secre-

tions who have recently had surgery or have a decreased level of consciousness with an inadequate cough reflex.

CARE OF TUBES

When an NTT, OTT, or tracheostomy tube is used, always use im-
plant-tested material with a high-volume low-pressure cuff.

Cut the tube off flush with the mouth or nose, to prevent kinking,
to decrease resistance, and to prevent excessive movement within the
trachea.

Take a chest x-ray after insertion and at least daily to verify positioning (see Chapter 18). When not visualized radiographically, the
carina can be expected to lie on a line corresponding to approximately
halfway down the aortic knob. Neck flexion and extension can cause
the tip of the ETT to move up to 2 cm.

Change a tube immediately if obstruction is suspected and cannot
be excluded (eg increased ventilatory pressures or difficulty in breathing). Simply passing a suction catheter successfully through the lumen of a tube does not guarantee that it is not obstructed. Viscous secretion can cause a ball-valve effect as the catheter passes through it.

TRACHEAL SUCTION

• Regular suctioning of any tube is necessary, but unfortunately the
procedure is always accompanied by hypoxia.

1. Pre-oxygenate with 100% oxygen before suction.

2. Use an ETT connector through which a suction catheter can be
passed without having to disconnect the patient.

3. Suction rapidly – do not leave the catheter down for more than
5 seconds at any one time.

4. Avoid mechanical damage – be gentle, and use soft tips with
lateral holes.

• Never suction active pulmonary oedema, and reduce suctioning of
hypoxic patients otherwise.

• Never actively suction the trachea while the patient is being extubated – that would cause hypoxia at a critical time. Suction around
the pharynx, and extubate at the height of inspiration so that the patient can clear secretions by exhaling or coughing.

ROUTINE CARE OF VENTILATED PATIENTS

Take at least hourly measurements of tidal volume, respiratory rate, and ventilator pressure. Ventilator alarms usually provide continuous monitoring of excessive pressure and notice of disconnection.

Assess lung abnormalities at least once daily with an upright chest x-ray (see Chapter 18).

The aim of ventilation is to maintain adequate gas exchange. Regular determinations of arterial blood gases, continuous pulse oximetry, and clinical assessment are essential (see p. 17).

FLUIDS

Fluid treatment can be perplexing in seriously ill patients. This topic is discussed in some detail later (see Chapter 4). Briefly, some of the difficulties faced are as follows:

• Conventional guides to fluid treatment (fluid-balance chart, CVP, urine output, arterial blood pressure, PAWP, pulse rate) are often misleading in a seriously ill patient (see p. 55).

• In patients who are not seriously ill, the normal compensation mechanisms, such as thirst and renal function, allow more room for error in fluid treatment. However, these mechanisms are often compromised in the critically ill. Such a patient cannot, therefore, compensate for poor fluid treatment.

The sequelae of poor fluid treatment, such as pulmonary oedema, hypotension, and renal failure, will compound the existing MOF.

The following are guidelines for routine fluid treatment for seriously ill patients:

COLLOID AND BLOOD PRODUCTS   Colloid and blood products are confined mainly to the intravascular space. Measurements in this space (eg blood pressure, pulse rate, urine output, CVP, PAWP) are much more easily accomplished than are measurements in the interstitial and intracellular spaces (eg tissue turgor, dry mucosa). The best method of assessing the intravascular volume is with a fluid challenge: Measure intravascular parameters before and after a challenge of 200–500 ml of colloid, as a guide to fluid requirement.

IT IS VITAL TO MAINTAIN INTRAVASCULAR VOLUME IN SERIOUSLY ILL PATIENTS AT ALL TIMES AND IS ESSENTIAL TO AVOID OVER-EXPANSION OF THE INTERSTITIAL SPACE.

CRYSTALLOID SOLUTIONS Crystalloid solutions will rehydrate the intracellular and interstitial spaces. Clinical assessment of these spaces is notoriously inaccurate, and the 'stress response' in the critically ill encourages salt and water retention, thus promoting peripheral and pulmonary oedema. Excessive administration of crystalloid solutions should therefore be avoided.

CLINICAL GUIDELINES
- Give packed cells or whole blood to keep haemoglobin above 10 g/dl.
- Titrate the colloid solution against intravascular measurements (eg CVP, blood pressure, pulse rate, urine output)
- Give 500–2,500 ml of water (5% dextrose) over 24 hours for a normal-sized adult, titrated empirically against the daily serum sodium concentration if the blood glucose is within normal limits.
- If patient is normovolaemic and has a stable cardiovascular system, only maintenance fluids are necessary (eg 4% dextrose and 0.2-N saline at 1,000–3,000 ml over 24 hours).
- Otherwise, limit saline-containing crystalloids, unless indicated by interstitial-space dehydration.

GASTRO-INTESTINAL-TRACT HAEMORRHAGE
(see p. 686)

Stress ulceration is related primarily to ischaemia and can be a complication of acute illness. A low gastric pH in seriously ill patients is associated with a higher incidence of gastric bleeding than is a gastric pH of 4 or more. That has, in the past, prompted many ICUs to institute prophylactic measures to prevent stress ulceration. However, if gastric juice has a pH greater than 4, there will be bacterial overgrowth, which will predispose to nosocomial infections. There are increasing indications that the incidence of stress ulceration in ICUs is decreasing. This is probably related to improved care for the seriously ill, particularly in regard to oxygenation and perfusion of the GIT.

Stress-ulcer prophylaxis probably should be given only to critically ill patients, those on IPPV for more than 48 hours, and those with recent GIT bleeding.

SUCRALFATE

Sucralfate protects against stress ulceration by mechanisms such as cytoprotection or pepsin adsorption, and it is probably as effective as antacids or H_2-receptor antagonists in preventing stress ulceration. Sucralfate reduces the need to monitor gastric pH, and because it does not cause alkalinity of the stomach, there is much less gastric colonization. Sucralfate is less effective when combined with antacids or H_2-receptor blockers.

The sucralfate dosage should be 1 g every 6 hours if taking oral fluids; otherwise, the same dosage suspended in 20 ml of sterile water and administered by a nasogastric (NG) tube, which should then be flushed with 10 ml of sterile water to prevent obstruction of the tube.

ALKALINIZATION OF GASTRIC pH

In at-risk patients (eg septicaemia, burns, MOF, underlying peptic ulcer) there may still be a place for gastric alkalinization.

TECHNIQUE　　Aspirate and measure the gastric pH using indicator paper, on a regular basis. Staff should handle the NG aspirate with care, as it is potentially contaminated with bacteria and fungi.

Gastric pH should be noted, with alkalinization measures taken accordingly:

- pH > 4: No measures need be taken.
- pH < 4: Use one of the following:

    (a) H_2-receptor antagonist – use intermittently in standard intravenous doses or as a continuous infusion, with intermittent boluses titrated against gastric pH measured regularly.

    (b) Antacid: Commence at 10 ml/h. Then decrease or increase by 20 ml/h each hour, in order to maintain pH > 4.

    (c) Combination: Either use H_2-receptor antagonists in standard intravenous doses as a background, with antacids given as required to keep gastric pH > 4, or use regular antacids as a background, with H_2-receptor antagonists added as necessary to keep gastric pH > 4.

NUTRITION

Many aspects of feeding critically ill patients remain unclear, even after more than two decades of research. These issues are discussed in more detail in Chapter 5. Some of the bottom-line messages are included here:

• Enteral feeding is preferable to intravenous nutrition (IVN) and should be used whenever possible. Enteral feeding is cheaper and more efficient, encourages GIT mucosal growth, and involves fewer complications.

• Many of the contraindications to enteral feeding, such as abdominal distension, gastric aspirate, and recent surgery, are only relative. Increasingly, feeding tubes are being used to bypass the stomach in order to facilitate feeding.

• Obligatory catabolism often occurs in the seriously ill, especially during the early, unstable period. Nutrition is therefore of doubtful benefit while a patient is being resuscitated. Moreover, IVN probably is not necessary until approximately 7–10 days after initial resuscitation.

DAILY NUTRITION

1. Use enteral nutrition (see p. 87) if the gut is working.

2. Use parenteral nutrition (see p. 89) if the substrates are being utilized and are within the limitations of fluid requirements. Do not try to achieve perfect nitrogen balance. Aggressive feeding of calories also is not necessary. Approximately 2,000 kcal/d is a realistic level for adults. Other components also need to be considered:

  • Trace elements (see p. 92), especially zinc, should be given empirically.
  • Multivitamin preparations.
  • Folic acid.
  • Vitamin K.

• Potassium, phosphate, magnesium, and calcium must be measured frequently (at least once each day) and supplemented if necessary.

AGE AND THE SERIOUSLY ILL

Elderly patients are becoming increasingly common in most ICUs. Age alone should not preclude admission to intensive care. A patient's level of functioning before hospitalization and the number of comorbidities probably are better predictors of outcome than is age.

• In general, the elderly have limited physiological reserves.

• There are increasing incidences of coexisting illnesses, such as diabetes, carcinoma, heart failure, and ischaemic heart disease.

• There tend to be increasing effects from tobacco- and alcohol-related diseases.

• There tends to be increased use of medications that can interact with the acute illness or with the medications used to treat the acute illness or impair the ability of the body to metabolize drugs.

• Central nervous system:
   ↑ predisposition to confusional states
  impaired thermoregulation
   ↓ neuronal numbers
   ↓ hearing and vision
   ↑ cerebral atrophy

• Respiratory system:
   ↓ functional residual capacity
   ↑ closing volume
   ↑ airway closure
   ↓ alveoli and lung mass from age 16 years
   ↑ emphysematous changes
   ↓ lung compliance
   ↑ alveolar–arterial gradient: $PaO_2 = 105 - 0.3$ (age in years) (mm Hg)
   ↓ vital capacity
   ↓ inspiratory reserve
   ↓ ventilatory drive to hypoxia and hypercarbia
   ↓ respiratory reflexes

- Cardiovascular system:
  - ↓ ability to increase heart rate
  - ↑ blood pressure (systolic pressure is approximately age + 100 mm Hg)
  - less compliant ventricles, and decreased ejection fraction and cardiac index
  - ↑ incidence of valvular dysfunction
  - ↑ incidence of arrhythmias
  - ↑ impedance of cardiovascular system
  - ↑ atheroma
  - ↑ blunting of sympathetic response
- Musculoskeletal system and skin:
  - ↓ muscle mass
  - ↓ mobility
  - ↓ elasticity of skin, and more prone to pressure necrosis
  - ↑ osteoporosis
  - ↑ incidence of joint dysfunction
- Renal system:
  - ↓ total body water
  - ↓ glomerular filtration rate (approximately half that of a 30-year-old by age 60 years)
  - ↑ benign prostatic enlargement
  - ↓ number of nephrons
- Gastro-intestinal tract and nutrition:
  - ↓ motility
  - ↓ fat stores
  - ↓ basal metabolic rate
  - ↓ hepatocyte numbers
  - ↓ gall-bladder emptying
  - ↑ glucose intolerance
- Social and ethical considerations:
  - Involve friends and family in decisions and discussion of the prognosis. Elderly patients have often discussed what they would like to happen in the event of a life-threatening illness.
  - Evaluate the patient's circumstances of living and support and the degree of independence before illness.

PATIENT REACTION TO INTENSIVE CARE

PATIENT

The reactions of patients in intensive care often involve anxiety, exhaustion, disorientation, and lack of communication. They are to be expected and are quite normal. Every effort must be made to modify these reactions.

• Explanation: Medical and nursing staff should try to explain each procedure and why it is being done, in addition to orienting the patient in time and place.
• Measures for sedation and pain relief should be taken only if necessary.
• Relatives and friends should be allowed unrestricted access, in limited numbers, to the patient. They should be encouraged to touch and talk to the patient.
• Speech aids and writing devices should be fully utilized if the patient is awake and unable to speak.

Despite the occurrence of what often resembles torture in an ICU – sleep deprivation, distressing and painful procedures, disorientation – most patients have complete amnesia about their time in an ICU. This may be related to the underlying illness or the use of sedation and pain-relieving drugs (see p. 110). However, there can be long-term social and psychological sequelae (eg depression, nightmares, and mood swings) after a severe illness and a stay in an ICU. These can last for many months or even years and will require dedicated support and honest explanation from health professionals, relatives, and friends.

RELATIVES

Relatives and friends often experience anxiety, stress, and sleep deprivation to similar degrees as the patient. This is one of the most traumatic times for any family. The patient may be critically ill for days or weeks. Relatives initially have a tendency to want to maintain a 24-hour vigil. That should be discouraged. Friends and relatives should be given an instruction pamphlet explaining that patients can remain seriously ill for days or even weeks and months. The relatives should be prepared for a marathon, not a 100-m dash. Although visiting at any time is to be encouraged, some sort of regular eating and sleeping pattern for the relatives should also be encouraged. The pamphlet should also contain a lay description of all the machines and tubes that may be supporting the patient, and what the staff hope to achieve with these devices. Relatives should be encouraged to talk to medical or nursing staff about any problems or questions they may have.

Relatives often have an insatiable need for reassurance and information. Such information must be consistent and straightforward. Discussing what the family 'line' will be, during the ward round, with medical, nursing and social-work staff, will help ensure this. A family conference is also a good way to communicate consistent information. If interpreters are required, use a formal, reliable service, not a family member; otherwise, information could become distorted or be censored during translation.

TROUBLESHOOTING

ROUTINE ASSESSMENT OF THE SERIOUSLY ILL IN THE ICU

Inquire about the patient's condition from the nursing staff. Obtain a general impression of the patient's condition, level of support, and monitoring from the end of the bed. The following is a checklist of some major points to be considered during routine assessment of the seriously ill in the ICU. Further details are available elsewhere (see p. 14).

Central nervous system
Assess the patient's level of consciousness in the light of
- intracranial abnormalities
- sedatives and other drugs.

Look for lateralizing neurological signs.

Respiratory system
Check airway, secretions, and chest drains.
Oxygenation: Assess F_{IO_2}, Pa_{O_2} or Sa_{O_2}, physical examination, and chest radiograph.
Ventilation: Assess ventilatory mode, Pa_{CO_2}, and inspiratory pressures.

Cardiovascular system

Determine blood pressure, pulse rate and rhythm, and peripheral perfusion.

Check for the presence of inotropes, vasopressors, vasodilators, and other cardiovascular drugs.

Fluid and renal

Urine output and other abnormal losses

Creatinine, urea, and electrolytes

Fluid input: volume and composition

Gastro-intestinal tract

Type of feeding and vitamins (Is it being tolerated?)

Examination of abdomen

Liver function tests

Haematology

Haemoglobin

Platelets

Clinical bleeding and coagulation profile

Microbiology

Temperature

White-cell count

Results of microbiological tests and culture

Type of antibiotics, dose, duration, and appropriateness

Drugs

Are they all still required?

Check drug levels.

Catheters, lines, and monitoring

Appropriateness and duration

Devise a plan of action based on this assessment

TROUBLESHOOTING

POST-OPERATIVE CARE FOLLOWING ABDOMINAL ANEURYSM REPAIR

Maintain the patient's NORMAL pre-operative arterial blood pressure.

Aggressive fluid replacement is crucial for the first 24 hours. Patients often require colloid or blood at 150–300 ml/h, as well as boluses, in order to maintain blood pressure and urine output. Maintenance fluid should also be given when the patient is stable.

Hypovolaemia commonly can cause a paradoxical hypertension in these patients and should be excluded before antihypertensive treatment is given.

Monitor post-operative myocardial ischaemia (eg 12-lead ECG, cardiac enzymes, symptoms, and ST/T-wave changes on continuous ECG).

Provide optimal pain relief (eg epidural or continuous IV narcotic).

Monitor intra-abdominal pressure if the abdomen feels tense (see p. 699). Increased pressure can severely compromise renal function and may require surgical intervention.

Prevent basal lung collapse by providing pain relief and physiotherapy, by nursing in the sitting-up position, and by using prophylactic continuous positive airway pressure (CPAP) if necessary.

Monitor distal blood flow in the limbs, and liaise closely with surgeons if it looks compromised.

Be aware of the possibility of intra-abdominal bleeding (eg excessive fluid requirements, decreasing haemoglobin, and increasing abdominal pressure). Liaise early with surgeons.

Encourage the surgeons to use a horizontal rather than vertical abdominal incision, as it is less painful and is accompanied by fewer respiratory complications.

TROUBLESHOOTING

ROUTINE POST-OPERATIVE MANAGEMENT FOLLOWING ELECTIVE VASCULAR SURGERY

These patients often have severe impairments of their underlying physiological reserves (eg previous myocardial infarction, ischaemic heart disease, chronic airway limitation, diabetes). As such, they are at risk for acute peri-operative events, such as myocardial ischaemia and stroke. The key to peri-operative management is to maintain excellent cardiorespiratory stability.

Ventilation   Elective post-operative ventilation is sometimes used, especially after laparotomies. Adequate pain relief, supplemental oxygen, and CPAP (see p. 367) may be as effective as elective ventilation.

Oxygenation   Normal oxygenation should be carefully maintained in order to prevent myocardial ischaemia and to facilitate wound healing. Oxygen supplementation is almost invariably required and is not usually a problem, even in the presence of severe chronic air-flow limitation (CAL) (see p. 447).

Blood pressure   These patients often are hypertensive and need to have their blood pressure maintained within their own 'normal' pre-operative limits. Hypotension usually responds to fluid replacement, but sometimes may require inotrope support. Remember that para-doxical hypertension often occurs in these patients when they are hypovolaemic.

Fluid replacement   Patients, especially those who have had vascu-lar surgery including a laparotomy, often require large amounts of fluid replacement for the first 12 hours post-operatively (eg 2–4 L).

Urine output   It is crucial to maintain urine output at or above 0.5 ml $\cdot$ kg^{-1} $\cdot$ h^{-1}. Fluids and low-dosage dopamine are usually suffi-cient to achieve this (see p. 645).

Pain relief   Recovery from surgery involving a lower limb or the carotid artery is not especially painful. However, it is important to provide adequate pain relief for patients following laparotomy, in or-der to ensure adequate ventilation and oxygenation. Horizontal ab-dominal incisions are less painful than the more traditional vertical ones. Techniques for pain relief include

- epidural analgesia (see p. 120)
- continuous or intermittent narcotic infusion

Routine post-operative monitoring   Routine post-operative moni-toring should include the following:

- determinations of blood pressure, pulse rate, respiratory rate, pulse oximetry, and temperature
- neurological assessment, especially after carotid surgery
- determinations of peripheral pulses and perfusion to test adequacy of grafts
- monitoring for bleeding around graft sites

TROUBLESHOOTING

POST-OPERATIVE CARE FOLLOWING CAROTID ENDARTERECTOMY

Maintain arterial blood pressure within the patient's normal pre-operative range.

Monitor the patient for post-operative myocardial ischaemia with routine 12-lead ECG, considering cardiac enzymes, symptoms, and ST/T-wave changes on continuous ECG recording. Treat myocardial ischaemia aggressively.

Early signs of cerebral ischaemia (eg focal neurological signs) should be reported to the surgeon immediately. A surgical cause is common, and surgical intervention is necessary.

Early signs of bleeding around the operative site should be taken seriously. Severe obstruction of the upper airways can occur rapidly, even without obvious signs such as stridor. Intubation is EXTREMELY DIFFICULT in these circumstances, and expert assistance is necessary.

FURTHER READING

Benjamin, B. (1993). Prolonged intubation injuries of the larynx: endoscopic diagnosis, classification and treatment. *Annals of Otology, Rhinology and Laryngology (Suppl.)* 102:1–15.

Cook, D. J., Fuller, H. D., Guyatt, G. H., Marshall, J. C., Leasa, D., Hall, R., Winton, T. L., Rutledge, F., Todd, T. J. R., Roy, P., Lacroix, J., Griffith, L., & Willan, A. (1994). Risk factors for gastrointestinal bleeding in critically ill patients. *New England Journal of Medicine* 330:377–81.

Dobb, G.J., & Cooms, L. J. (1987). Clinical examination of patients in the intensive care unit. *British Journal of Hospital Medicine* 5:102–8.

Grover, E. R., & Bihari, D. J. (1992). The role of tracheostomy in the adult intensive care unit. *Postgraduate Medical Journal* 68:313–17.

Hazard, P., Jones, C., & Benitone, J. (1991). Comparative clinical trial of standard operative tracheostomy with percutaneous tracheostomy. *Critical Care Medicine* 19:1018–24.

Soni, N. L. (ed.) (1989). *Anaesthesia and Intensive Care: Practical Procedures.* London: Butterworth.

Tryba, M. (1994). Stress ulcer prophylaxis – quo vadis? *Intensive Care Medicine* 20:311–13.

3

ECONOMICS, OUTCOME, AND ETHICS IN INTENSIVE CARE

No book should discuss critically ill patients without addressing the issues of economics, outcome, and ethics. Certain questions must continuously remain on the agenda: For whom is intensive care appropriate? Is the cost justified? How long should treatment be continued? In what manner should treatment be withdrawn? Economics and ethics can no longer be kept separate. No matter how wealthy a society is, today it has a finite health budget. Economic considerations will therefore increasingly dictate the limits of therapy, and ethical considerations must be evaluated within those limits.

COSTS OF INTENSIVE CARE

The cost of providing intensive care is high – at least three times the cost of providing normal hospital care. Approximately 15% of hospitalized patients account for as much of the health budget as do the other 85%. Among that 15% of patients, treatment for chronic diseases, outside of intensive care, accounts for most of that half of the budget.

COST CONTAINMENT

There is no longer a blank cheque for medical care. We are all having to become aware of the increasing costs of medical care and the limitations they impose upon our practice. In certain cases we can no longer assert our traditional right to do what we think is best for our patients, regardless of cost. Rather than become self-righteous about these new limitations, we must responsibly meet the practical challenge of a finite health budget. Some of the measures required are discussed next.

Management principles

Many doctors working in intensive care are familiarizing themselves with the principles of good management, including how best to manage manpower within the intensive care unit (ICU), how to apply cost–benefit concepts to patient treatment, and how to manage budgets efficiently. These and other principles will become increasingly important in our everyday practice (see Chapter 1).

High technology

Unless a technology has been shown to be effective and to be justified by economic appraisal, it might be regarded as unethical to use it. This can raise difficult dilemmas in the face of physicians' traditional obsession with clinical freedom and their often naive attitudes toward more aggressive marketing strategies. Many commercial strategies exploit the human desire to have the latest complex piece of machinery, or to be seen using the latest drug. Physicians are becoming more skeptical and better educated about these matters, but unless we take an informed initiative in this area, decisions will be indirectly or directly imposed on us by people who are less well informed.

Efficiency

Labour costs account for the greater part of an ICU budget. As this is a relatively constant feature, strategies such as rapid turnover of patients and more efficient work practices can enable a greater number of patients to be dealt with by the same number of staff.

Drugs and equipment

Continuous monitoring and appraisal of one's own practice in intensive care can reduce costs.

INVASIVE MONITORING Invasive monitoring is expensive in terms of both labour and material costs. There is widespread feeling that invasive haemodynamic monitoring has been over-used and that in the future there will be more reliance on non-invasive and simpler continuous monitoring (see Chapter 21).

VENTILATORY TECHNIQUES Although many ICUs are relying on increasingly sophisticated and expensive ventilators, among others there is a new tendency to use simple and efficient devices that provide continuous positive airway pressure (CPAP) to support spontaneous respiration (see p. 367). In many cases this is cheaper and more effective than artificial ventilation.

MATERIALS Many volumetric infusion devices utilize dedicated plastic giving sets that are very expensive. Infusion syringe pumps perform the same function and utilize inexpensive and universal plastic giving sets.

DRUGS Clinicians and nursing staff should be aware of the costs of individual drugs, as well as the amounts of drugs used by their own ICU. Areas of high cost can then be examined.

THE LATEST-IS-BEST PHENOMENON Money for research is becoming increasingly difficult to find. It is no surprise, therefore, that research is often financed by companies that are marketing new devices or drugs. Publications and marketing techniques associated with newer drugs and equipment tend to focus one's alternatives in that direction: In other words, commerce can set the agenda for our research and therefore influence the current interests of practising clinicians. Often an older and cheaper drug may be just as effective (eg when choosing an inotrope in intensive care, many clinicians limit their choice to dobutamine or dopamine, rather than considering adrenaline or noradrenaline. Similarly, morphine and pethidine are much cheaper than fentanyl and phenoperidine. Antibiotics account for a large part of the budget in intensive care, and the newer ones are not necessarily better, but almost invariably are more expensive.

PREVENTIVE MEDICINE It is sobering to consider that the presence or absence of medical care accounts for only 10% of the differences in mortality among all societies. Genetics, health habits, and social class account for the majority of the differences.

Although many clinicians in intensive care tend to see a strict boundary between preventive medicine and their own practice, it does not take much imagination to see the enormous impact of preventable diseases in our own specialty: alcohol-related admissions (eg self-poisoning, road-traffic trauma, oesophageal varices), smoking-related diseases (coronary artery disease, peripheral vascular disease, respiratory disease), and other forms of drug abuse.

SEVERITY SCORING AND OUTCOME PREDICTION

The basic question whether or not ICUs are justified is difficult, if not impossible, to answer. Randomized controlled trials involving critically ill patients are almost impossible to perform because, like many areas of modern medicine, the practice in question has become an accepted and standard mode of treatment. Attention has been focused, therefore, on scoring the severity of illness. Such measurements are used to predict outcomes and as a form of quality assurance.

There are many ways of measuring illness severity. One of the first and most commonly used is the Glasgow coma scale (GCS), which measures a patient's level of consciousness (see p. 586). There are other scales that specifically measure the severity of trauma (see p. 257). One of the earlier measures of illness severity used in intensive care was the therapeutic intervention scoring system (TISS). However, TISS provides a measure of treatment, and that assumes that treatment and monitoring are directly related to illness severity. That obviously is not always an accurate assumption, because there is a wide range of different treatments delivered by different units for the same disease state. For example, there is wide variation between units with regard to the use of invasive monitoring. TISS may, in fact, be a more accurate indicator of other outcomes, such as the nursing work load, rather than a marker of illness severity.

APACHE SCORE   The Acute Physiology and Chronic Health Evaluation (APACHE) scoring system probably is the one most widely used in ICUs throughout the world. Currently, the APACHE II system is most commonly used, but a more recent and more complicated version, APACHE III, is also available.

The APACHE II system uses basic physiological data to assess the severity of illness and to stratify patients prognostically on the basis of risk of death. It uses 12 physiological variables that are weighted for the severity of the abnormality to yield an acute physiological score (APS) (Table 3.1). The APS is derived from the worst physiological

TABLE 3.1   APACHE II: A SEVERITY-OF-DISEASE CLASSIFICATION SYSTEM

APS points
TEMPERATURE (rectal)
MEAN BLOOD PRESSURE
HEART RATE (ventricular response)
RESPIRATORY RATES (total non-ventilated or ventilated rate)
OXYGENATION (A-a)Do_2 OR Pao_2
ARTERIAL pH
SERUM SODIUM
SERUM POTASSIUM
SERUM CREATININE
HAEMATOCRIT (%)
WHITE-BLOOD-CELL COUNT
NEUROLOGICAL STATE (Glasgow coma scale)

A. TOTAL ACUTE PHYSIOLOGY SCORE (APS)
  Sum of the 12 individual variable points

B. AGE POINTS
  Assign points as follows:

AGE (years)	Points
≤44	0
45–54	2
55–64	3
65–74	5
≥75	6

C. CHRONIC HEALTH POINTS
  If the patient has a history of chronic disease (ie a history of severe insufficiency) or is immunocompromised, then assign points as follows:
  (a) for non-operative or emergency post-operative patients, 5 points
  (b) for elective post-operative patients, 2 points

values, either on admission or during the first 24 hours after admission. This score is then added to a chronic health evaluation (CHE), which attempts to score the state of health of the patient just before admission. This takes into account age and the presence of any chronic health problems. The assumption is that age and chronic health problems reflect a diminished physiological reserve.

There is a direct relationship between the total APACHE II scores and hospital death rates. However, this risk of death also varies according to various disease categories. For example, diabetic ketoacidosis is associated with severe acute physiological abnormalities and a high APACHE II score. However, the same score in a patient with severe trauma would indicate a higher risk of death. Therefore, a diagnostic-category weight reflecting the risk of death for each disease category must also be taken into account. The APACHE II score and diagnostic weight are used to derive the risk of death.

The figure predicting death can be used as an estimate only for large groups; it is not accurate enough to predict death in an individual patient.

The use of these scores can be quite valuable in comparing standardized mortality rates (SMRs). The SMRs can be used by ICUs to compare their own performances at various points in time and to compare SMRs between units. This is currently one of the best ways of measuring a unit's performance.

SAPS SYSTEM   The simplified acute physiology score (SAPS II) was derived from a large, heterogeneous patient population using logistic regression. It incorporates age, the presence of chronic disease, and the type of admission, as well as data from 12 physiological measurements and investigations. The worst value during the first 24 hours is considered, and weighted points are assigned according to severity and the particular variable (eg 0 to 3 for temperature abnormalities, and 0 to 26 for GCS abnormalities). An equation based on the multiple-logistic-regression model is then used to predict hospital mortality. Unlike the APACHE score, the SAPS II score is not weighted for individual diagnosis. It is also easy to calculate.

MPM II SYSTEM   The mortality probability model (MPM II) is based on a series of models, rather than a single model that is applied repeatedly over all ICU admissions. It is used to estimate hospital mortality, and it is also a quality-assurance tool to compare outcomes between various ICUs.

LONG-TERM OUTCOME   Probably even more important than survival is the quality of that survival. It is now becoming possible to quantify a patient's quality of life and to use that measurement to determine the efficacy of an intervention.

The measurement of a patient's quality of life (QOL) is in its infancy, and there is, as yet, no universally accepted and validated scale. Measurement of QOL takes into account factors such as physical capabilities, pain, ability to work, and social interactions. A QOL rating is usually expressed as a fraction between 0 and 1, where 0 is death and 1 is a full life. Interestingly, there are some states of ill health that are considered worse than death, and they are assigned negative values. From the QOL we have derived the concept known as the quality-of-life-adjusted year (QALY). This is calculated as the total number of years over which a particular health intervention is used multiplied by the QOL fraction. For example, if a patient lived for 10 years with a full QOL score of 1, then the intervention is said to have generated 10 QALYs (10 × 1.0). If the patient lived for 10 years, but was racked with pain and confined to bed, with a QOL score of, say, 0.5, the intervention is said to have generated 5 QALYs (10 × 0.5).

If the cost of the intervention can be determined, then the ratio cost/QALY can be determined. Thus, various health interventions can be compared for effectiveness. The concept of the QOL measurement adds another dimension to the field of outcome measurements.

WHO SHOULD RECEIVE INTENSIVE CARE?

This is never an easy decision, and it is not amenable to strict rules. Some of the factors that need to be considered are discussed next.

UNDERLYING DISEASES   Incurable cancer is often cited as a contraindication to admitting a patient to intensive care. However, at the time of such consideration it is not always known whether or not the cancer is incurable, and even if it is, a short stay in intensive care after a palliative operation may guarantee that the patient will at least be able to leave the hospital.

AGE   An age limit could preclude many of the world's current political leaders from admission to an ICU. Whether that would be a good thing or a bad thing is another matter. A strict age limit probably would be as irrelevant as many other single factors in assessing any-one's right to intensive care. Some elderly patients can benefit from a short, effective stay in intensive care. On the other hand, there is often enormous pressure to admit young patients who are hopelessly ill. This is related more to emotional reasons than to logic.

REVERSIBILITY OF ILLNESS   It could be argued that anyone with an acute, reversible pathological condition should be admitted to an ICU. The problem is that the reversibility of such conditions often is not known at the time of admission. A practical approach, then, depending on the availability of beds and the staffing situation, is to admit most patients for a 'short, sharp burst' of intensive care. Thereby, acute physiological abnormalities can be reversed while the staff observes RATE OF RESPONSE OF THE PATIENT.

Depending, then, on the slope of this empirical response curve, and together with other factors, such as age and underlying disease, a decision can be made to

(a) continue management without reservation,

(b) continue management with reservations, or

(c) discontinue treatment and allow the patient to die with dignity.

This flexible policy will allow efficient use of scarce ICU resources, on the understanding that if the patient is not responding rapidly and has other adverse features, then treatment can be ceased at any point. A careful assessment should be made at least daily, involving all relevant parties in the decision-making process. That will preclude a mindless policy of blindly continuing treatment and support until the patient dies in spite of every effort.

DISCONTINUATION OF TREATMENT

It has become clear that when a patient is brain dead, active management should be ceased, as there is no hope of survival (see p. 618). Although this is no longer a problem in intensive care, we now recognize that there is a group of patients with irreversible diseases for whom we are prolonging the dying process. At the same time, we have to accept that we will never be 100% sure of a given patient's probability of death. In the past, that consideration prompted us to sustain the lives of all patients with every available means until death finally supervened. That approach caused suffering for both patients and relatives, in addition to attracting criticism from many of our colleagues and from society.

Increasingly we are coming to realize that keeping one patient alive in such a manner is at some cost to another patient. Economic pressure is forcing a wider-ranging ethical debate. The desirability of attempting to restore health does not imply that it is ethically justified to prolong life at any cost. 'Dying' is a diagnosis commonly overlooked or evaded. The decision to withhold life-sustaining treatment from hopelessly ill patients involves an ethical dilemma and legal uncertainties. Each ICU has to solve these problems in its own way. Some guidelines used within our own unit are as follows:

1. No matter how many people or committees are involved in the decision to cease active management, we attempt never to make the relatives feel that it is their decision. We take complete responsibility for that decision, while involving them fully in all other aspects of the dying process.

2. All members of the medical and nursing team in the ICU looking after a given patient are involved in the decision to withdraw active management.

3. The patient must be allowed as much dignity in the dying process as during the living process. The challenge is to ensure that the patient dies pain-free and that the needs of the relatives are attended to, and meeting that challenge can be as rewarding as any other aspect of intensive care medicine.

3. Because of the controversies surrounding the use of life-support machines, we usually continue ventilatory support in most patients. Usually this is not a major problem, as many seriously ill patients can breath spontaneously. If the brain-stem is intact, the terminal event usually is cadiovascular collapse or hypoxia, rather than hypoventilation. When it is decided that active management is no longer appropriate, all support measures are ceased, and every attention is paid to the patient's comfort during the dying process. If the patient is unconscious, feeding is stopped, drugs (apart from sedation and pain relief) are discontinued, observations and monitoring are stopped, and the patient's appearance is attended to. Pain is treated without causing cessation of breathing. The patient is made to look comfortable and at peace. Dignity is preserved. Where possible, privacy is ensured, so that relatives can, if they wish, be with the patient when death occurs.

Where a patient is conscious and able to communicate, the prognosis must be discussed openly and honestly. The principles of palliative care and management of the dying process for these patients are the same as for other terminally ill patients

5. If possible, we prefer to manage the dying process within the ICU. However, often there are constraints involving staffing levels and bed status. When it is expected that the dying process may be prolonged, the patient may have to be transferred to a general ward.

TROUBLESHOOTING

MANAGEMENT OF THE DYING PATIENT

Periodically in any ICU it will become obvious that further active management of a given patient is futile. The following are some guidelines for dealing with that difficult situation.

Consensus The medical and nursing staff responsible for the patient's management must reach a consensus that further active management is futile.

Involvement of the relatives Various ICUs will have different policies with regard to the involvement of relatives. Our own policy is to be honest about the hopelessness of continuing treatment, but not to hint in any way that the decision is one that the relatives must make.

Change in management direction Once it has been decided that there is no point in continuing active treatment, several principles become clear:
- Every effort must be made to guarantee that the patient can die with dignity and without pain.
- Careful consideration should be given to cessation of all support, apart from pain relief and basic procedures related to cleanliness and appearance.
- Ventilatory support often can be continued under these circumstances, even if the F_{IO_2} is reduced. This allows large amounts of nar-

> cotics to be used, without directly impairing the patient's airway or respiration.
>
> • Nursing and medical efforts should be redirected toward supporting the patient's relatives and friends.

FURTHER READING

Bayliss, R. I. S. (1982). Thou shalt not strive officiously. *British Medical Journal* 285:1373–5.

Birnbaum, M. L. (1986). Cost-containment in critical care. *Critical Care Medicine* 14:1068–77.

Buist, M. (1994). Intensive care unit resource utilisation. *Anaesthesia and Intensive Care* 22:46–60.

Cohen, C. B. (1982). Interdisciplinary consultation on the care of the critically ill and dying: the role of one hospital ethics committee. *Critical Care Medicine* 10:776–84.

Daffurn, K., Kerridge, R., & Hillman, K. (1992). Active management of the dying process. *Medical Journal of Australia* 157:701–4.

Dragsted, L. (1991). Outcomes from intensive care. *Danish Medical Bulletin* 38:365–74.

Gregory, G. A. (1983). Who should receive intensive care? *Critical Care Medicine* 11:767–8.

Hampton, J. R. (1983). The end of clinical freedom. *British Medical Journal* 287:1237–8.

Jennett, B. (1984). Economic appraisal. *British Medical Journal* 288:1781–2.

Kerridge, R., Brooks, R., Bauman, A., & Hillman, K. (1994). Quality of life after intensive care. In *Yearbook of Intensive Care and Emergency Medicine,* ed. J. L. Vincent, pp. 827–38. Berlin: Springer-Verlag.

Knaus, W. A., Draper, E. A., Wagner, P., & Zimmerman, J. E. (1985). APACHE II: a severity of disease classification system. *Critical Care Medicine* 13:818–29.

Knaus, W. A., Wagner, D. P., Draper, E. A., Zimmerman, J. E., Bergner, M., Bastos, P. G., Sirio, C. A., Murphy, D. J., Lotring, T., Damiano, A., & Harrell, F. E. (1991). The Apache III prognostic system. *Chest* 100:1619–36.

Le Gall, J. R., Lemeshow, S., & Saulnier, F. (1993). A new simplified physiology score (SAPS II) based on a European–North American multicentre study. *Journal of the American Medical Association* 270:29057–8.

Lemeshow, S., & Teres, D. (1994). The MPM II system for ICU patients. In *Yearbook of Intensive Care and Emergency Medicine,* ed. J. L. Vincent, pp. 805–15. Berlin: Springer-Verlag.

McIntyre, N., & Popper, K. (1983). The critical attitude in medicine: the need for a new ethics. *British Medical Journal* 287:1919–23.

Meisel, A., Grenvik, A., Pinkus, R. L., & Snyder, J. V. (1986). Hospital guidelines for deciding about life-sustaining treatment. Dealing with health 'limbo'. *Critical Care Medicine* 14:239–46.

Ninos, N. P. (1988). Humanism and technology. *Critical Care Medicine* 16:1252–3.

Slatyer, M. A., James, O. F., Moore, P. G., & Leeder, S. R. (1986). Costs, severity of illness and outcome in intensive care. *Anaesthesia and Intensive Care* 14:381–9.

Smith, T. (1984). Taming high technology. *British Medical Journal* 289:393–4.

4

FLUID AND ELECTROLYTE REPLACEMENT

- Rapid and continual replacement of the circulating volumes is one of the commonest and most important manoeuvres in intensive care.
- The intravascular space should be continually resuscitated against 'hard' and easily measurable end points, while the interstitial and intracellular fluid spaces are maintained using 'softer' end points.
- Serum potassium, magnesium, and phosphate values should be measured at least daily and corrected.

ASSESSMENT OF BODY FLUID SPACES

Body fluid is distributed to three compartments – the intravascular space (IVS), the interstitial space (ISS), and the intracellular space (ICS) (Figure 4.1). The IVS and ISS together contain the extracellular fluid (ECF). The fluid in each space has a unique composition and function. The function of the IVS fluid is to carry gases, nutrients, and metabolites to and from cells. The ISS bridges the gap between the cells and the capillaries. It also carries the lymph system, which transports protein, other solutes, and fluid back into the circulation. Dehydration results in depletion of the ISS fluid, whereas oedema occurs when there is excessive fluid. Oedema is common in the seriously ill and can cause serious complications (see p. 62). The ISS fluid consists largely of sodium and water, and the ICS fluid consists mainly of potassium and water.

Assessment of the ISS is more difficult than assessment of the IVS. There are many reasonably accurate measurements, such as blood pressure, pulse rate, urine output, and cardiac filling pressures, that can reflect the volume of the IVS, whereas measurements reflecting the ISS and ICS, such as tissue turgor and the extent of dry mucosa, are relatively 'soft' in comparison.

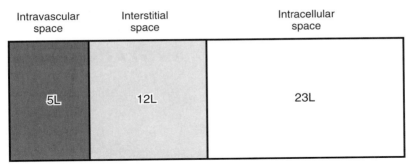

FIGURE 4.1   Volumes of the body's fluid compartments.

Before any decision about fluid replacement is made, one must determine which fluid space is depleted; then the most appropriate fluid for replenishing that particular space should be given (see p. 61).

- IVS volume: approximately 70 ml/kg in adults
- ISS volume: approximately 200 ml/kg in adults
- ICS volume: approximately 330 ml/kg in adults

Table 4.1 lists the causes of hypovolaemia.

ASSESSMENT OF THE IVS

Pulse rate

Tachycardia is a good indicator of hypovolaemia in the young when there are no other complicating factors. However, interpretation can be difficult, as tachyarrhythmias due to underlying disease, such as sepsis, pain and anxiety, or drug administration, can commonly affect heart rate in the seriously ill. Underlying cardiac disease, especially in the elderly, can also complicate the interpretation of tachycardia as an indicator of hypovolaemia.

Arterial blood pressure

Hypotension often means hypovolaemia, whereas hypertension is rarely caused by hypervolaemia. In fact, hypovolaemia can paradoxically cause hypertension, especially in patients who previously have

TABLE 4.1   CAUSES OF HYPOVOLAEMIA

1. Blood loss
2. Water and electrolyte loss, eg
   GIT losses
   Excessive diuresis
   Excessive sweating
3. Plasma loss, eg
   Burns
4. Vasodilation causing relative hypovolaemia, eg
   Sepsis
   Drugs

been hypertensive, in children, or in the presence of autonomic dysfunction (eg tetanus, poliomyelitis, Guillain-Barré syndrome). However, there is a reasonably steady relationship between arterial blood pressure and intravascular volume in seriously ill patients in intensive care. The pressure must be interpreted in light of any artificial support by inotropes and vasopressors. Intravascular volume 'tracks' blood pressure more accurately in the elderly than in fit young patients, where it tends to be compensated for by an active response to sympathoadrenal activity, until dangerous levels of hypovolaemia have been reached.

Central venous pressure

Central venous pressure (CVP) is a reflection of only right-side cardiac filling pressures; it is not an accurate indicator of left-side cardiac pressures.

Lung abnormalities, artificial ventilation, and positive end expiratory pressure (PEEP) can cause increases in pulmonary artery pressure and right-side heart pressures even in the presence of normal or low blood volumes (Figure 4.2).

Excessive sympathetic tone accompanying hypovolaemia also can artificially increase CVP. Thus, CVP in the presence of hypovolaemia can be low, normal, or high. Similarly, after fluid correction, it may increase, decrease, or remain the same.

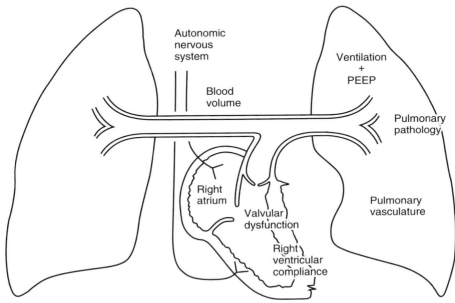

FIGURE 4.2 Determinants of CVP other than blood volume (keep in mind that there may be inherent inaccuracies in the measuring of CVP, as well as the possible effects of drugs).

CVP IS, AT BEST, USEFUL TO INDICATE A TREND, AND THEN ONLY WHEN IT IS CONSISTENT WITH OTHER MEASUREMENTS OF INTRAVASCULAR VOLUME.

Pulmonary artery wedge pressure

The pulmonary artery wedge pressure (PAWP), measured with a pulmonary artery catheter, is a reflection of left-side filling pressure in the heart and thus is a more accurate indicator of the systemic circulation than is CVP. As with CVP measurement, technical errors can be common.

There is little relationship between left ventricular end-diastolic volume and PAWP in seriously ill patients. This is largely because of the unpredictable relationship between left ventricular pressure and volume, or compliance, in the presence of critical illness such as multitrauma and septicaemia.

The PAWP may be difficult to interpret in artificially ventilated patients, because it increases in the presence of increased intrathoracic pressure, such as PEEP, continuous positive airway pressure (CPAP), or intermittent positive-pressure ventilation (IPPV).

Thus, PAWP is useful to indicate a trend, rather than as an absolute reading, and is useful in association with, rather than in isolation from, other indications of intravascular volume.

Peripheral perfusion

The ratio between core temperature and peripheral temperature reflects peripheral perfusion. The temperatures in the extremities provide a rapid means for estimating peripheral perfusion. They cannot, of course, allow one to differentiate between hypovolaemia and poor cardiac function.

Urine output

Hourly urine output offers an accurate and easy means for assessing peripheral perfusion and circulating volume. However, it can be affected by drugs, including diuretics, as well as by the underlying renal function.

Tonometry

The problem with many of our current measurements of circulating volume is that they do not reflect the adequacy of blood flow to the tissues. Tonometry indirectly measures blood flow in the mucosa of the gastro-intestinal tract (GIT). The technique is described in more detail later (see p. 493). Tonometry was one of the first measurements to give us information about tissue perfusion in a non-invasive way. Although it has disadvantages, such as the lack of a continuous readout, it heralds a new direction in monitoring that almost certainly will become more popular.

Fluid challenge

THE INTRAVASCULAR COMPARTMENT IS MOST ACCURATELY AS-SESSED BY USING THE FLUID-CHALLENGE TECHNIQUE: Measure all available indicators of the IVS before and after rapidly infusing a fluid bolus (200–500 ml). If they all rapidly improve, consideration should be given to a further bolus. If minimal improvement occurs, the circulating volume is close to being optimally filled.

ASSESSMENT OF THE ISS AND ICS

The ISS and ICS usually are assessed together, because it is difficult to distinguish between them on clinical grounds. Although they contain the majority of the body's water, the ISS and ICS are far less accessible to estimation than is the IVS.

Fluid-balance charts

A fluid-balance chart, at best, provides only a guideline to fluid needs. Limited ins and outs are recorded on a fluid-balance chart (eg gastric aspirate, urine output, oral and intravenous intakes). The recorded fluid balance can represent less than half of the fluids actually lost or gained, as many of the fluids are inaccessible to measurement (eg insensible loss, water of oxidation, GIT losses from an ileu, and wound oedema).

Unless the electrolyte and protein concentrations of lost body fluids are known, we cannot know from which body space a fluid was lost, nor, therefore, the most appropriate fluid with which to replace that loss.

History

A history of fluid losses (eg diarrhoea, gastric contents, diuresis, excessive sweating, wound and fistula losses, hyperventilation) will provide information on the magnitude and composition of the lost fluid. For example, pancreatic fluid and bile will have electrolyte concentrations similar to those of ISS fluid, whereas gastric losses and fluid from an osmotic diuresis will have comparatively lower sodium con-

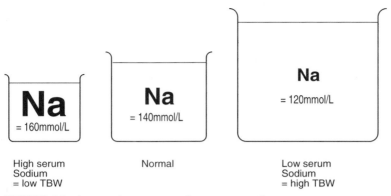

High serum
Sodium
= low TBW   Normal   Low serum
                                                       Sodium
                                                       = high TBW

FIGURE 4.3   Interpreting serum sodium concentrations.

centrations and higher potassium concentrations, indicating fluid losses from the ICS as well as from the ISS.

Serum sodium

The serum sodium concentration is the single most important indicator of total body water (TBW), as it usually is a reflection of body water changes rather than the absolute amount of body sodium. Thus, hyponatraemia usually represents excessive body water, and hypernatraemia usually represents depleted body water (Fig. 4.3).

Chest x-ray

A chest x-ray will provide an accurate indication of lung water, which is equivalent to the ISS of lung tissue. Regular chest x-rays constitute an efficient and accurate predicator of lung water. However, the lung water usually is the result of an underlying abnormality, such as cardiogenic pulmonary oedema or adult respiratory distress syndrome (ARDS), rather than simple fluid overload. However, there is a direct relationship between intravascular pressures and the amount of lung water in a patient with either ARDS or cardiogenic pulmonary oedema.

Dry mucosa

The extent of dry mucosa is difficult to interpret in intensive care, as such patients usually are unconscious or have a high rate of gas flow from an oxygen mask.

Tissue turgor

Tissue turgor is an estimate of both the ISS and ICS volumes. It varies enormously with age. It provides an empirical guide, at best, allowing one to estimate the extremes of 'very dry' (dehydration) or 'very wet' (oedema).

FLUID REPLACEMENT

Fluid replacement in the critically ill must be precise, as these patients often will have lost the normal mechanisms for fluid control, such as thirst and normal renal function, and thus they cannot compensate for excessive or inadequate fluid volumes.

PRIORITIES IN FLUID REPLACEMENT

1. THE FIRST PRIORITY, AND ONE OF THE MOST IMPORTANT AND COMMON MANOEUVRES IN INTENSIVE CARE, IS TO CONTINUALLY ASSESS AND CORRECT THE INTRAVASCULAR VOLUME. Replacement of lost IVS fluid is essential in order to maintain normal tissue perfusion.

2. Maintain adequate haemoglobin concentration, to ensure adequate oxygenation.

3. Replace electrolytes, in order to maintain the distribution and volume of body water, as well as to maintain cellular function (eg sodium, potassium, calcium, magnesium, phosphate) (see p. 72).

4. Replace water, to maintain the ISS and ICS.

INTRAVASCULAR SPACE

Once measurements have verified hypovolaemia, a fluid that will be retained within the circulating volume is the most efficient form of replacement (eg colloid or blood). Crystalloid solutions (eg isotonic saline, Ringer's lactate) are distributed throughout the whole ECF and therefore are not as efficient for correcting intravascular deficits as are colloid solutions. Where possible, colloid or blood should be titrated against the indicators of intravascular volume – blood pressure, pulse rate, CVP, PAWP, urine output, peripheral perfusion.

In practice, all of these measurements of intravascular volume have shortcomings, and they are more useful when taken in conjunction with a FLUID CHALLENGE. Appropriate readings should be taken before and after a challenge of 200–500 ml of rapidly infused fluid, for adults, or aliquots of 20 ml/kg, for children.

INTERSTITIAL SPACE

Most of a crystalloid solution will be distributed to the ISS, not the IVS. Thus, crystalloids are the most useful fluids for rehydrating the ISS. However, it is rare to have a depleted ISS in a seriously ill patient. In fact, oedema or expansion of the ISS usually is a much greater problem. Crystalloid solutions should therefore be used cautiously when correcting hypovolaemia.

Pulmonary and peripheral oedema

Because crystalloids are distributed mainly to the ISS, rather than the IVS, they can cause pulmonary and peripheral oedema in subclinical and overt forms. Pulmonary oedema causes decreases in oxygenation and lung compliance, and peripheral oedema decreases cellular perfusion and oxygen consumption.

Salt-containing solutions (eg isotonic saline or Ringer's lactate solution) should be used judiciously for the correction of hypovolaemia, especially when large volumes are contemplated. Often the ISS is already over-expanded in the seriously ill, as a result of the salt and water retention that accompanies the stress response.

INTRACELLULAR SPACE

Assessment of the ICS is clinically difficult. Most of the body's water contained within the ICS, and SERUM SODIUM CONCENTRATION IS THE MOST IMPORTANT CLINICAL INDICATION OF TBW STATUS. Hyponatraemia usually indicates excessive TBW, and hypernatraemia usually indicates inadequate TBW. Thus, water (usually in the form of 5% dextrose) can be titrated in an empirical fashion against serum sodium.

Although water losses in the seriously ill can be substantial, water gains due to secretion of antidiuretic hormone (ADH) and due to catabolism are not insignificant. As a guideline, 500–2,000 ml of 5% dextrose per 24 h (20–100 ml/h) usually will be sufficient water replacement in the seriously ill.

APPROACH TO FLUID REPLACEMENT IN THE CRITICALLY ILL

ONE SHOULD NOT USE RIGID AND INFLEXIBLE REGIMENS AND FORMULAE FOR FLUID REPLACEMENT. EACH PATIENT SHOULD BE CAREFULLY ASSESSED, AND THE RIGHT TYPE OF FLUID IN THE RIGHT AMOUNT SHOULD BE PRESCRIBED FOR THAT PARTICULAR TIME IN THE COURSE OF THAT PATIENT'S ILLNESS.

No matter what the origin of the fluid problem (eg shock, dehydration, excessive GIT losses, diabetic ketoacidosis, polyuria), the general principles for fluid and electrolyte replacements are the same:

1. CORRECT THE CIRCULATING VOLUME WITH COLLOID OR BLOOD. Restore organ perfusion and the oxygen-carrying capacity of the blood AS SOON AS POSSIBLE. Often a continuous infusion of colloid (50–200 ml/h) is required in the seriously ill in order to maintain a normal circulating volume. In disorders such as septicaemia or pancreatitis, higher infusion rates are sometimes required.

2. Rehydrate the interstitial and intracellular compartments, as appropriate in view of the patient's clinical status and biochemistry (eg serum electrolyte composition). This is usually achieved by titrating 5% dextrose empirically against the serum sodium concentration. An empirical hourly rate (20–100 ml/h is usually sufficient) can be charted once each day according to the daily serum concentration. More may be necessary in the presence of large fluid losses and hypernatraemia.

3. If a patient is relatively stable, a solution containing sodium and water can be used as maintenance fluid. Such solutions usually contain dextrose and saline in varying amounts to achieve isotonicity (Table 4.2). The sodium concentration is usually between 30 and 70 mmol/L. Such a maintenance solution should be given at a rate between 50 and 150 ml/h (1,200–3,000 ml/d). Compositions of commonly used intravenous fluids are given in Table 4.3.

4. If there are excessive losses from one particular part of the body,

TABLE 4.2 COMPOSITIONS OF COMMONLY USED IV SOLUTIONS

	Na (mmol/L)	K (mmol/L)	Ca (mmol/L)	Mg (mmol/L)	Cl (mmol/L)	Lactate (mmol/L)	Dextrose (g/100 ml)	pH	Osmolality
0.9% NaCl	154	—	—	—	154	—	—	5.0	308
0.45% saline (N/2)	77	—	—	—	77	—	—	5.2	154
Hartmann's solution (Ringer's lactate)	131	5	1	1	112	29	—	5.2	280
4.0% dextrose in 0.18% NaCl	31	—	—	—	31	—	4.0	4.0	282
5.0% dextrose	—	—	—	—	—	—	5.0	4.0	278
2.5% dextrose in 0.45% saline (N/2)	75	—	—	—	75	—	2.5	4.0	280
3.75% dextrose in 0.225% NaCl (N/4)	37.5	—	—	—	37.5	—	3.75	4.0	280

Source: From Hillman (1990), with permission.

TABLE 4.3 VOLUMES AND ELECTROLYTE CONCENTRATIONS OF VARIOUS BODY FLUIDS

	Volume (L/d)	Sodium (mmol/L)	Potassium (mmol/L)	Chloride (mmol/L)	Bicarbonate (mmol/L)
Saliva	1–2	30	20	35	15
Gastric juice	2	50	10	150	—
Bile	1.5	140	5	100	30
Pancreatic fluid	1.0	140	5	30	120
Small-intestine fluid	3.5–4.0	100	5	100	25
Large-intestine fluid	0.5	80	15	50	—
Diarrhoeal fluid		80	30	60	25
Sweat	0–3	50	10	50	—

then extra infusion of fluid of the appropriate composition will be required. For example, fluid losses from diarrhoea, from a small-bowel fistula, and from an osmotic diuresis will all have different electrolyte concentrations (Table 4.3). Moreover, the amount recorded as draining from a particular site may represent only a small percentage of the real losses. For example, whereas a fistula from the bowel may drain a substantial amount, fluid can also be lost into the intra-abdominal cavity and thus not recorded. As a general rule, we assume that losses are actually greater than those recorded.

PERI-OPERATIVE FLUIDS

The principles of fluid replacement are the same in the peri-operative period as for critically ill patients, no matter what the cause of the fluid loss or from which space it occurs.

1. Rapidly and aggressively correct hypovolaemia with blood or colloid.

2. Maintain TBW by infusing 5% dextrose at a rate to maintain the serum sodium concentration within normal limits.

3. When the patient becomes stabilized, a maintenance fluid can be used:

Adults: 4% dextrose at 20–40 ml · kg^{-1} · d^{-1} plus 0.18% NaCl, or a similar combination of dextrose and saline

Paediatrics: 4% dextrose at 60–80 ml · kg^{-1} · d^{-1} plus 0.18% NaCl, or a similar combination of dextrose and saline

4. Replacement fluid: Most body secretions (eg urine, gastric fluid, large-intestine fluid) contain relatively low concentrations of sodium. A dextrose/saline combination (Na at 30–70 mmol/L) can be used to replace excessive losses of most body fluids. Some body fluids (eg bile and pancreatic juice) contain higher amounts of sodium and may need crystalloids (eg isotonic saline or Ringer's lactate) in order to replace losses.

MANIPULATION OF FLUID SPACES

The distribution of infused fluid can be predicted on the basis of its colloid oncotic pressure and sodium content. For example, fluid with a colloid oncotic pressure the same as that of plasma will largely remain in the IVS. Isotonic saline will largely remain within the ECF. A 5% dextrose solution will be distributed equally over all three body fluid compartments. Dextrose/saline-containing solutions will be distributed over all three compartments; the amount going to the ECF is dependent on the sodium concentration in that fluid. Artificial elimination of fluid from the body spaces, such as via haemofiltration, follows the same principles. The IVS is more amenable to manipulation than are the ISS and ICS. For example, the circulating volume can be artificially vasodilated or vasoconstricted with drug combinations.

Intravascular space

• Replace fluid losses with blood or colloid.

• The size of the intravascular compartment can also be manipulated by drugs that act either directly on smooth muscle or indirectly via the autonomic nervous system and adrenergic receptors – vasodilators and vasopressors.

Interstitial and intracellular spaces

• Assessment of these spaces is more difficult than is that of the IVS.
• Use isotonic saline to replace ISS losses; use water in an isotonic form to replace losses from the ICS.
• Excess fluid in the ISS and ICS can be removed by dialytic techniques, such as haemodialysis and ultrafiltration, or with drugs, such as diuretics or aldosterone and angiotensin antagonists.

Fluid manipulation across body spaces

Fluids can be encouraged to move from one compartment to another by a combination of strategies. For example, a patient with peripheral oedema in the presence of hypovolaemia and hypotension can be given a solution containing colloid osmotic particles, which will exert an oncotic pressure, causing the interstitial fluid to move into the IVS. Simultaneously, a diuretic or ultrafiltration can be used to decrease the ISS. Similarly, glucose, insulin, and potassium can be given to move water into the ICS (Figure 4.4).

By considering each fluid compartment separately, one can devise the right fluid for each space, or, alternatively, the right strategy when there is excessive fluid in any individual space.

COLLOID OR CRYSTALLOID?

This is largely an irrelevant question. The controversy as to whether crystalloid or colloid solutions should be used arose because of the false assumptions that both fliuds performed the same function, that they were distributed to the same body fluid spaces, and that the same measurements could be used as guidelines to their use. None of those assumptions was true. Using blood or colloid is the most efficient way of replacing intravascular volume, because the majority of it will be distributed to that space. Crystalloid, on the other hand, will mainly be distributed to the ISS.

When measurements of the IVS are used for fluid replacement (eg

Manipulation of fluid compartments

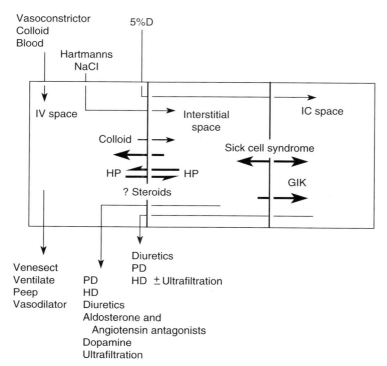

FIGURE 4.4 Representation of the different fluid compartments and how they can be manipulated. Following access through vascular cannulation, the various fluids are distributed mainly to one compartment or another. Similarly, by the use of various drugs or techniques, fluid can be removed from the fluid compartments. Fluid can also be encouraged to move from one compartment to another. The following key is used:

PD   peritoneal dialysis
HD   haemodialysis
GIK   glucose, insulin, and potassium
HP   hydrostatic pressure
PEEP   positive end-expiratory pressure
IC   intracellular
IV   intravascular

(From Hillman, 1990, with permission.)

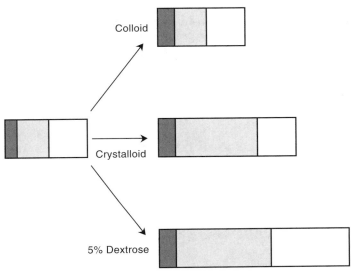

FIGURE 4.5 Correction of hypovolaemia with various fluids. The box on the left represents a hypothetical hypovolaemic patient. It can be seen that with the use of 5% dextrose to resuscitate the patient, massive expansions of the ICS and ISS will also occur. Similarly, with the use of a crystalloid, there will be significant expansion of the ISS. It is more efficient to use a colloid as the fluid, as less is required, and there are fewer complications because of less oedema.

blood pressure, pulse rate, CVP, PAWP), then a fluid that will be largely distributed to that space should ideally be used (eg blood or colloid solutions). As crystalloid solutions are distributed mainly to the ISS, they should be titrated against the assessment of that space (eg tissue turgor).

Crystalloid solutions (solutions containing isotonic amounts of sodium) are mainly distributed to the ISS, not to the IVS, and therefore are inefficient for intravascular volume replacement. In excessive amounts, crystalloids can cause pulmonary, peripheral, and perhaps even cerebral oedema (Figure 4.5).

Critically ill patients are stressed, and because of associated neuroendocrine responses, they retain sodium and water. This protects the ISS more than the ICS or IVS, exacerbating peripheral and pulmonary oedema.

The ISS should be kept 'dry' for optimum gas exchange in the lungs and for exchange of gases, substrates, and metabolites at a capillary level. Moreover, optimum lymphatic function depends on a 'dry' ISS. This is difficult to achieve when crystalloid solutions are used in the seriously ill.

COLLOID OR BLOOD SHOULD BE USED TO REPLENISH THE IVS ON THE BASIS OF INTRAVASCULAR MEASUREMENTS. CRYSTALLOID AND HYPOTONIC SOLUTIONS SHOULD BE USED TO MAINTAIN THE OTHER FLUID SPACES ON THE BASIS OF BIOCHEMICAL AND CLINICAL ASSESSMENT.

SPECIAL PROBLEMS

SYNDROME OF INAPPROPRIATE SECRETION OF ANTIDIURETIC HORMONE

Hyponatraemia is common in ICUs, and there are many causes (see p. 73). The syndrome of inappropriate secretion of antidiuretic hormone (SIADH) is usually a diagnosis of exclusion. Increased serum osmolality, stress, and hypovolaemia will cause release of ADH, which in turn causes water retention. All of these conditions are common in the seriously ill. Hypovolaemia will cause ADH release even if the patient is hypo-osmolar. MOST ADH RELEASE IN THE CRITICALLY ILL IS APPROPRIATE.

Inappropriate ADH release implies that ADH is released in the face of a normal initial intravascular volume and osmolality.

Inappropriate ADH release is rare and is associated with acute infections, acute psychiatric conditions, carcinoma, neurological disorders, endocrine disorders, and some drugs.

APPROACH

• Correct any reversible aspect of the primary disease.

• Correct any abnormalities of the circulating volume and serum osmolality; then reduce water intake according to the clinical state, serum osmolality, and serum sodium concentration.

• Administer demeclocycline (600–1,200 mg/24 h); lithium and frusemide have been used in resistant cases.

TABLE 4.4 COMPARISON OF SIADH AND DIABETES INSIPIDUS

	SIADH	**Diabetes insipidus**
Pathophysiology	ADH release inappropriate to the volume/osmolar state	Too little ADH, or insensitive to ADH
Alerting sign	Hyponatraemia	Polyuria
Serum osmolality	<275 mOsm/L	>310 mOsm/L
Urine osmolality	>100 mOsm/L	<200 mOsm/L
Urinary sodium	>20 mmol/L	>20 mmol/L

DIABETES INSIPIDUS

This syndrome is characterized by polyuria, thirst, and polydipsia secondary to plasma hyperosmolality and results when there is an absolute or relative deficiency of ADH (Table 4.4).

NEPHROGENIC The nephrogenic form is rare – the renal concentrating mechanism is not responsive to ADH.

NEUROGENIC The neurogenic form is common – often follows neurosurgery, head injury, or other cerebral insults. It results in polyuria that often is severe.

Diagnosis

Take a history and conduct a physical examination. Determine

• urine volume and osmolality
• plasma osmolality
• glucose, electrolyte, and calcium concentrations

In diabetes insipidus, the plasma osmolality is usually greater than 310 mOsm/kg (often >350), whereas the urine osmolality is usually less than 200 mOsm/kg (often <100).

In the acute setting, a therapeutic trial of desmopressin acetate (DDAVP) may be indicated: In patients with neurogenic diabetes insipidus, urine output, as well as urine and plasma osmolarities, will be corrected. In patients with nephrogenic diabetes, the polyuria will not respond to DDAVP. Water-deprivation tests are more suitable for ambulant patients with chronic diabetes insipidus, rather than those in an ICU.

Management

Exclude other causes of polyuria (eg associated with hyperglycaemia, mannitol, or other diuretics). Correct hypovolaemia with colloid, and replenish other body spaces as appropriate (see p. 61).

IT IS PARTICULARLY IMPORTANT TO TREAT POLYURIA IN AN UN-CONSCIOUS PATIENT, BECAUSE THE THIRST MECHANISM IS IM-PAIRED, AND DEHYDRATION MIGHT OTHERWISE OCCUR.

Use DDAVP parenterally rather than nasally in the acute situation. Give 1–5 units IM every 4–6 hours, according to control of polyuria. DDAVP is a potent drug, and care must be taken to avoid overdose and water intoxication. Alternatively, use a continuous intravenous infusion of vasopressin (1–2 units per hour initially, and then titrate against urine output). When using vasopressin, beware of myocardial ischaemia, which can be reversed by nitrates. Other complications include diarrhoeae, nausea, and abdominal cramps.

Measure the urinary electrolytes, and replace the urinary losses with the most appropriate solution – usually a dextrose/saline solution. Maintain the plasma osmolarity and serum sodium concentration within normal ranges.

ELECTROLYTES

SODIUM

Sodium is the principal extracellular ion. Its turnover is approximately 150 mmol/24 h. The normal kidney will slowly (over 3–5 days) adjust to widely varying sodium intakes.

Stressed and seriously ill patients have a neuroendocrine adaption to retain water and sodium. Excessive sodium as a result of replacement and retention is common and will cause ECF expansion, with pulmonary and peripheral oedema (see p. 62).

Hyponatraemia

Hyponatraemia does not necessarily imply hypo-osmolality, nor sodium depletion. Hyponatraemia can occur with decreased, normal, or even increased total body sodium. In the seriously ill, hyponatraemia is commonly due to excess body water, but rarely due to too little sodium. Clinical evaluation of the patient's fluid status will assist in the diagnosis. Hyponatraemia can occur with any acute illness, in association with liver disease and alcoholism, or as a result of water intoxication.

Rarely, hyponatraemia can be spurious, as a result of hyperlipidaemia or hyperproteinaemia. It can also occur in association with hyperglycaemia as a result of intracellular water moving into the extracellular space (see p. 731).

Hyponatraemia is rarely a problem in chronic states, as long as the serum sodium concentration is above 120 mmol/L.

Symptoms are related to the rate of change as well as to the absolute level – mild (weakness, dysarthria, and confusion) or severe (seizures, coma, central pontine myelinolysis, and cerebral oedema). Rapid correction of the hyponatraemia may also precipitate these symptoms.

TREATMENT The goals of treatment in acute hyponatraemia are to reduce excessive water and increase the plasma sodium concentration.

• CORRECTION OF HYPONATRAEMIA MUST BE SLOW, UNLESS THE PATIENT IS IN COMA OR IS HAVING CONVULSIONS. Permanent cerebral damage can occur secondary to rapid correction.

• Treat any underlying cause (eg cardiac failure).

• Aim to increase the serum sodium by no more than 10 mmol/24 h, even when a level of 120 mmol/L has been reached.

• Correction to more than 130 mmol/L is rarely necessary.

• In symptomatic cases (eg seizures or coma), consider using hypertonic solution (514 mmol/L) in conjunction with a diuretic such as mannitol or frusemide. Initially correct the serum sodium concentration to no more than 120 mmol/L.

• Water restriction will reverse most cases of mild hyponatraemia (>125 mmol/L) in patients who are asymptomatic.

Hypernatraemia

Hypernatraemia is almost always due to a deficit in body water (eg from GIT losses, skin losses, or osmotic diuresis). It is rarely due to excess total body sodium. Hypernatraemia can cause central nervous system symptoms.

TREATMENT

• Correct the underlying cause.

• A slow rehydration with 5% dextrose (100–200 ml/h) will correct most cases.

• Rarely, dialysis may be necessary.

POTASSIUM

Potassium is the principal intracellular ion. It is an important determinant of the resting membrane potential. Its turnover is approximately 50–100 mmol/24 h.

Unlike the case for sodium, the body's mechanisms for retaining potassium are underdeveloped. Small shifts in serum concentrations can be dangerous.

Hypokalaemia

Hypokalaemia is common in the ICU.

HYPOKALAEMIA IS A POTENT CAUSE OF BOTH SUPRAVENTRICULAR AND VENTRICULAR ARRHYTHMIAS.

Hypokalaemia can also cause coma and neuromyopathy.

Acute hypokalaemia is more arrhythmogenic than is the chronic form. The ECG changes include flat or inverted T waves, ST-segment depression, and U waves (Figure 4.6).

Many patients on long-term diuretics or oral theophylline preparations will be hypokalaemic on admission. Hypokalaemia also accompanies drugs with β_2-agonist activity (eg adrenaline, salbutamol).

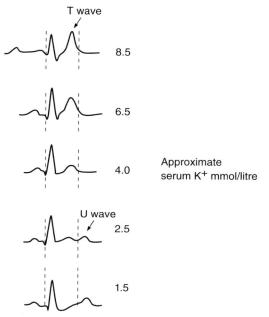

FIGURE 4.6 ECG changes resulting from alteration of the serum potassium concentration. (From Hutton & Cooper, 1985, with permission.)

CAUSES

Losses

• **THE KIDNEY IS THE MAIN SOURCE OF CLINICALLY SIGNIFICANT HYPOKALAEMIA IN THE SERIOUSLY ILL.**

• diuretics (eg frusemide or mannitol), diabetic ketoacidosis, and diabetes insipidus.

• GIT loss (eg diarrhoea) and excessive nasogastric losses.

Intracellular shift

• Correction of metabolic acidosis
• Insulin-treated hyperglycaemia
• Aminophylline
• Catecholamine with β_2 activity

TREATMENT

• Cardiac arrhythmias, including supraventricular and ventricular, are more common with hypokalaemia, even at the lower limits of 'normal'.

• Keep the serum potassium concentration higher than 4 mmol/L.

• Intravenous potassium (5–40 mmol/h) should be given via a central line, with the rate readjusted regularly and with frequent monitoring of the serum concentration, until the hypokalaemia is corrected.

Hyperkalaemia

The ECG changes include T-wave elevation, prolongation of the PR interval, widening of the QRS complex, and deepening of the S wave (Figure 4.6). Patients are prone to cardiac tachyarrhythmias, peripheral paraesthesia, profound muscle weakness, and eventually asystole.

CAUSES

• Failure of excretion, renal insufficiency

• Cellular damage and potassium release: crush injury, burns, rhabdomyolysis, haemolysis, succinylcholine administration

• Potassium shift from cells as a result of severe acidosis

TREATMENT

1. Protect the heart from life-threatening arrhythmias. Treat any life-threatening arrhythmias.

    • Calcium: 10 ml of 10% solution (calcium chloride)

    • Sodium bicarbonate: 100 mmol (100 ml of 8.4% solution) – also drives potassium intracellularly

2. Shift potassium intracellularly.

    • Glucose: 100 ml of 50% glucose, with 20 units of soluble insulin. By driving potassium intracellularly, this acts as a temporary measure.

3. Remove potassium.

    • Ion-exchange resin: calcium resonium, 30–60 g, 2–6-hourly, either orally or rectally, will decrease the serum potassium.

• Dialysis may be urgently required in severe or resistant hyper-kalaemia.

CHLORIDE

Chloride is the principal anion in the body. Its concentration varies in different body fluid spaces. The chloride concentration is largely dependent on the concentration of other organic anions:

• Plasma, 104 mmol/L
• Interstitial fluid, 117 mmol/L
• Cells vary from 2 mmol/L in skeletal muscle to 90 mmol/L in erythrocytes

The turnover of chloride is approximately 135 mmol/d. The plasma concentration of chloride tends to vary in the same direction as that of sodium and in the opposite direction to that of bicarbonate (ie increased sodium is associated with increased chloride, and increased bicarbonate is associated with decreased chloride).

Hypochloraemia (serum concentration < 95 mmol/L)

Hypochloraemia accompanies losses from the GIT and kidneys; it can be caused by dilution and accompanies certain disease states.

CAUSES
• Large gastric aspirate
• Metabolic alkalosis
• Respiratory acidosis (chronic)
• Over-hydration with hypotonic solutions
• Diuretic therapy
• Inappropriate ADH release
• Burns

TREATMENT The treatment is the same as for hyponatraemia. Remember to correct the serum potassium concentration.

Hyperchloraemia (serum concentration $>$ 110 mmol/L)

Hyperchloraemia in intensive care often accompanies respiratory alkalosis, hypovolaemia, and metabolic acidosis. Artifactual readings may be due to sampling blood close to an intravenous line or may be secondary to replenishment with hyperosmolar solutions containing chloride.

CAUSES

- Hyperchloraemic metabolic acidosis
- Respiratory alkalosis
- Dehydration and hypovolaemia
- Renal disease
- Diabetes insipidus
- Hypertonic saline infusion
- Bromide intoxication

TREATMENT   Chloride disturbances often are markers of other abnormalities in the seriously ill, and usually no specific treatment is indicated. However, it is important to determine the cause of the abnormal chloride concentration and treat the underlying disease.

CALCIUM

Calcium is an essential component of a 'universal messenger system'. Calcium is essential for the integrity of cell membranes (muscles, nerves), as well as for a range of other functions: complement activity; clotting; secretion of exocrine, endocrine, and neurocrine products; transport and secretion of fluids and electrolytes; growth of cells.

About 99% of the body's calcium is found in bones and teeth. Only a small amount is present in body fluids and cells. Circulating calcium can exist in either the protein-bound form (about 45%), where it is mainly bound to albumin, in the form of non-ionized salts with phosphate, sulphate, and citrate (5–10%), or in the active form, as ionized calcium (about 50%). Acidosis decreases its protein binding (increasing ionized calcium), and alkalosis increases its protein binding (decreasing ionized calcium). A low serum concentration of albumin will also affect the total calcium concentration. Mesurement of ionized calcium is therefore necessary to evaluate the physiologically active fraction.

Circulating calcium is closely regulated by parathyroid hormone (PTH) and vitamin D through their effects on bone, kidney, and the GIT. The influence of severe illness on calcium homeostasis is not clear. Normally, calcium is controlled within narrow limits by a complex and efficient feedback system. Its daily turnover is approximately 5–15 mmol.

Hypocalcaemia

Hypocalcaemia is very common in the ICU – predisposing factors being sepsis, alkalaemia, chelation (eg citrate in blood products), and renal failure. It can also result from acute deposition of calcium into soft tissue (eg following rhabdomyolysis), as well as from PTH deficiency, hypomagnesaemia, vitamin D deficiency, acute pancreatitis, or anticonvulsant treatment (phenytoin, phenobarbital).

Always measure the ionized calcium concentration, not the total serum calcium, because correlation between the two is poor.

Hypocalcaemia can cause increased neuronal membrane irritability and tetany, central nervous system symptoms such as seizures, and even heart failure and arrhythmias.

The ECG changes include a prolonged QT interval as a result of a prolonged ST segment.

TREATMENT

• Correct the serum magnesium and phosphate concentrations.

• Give 10 ml of 10% calcium chloride solution (IV) over 10 minutes. Beware of treating hypocalcaemia in patients with rhabdomyolysis, as it can predispose to precipitation of calcium in muscle and soft tissues.

• A vitamin D supplement may also be required.

Hypercalcaemia

Hypercalcaemia is commonly associated with hyperparathyroidism (usually mild, <3.5 mmol/L) or malignancies (can be severe, >4.0

TABLE 4.5 CAUSES OF HYPERCALCAEMIA

Primary hyperparathyroidism – confirmed by measurement of serum PTH

Underlying malignancy – assays of PTH-related protein are available

Non-parathyroid endocrine disorders (eg thyrotoxicosis, phaeochromocytoma, adrenal insufficiency)

Granulomatous diseases (eg sarcoidosis, tuberculosis)

Drugs (eg thiazide diuretics, lithium)

Miscellaneous (eg immobilization, milk alkali syndrome, vitamin A and D intoxication, IVN, acute and chronic renal insufficiency)

mmol/L) (Table 4.5). Distinguishing between the two causes usually is not difficult, and the diagnosis is readily confirmed by measurement of serum PTH.

Hypercalcaemia can result in muscle weakness, polydipsia, and polyuria, as well as GIT symptoms (anorexia, nausea, vomiting, constipation) and central nervous system disturbances (lethargy, depression).

TREATMENT

Guidelines

1. Resuscitate (airway, breathing, circulation).

2. Identify and treat the underlying disorder. The following measures are only temporary, and the underlying disorder must be addressed (Table 4.5).

3. Correct other obvious fluid (eg dehydration) and electrolyte problems.

4. Enhance renal excretion: calciuresis with 2.5–4 L of isotonic saline daily, plus a loop diuretic (eg frusemide at 10–50 mg IV 2-hourly).

Avoid thiazide diuretics, as they can enhance calcium reabsorption from the distal tubule.

Hydration and calciuresis with normal saline and diuretic are adequate for most cases of moderate hypercalcaemia, constituting the first line of management even in severe cases.

SEVERE OR REFRACTORY HYPERCALCAEMIA Give calcitonin at 4 units per kilogramme IV, then 4 units per kilogramme IM at 12–24-

hour intervals. Calcitonin acts rapidly and is relatively safe. It is the drug of first choice in severe hypercalcaemia (>4.0 mmol/L) or if the patient is symptomatic. Calcitonin acts as an osteoclast inhibitor and also increases renal excretion of calcium.

Give mithramycin at 25 μg/kg IV over 4–6 hours, repeated every 24–48 hours if there is no hepatic or renal dysfunction, thrombocytopenia, or coagulopathy. Mithramycin is a useful drug for severe hypercalcaemia, as it is rapid-acting.

Diphosphonates inhibit osteoclasts and accelerate bone resorption. These can be considered when mithramycin is contraindicated or when the need to reduce the calcium levels is less urgent (eg etidronate at 7.5 mg/kg IV over 8 hours for 3–7 days). Diphosphonates together with hydration will reduce calcium concentrations in 90% of patients with malignancies.

The place of gallium nitrate is not clear. It appears to be as potent as the diphosphonates and mithramycin, but less toxic than the latter.

Other measures
• Corticosteroids (eg prednisolone, 60 mg/24 h) should be considered in the presence of severe hypercalcaemia, especially if an underlying malignancy is suspected.
• Give phosphate, 50 mmol over 12 hours, only as an emergency measure. This treatment can cause precipitation of calcium salts. Phosphate should be limited to patients with life-threatening hypercalcaemia in whom other measures have failed.
• Haemodialysis, using a low-calcium dialysate, should also be considered in severe unresponsive cases. This treatment can be dangerous, as it can cause precipitation of calcium salts. It should be limited to patients with life-threatening hypercalcaemia when other measures have failed.

MAGNESIUM

Magnesium is the second most common intracellular cation and is essential for many enzyme systems. The average daily requirements are approximately 3 mmol/d. Often, more is required in the critically ill (eg 10–20 mmol/24 h).

Hypomagnesaemia

ALWAYS THINK OF HYPOMAGNESAEMIA WHEN THERE IS HY-
POKALAEMIA, ESPECIALLY IN THE PRESENCE OF POLYURIA (eg diuretics, diabetes). Hypomagnesaemia is often seen in association with
chronic diuretic treatment, alcoholism, malnutrition, or intravenous
nutrition without magnesium supplements. Significant losses of magnesium can also occur with diarrhoea, ileus, or gastric suction, as well
as from other GIT losses.

Hypomagnesaemia is common in the seriously ill and is often unrecognized. The most important sequelae are ventricular and
supraventricular arrhythmias, neuromuscular excitability, GIT and
central nervous system abnormalities, and heart failure. It is difficult
to separate the clinical syndrome of hypomagnesaemia from hypokalaemia and hypocalcaemia, as they often occur together. Moreover, there is no direct relationship between intracellular and extracellular magnesium concentrations.

TREATMENT

- Give magnesium: 20 mmol diluted in 100 ml of 5% dextrose IV over
30 minutes; repeat as necessary until the condition is corrected.
- Use a maintenance dosage, with daily monitoring.

Hypermagnesaemia

Hypermagnesaemia is rare in intensive care. Sometimes it is seen in
association with renal insufficiency or occurs as a result of magne-
sium-containing antacids. It is associated with impaired neuromuscular activity and depression of the central nervous system and cardiovascular system. It can be associated with magnesium treatment
(eg pre-eclampsia).

TREATMENT

- Give calcium, 5 mmol IV, or isotonic saline plus 5 mmol calcium per
litre, 6-hourly
+
frusemide, 20 mg IV, 4-hourly

• Use haemodialysis if the condition is resistant and is associated with symptoms.

PHOSPHATE

Phosphate is a major intracellular anion – an important buffer and an integral part of the adenosine triphosphate (ATP) phospholipids. The daily requirements are at least 20 mmol/24 h.

Hypophosphataemia

Hypophosphataemia is common in the ICU. Hypophosphataemia can cause SEVERE RESPIRATORY AND MUSCLE WEAKNESS, AS WELL AS CENTRAL NERVOUS SYSTEM DEPRESSION. It can mimic polyneuritis and lead to profound coma. It can also cause erythrocyte and leukocyte dysfunction, predisposing to infection, as well as myocardial dysfunction and rhabdomyolysis. Hypophosphataemia is commonly associated with chronic alcoholism, acute severe asthma, malnutrition, and diabetic ketoacidosis.

TREATMENT

• Give 20–60 mmol of phosphate over 6 hours as an intravenous infusion, repeated as necessary.
• Up to 10 mmol/h can be given safely, followed by up to 20–60 mmol/24 h to maintain a normal concentration, according to daily measurements.

Hyperphosphataemia

Hyperphosphataemia is usually seen in the presence of renal failure or in association with hypercatabolic states, chemotherapy, or cell destruction (eg rhabdomyolysis).

TREATMENT

• The only reliable way to decrease the serum phosphate concentration is to restore renal function or use dialysis. Commence oral aluminium hydroxide (30 ml every 8 hours) or calcium carbonate (600 mg every 8 hours).

FURTHER READING

Bidani, A. (1986). Electrolyte and acid–base disorders. *Medical Clinics of North America* 70:1013–36.

Bilezikian, J. P. (1992). Management of acute hypercalcaemia. *New England Journal of Medicine* 326:1196–203.

Black, R. M. (1989). Diagnosis and management of hyponatraemia. *Journal of Intensive Care Medicine* 4:205–20.

Blevins, L. S., & Wand, G. S. (1992). Diabetes insipidus. *Critical Care Medicine* 20:69–79.

Chernow, B., & Zaloga, G. P. (1984). Ions for society members: sulphate, chloride, calcium and magnesium. In *Critical Care: State of the Art,* vol. 5, ed. W. C. Shoemaker, pp. K1–42. Fullerton, CA: Society of Critical Care Medicine.

Edelmann, C. M. (1982). Fluid and electrolyte problems in the child. In *Critical Care: State of the Art,* vol. 3, ed. W. C. Shoemaker & W. L. Thompson, pp. M1–36. Fullerton, CA: Society of Critical Care Medicine.

Hillman, K. M. (1990). Fluids and electrolytes. In Scurr C, Feldman S, Soni N, eds. *The Scientific Foundations of Anaesthesia and Intensive Care: The Basis of Intensive Care,* 4th ed., ed. C. Scurr, S. Feldman, & N. Soni, pp. 448–62. Oxford: Heinemann.

Hutton, P., & Cooper, G. (1985). *Guidelines in Clinical Anaesthesia.* London: Blackwell.

Kaufman, B. S. (ed.) (1992). Fluid resuscitation of the critically ill. *Critical Care Clinics* 8:235–459.

Koch, S. M., & Taylor, R. W. (1992). Chloride ion in intensive care medicine. *Critical Care Medicine* 20:227–40.

Oh, M. S., & Carroll, H. J. (1992). Disorders of sodium metabolism: hypernatraemia and hyponatraemia. *Critical Care Medicine* 20:94–103.

Schrier, R. W. (ed.) (1986). *Renal and Electrolyte Disorders,* 3rd ed. Boston: Little, Brown.

Shoemaker, W. C. (1982). Fluid and electrolyte problems in the adult. In *Critical Care: State of the Art,* vol. 3, ed. W. C. Shoemaker & W. L. Thompson, pp. N1–96 Fullerton, CA: Society of Critical Care Medicine.

Walmsley, R. N., & White, G. H. (1988). *A Guide to Diagnostic Clinical Chemistry,* 2nd ed. London: Blackwell.

Worthley, L. I. G. (ed.) (1986). Fluids and electrolytes. *Anaesthesia and Intensive Care* 5:284–371 (symposium issue).

5

NUTRITION AND METABOLISM

- Giving substrates to a severely catabolic patient does not guarantee their utilization.
- Enteral feeding is safer, cheaper, and more beneficial than parenteral feeding.
- The usual contraindications to enteral feeding, such as recent surgery and an ileus, are relative, not absolute.

METABOLIC RESPONSES TO ILLNESS AND SUBSTRATE UTILIZATION

Nutritional support for the critically ill is aimed at preventing malnutrition and its consequences, particularly for the immune system. Malnutrition is associated with suppression of several functions: cell-mediated immunity, complement activity, and the bactericidal function of neutrophils. It also decreases wound healing.

The metabolic consequences of starvation in a normal person are well known. It results in a decrease in metabolic rate, reduced glucose utilization in the central nervous system (CNS), and increases in fat utilization and ketone production. Carbohydrate in the form of glycogen will meet the needs of a fasting person for the first 12 hours, after which glucose must be derived from protein breakdown. To preserve protein, fat will increasingly be utilized, so that by the 17th day of fasting, fat will account for more than 90% of the energy supply.

That scenario has little relevance to a critically ill, 'stressed' patient. There are vast differences between a stressed (eg having injury and sepsis) patient and a starved normal person. 'Stress,' in this sense, loosely refers to a patient's metabolic responses to insults such as injury or sepsis. It is important to define the term more precisely when trying to determine its effects on nutritional needs.

Stress leads to hypermetabolism, proteolysis, increased lipolysis, sodium and water retention, and gluconeogenesis. There is marked wasting of muscle bulk. Afferent nerve fibres, and possibly chemical mediators such as cytokines, convey stimuli to the hypothalamus, causing a neuroendocrine response characterized by increased sympathetic activity and enhanced secretion of cortisol, glucagon, and growth hormone, all of which are hormones that counteract the effects of insulin. An initial suppression of insulin release is followed by insulin resistance. Not only is the neuroendocrine system active in these processes, but chemicals such as monokines and lymphokines also play important roles.

Stressed patients do not respond well to nutritional manipulation, and the more severe the stress response, the more difficult it is to guarantee substrate utilization.

Late stress (as contrasted with the first 48 hours after injury) is often associated with sepsis, which is characterized by decreased utilization of fat and glucose. Nutritional support can be even less effective at this stage.

Tissue atrophy is a marked feature in a bedridden patient, especially seriously ill patients who can barely move. The wasting of a limb encased in a full-length plaster cast is significant even in a mobile, well-nourished patient. It is not surprising, therefore, to find that disuse atrophy accounts for much muscle wasting and that this is unaffected by substrate availability. Wasting is probably exacerbated by long-term use of muscle relaxants.

NUTRITIONAL ASSESSMENT

As in many areas of nutrition in the ICU, there is little information available on simple and effective ways to assess current nutritional status and needs. Commonly used parameters include

- premorbid history (eg length of starvation period)
- patient's weight
- anthropometric determinations (eg triceps skin fold)
- biochemical markers (eg serum albumin, transferrin, cholesterol, and retinol-binding protein)

These measurements have inherent inaccuracies. Metabolic-measurement carts are sometimes used to estimate oxygen consumption, thus indirectly giving some information on caloric requirements. However, such carts are expensive and difficult to use, and the information is not easily interpreted.

Many ICUs do not use any formal measurements of nutrition, but simply assume that certain amounts are required.

Clinical examination using the Hansel-and-Gretel squeeze test (the shortsighted witch squeezed Hansel's finger to assess his weight gain) is simple and practical.

ENTERAL NUTRITION

Whenever possible, enteral feeding should always be used in SERIOUSLY ILL PATIENTS. If the patient has an intact or partially intact gastro-intestinal tract (GIT), it should be used. The only absolute contraindications to enteral feeding are

- complete bowel obstruction
- mesenteric ischaemia

Other conditions may allow some enteral feeding, perhaps supplemented by intravenous nutrition (IVN):

- partial bowel obstruction
- severe diarrhoea
- severe pancreatitis

After an acute insult (eg trauma or surgery), gastric and colonic atony occurs, but small-bowel motility is restored quickly (within 12 hours), and so early feeding may be possible with duodenal or jejunal tube placement. Bowel sounds are not good indicators of when to start enteral nutrition; gas is present mainly in the stomach and colon, not in the small bowel. The presence or absence of bowel sounds is not indicative of small-bowel activity.

Enteral nutrition has many real advantages. Compared with IVN, it

- is cheap
- has fewer complications
- limits mucosal atrophy
- improves motility
- maintains the integrity of the GIT mucosa and may help prevent bacterial translocation

- prevents stress ulceration
- reduces the hypermetabolic response to trauma by 20%

IVN will not maintain the integrity of the gut mucosal barrier as enteral nutrition does – an advantage for enteral nutrition as important as its nutritive values.

The disadvantages of enteral nutrition relate mainly to whether or not nutrients are being absorbed and to the problem of diarrhoea. There is a small risk for passive regurgitation and aspiration. If in doubt, put methylene blue in the feeds.

The type of food used probably is not of great importance for the majority of patients. Most feeds have the following characteristics:

- isomolar composition
- 1 kcal/ml
- protein content < 20% of total calories
- long-chain triglycerides ± medium-chain triglycerides
- some vitamins and trace elements

Glutamine is the preferred substrate for enterocytes, and adding glutamine to enteral nutrition may reduce bacterial translocation. Short-chain fatty acids may confer a similar advantage on colonocytes.

CLINICAL GUIDELINES

Start with the ordinary nasogastric tube. If that is unsuccessful, consider duodenal or jejunal placement of a small-bore tube:

- Begin with 30 ml/h. Remember that gastric juice is produced at a rate of approximately 1,000 ml/24 h, and take this into account in assessing aspirated volumes.
- Opiates may decrease gastric motility.
- Metoclopramide has not been shown to hasten feeding.
- Continuous infusion is better tolerated than bolus feeding.
- Diarrhoea can be a problem (see p. 700); usually it is partially osmotic and partially due to malabsorption. Do not stop feeding, as the problem will recur when you start again. Bulking agents may help. Bloody diarrhoea points to mesenteric ischaemia.

INTRAVENOUS NUTRITION

Parenteral nutrition should be considered only for patients who cannot tolerate food enterally. It is effective in patients with isolated GIT abnormalities, but its place in the seriously ill is far from clear. It is probably no coincidence that there has been an enormous amount of information published on the subject of IVN and that it is an aggressively marketed and expensive product.

During the acute phase of critical illness (as contrasted with isolated GIT disorders), we still know little about what portions of the substrates in IVN are actually used for metabolism and anabolism. Nor do we know to what extent the catabolic process is obligatory and whether or not it is affected by IVN. Although IVN can improve some biochemical indices, we do not know if IVN actually influences outcomes in patients with serious illnesses.

CLINICAL GUIDELINES

Some of the best available guidelines for IVN are discussed next, but the bottom-line messages are far from clear.

Indications

IVN supplementation may be indicated in the following conditions:

- when enteral feeding is not possible or is inadequate
- hypermetabolic states (eg burns, sepsis, multitrauma)
- abnormalities of the GIT that would limit enteral feeding (eg high-output fistulae, malabsorption syndrome, chronic pancreatitis, inflammatory bowel disease, prolonged obstruction)
- severe pre-operative malnutrition
- anticipated nutritional deficiency lasting longer than 10 days (eg small-bowel fistula)

Protein metabolism

The main goal of nitrogen supply is to limit muscle catabolism and supply the liver with amino acids to synthesize proteins – especially those involved in the immune system:

Normal protein requirement: 0.4 g $\cdot$ kg^{-1} $\cdot$ d^{-1}
Recommended in the ICU: 0.7–2.0 g $\cdot$ kg^{-1} $\cdot$ d^{-1}

(1 g of nitrogen approximately equals 6.25 g of protein or 7.5 g of amino acids.)
    Use synthetic L-amino acid mixtures:

Essential: non-essential ratio approximately 2:5
Branched-chain: total amino acid ratio approximately 1:4

Branched-chain amino acids (leucine, isoleucine valine) are metabolized mainly by skeletal muscle. There is no good evidence for their use at high levels in hypermetabolic states.
    Give albumin separately, as needed.

Energy metabolism

Lipid and glucose are equally effective for nitrogen sparing. Stressed patients (apart from those with burns) are not as hypermetabolic as was once thought. Energy expenditure in patients with septicaemia is 1.5–1.7 times the normal level. They therefore do not require large amounts of calories. This is due to the fact that while the basal energy requirements are increased, the energy actively expended is reduced. Whereas exogenous substrates do not prevent gluconeogenesis, they may reduce it. The clearing of blood glucose does not necessarily mean that the glucose has been oxidized or utilized in metabolic pathways. Using insulin to decrease the blood sugar concentration by moving it intracellularly does not necessarily guarantee utilization.
    The recommended non-protein calories for patients in intensive care – approximately 2,000–2,500 kcal (8,500–10,500 kJ) per 24 hours or 30–35 kcal $\cdot$ kg^{-1} $\cdot$ d^{-1} (126–147 kJ $\cdot$ kg^{-1} $\cdot$ d^{-1}) – are as follows:

500 ml of 50% dextrose = 1,000 kcal (4,200 kJ)
500 ml of 20% intralipid = 1,000 kcal (4,200 kJ)

The caloric requirements increase as the metabolic rate of the patient increases (eg patients with burns may require up to 70 kcal $\cdot$ kg^{-1} $\cdot$ d^{-1}).

LIPID OR GLUCOSE?   Calories are usually supplied as glucose (3.4 kcal/g) or fat (9 kcal/g). Fat minimizes oxygen consumption and carbon dioxide production, whereas excess glucose can markedly increase both. Fat is probably cleared well in most seriously ill patients, but serum lipid should be monitored during IVN. Whether or not lipid solutions cause immunosuppression or changes in pulmonary vascular tone is not clear. Clearance is helped by a slow infusion rate – 500 ml over 24 hours.

Hyperglycaemia can be due to stress, administration of steroids or catecholamines, diabetes, or sepsis. Glucose is not well tolerated in the seriously ill. Hyperglycaemia and hepatic steatosis can occur if excessive glucose is administered. A non-diabetic patient should not require an insulin infusion to maintain a normal blood sugar – reduce the glucose infusion rate if necessary. Furthermore, insulin stimulates lipogenesis.

Some lipid is needed to prevent fatty acid deficiency.
Excessive glucose or lipid can disturb liver function.
Lipid solutions are approximately 5 times more expensive than dextrose solutions.

Lipid solutions often are not tolerated late in sepsis and can cause lipidaemia. Exogenous lipid should be withheld in these circumstances.

As a general recommendation, fat should contribute no more than 20–35% of non-protein calories.

Electrolytes (see Chapter 4)

Acute illness often leads to deficits in magnesium, phosphate, and potassium. Their concentrations should be measured daily, and supplements should be given as necessary.

Vitamins

The exact vitamin requirements of the seriously ill have not been well documented. Recommendations are given in the form of theoretical estimates for each day, or, more practically, there is regular administration of a commercial preparation.

A preparation of water-soluble vitamins should be given daily. Vitamins A, D, and K should be added intramuscularly if not included otherwise. One litre of lipid solution per week will provide adequate vitamin E.

Intramuscular injection of folinic acid at 5 mg/d is necessary for the seriously ill. This is much higher than the recommended doses for normal patients, probably because of rapid cell turnover. Fat-soluble vitamins (except for vitamin K) probably are not necessary in the short term (less than 2 weeks).

Guidelines for Daily Vitamin Requirements

A (retinol)	1–3.5	mg
D (ergocalciferol)	5–10	μg
E (α-tocopherol)	2–10	mg
K	0.5–1.5	mg
biotin	60	μg
B_1 (thiamine)	3–50	mg
B_2 (riboflavin)	4–10	mg
niacin	40–100	mg
B_6 (pyridoxin)	4–15	mg
B_{12}	5–150	μg
pantothenate	10–25	mg
C	100–500	mg

Trace elements

Humans need trace amounts of iron, aluminium, zinc, copper, chromium, selenium, iodine, and cobalt. Vanadium, fluoride, iodide, manganese, silicon, and molybdenum probably should also be replaced over the long term (more than 3 months).

Zinc is important in many enzyme systems and is the only trace element that must be included in IVN in the short term (less than 2 weeks).

High concentrations of aluminium can occur in association with antacid treatment and excessive administration of plasma protein solutions.

Information on trace elements is sparse. Most sources emphasize the importance of trace elements, but stop short of recommending practical guidelines as to how much of each should be given and when they should be commenced. One of the difficulties is monitoring and interpreting the concentrations. Some trace elements occur as contaminations in intravenous fluid and in blood products. Over the long term (more than 2 weeks), consideration should be given to adding trace elements to IVN regimens, especially in the face of abnormal GIT losses and malnutrition.

Guidelines for daily trace-element replacement

zinc (Zn)	50–200	μmol
iron (Fe)	20–70	μmol
manganese (Mn)	3–35	μmol
copper (Cu)	5–70	μmol
fluoride (F)	20	μmol
iodide (I)	1–7	μmol
molybdenum (Mo)	0.2	μmol
selenium (Se)	0.4–2.5	μmol
chromium (Cr)	0.2–0.3	μmol

Monitoring

Formal assessment of nutritional status (eg muscle power, nitrogen balance, anthropometric parameters) usually is not required in seriously ill patients, nor are serum albumin and immune-status tests (eg anergy) accurate guides to nutritional status. Because indirect calorimetry is expensive and difficult to interpret, it is not practical for many ICUs.

Basic monitoring of IVN

Daily
  fluid balance
  serum electrolytes
  serum urea/creatinine
  arterial blood gases
  blood glucose
Twice weekly
  liver function tests
  calcium, phosphate, magnesium
  complete blood count
  prothrombin time
Special
  serum/urine osmolalities

serum lipids
serum urate
serum zinc and copper
serum B_{12} and folate
iron studies
microbiological cultures as necessary

Recommendations

There have been more obscure and mysterious 'facts' and fewer bottom-line messages written about IVN than about almost any other aspect of intensive care. The recommendations often do not match the reality of the clinical situation. In the absence of more precise knowledge, KEEP IT SIMPLE AND CHEAP. Fat and carbohydrate should be given in roughly equal proportions to supply no more than the patient's measured or estimated energy needs. A positive nitrogen balance is unlikely to be achieved in catabolic patients lying immobile in bed. Nutrition should support metabolic pathways, without forcing them in abnormal and possibly detrimental directions. In the light of that advice, the following is an example of a standard IVN regimen for 24 hours:

• Amino acid solution: 1,000 ml of 5% balanced essential and non-essential L-amino acids ($0.7 \text{ g} \cdot \text{kg}^{-1} \cdot \text{d}^{-1}$)

• dextrose: 30% solution, 1,000 ml

• soya bean emulsion, 20%, 500 ml (eg Intralipid, a mixture of triglyceride, 20%, phospholipid, 12%, and glycerol, 2.25%)

+

appropriate amounts of sodium, potassium, calcium, magnesium, phosphate, zinc, and trace elements

+

appropriate vitamins

Over 24 hours, this regimen will provide

2,500 ml of fluid
12,000 kJ of energy (approximately)
500 g of carbohydrate

TABLE 5.1 POTENTIAL COMPLICATIONS OF IVN

Complications associated with central-line insertion (eg thrombosis, infection, pneumothorax, haemorrhage)
Hyperlipidaemia and hypertriglyceridaemia
Electrolyte disturbances
Hyperosmolality
Hyperglycaemia
Acid–base disturbances
Vitamin and trace-element deficiencies
Hypercarbia
Fatty liver

100 g of protein (approximately, depending on the preparation)
100 g of fat

IVN should not be commenced until the patient is fully resuscitated. It works best when patients are metabolically normal. However, that is rarely the case in the seriously ill, and thus the guidelines are empirical.

Amino acid and dextrose solutions are hypertonic and should be delivered through a central line. Most lipid solutions are isotonic.

The most important practical limitation to IVN concerns fluid. Seriously ill patients often have neuroendocrine systems adapted to retain salt and water, or they may have renal insufficiency, which can limit water excretion. Both can predispose to water retention.

Pulmonary and peripheral oedema will accompany water retention, especially in combination with excessive fluid administration. Seriously ill patients with normal renal function often cannot tolerate more than 1,000 ml of water per day (see Chapter 4). Haemofiltration (see p. 655), with or without dialysis, can make more 'space' for fluid. It may be useful in conjunction with IVN.

Individual ICUs should establish their own protocols for IVN delivery, as well as for insertion of central venous lines, catheter dressing and care, and routine monitoring of the biochemistry. Until we know more, the guidelines for IVN use will remain largely empirical. Potential complications from IVN are listed in Table 5.1.

NUTRITION FOR SPECIFIC ORGAN FAILURE

Acute renal failure

Acute renal failure is associated with hypermetabolism – a measured energy expenditure of 20–50% above normal. Provisions for adequate nutrition are hampered by volume restrictions, electrolyte problems, and rising concentrations of blood urea. Special IVN solutions and manipulations of feeding regimens (eg increasing the calorie-to-nitrogen ratio) can limit the increase in blood urea.

Early dialysis or filtration will solve the electrolyte, urea, and volume-overload problems. Amino acids, glucose, and vitamins are all removed by dialysis.

Hepatic failure

There is a lot of confusion in this area, mainly concerning support for patients with acute and chronic liver failure. As a bottom line, whereas administration of branched-chain amino acids will increase the number of people who will awaken from hepatic encephalopathy, they can confer no morbidity/mortality advantage over balanced, standard amino acid solutions. Fat solutions probably should be restricted to 125–250 ml of 20% emulsion per day. Hypertonic glucose should supply the bulk of the calories.

Pre-operative nutrition

The advantages of increasing the pre-operative nutrition outweigh the disadvantages (eg catheter-related sepsis) only for a very small population of severely malnourished patients.

TROUBLESHOOTING

FAILURE OF ENTERAL FEEDING

Aspirated secretions   The stomach produces gastric secretions at a rate of 40 ml/h.

Feeding has failed when the aspirate is greater than 100 ml/h or is greater than double the amount of feed put into the stomach.

If the amounts of aspirated secretions are high, do not cease feeding; simply reduce to 10–20 ml/h. Enteral feed acts as gastric protection.

Metoclopramide, cisapride, or low-dosage dopamine may assist GIT function.

High doses of narcotics may slow GIT activity. As an alternative, consider epidural analgesia for pain relief.

Detection of bowel sounds is not necessary before feeding starts or for effective feeding.

Bypassing the stomach: Nasoduodenal or nasojejunal tubes can be used for early feeding. If the patient requires a laparotomy, consider inserting a feeding jejunostomy.

Vomiting   Stop feeding, and check for the reason (eg bowel obstruction, gastric dilation, drug effects)

Diarrhoea   Continue feeding at the same rate; do not stop. If feeding is stopped, diarrhoea will only recur when feeding is started again.

Check for *Clostridium difficile* toxin.

Fibre, bulking agents, codeine, or Lomotil may help.

FURTHER READING

Babineau, T. J., & Blackburn, G. L. (1994). Time to consider early gut feeding. *Critical Care Medicine* 22:191–3.

Berger, R., & Adams, L. (1989). Nutritional support in the critical care setting. *Chest* 96:139–47, 372–9.

Cerra, F. B. (1987). Hypermetabolism, organ failure and metabolic support. *Surgery* 101:1–14.

Heyland, D. K., Cook, D. J. U., & Goyatt, G. H. (1993). Enteral nutrition in the critically ill patient: a critical review of the evidence. *Intensive Care Medicine* 19:435–42.

Jeejeebhoy, K. N. (1984). Nutrition in critical illness. In *Critical Care: State of the Art,* vol. 5, ed. W. C. Shoemaker, pp. B1–74. Fullerton, CA: Society of Critical Care Medicine.

Maynard, N. D., & Bihari, D. J. (1991). Postoperative feeding. *British Medical Journal* 303:1007–8.

Minard, G., & Kudsk, K. A. (1994). Is early feeding beneficial? How early is early? *New Horizons* 2:156–63.

Nitenberg, G. (1993). Enteral and parenteral nutrition. In *Pathophysiologic Foundations of Critical Care,* ed. M. R. Pinsky & J.-F. Dhainant, pp. 42–81. Baltimore: Williams & Wilkins.

Phillips, G. D. (1985). Total parenteral nutrition in acute illness. *Anaesthesia and Intensive Care* 13:288–99.

Phillips, G. D., & Odgers, C. L. (eds.) (1986). *Parenteral and Enteral Nutrition.* London: Churchill Livingstone.

Powell-Tuck, J. (1993). Glutamine, parenteral feeding and intestinal nutrition. *Lancet* 342:451–2.

Streat, S. J., & Hill, G. L. (1987). Nutritional support in the management of critically ill patients in surgical intensive care. *World Journal of Surgery* 11:194–201.

Teich, S., Sharpe, S., & Chernow, B. (1985). Endocrine function in the critically ill. *Clinical Anaesthesiology* 3:999–1026.

Weissman, C. (1990). The metabolic response to stress: an overview and update. *Anaesthesiology* 73:308–27.

6

ACID–BASE BALANCE

- Arterial blood gases reflect oxygenation (Pa_{O_2}), ventilation (Pa_{CO_2}), and acid–base status.
- In general, the pH value reflects the primary disorder, not the compensation.
- Specific therapy is rarely required – correct the underlying disorder.

Acid–base disturbances affect the basic molecules of metabolism – enzymes. Severe alkalosis is as harmful as is severe acidosis. Acid–base homeostasis depends on chemical reactions involving buffers, in combination with intact renal and respiratory functions. There is no neural or endocrine control. Before considering any acid–base disorder, the hydrogen-ion concentration or pH value (Table 6.1), Pa_{CO_2}, and bicarbonate concentration must be determined. Most intensive care units (ICUs) now have facilities for 24-hour blood-gas analysis that can readily provide information on arterial pH, blood gases, and derived information. It is also important to remember, when interpreting arterial blood gases, that an immediate reaction with body buffers is followed by a compensatory respiratory response and/or renal adaption.

Although in the following guidelines we consider metabolic and respiratory disorders separately, severely ill patients often have combined disturbances, whose interpretations can be complicated by the presence of artificial ventilation and drugs. It is vital to consider the underlying cause of the disorder before actively treating acidosis or alkalosis.

Table 6.2 provides guidelines for blood-gas analysis.

TABLE 6.1   VARIATION OF [H$^+$] WITH pH

pH units	Hydrogen-ion concentration (nmol/L)
3.0	1,000,000
6.0	1,000
7.0	100
7.1	80
7.4	40
7.7	20
8.0	10
9.0	1

TABLE 6.2   INTERPRETATION OF ARTERIAL BLOOD-GAS FINDINGS

1. Look at PaO_2. Rapidly correct it if it is abnormal.
2. Look at the pH value:
   Acidosis: H$^+$ > 44 nmol/L, pH < 7.35
   Alkalosis: H$^+$ < 35 nmol/L, pH > 7.45
3. Is the acidosis respiratory or metabolic?
   Respiratory: PaCO_2 > 45 mm Hg (>6 kPa)
   Metabolic: HCO_3 < 22 mm Hg (<2.9 kPa)
4. Is the alkalosis respiratory or metabolic?
   Respiratory: PaCO_2 < 35 mm Hg (<4.7 kPa)
   Metabolic: HCO_3 > 26 mm Hg (>3.5 kPa)
5. Is there any compensation? The compensation is the opposite of the original disorder (eg the compensation for metabolic acidosis is respiratory alkalosis).

BODY pH REGULATION

BUFFERS

Although many reactions in the body can influence the hydrogen-ion concentration, the pH value remains remarkably stable. This is achieved initially by the body's natural buffers, and then by renal and respiratory adjustments of bicarbonate and PaCO_2 (Figure 6.1). Buffers are present in both extracellular fluid and intracellular fluid.

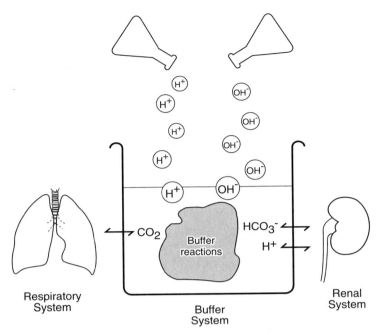

FIGURE 6.1 The body's ability to regulate acid–base balance depends on the lungs, kidneys, and chemical buffers.

Their effectiveness will depend on the buffer concentration, the pK_a (the pH of a system when the acid and its anion are in equal concentrations), and whether or not the buffers can be influenced by renal and respiratory functions (Fig. 6.1).

BICARBONATE–CARBONIC ACID   The carbonic acid–bicarbonate (H_2CO_3/HCO_3) buffer system plays a central role in acid–base balance because of its prevalence and its relation to physiological regulatory mechanisms. The pK_a value (6.1) of this buffering system is well outside the body's normal pH value of approximately 7.4. Its buffering capacity would therefore appear to be poor. However, this system is influenced by both renal and respiratory mechanisms, which markedly increases its effectiveness. Renal mechanisms regulate the bicarbonate concentration, and respiratory mechanisms adjust the $Paco_2$. It thus becomes the most important of the body's buffering systems – all other systems adjust according to this pair.

OTHER BUFFERS

Haemoglobin: Haemoglobin handles carbonic acid by utilizing the imidazole group of histidine. By virtue of the large numbers of imidazole groups, haemoglobin provides a large buffering capacity.

Protein: Both extracellular and intracellular proteins are efficient buffering systems.

Phosphate: Phosphate has an effective pK_a (6.8) and is an important source of intracellular buffering.

RENAL RESPONSE

Compared with the respiratory contribution to acid–base balance, the renal response to pH disturbances is slow and works through bicarbonate, rather than carbonic acid. The kidney can adjust to excreting large acid loads (up to 600–700 mmol of H^+ per day). Mechanisms include excretion of titratable acid, excretion of ammonia, secretion of hydrogen ion, and excretion and reabsorption of filtered bicarbonate.

RESPIRATORY RESPONSE

Normal CO_2 production is about 13,000 mmol/d. The ventilatory response to changing CO_2 levels is rapid and precise.

ACIDOSIS

RESPIRATORY ACIDOSIS

Respiratory acidosis is initiated by an increase in carbon dioxide tension (Pa_{CO_2}). The immediate consequence is an increase in plasma acidity. There is an initial small increase in plasma bicarbonate concentration, and if the hypercapnia becomes more chronic, renal absorption of bicarbonate results in a further increase in plasma bicarbonate concentration.

Clinical manifestations

Acute hypercapnia induces peripheral vasodilatation, stimulates the sympathetic nervous system, and increases cardiac output. Cerebral dysfunction occurs as hypercapnia becomes more severe.

Causes

INADEQUATE CO_2 REMOVAL (see also hypoventilation, p. 426, and acute respiratory failure, p. 353)

- obstructed airway
- lung abnormalities (eg chronic airway disease)
- central or neuromuscular abnormalities (eg drug-induced hypoventilation, Guillain-Barré syndrome, exhaustion as a result of acute respiratory failure)
- mechanical failure – related to inefficient action of the muscles of respiration (eg kyphoscoliosis, obesity, pain, flail chest, pneumothorax)
- an increase in dead space, relative to tidal volume

EXCESS CO_2 PRODUCTION (eg hypermetabolism, excessive parenteral glucose, or rapid injection of sodium bicarbonate, which forms CO_2)

Treatment

1. CORRECT ANY UNDERLYING CAUSE (eg obstructed airway or excessive opiates)

2. ARTIFICIALLY VENTILATE (especially patients with hypoventilation and acute hypercarbia)

EXCEPTIONS Many patients who have acute respiratory failure and who are being artificially ventilated are deliberately under-ventilated with low tidal volumes to limit peak inspiratory pressures. This technique is called elective hypoventilation or permissive hypercarbia (see p. 360). High inspiratory volumes and pressures can cause complications, such as cardiovascular impairment and pulmonary barotrauma (see p. 465).

Artificially ventilated patients with chronic lung disease and hypercarbia who have acute exacerbations of their disease should be ventilated only to correct the $Paco_2$ to their 'normal' levels. Values lower than that can alter the pH of the cerebrospinal fluid (CSF) and make it difficult to wean the patient.

METABOLIC ACIDOSIS

Metabolic acidosis is initiated by a reduction in plasma bicarbonate concentration, which then causes an increase in plasma acidity. That is followed by compensatory hyperventilation and a reduction in Pa_{CO_2}.

Clinical manifestations

• respiratory system: compensatory hyperventilation or Kussmaul respiration
• cardiovascular system: possible myocardial depression, arterial vasodilatation, and direct venoconstriction
• oxygen transport: rightward shift in oxyhaemoglobin dissociation curve, making dissociation easier

Causes

EXCESSIVE HYDROGEN-ION PRODUCTION OR ADMINISTRATION (eg lactic acidosis, ketoacidosis, salicylic acid, lysine, ammonium chloride, and synthetic amino acids)

LOSS OF BICARBONATE [eg small-bowel loss (especially pancreatic fistulae), diarrhoea, renal tubular acidosis, carbonic anhydrase inhibition]

FAILURE TO EXCRETE HYDROGEN ION (eg sulphate and phosphate acids associated with renal failure and renal tubular acidosis)

Metabolic acidoses are usually split into categories, depending on the anion gap (Table 6.3). The positively charged ions (sodium and potassium) and the negatively charged ions (bicarbonate and chloride) usually have a gap of less than 18 mmol/L, made up mainly of protein. In the presence of metabolic acidosis, unmeasured anions (eg lactate in septic shock) add to the gap.

Treatment

The most common cause of acidosis in the ICU is lactic acidosis resulting from inadequate perfusion and oxygenation. Although acido-

TABLE 6.3 ANION GAP

---

1. Calculate: $(Na^+ + K^+) - (Cl^- + HCO_3^-)$
2. High-anion-gap metabolic acidosis (>18 mmol/L)
   Sepsis entails the presence of lactate
   Renal failure involves phosphate and sulphate
   Diabetic ketoacidosis involves acetoacetate and β-hydroxybutyrate
   Presence of methanol, ethanol, ethylene glycol involves formate, lactate, oxalate
3. Low-anion-gap metabolic acidosis (<18 mmol/L)
   Renal tubular acidosis entails loss of HCO_3 in urine
   Gastro-intestinal losses cause loss of HCO_3 from the gut

---

sis causes negative inotropic effects in vitro, it is not necessary to correct the arterial pH to 'normal' in the clinical setting, as even with severe acidosis the effect on myocardial contractility may not be as depressant as was once thought. A pH of 7.20 (H^+ at 63.1 nmol/L) is well tolerated.

- **CORRECT** reversible causes such as diabetic ketoacidosis (see Chapter 30).
- **RESTORE** adequate **CIRCULATION** and **OXYGENATION**.
- **ALKALI:** Usually the foregoing measures are sufficient, and bicarbonate is not necessary. Treatment of the acidosis per se is not as important as treatment of the cause of the acidosis. The bicarbonate may 'buy time' while waiting for definitive treatment.
- Dialysis may be required for intractable acidosis or where renal failure is anticipated.

COMPLICATIONS OF BICARBONATE TREATMENT Excessive bicarbonate is sometimes given to seriously ill patients, especially during cardiopulmonary resuscitation (CPR). This can be dangerous in itself, and it often results in rebound alkalosis (see p. 150) and hypernatraemia. During CPR, give bicarbonate only for severe acute acidosis (eg pH < 7.0): Start with 1 mmol/kg, wait 20 minutes, repeat arterial blood-gas determinations, and give another 1 mmol/kg if needed. Correcting the metabolic acidosis using formulae based on base deficits and weight is inaccurate and causes over-correction. If bicarbonate is necessary, it should be given as a slow infusion, rather than as a bolus. This allows adequate time for elimination of the CO_2 generated from the reaction between the hydrogen ion and bicarbonate. Overcorrection with sodium bicarbonate can result in

- sodium and osmolar loading
- reduced availability of calcium
- reduced oxygen availability, by shifting the oxyhaemoglobin curve to the left
- a paradoxical decrease in intracellular pH

ALKALOSIS

RESPIRATORY ALKALOSIS

Respiratory alkalosis is a result of a reduction in Pa_{CO_2} that alkalinizes the body fluids. With changes in renal absorption of bicarbonate, the degree of alkalinization is gradually modified.

Causes

Hypocarbia and alkalosis are commonly associated with the early stages of acute respiratory failure (see Chapter 17), liver failure, and central nervous system disorders. However, another common cause in the ICU is inadvertent or deliberate hyperventilation.

Hypocarbia can also occur with hypometabolism and decreased CO_2 production, such as after barbiturate overdose, brain death, or hypothermia.

Clinical manifestations

As with respiratory acidosis, central nervous system dysfunction is the most prominent clinical feature of respiratory alkalosis. Acute hypocapnia decreases cerebral blood flow, causing lightheadedness, confusion, and even seizures.

Treatment

- CORRECT any underlying cause.
- DECREASE the minute volume of the ventilator.

METABOLIC ALKALOSIS

Metabolic alkalosis is initiated by an increase in plasma bicarbonate. This gives rise to a compensatory decrease in alveolar ventilation. Alkalosis will disturb enzyme activities and body functions to the same extent as acidosis. Metabolic alkalosis occurs commonly in the ICU and often is iatrogenic in origin.

Clinical manifestations

Central nervous system manifestations include lethargy, confusion, muscle twitching, and seizures. Hypokalaemia occurs as potassium shifts into cells.

Causes

LOSS OF ACIDS

• from the gastro-intestinal tract: nasogastric suctioning and vomiting, diarrhoea, villous adenoma
• from the kidney: diuretics, hypermineralocorticoid states such as occur with corticosteroid use or hyperaldosteronism, Conn's syndrome, Cushing's syndrome

GAIN IN ALKALI

• antacid treatment, milk alkali syndrome, excessive bicarbonate administration, metabolism of organic anions (lactate, citrate, acetate)
• compensation for respiratory acidosis

Treatment

• Correct any reversible cause.
• Correct factors that maintain the alkalosis:
  decreased extracellular fluid
  hypokalemia, hypomagnesaemia, hypochloraemia
  mineralocorticoids
  stress
• Drugs
  Give acetazolamide, 500 mg IV once or twice daily

If still alkalotic, give HCl (0.1 mol) at a rate of 0.2 mmol [H$^+$] per kilogramme per hour until pH returns toward normal (only in cases of severe, resistant alkalosis).

Avoid ammonium chloride and arginine hydrochloride infusions, as they both require hepatic conversion and good renal function for full activity and are more difficult to titrate against pH.

MIXED DISORDERS

Many acid–base disturbances in the ICU are mixed (eg a patient with chronic lung disease who retains CO_2, has a myocardial infarct, and develops shock and acidosis). Useful points for interpretation are included in the following troubleshooting section.

It must be remembered that there can be variations from these predictions and that the predicted changes do not necessarily exclude mixed or complex disorders (eg acute hypocapnia superimposed on chronic respiratory acidosis could mimic the findings of uncomplicated metabolic alkalosis). Careful analysis of the history, clinical findings, and response to treatment will usually allow one to sort out these dilemmas.

TROUBLESHOOTING

ARTERIAL BLOOD-GAS TRICKS

Arterial or venous?   There is no infallible rule for quickly telling if the sample is arterial or venous. Assume that it is arterial, and check against the oximetry findings.

Primary disorder or compensation?   In general, the pH reflects the primary disorder, not the compensation.

Metabolic acidosis   The two figures in the fractional part of the pH value should equal the Pa_{CO_2} if the disorder is fully compensated (pH range 7.10–7.30: If pH is 7.25, Pa_{CO_2} should be 25 mm Hg).

Respiratory acidosis
Acute: The HCO_3 concentration will increase 1 mmol/L for each increase in Pa_{CO_2} of 10 mm Hg (1.3 kPa).

Chronic: The HCO_3 concentration will increase 4 mmol/L for each increase in $Paco_2$ of 10 mm Hg (1.3 kPa).

Metabolic alkalosis $Paco_2$ will increase 7 mm Hg (1.0 kPa) for each increase in HCO_3 concentration of 10 mmol/L.

Respiratory alkalosis The HCO_3 concentration will decrease 2 mmol/L for each decrease in $Paco_2$ of 10 mm Hg (1.3 kPa).

Results Results may not be accurate below a temperature of 35°C.

FURTHER READING

Adams, A. P., & Hahn, C. E. W. (eds.) (1982). *Principles and Practice of Blood-Gas Analysis,* 2nd ed. London: Churchill Livingstone.

Arieff, A. I. (1991). Indications for use of bicarbonate in patients with metabolic acidosis. *British Journal of Anaesthesia* 67:165–77.

Bihari, D. J. (1986). Metabolic acidosis. *British Journal of Hospital Medicine* 35:89–95.

Davenport, H. W. (ed.) (1974). *The ABC of Acid–Base Chemistry,* 6th ed. University of Chicago Press.

Kurtman, N. A., & Battle, D. C. (eds.) (1983). Acid–base disorders. *Medical Clinics of North America* 67:751–932 (symposium issue).

Masaro, E. J. (1982). An overview of hydrogen ion regulation. *Archives of Internal Medicine* 142:1019–23.

Riley, L. J., Ilson, B. E., & Narins, R. G. (1987). Acute metabolic acid–base disorders. *Critical Care Clinics* 5:699–723.

Rimmer, J. M., & Gennari, F. J. (1987). Metabolic alkalosis. *Journal of Intensive Care Medicine* 2:137–50.

Worthley, L. I. G. (1977). Hydrogen ion metabolism. *Anaesthesia and Intensive Care* 5:347–60.

7

SEDATION, ANALGESIA, AND MUSCLE RELAXANTS

- Make sure that sedation is for the good of the patient, not for the benefit of the staff.
- Optimal pain relief is every patient's right in intensive care.
- Muscle relaxation is rarely required in the critically ill.

ASSESSING THE NEED FOR SEDATION

The words 'sedation' and 'sedatives' are used here in the broadest sense (ie in the sense of producing a sleep-like state). Drugs such as opiates obviously have other properties, such as providing pain relief (Table 7.1). DRUGS SHOULD NEVER BE USED AS SUBSTITUTES FOR SYMPATHETIC EXPLANATION AND REASSURANCE. This is particularly important when patients are emerging from coma – pathological or drug-induced. It is often tempting to sedate these patients in order to make them look 'tidy' and to facilitate management for the staff. Explanation and reassurance will often make sedation unnecessary. Nor should sedation be used when the cause of agitation or confusion is unknown. Withdrawal from alcohol or drugs, hypoxia, electrolyte disorders, and many other abnormalities can cause confusion and agitation. These must be excluded before one resorts to sedation.

Patients should be allowed to sleep whenever possible. Sleep is important for optimum physiological functioning and immune competence. Drugs do not necessarily ensure that a patient will get adequate sleep. Sleep deprivation is to be avoided, even if it means a less rigorous approach to routine tests, monitoring, and treatment.

When a patient's pain is not amenable to regional or epidural analgesia, liberal pharmacological pain relief should be provided. Patients should not suffer pain in an intensive care unit (ICU). Opiates used in the right dosages do not necessarily inhibit spontaneous respiration.

TABLE 7.1 SEDATION IN INTENSIVE CARE

1. **Assess need**

   Sedation should not be a substitute for explanation and reassurance by medical and nursing staff.

   Adjust ventilatory strategies to encourage spontaneous breathing, instead of sedating and paralysing patients to make them conform with the ventilator.

2. **Pain relief and sedation**

   Local analgesia: If possible, use an epidural or regional local anaesthetic technique for pain relief.

   Opiate: Use either intermittent doses or continuous intravenous infusion (eg morphine infusion at 2–20 mg/h for pain relief as well as sedation).

   Benzodiazepines: Either add intermittent p.r.n. intravenous doses of benzodiazepine if anxiolysis is inadequate (eg diazepam, 5–10 mg) or include a benzodiazepine with the opiate infusion in order to guarantee anxiolysis (eg 50 mg of midazolam with 250 mg of morphine diluted in a 50-ml infusion pump, 1–5 ml/h).

Sedation should not be used to facilitate positive-pressure ventilation in cases in which patients could otherwise breathe spontaneously, facilitated by techniques such as continuous positive airway pressure (CPAP) or intermittent mandatory ventilation (IMV) (see Chapter 20).

The pharmacokinetics of drugs used in the ICU can be unpredictable because of factors such as depressed hepatic and renal functions, as well as an increased volume of drug distribution. Drugs should be titrated against clinical end points such as pain relief and sedation, rather than prescribed in absolute dosages.

FEATURES OF THE MAIN SEDATIVE GROUPS

OPIATES

- Pain relief, euphoria, and drowsiness.
- Predictable cardiovascular and respiratory depressions.
- Relatively inexpensive.
- Dependence, despite high dosages, is rare.

- Tolerance and increased plasma clearance can gradually occur.
- May contribute to the ileus and pseudo-obstruction (see p. 696) commonly seen in seriously ill patients.
- Variable actions, and usually affected by both renal and hepatic functioning.
- No clinical evidence of immune depression.
- No direct effect on intracranial pressure (ICP).

BENZODIAZEPINES

- Provide sedation, anxiolysis, and amnesia and contribute to muscle relaxation.
- Variable responses.
- Unpredictable cardiovascular and respiratory depressions, especially with bolus doses.
- Variable durations of action (eg very prolonged action of diazepam). This may or may not be a disadvantage in the ICU (though it is a problem for their use in anaesthesia).
- Well-documented incidence of withdrawal symptoms, such as seizures, after long-term use (more than 1 week) of short-acting drugs such as midazolam.
- Thrombophlebitis in small veins with some agents.

BARBITURATES

- Long-acting and cumulative – difficult to assess neurological status.
- More cardiovascular depression than with other agents.
- Possible depression of immune system.
- Inhibit epileptic activity.
- Reduce ICP.

KETAMINE

- Minimum cardiovascular and respiratory effects.
- Analgesia as well as sedation.

- Incidence of unpleasant dreams and psychological disturbances.
- Increases ICP.

PROPOFOL

- Short-acting, rapidly metabolized intravenous anaesthetic agent in the form of an emulsion.
- Expensive.
- Rapid metabolism and lack of accumulation may make it suitable for use as a continuous infusion in the ICU, especially as an adjunct in the management of coma. It is sometimes used to cover the period of agitation as longer-acting agents gradually wear off.
- May unacceptably depress the cardiovascular system.
- Experience with this drug is limited in the ICU, and possible complications such as immunosuppression have not been excluded.

CHLORMETHIAZOLE

- Short-acting.
- Minimal cardiorespiratory depression.
- Inhibits epileptic activity.
- Thrombophlebitis in small veins.
- Bronchorrhoea.
- Causes haemolysis, even at relatively low dosages.

Because of its haemolytic side effects, it must be given in low concentrations (0.8%). Its use in the ICU is limited by the potentially large fluid load needed to maintain sedation with that concentration.

NITROUS OXIDE

- Needs special apparatus for delivery and scavenging.
- Good analgesia and sedation.
- Interferes with bone-marrow function, even with short-term exposure, and should be avoided, if possible, in the ICU.
- Causes increase in ICP.

OTHER VOLATILE ANAESTHETIC AGENTS

- Special apparatus needed for delivery.
- Expensive.
- Unknown effects over the long term.
- Potential problems with scavenging.

CHOICE OF DRUG

Assess whether the proposed sedation is for the benefit of the patient or the staff. It can be tempting to use excessive sedation in order to maintain and control artificial ventilation, instead of weaning the patient to CPAP as soon as possible.

WHEN SEDATION IS NECESSARY, OPIATES AND BENZODIAZEPINES REMAIN THE MAINSTAYS FOR SEDATION IN INTENSIVE CARE.

Pain relief

Where possible, use an epidural analgesic, or regional local anaesthetic blocks, rather than pharmacological techniques. They permit greater patient cooperation and facilitate spontaneous breathing. If that is not possible, titrate an intravenous narcotic infusion against pain.

Anxiolysis

If a patient needs more sedation, or if it is believed that anxiolysis or amnesia is also necessary, benzodiazepines can be used in addition to, or instead of, narcotics.

Liver and renal dysfunctions

Benzodiazepines and narcotics should be titrated against the end points of pain relief and sedation, rather than given at absolute dosages. This is especially important when drug metabolism is compromised in the presence of renal or hepatic failure. Drugs such as morphine, which traditionally have been thought to be inactivated by the liver, have significantly prolonged actions in the presence of renal failure. In a patient with acute liver failure, sedation often is not needed, because of the accompanying encephalopathy. These patients often have cerebral oedema and elevated ICPs; sedative drugs that cause increases in ICP should therefore be avoided.

Immune depression

As the risk of immune depression is possible with anaesthetic induction agents, their use should be confined to cases of severe increases in ICP that are refractory to conventional treatment, status epilepticus unresponsive to conventional treatment, and short-term procedures requiring anaesthesia in the ICU.

Nitrous oxide

Nitrous oxide causes marrow dysfunction, even after short-term use, and should no longer be used routinely in seriously ill patients.

Tolerance

Because of enzyme induction, sedation invariably will have to be increased over time. At the end of a number of weeks, the drug requirement, especially when narcotics are being used, can be extremely high.

Choice of narcotics

All the opiates have effective pain-relieving and sedative properties. Each ICU will have its favourite opiate. If the differences among them are marginal, cost should be considered. Pethidine, papaveretum, and morphine cost approximately the same; fentanyl and phenoperidine are at least eight times as expensive. Pethidine probably should be avoided in the ICU, as it can accumulate in the form of norpethidine and at high dosages can cause epileptiform activity, irritability, and hallucinations.

Choice of benzodiazepines

Although diazepam has been used extensively in ICUs for many years, it can have very prolonged actions, especially in the presence of hepatic and renal dysfunctions. Because the metabolites of diazepam are pharmacologically active, that may further explain its cumulative effects. Lorazepam, oxazepam, clonazepam, and temazepam are intermediate-acting benzodiazepines, whereas midazolam and triazolam are short-acting benzodiazepines that have an established place for short procedures and may be useful in intensive care. However, seriously ill patients do not metabolize drugs in the same way as normal patients, and so-called short-acting benzodiazepines also accumulate over the long term. Whereas long-acting benzodiazepines may not be suitable for a short anaesthetic procedure, they may be satisfactory for use in long-term seriously ill patients. Moreover, the long-acting benzodiazepines usually are less expensive than the short-acting varieties.

MODE OF DELIVERY

Sedatives should be given intravenously in the ICU – they will be more reliably absorbed. The drugs can be given either on an as-required basis or via a continuous intravenous infusion.

Continuous intravenous infusions

Infusions should be titrated against an end point (eg pain relief or anxiolysis). This is an easy, effective, and flexible technique for drug delivery. Moreover, less total drug is required. Aggressive marketing has popularized the use of volumetric infusion pumps for continuous intravenous infusions. The simple motorized infusion syringe pump may have more advantages: It is cheaper and does not require dedicated and expensive giving sets; it is easy to operate and can use high concentrations of drugs in standard syringes; it is small and can be more easily placed in the overcrowded area around a patient's bed. The high degree of accuracy claimed by the manufacturers of volumetric infusion pumps is not necessarily an advantage when titrating against physiological end points such as pain relief or anxiolysis. The infusion syringe systems are accurate enough to titrate drugs against finer physiological end points, such as pulmonary artery wedge pressure or blood pressure.

MULTILUMEN CENTRAL VENOUS LINES   These catheters are often used for patients who require multiple continuous infusions of intravenous drugs. Together with multiple three-way taps, they facilitate drug delivery, remove the danger of inadvertent drug surges, and eliminate the need to cease drug infusions while central venous pressure measurements are performed.

COMPLICATIONS OF SEDATION

AIRWAY OBSTRUCTION AND LOSS OF COUGH REFLEX

All sedatives will cause decreases in a patient's level of consciousness, with depressed upper-airway reflexes and possible airway obstruction. This is not a problem when a patient has an artificial airway. If there is any doubt about the patency of the airway, sedation should be avoided until it is secured.

RESPIRATORY DEPRESSION

Opiates, particularly, cause respiratory depression. Because of the high numbers of trained staff in ICUs and the predictable nature of respiratory depression, this does not present the same problem that it might on a general ward with fewer nursing staff. Opiates should be titrated against pain relief and respiratory depression.

CARDIOVASCULAR DEPRESSION

Like respiratory depression, this well-documented side effect of many sedative drugs is not necessarily a contraindication to their use in an ICU. Hypotension usually is related to vasodilatation, rather than cardiac depression; it is dosage-dependent and predictable and is easily reversed with a fluid infusion. Even in the presence of severe multiorgan failure and hypotension, drugs such as benzodiazepines and opiates can be used to sedate patients as long as the intravascular volume is optimal.

IMMUNE DEPRESSION

It has been suspected for some years, on an anecdotal and limited scientific basis, that there is an association between excessive use of intravenous anaesthetic agents (eg thiopentone, Althesin, and etomidate) and overwhelming bronchopneumonia or septicaemia. All of these drugs have been shown to suppress immune responses in vitro. The use of etomidate has been associated with suppression of endogenous corticosteroid production and an increase in mortality secondary to septicaemia.

Nitrous oxide and volatile anaesthetic agents have also been implicated in suppressing immune responses. Other sedatives such as narcotics and benzodiazepines have not, as yet, been associated with immune depression in the clinical setting.

ALLERGIC REACTIONS

Even mild allergic reactions are quite rare with the commonly used sedative drugs.

ADDICTION AND DEPENDENCE

Whereas narcotics often are grudgingly dispensed in meagre doses on general wards, for fear of dependence, they are often used in "industrial" doses for long periods in the ICU. Despite that, addiction or psychological dependence is rare. Physical withdrawal symptoms are only rarely seen when narcotics and benzodiazepines are used in large amounts over long periods. Such symptoms can be modified by gradually reducing the dosage.

Similarly, physical and psychological withdrawal symptoms have not been reported often for the other commonly used sedatives. It is possible that there are degrees of withdrawal reactions for many sedative drugs that have been disguised by the concurrent illness and gradual drug withdrawal. Pre-existing psychosocial circumstances and an active decision to take the drug may be more important in the development of drug dependence.

Long-term use of short-acting benzodiazepines (eg midazolam for 2–3 weeks) can provoke epileptic seizures on their withdrawal. Patients thought to be at risk should be changed to long-acting benzodiazepines (eg diazepam for 3–4 days) prior to stopping benzodiazepines altogether.

CHANGES IN INTRACRANIAL PRESSURE

Simply sedating a patient (preventing movement, especially coughing and straining) will decrease the ICP. There are also some sedatives that can independently reduce the ICP. These are mainly intravenous anaesthetic induction agents, such as thiopentone. Most volatile anaesthetic agents, as well as nitrous oxide and ketamine, will increase the ICP and should be avoided in the presence of intracranial abnormalities that are likely to increase the ICP.

PHLEBITIS

Many of the commonly used sedatives, apart from opiates, cause phlebitis; this is usually overcome by delivering the drug through a central venous catheter.

MUSCLE RELAXANTS

Muscle relaxants are most commonly used in an ICU to facilitate ventilation. Sometimes this is necessary, as in patients with severe hypoxia or high ICP. However, most patients, when given judicious analgesia with or without sedation and with appropriate ventilatory support (eg IMV or CPAP), will not require muscle relaxation for ventilation.

Muscle relaxants also prevent assessment of neurological status and detection of epilepsy, and they can preclude spontaneous breathing in the event of a disconnection from ventilatory support. Muscle relaxants should never be used without adequate sedation.

Muscle relaxants have also been implicated in the aetiology of polyneuropathy in the critically ill (see p. 631).

MODE OF DELIVERY AND MONITORING

Muscle relaxants can be given as a continuous infusion or in intermittent doses. Excessive amounts should be avoided, as unpredictable rates of drug metabolism and excretion can lead to prolonged paralysis. Neuromuscular blockade can be monitored clinically using end points such as patient movement, respiratory effort, or coughing. Prolonged neuromuscular blockade should be monitored by measuring the muscle responses to peripheral nerve stimulation. This may avoid prolonged weakness after the use of neuromuscular blocking agents.

CHOICE OF DRUG

• Pancuronium is relatively inexpensive and has little effect on cardiovascular stability, but it can potentiate tachyarrhythmias. The dose is usually 0.1 mg/kg as an intubating dose, and 2 mg IV as a bolus dose to maintain relaxation.

• Vecuronium (0.08–0.1 mg/kg as an intubating dose, 75–100 μg · kg^{-1} · h^{-1} for infusion) may also be suitable for use in the ICU, as it has a short half-life. It has no cardiovascular side effects and is eliminated by both renal excretion (10–20%) and hepatic metabolism. Accumulation of 3-desacetylvecuronium may be responsible for the decreased infusion rates needed with long-term vecuronium use, especially in the elderly.

• Atracurium (0.5 mg/kg IV as an intubating dose) is expensive, but it has the advantage of not being dependent on renal or hepatic function for degradation and has a relatively short action. However, atracurium may not be suitable for long-term use in the ICU, as laudanosine (a metabolite of atracurium) may accumulate, causing seizures at high concentrations.

• Newer drugs such as mivacurium, doxacurium, and pipercuronium may have a future role in the ICU.

OTHER FORMS OF PAIN RELIEF

REGIONAL OR EPIDURAL ANALGESIA USING LOCAL ANAESTHETICS

Regional or epidural analgesia is eminently suitable for seriously ill patients. The local anaesthetic agents and opiates used are relatively safe and provide excellent pain relief. The techniques are specialized and, like all other procedures, are best performed by experienced operators. Both regional and epidural analgesia can be provided by continuous infusion techniques or by intermittent boluses with long-acting agents. They should be considered for relief of pain associated with

- flail chest
- fractured ribs
- post-operative states, especially following laparotomy and thoraco-tomy
- pelvic and limb injuries

Complete thoracic and abdominal pain relief will aid deep breathing, coughing ability, and physiotherapy and may improve oxygenation and obviate artificial ventilation.

EPIDURAL ANALGESIA

Exclude any patient with an unstable cardiovascular system, spinal trauma, overlying skin infection, coagulopathy, previous laminectomy, or head injury, as well as any patient who is unconscious, unwilling, or uncooperative.

Analgesia should provide sensory blockage to the painful area, but no higher than T4.

The level of insertion should be at the lower limit of the site that needs blocking. Lumbar epidurals with large volumes of dilute local anaesthetic are rarely successful if a high thoracic block is needed. Ensure that the patient is normovolaemic and fluid-loaded before using local anaesthetic agents, as sympathetic blockade may unmask hypovolaemia.

Techniques

Many different protocols are used, and each unit should develop its own. The following are several established techniques that can be adapted; the variations have to do with such issues as continuous or intermittent, with or without narcotics, long-acting or short-acting agents.

LOCAL ANAESTHETICS

- bolus dose: bupivacaine, 0.5%, plain or with a 1 : 20,000 solution of adrenaline, 5–8 ml, depending on level of analgesia required.
- continuous infusion: bupivacaine, 0.125–0.25%. Start immediately after the bolus dose. The infusion rate will depend on the level of analgesia required.

Continuous infusions will provide more satisfactory pain relief and less severe cardiovascular effects. The recommended amounts of bupivacaine to avoid toxicity are

- no more than 2 mg/kg as a bolus
  or
- no more than 400 mg/d.

Tachyphylaxis can occur with the use of bupivacaine, necessitating more frequent increases in dosage.

LOCAL ANAESTHETICS ± NARCOTICS Mixtures of narcotics and local anaesthetics are very successful. Bupivacaine concentrations tend to vary between 0.125% and 0.2%. Fentanyl is the commonest narcotic used, and its concentrations range between 2 and 4 μg/ml. The 'mixture' we use is

bupivacaine, 0.5%, 20 ml ⎫
fentanyl, 200 μg   ⎬ given at 5–8 ml/h
normal saline, 26 ml   ⎭

This mixture gives

bupivacaine concentration, 0.2%
fentanyl, 4 μg/ml

Commercial packs are also available.

Epidural narcotics alone offer little advantage over intravenous narcotics.

In the ICU, epidural and systemic narcotics are often used together (eg for flail chest plus fractured upper limbs), as the patient can be closely watched for respiratory depression. If that occurs, a small dose of naloxone (50–100 μg IV) will reverse the respiratory depression. Decrease the epidural infusion rate or decrease the narcotic concentration in the solution.

Pruritus, nausea, and vomiting can also be reversed with 50–100 μg of naloxone intravenously while continuing the epidural infusion.

INADEQUATE PAIN RELIEF Check the delivery system for leakages or mechanical faults. Check the epidural concentration; a bolus of 2–4 ml of infusion solution plus a higher infusion rate may be required.

INTRAPLEURAL ANALGESIA

Pain relief can be provided by administration of local anaesthetic agents into the pleural space. This can be achieved by a single injection (eg 10–20 ml bupivacaine, 0.5%, with adrenaline, 5 μg/ml) or by continuous infusion via a catheter in the pleural space. This technique is particularly suitable for post-operative thoracic or upper-abdominal wounds.

TROUBLESHOOTING

THE CONFUSED PATIENT IN THE ICU: APPROACH

Rapidly exclude reversible factors:

hypoxia
hypercarbia
hypotension
hypertension
rarer causes (electrolyte disturbances, hypoglycaemia, renal or liver failure, vitamin and co-factor deficiencies, generalized sepsis, and intracranial abnormalities)

History Elicit past history of disease and drugs, particularly alcohol and sedative dependence.

Relieve pain

Reassure Encourage visitors and staff to talk to the patient, explaining the underlying disease and orienting the patient as to time and place.

Sleep Encourage sleep, with as little disturbance as possible to the patients while they are sleeping.

Secure lines Secure lines and tubes to minimize patient interference.

Restraint Bed rails, finger tapes, and even manacles may be necessary.

Sedation Additional sedation may be necessary when reasonable causes have been excluded and other measures have failed.

Psychiatric consultation Psychiatric consultation may help in some cases when patients become more co-operative.

TROUBLESHOOTING

THE CONFUSED PATIENT IN THE ICU: CAUSES

Metabolic   Uraemia, electrolyte abnormalities, vitamin and co-factor deficiencies, hypoglycaemia and hyperglycaemia

Global hypoperfusion or hypoxia

Drugs
Withdrawal from alcohol, sedatives, opiates, hypnotics, barbiturates
Idiosyncratic reaction to sedation
Direct effect (eg ketamine or breakdown products of pethidine)
Drug overdose (eg hallucinogenics, tricyclic antidepressants, phe-
    nothiazines, theophylline, and anticholinergics)

Systemic infection   (eg septicaemia)

Pain   (eg full stomach or bladder)

Fever

Underlying chronic disease
Psychiatric (eg psychosis, schizophrenia)
Chronic organic brain disease (eg collagen disease)
Endocrine disease, thyroid and parathyroid disorders

Intracranial problem   (eg trauma, infection, epilepsy, stroke, tumour, abscess, haematoma)

Acute post-cardiac-bypass confusional state

Fat emboli

Hypertensive encephalopathy

'ICU psychosis'   A DIAGNOSIS OF EXCLUSION, due to a combination of disorientation, drugs, sleep deprivation, etc. The elderly and very young are prone to confusional states in the ICU.

FURTHER READING

Crankshaw, D., & Purcell, G. (eds.) (1987). Opioids, hypnotics and muscle re-laxants: an update on pharmacokinetics and techniques of administration. *Anaesthesia and Intensive Care* 15:5–96 (symposium issue).

Murphy, D. F. (1993). Interpleural analgesia. *British Journal of Anaesthesia* 75:426–34.

O'Connor, M. F., & Roizen, M. F. (1993). Use of muscle relaxants in the intensive care unit. *Journal of Intensive Care Medicine* 8:34–46.

Pollack, M. H., Stern, T. A. (1993). Recognition and management of anxiety in the intensive care unit. *Journal of Intensive Care Medicine* 8:1–15.

Pollard, B. J., Bion, J. F. (eds.) (1992). Neuromuscular blocking agents in intensive care. *Intensive Care Medicine* 19:S35–98 (symposium issue).

Stevens, D. S., & Edwards, W. T. (1990). Management of pain in the critically ill. *Journal of Intensive Care Medicine* 5:258–91.

Topulos, G. P. (1993). Neuromuscular blockade in adult intensive care. *New Horizons* 1:447–62.

8

SHOCK AND ANAPHYLAXIS

- Ischaemia and shock merge. Even minor ischaemia can adversely affect cellular function.
- 'Normal' vital signs and monitoring may not ensure adequate oxygen delivery.
- Hypovolaemia (relative or absolute) is the commonest cause of ischaemia and the easiest to correct.

GENERAL FEATURES OF SHOCK

Shock can be defined as a state of inadequate cellular sustenance associated with inadequate or inappropriate tissue perfusion resulting in abnormal cellular metabolism. This can occur as a result of inadequate oxygen delivery, maldistribution of blood flow, a low perfusion pressure, or, as usually is the case, a combination of all three. Shock is associated with oxygen debt, anaerobic metabolism, and tissue acidosis.

Shock predisposes to multiorgan failure (MOF) (see Chapter 9), manifested by coma, ileus, diarrhoea, liver malfunction and jaundice, renal insufficiency, coagulopathy, and adult respiratory distress syndrome (ARDS).

The common denominator and earliest manifestation of shock is reduced oxygen consumption ($\dot{V}o_2$). This is caused by low flow in haemorrhagic or cardiogenic shock, by a cellular or metabolic deficit in septic shock, and by maldistribution of flow in all types of shock.

The term 'compensated shock' suggests that the blood pressure is maintained at the expense of peripheral shutdown and ischaemia to many tissues.

It is becoming increasingly recognized that compensated shock is difficult to detect clinically, but can have deleterious effects. Measurements of parameters such as blood pressure, pulse rate, and urine output may be normal in these circumstances, because of redistribution of blood flow to vital organs, such as the brain and heart, and away from the so-called non-vital organs, such as skin and the gastro-intestinal tract (GIT). It may be appropriate to employ measurements of tissue perfusion, such as monitoring the pH of the gastric mucosa (tonometry) (see p. 493), as well as global measurements of oxygen delivery (see p. 376). The state of compensated shock is associated with relatively normal estimates of global oxygen delivery in the presence of ischaemia in many tissues. Compensated shock is associated with inadequate resuscitation and with high rates of morbidity and mortality. For example, decreased splanchnic blood flow is associated with potentially serious sequelae, such as bacteraemia, endotoxaemia, and MOF (see p. 137). Oxygen free radicals and other damaging substances are produced during hypoperfusion. The threshold of oxygen delivery at which this occurs has not been defined, and each tissue may have a different threshold. There is an increasing tendency to 'hyper-resuscitate' patients suspected of having hypoperfusion or compensated shock in order to provide adequate oxygen delivery to all cells.

CLASSIFICATION OF SHOCK

There are many classifications of shock, some based on clinical entities, and some based on pathophysiology. This is somewhat unreal, as there is large overlap between some of the groups, especially in their more severe forms, and one or more processes may be involved simultaneously (Table 8.1). All forms of shock can eventually result in profound cellular dysfunction and death – so-called irreversible shock. Irreversibility is difficult to define and may depend on the individual hospital as much as on the clinical state.

The following is a clinically useful scheme for determining causes of shock:

- Hypotension is often the first sign of shock.
- Blood pressure = cardiac output × systemic vascular resistance (SVR).
- Firstly, determine whether the problem is mainly one of decreased SVR or one of decreased cardiac output.
- If cardiac output is decreased, is that associated with a high or a low filling pressure?

TABLE 8.1 CLASSIC HAEMODYNAMIC PATTERNS IN SHOCK

Type of shock	Cardiac output	Left ventricular volume	Systemic vascular resistance
Hypovolaemic	↓	↓ ↓	↑ ↑
Cardiogenic	↓ ↓	↑ ↑	↑
Septic	↑ ↑	↓ ↓	↓ ↓ ↓
Anaphylactic	↓	↓ ↓	↓ ↓
Neurogenic	↓	↓ ↓	↓ ↓ ↓

Hypovolaemic shock

Hypovolaemic shock is related to decreased intravascular volume, secondary to loss of

- blood (eg trauma)
- plasma (eg burns)
- water and electrolytes (eg vomiting, diarrhoea)

Cardiogenic shock

Cardiogenic shock is related to 'pump' failure from many causes:

- valve dysfunction
- papillae rupture
- myocardial infarct
- arrhythmias
- tamponade
- pulmonary embolus

Septic shock

Septic shock involves both central and peripheral problems:

- peripheral circulation failure (eg redistribution, shunts)
- leaky capillaries in both the periphery and lungs
- depressed myocardial contractility

Anaphylactic shock

Anaphylactic shock is related to vasodilatation:

- leaky capillaries, leading to loss of intravascular volume
- severe bronchospasm, leading to high intrathoracic pressures with artificial ventilation, and further decreased venous return

Neurogenic shock

Neurogenic shock involves loss of sympathetic tone, leading to vasodilation.

ADVERSE EFFECTS OF SHOCK

Kidney: oliguria and renal failure.
Central nervous system: confusion and restlessness, with permanent damage in the presence of severe and prolonged ischaemia.
Gastro-intestinal tract: stress ulceration, ileus, diarrhoea, and ischaemia. Ischaemia of the GIT encourages bacterial translocation, endotoxaemia, and MOF.
Liver: elevation of hepatic transaminases and bilirubin.
Lung: ARDS.
Myocardium: may be impaired in severe ischaemia.
Other tissue damage: Other systems (eg skin, muscle, immune system) are almost certainly involved as well, but the end points of damage are difficult to measure.

MANAGEMENT

Like all acute situations in the ICU, diagnosis and treatment go hand in hand. Airway, breathing, and circulation must be secured first.

Airway

If in any doubt, intubate.

Breathing

Always maintain a high inspired oxygen fraction (F_{IO_2}) in shock patients, even if respiratory function appears normal, in order to enhance oxygen delivery and to compensate for V̇/Q̇ inequalities and the hypoxia that accompanies low-flow states.

Use artificial respiratory support – continuous positive airway pressure (CPAP), intermittent mandatory ventilation, and intermittent positive-pressure ventilation – where necessary (see Chapter 20). Apply other principles of treatment for acute respiratory failure as necessary (see Chapter 17).

Circulation

HYPOVOLAEMIA IS THE COMMONEST CAUSE OF SHOCK AND THE MOST EASILY REVERSED.

After hypovolaemia has been corrected, cardiac function should be optimized.

FLUID Simple measurements should be used initially to monitor resuscitation (eg blood pressure, pulse rate, skin perfusion, urine output) (see Chapter 21). As the intravascular volume is corrected, it can be find-tuned using more complex, time-consuming measurements of parameters such as central venous pressure (CVP), pulmonary artery wedge pressure (PAWP), cardiac output, and tissue pH. A fluid challenge, using 200–500-ml aliquots titrated against the relative changes in all relevant intravascular volume measurements, rather than a single absolute measurement, is the most accurate way of replacing intravascular fluid (see Chapter 4).

INOTROPES If hypotension persists despite volume replacement, inotrope support and/or a vasopressor may be needed. A particular drug or combination of drugs at a certain concentration will suit a particular patient at a particular time in that illness. The principles of choosing an inotrope are outlined elsewhere (see p. 520).

A useful first choice for hypotension that is not responsive to fluid is adrenaline (4 mg in 100 ml of 5% dextrose), titrated against blood pressure, together with low-dosage dopamine (2–4 $\mu g \cdot kg^{-1} \cdot min^{-1}$) to spare renal and mesenteric blood flow.

ADEQUATE HAEMOGLOBIN CONCENTRATION Red blood cells must be rapidly replaced in actively bleeding patients. If necessary, group-specific blood, which normally can be obtained more quickly than cross-matched blood, should be used in severe bleeding to ensure adequate oxygenation of tissues (see p. 372).

Reversible elements

RAPID CORRECTION OF REVERSIBLE AND TREATABLE FACTORS IS THE MOST IMPORTANT STEP IN THE MANAGEMENT OF SHOCK.

Correct any reversible factors (eg bleeding, bacteraemia, intra-abdominal sepsis, pulmonary embolism, pericardial tamponade, rupture of heart valve).

Fine tuning of shock

Ischaemia merges with shock, and compensated shock represents inadequate resuscitation. After the patient has initially been resuscitated, evidence of residual ischaemia must be monitored and corrected. Simple matching of global oxygen delivery (Do_2) to $\dot{V}o_2$ may not ensure adequate tissue oxygenation.

Evidence of ischaemia can be detected clinically (eg cold peripheries and oliguria) and by more sophisticated measurements, such as those of oxygen delivery and consumption (see p. 376), serum lactate (see p. 504), and GIT mucosal pH, as measured by a gastric tonometer (see p. 493).

SPECIFIC FORMS OF SHOCK

Hypovolaemic shock (see p. 56), cardiogenic shock (see p. 555), septic shock (see p. 182), and neurogenic shock (see p. 281) are discussed in more detail elsewhere. Only anaphylactic shock will be discussed in detail here.

ANAPHYLAXIS

Both anaphylactic reactions and anaphylactoid reactions are characterized by sudden and dramatic changes in vascular tone, permeability, and bronchial hyper-reactivity. The clinical manifestations of anaphylactoid reactions and anaphylactic reactions are identical.

Anaphylactic reactions are usually attributed to participation of IgE antibodies (ie previous exposure to the agent), whereas the mechanism of anaphylactoid reactions has not yet been identified.

CLINICAL MANIFESTATIONS

- **Skin:** erythema, urticaria, pruritus, angioedema
- **Respiratory:** bronchospasm, laryngeal oedema
- **Gastro-intestinal:** vomiting, abdominal cramps, diarrhoea
- **Cardiovascular:** hypotension, tachycardia, arrhythmias, vasodilation
- **General:** apprehension, metallic taste, coughing, paraesthesias, arthralgia, clouding of consciousness, and clotting abnormalities

These changes are variable; some or all of them may occur. The changes usually occur within seconds.

MANAGEMENT

Adrenaline

Adrenaline is the drug of choice for anaphylaxis:

- Initially give 10 ml of 1 : 10,000 (1 mg) adrenaline intravenously over 1–5 minutes.
    OR
- Give 1 ml of 1:1,000 (1 mg) adrenaline subcutaneously while intravenous access is being obtained. Repeat adrenaline doses as necessary.

Plasma expansion

Because of vasodilatation and leakage of plasma protein, plasma solution or colloid should be used to correct the volume of the intravascular compartment. It must be given rapidly, and large volumes may be required. Filling pressures (CVP and PAWP) and haematocrit can be used to fine-tune intravascular volume replacement when a patient is stable.

Bronchospasm

Apart from adrenaline, other measures that are used for asthma may be necessary (eg salbutamol) (see p. 438).

Oxygen

Oxygen, via a face mask, should always be given. Intubation and ventilation may be necessary for severe bronchospasm. The same ventilatory techniques as for severe asthma should be used (see p. 443).

Drugs

Steroids are of no proven benefit after anaphylaxis has occurred. Antihistamines similarly are of no proven benefit acutely.

Monitoring

• Patients should be monitored closely in the ICU until stable. Fine tuning of the cardiorespiratory system can be accomplished after resuscitation.
• Continuous ECG monitoring.
• Monitor blood pressure and blood gases.

Further management

Take blood for determination of complement and antibody concentrations, in order to identify possible precipitating agents (eg anaesthetic agents). Skin testing at a later date may further clarify the causative agent.

Counsel the patient and relatives about future reactions to the same stimulus. Inform relevant medical practitioners of the event, and consider a hyposensitization programme.

FURTHER READING

Billhardt, R. A., & Rosenbush, S. W. (1986). Cardiogenic and hypovolaemic shock. *Medical Clinics of North America* 70:853–76.

Bochner, B. S., & Lightenstein, L. M. (1991). Anaphylaxis. *New England Journal of Medicine* 324:1785–90.

Fiddian-Green, R. G., Haglund, U., Gutierrez, G., & Schoemaker, W. C. (1993). Goals for resuscitation of shock. *Critical Care Medicine* 21:S25–31.

Fisher, M. M. (1986). Clinical observations on the pathophysiology and treatment of anaphylactic cardiovascular collapse. *Anaesthesia and Intensive Care* 14:17–21.

Houston, M. C., Thompson, W. L., & Robertson, D. (1984). Shock: diagnosis and management. *Archives of Internal Medicine* 144:1433–9.

King, E. G., & Chin, W. D. N. (1985). An overview of pathophysiology and general treatment goals. *Critical Care Clinics* 1:547–61.

Mizock, B. A., & Falk, J. L. (1992). Lactic acidosis in critical illness. *Critical Care Medicine* 20:80–93.

9

MULTIORGAN FAILURE

- Early aggressive resuscitation may prevent multiorgan failure (MOF).
- The clinical presentation of MOF is determined by the host's response, not by the triggering factor.
- Aggressive investigation and treatment of the cause are the most important steps.

Multiorgan failure (MOF) is considered to be a discrete entity or syndrome in the critically ill. It is a process, rather than an event, and it develops over time in response not only to an initial stimulus, such as sepsis, multitrauma, inflammation, severe burns, major surgery, or shock, but also to the host's response to that particular stimulus. In fact, the host's response may be a more important determinant of the development of MOF than is the initial stimulus.

So-called multiorgan failure may not be total failure of every individual organ, but rather relative dysfunction. Failure or dysfunction of certain organs can be difficult to quantitate, and so the extent of system disintegration may be underestimated. For example, renal function is estimated on the basis of relatively firm end points, such as a rising serum creatinine concentration or oliguria, whereas there is no equivalent biochemical test for gastro-intestinal-tract (GIT) function, and thus softer clinical end points must be used. Patterns of organ dysfunction are variable from one patient to another.

MANIFESTATIONS OF MULTIORGAN FAILURE

RESPIRATORY SYSTEM Adult respiratory distress syndrome (ARDS) is usually defined as hypoxia in the appropriate clinical setting, with bilateral pulmonary infiltrates and a normal left atrial pressure.

CARDIOVASCULAR SYSTEM   Peripheral dilatation, high cardiac output, supraventricular arrhythmias, impaired contractility, or low-output cardiac failure.

CENTRAL NERVOUS SYSTEM   Clouding of consciousness and coma (see p. 583).

RENAL SYSTEM   Acute renal failure, with impaired glomerular filtration and tubular function.

GASTRO-INTESTINAL TRACT   Stress ulceration, decreased gastric emptying, ileus, and diarrhoea.

HEPATOBILIARY SYSTEM   Increase in bilirubin, and increases in liver enzymes.

PANCREAS   Mild to moderate pancreatitis (see p. 678).

HAEMATOLOGICAL   Coagulopathies, thrombocytopenia, as well as impairment of bone-marrow function.

METABOLIC   Oxygen consumption may rise or fall, increased energy expenditure, increased gluconeogenesis from protein and consequent hyperglycaemia, increased fat oxidation, failure to prevent catabolism by nutritional support.

OTHER FACTORS   Other organs and tissues probably are also involved (eg skin, muscle, bone), but those dysfunctions are even more difficult to measure and define.

PATHOPHYSIOLOGY

Multiorgan failure is generally considered to be a syndrome with many causes, but a similar final common pathway. Animal studies have demonstrated that the physiological alterations associated with MOF are produced by a complex cascade of more than 100 separate molecular mediators, including cytokines, eicosanoids, complement components, platelet activating factor (PAF), and intermediates of nitrogen and oxygen metabolism. These mediators have overlapping biological effects and are released from host cells, mainly macrophages, in response to a variety of stimuli. Experimental administration of some of these mediators, including tumour necrosis factor (TNF), interleukin-1 (IL-1), IL-2, and IL-6, produces a picture that in many ways simulates MOF. The levels of mediators in the circulation do not correlate with the clinical responses. The responses of mediators to insults have important biological functions related to survival, as well as to injurious sequelae.

The pathogenesis of MOF may be more closely related to an uncontrolled host response to an initiating stimulus, such as sepsis, than to uncontrolled infection and unchecked bacterial multiplication. Thus, MOF probably results from a systemic inflammatory response, rather than a pure infection. Although MOF was initially thought to be triggered by bacteria, it is now apparent that many stimuli, including tissue ischaemia, can initiate the inflammatory response. The clinical findings and mediator responses do not allow one to differentiate between infectious and non-infectious causes of MOF. In addition to the ischaemic injury, reperfusion of the ischaemic areas will result in additional injury, mediated by inflammatory cells. Ischaemia of the mucosa of the GIT may also play an important role in MOF. The intestinal mucosal barrier is particularly vulnerable during ischaemia because of an increased demand for oxygen during sepsis in the face of a decreased oxygen supply. The compromised mucosa is unable to prevent translocation of bacteria, which leads to further stimulation of inflammatory mediators throughout the body. It has been suggested that the compromised GIT mucosa is the 'motor' of MOF.

The antecedents of the syndrome – trauma, burns, inflammation, major surgery, ischaemia, shock, and infection – are associated with a complex spectrum of immunological abnormalities. The result is a dynamic process due to the interplay of the initial stimulus and the host reaction. Management must therefore be directed to restoration of normal physiological status as rapidly as possible, rather than relying on simplistic solutions such as broad-spectrum antibiotics. In the future, there is the possibility of specific treatments directed against the many mediators of MOF. These include TNF, IL-1, IL-10, interferon-γ, transforming growth factors β (TGF-β), prostaglandins, PAF, and nitric oxide (NO).

MANAGEMENT

Treatment of sepsis is often considered the model for management of MOF. The principles of management for sepsis are the same for MOF and are discussed in detail elsewhere (see p. 137). The following are guidelines for the management of MOF.

Prevention

• Rapid resuscitation: Restore the circulating blood volume, arterial blood pressure, and blood flow; maintain oxygen delivery to the cells.

• Prevention of sepsis (see p. 192).

• Rapid diagnosis and treatment of sepsis (see p. 192).

• Reduce GIT colonization, and avoid alkalinization of the gastric contents (see p. 32).

Support

• Maintain oxygen delivery (Do_2) to the cells (see Chapter 17):

adequate arterial oxygenation
adequate haemoglobin concentration
adequate cardiac output

• There may be an abnormal relationship between Do_2 and consumption ($\dot{V}o_2$) in patients with MOF. Even at high rates of Do_2, there may be a dependence of $\dot{V}o_2$ on Do_2. The more oxygen supplied, the more that is utilized (see p. 376). It is probably reasonable to aim for higher rather than 'normal' Do_2 in patients with MOF (see p. 376).

• Maintain adequate perfusion pressure.

• Minimize peripheral oedema, to encourage capillary blood flow and oxygen consumption.

• Avoid high intrathoracic pressures associated with artificial ventilatory support, to encourage extrathoracic organ blood flow.

• Low-dosage dopamine to encourage renal and mesenteric blood flow may be beneficial.

• Take measures to prevent stress ulceration (see p. 31).

• Replace coagulation factors and platelets.

• Use enteral feeding where possible. Otherwise, use parenteral nutrition (see p. 87).

Definitive treatment

AGGRESSIVELY INVESTIGATE AND REMOVE OR TREAT THE SOURCE OF SEPSIS OR OTHER CAUSES OF THE MOF. THIS IS THE MOST IMPORTANT STEP, THE DEFINITIVE TREATMENT.

DRUGS Drugs such as steroids, non-steroidal anti-inflammatory agents, heparin, branched-chain amino acids, desferrioxamine, allopurinol, prostaglandins, and monoclonal antibodies have all been tried or are currently being investigated for use in patients with MOF. As yet, none can be unequivocally recommended.

OUTCOME

There have been few large and epidemiologically sound studies of MOF, and thus far it has been difficult to define the syndrome and determine what constitutes organ failure. More extensive trials will be required before we shall have precise information on how the high mortality associated with this syndrome can be reduced. However, we know that it is not only the number of failing organ systems that determines the outcome, but also the degree of dysfunction with each system.

FURTHER READING

Bihari, D. (1988). Oxygen delivery and consumption in the critically ill: their relation to the development of multiple organ failure. In *Shock and the Adult Respiratory Distress Syndrome,* ed. W. Kox & D. Bihari, pp. 95–121. Berlin: Springer-Verlag.

Bihari, D., & Semple, S. J. G. (1987). Multiple organ failure in the critically ill. *Medicine International* 2:1586–90.

Cerra, F. B. (1987). The hypermetabolism–organ failure complex. *World Journal of Surgery* 11:73–81.

Clarke, G. M. (1985). Multiple system organ failure. *Clinical Anaesthesiology* 3:1027–53.

Hayes, M. A., Timmins, A. C., Yau, E. H. S., Palazzo, M., Hinds, C. J., & Watson, D. (1994). Elevation of systemic oxygen delivery in the treatment of critically ill patients. *New England Journal of Medicine* 1330:1717–22.

Mainous, M. R., & Deitch, E. A. (1992). Bacterial translocation and its potential role in the pathogenesis of multiple organ failure. *Journal of Intensive Care Medicine* 7:101–8.

Pinsky, M. R., & Matuschak, G. M. (eds.) (1989). Multiple systems organ failure. *Critical Care Clinics* 5:1 (symposium issue).

Shoemaker, W. C., Appel, P. L., Kram, H. B., Waxman, K., & Lee, T. (1988). Prospective trial of supranormal values of survivors as therapeutic goals in high-risk surgical patients. *Chest* 94:1176–86.

Williams, J. G., & Maier, R. V. (1992). The inflammatory response. *Journal of Intensive Care Medicine* 7:53–66.

10

CARDIOPULMONARY RESUSCITATION

- Immediate cardioversion is the best treatment for ventricular fibrillation.
- Pupil size and reactions are unreliable indicators of cerebral function during cardiopulmonary resuscitation.
- Up to half of all patients who experience in-hospital cardiac arrest had major physiological abnormalities beforehand. These should be identified and treated.

INITIAL MANAGEMENT IN THE HOSPITAL SETTING

Firstly, determine that the patient is indeed unconscious: Shake the patient, and attempt to communicate. Call for help, and lie the patient flat.

IDENTIFY THE CARDIAC RHYTHM IMMEDIATELY.

- If ventricular fibrillation (VF) is the first rhythm encountered, three sequential countershocks should be delivered as soon as possible, at energy settings of 200 J, 200 J, and then 360 J (Figure 10.1).
- If the rhythm is other than VF, immediately proceed to that specific treatment protocol (Figures 10.2–10.5).
- **IF THE RHYTHM CANNOT BE IDENTIFIED IMMEDIATELY,** gain control of the airway, commence basic cardiopulmonary resuscitation (CPR), and establish intravenous access while waiting for rhythm-monitoring equipment to arrive.

AIRWAY

The three basic airway manoeuvres are head tilt, chin lift, and jaw thrust. The airway must be cleared of any foreign matter or obstruction with finger sweeps or suction. Initially use mouth-to-mask or

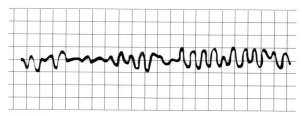

FIGURE 10.1   Ventricular fibrillation is the rhythm in 80–90% of non-traumatic cardiac arrests.

IMMEDIATE DEFIBRILLATION is the best treatment

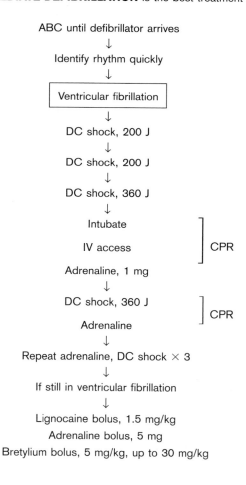

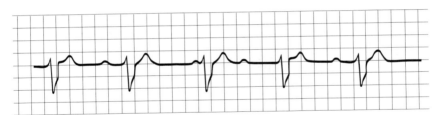

FIGURE 10.2   Bradycardia.

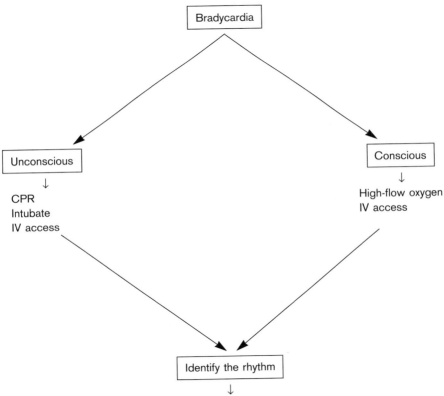

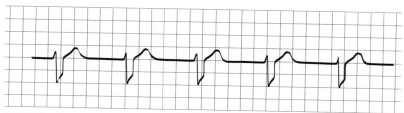

FIGURE 10.3 Pulseless electrical activity (PEA).

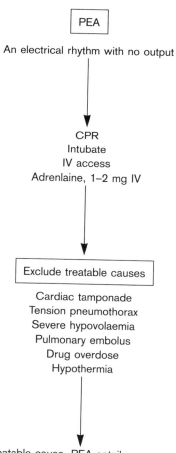

PEA

An electrical rhythm with no output

CPR
Intubate
IV access
Adrenlaine, 1–2 mg IV

Exclude treatable causes

Cardiac tamponade
Tension pneumothorax
Severe hypovolaemia
Pulmonary embolus
Drug overdose
Hypothermia

If there is no treatable cause, PEA entails a very poor prognosis

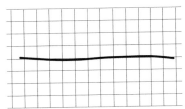

FIGURE 10.4 Asystole is not a rhythm. It is the baseline electrical activity of a dead heart.

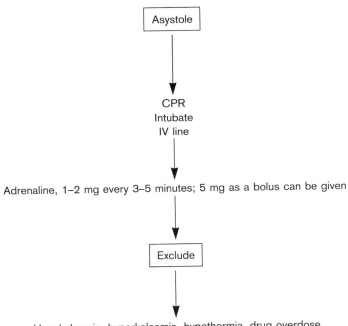

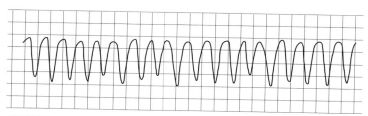

FIGURE 10.5   Ventricular tachycardia.

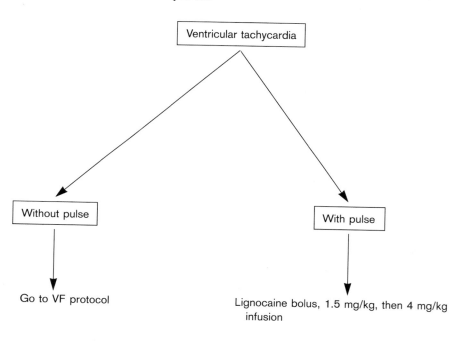

bag-and-mask ventilation. Intubation with an endotracheal tube (ETT) will give better control of the airway. If intubation is difficult, do not persevere – ensure adequate ventilation and oxygenation with a simpler technique.

VENTILATION

For most nursing and medical staff, the use of self-inflating bags probably is not as efficient as mouth-to-mask techniques with entrained oxygen. When using mouth-to-mask ventilation, pause to allow chest compression. The period of lung inspiration should be 1.5–2.0 seconds per breath. This will increase the likelihood of lung inflation, rather than gastric distension.

If the patient is intubated, ventilate the lungs and massage the heart independently at the recommended rates. Occasional synchrony between massage and ventilation is not necessarily deleterious.

CIRCULATION

Check for a carotid or femoral pulse. If there is no pulse or only a weak pulse and the blood pressure is too low to be measured, start external chest compression (Figure 10.6).

Measure two finger breadths up from the xiphisternum. Place the heel of your hand on the lower third of the sternum. Place your other hand on top of the first, keeping the heel of the hand on the chest and the fingers off.

With your shoulders directly over the patient, use your body weight (not your arm muscles) to depress the sternum.

- Compress at a rate of 80–100 times per minute.
- Depress the sternum 4–5 cm each time.
- Use equal compression and relaxation times.

Upstroke

Downstroke

$1\frac{1}{2}$ — 2 inches
38 — 50mm

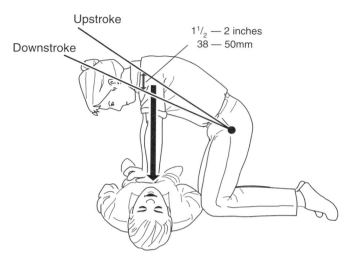

FIGURE 10.6 External cardiac compression.

Effective CPR will give a cardiac output that will be 25–30% of normal, a systolic blood pressure of 60–80 mm Hg, and a diastolic pressure of approximately 40 mm Hg. Cardiac output will decline with time. After 15 minutes, it will be only 15% of normal.

The 'chest thump' as an initial manoeuvre to convert VF is probably of no value.

INTRAVENOUS ACCESS

The initial intravenous access should be via a large peripheral vein (eg antecubital fossa). Central lines are not required; their insertion would only interrupt the performance of external chest compression. Intravenous fluids usually are not required during CPR, but a slow-running drip will facilitate drug infusion.

If intravenous access cannot be gained, some drugs, including adrenaline and lignocaine, can be administered via the ETT. Dosages up to 10 times normal should be used. Sodium bicarbonate and calcium should not be administered via the ETT. INTRACARDIAC DRUGS SHOULD NOT BE USED.

DEFIBRILLATION

Defibrillation depolarizes the myocardium and allows the most rapid natural pacemaker, the sinoatrial node, to drive the heart's rhythm. Immediate defibrillation is the treatment of choice for VF or pulseless ventricular tachycardia (VT) (Figure 10.5). If VF or VT without an output is the first rhythm encountered, up to three sequential countershocks of 200 J, 200 J, and then 360 J should be delivered, with no CPR in between. If the countershock can be delivered within 3 minutes, up to 80% of patients will revert. After 5 minutes, defibrillation rarely results in spontaneous reversion. This emphasizes the importance of early countershock. The use of sequential shocks without a pause for CPR takes advantage of the accumulated decrease in transthoracic impedance. More current is therefore applied to the heart. However, excessive current can damage the heart. Energy levels of more than 360 J are seldom required. Repeated shocks may be necessary, but check that the physiological environment is satisfactory (eg adequate oxygenation, as well as adequate potassium and magnesium concentrations).

The defibrillator operator is responsible for determining that staff members are clear of the bed at the time of defibrillation.

Staff members must familiarize themselves with their hospital's machines and have some basic knowledge about troubleshooting. The commonest reasons for defibrillator malfunction include batteries without sufficient charge, poor contact with the patient, and inadvertent use of the synchronization mode. This mode should be used only for supraventricular arrhythmias.

DRUGS

Drug treatment often must remain empirical during CPR. It is impossible to cite exact dosages for drugs.

Adrenaline

Adrenaline has consistently been shown to be one of the most beneficial drugs during CPR. Its vasoconstrictor action diverts the blood flow, increasing the flow to vital organs and increasing coronary and cerebral perfusion pressures. Adrenaline is the first-line drug for use in patients who have VF unresponsive to defibrillation, asystole, and pulseless electrical activity (PEA).

Although no optimal dose of drug can be stated, large doses (eg 5-mg bolus IV) can be used if smaller doses are unsuccessful. It must be emphasized that adequate chest compression is critical if one is to gain the full beneficial effects of vasoconstrictors.

GUIDELINES
- 1–2 mg IV every 3–5 minutes
  OR
- 8 mg in 100 ml of 5% dextrose as a continuous infusion during CPR

Other inotropes

Combinations of other drugs, such as dobutamine, dopamine, noradrenaline, and isoprenaline, may have a place in fine-tuning cardiovascular function after spontaneous circulation has been re-established.

Sodium bicarbonate

The indications for the use of sodium bicarbonate in CPR are few; they include pre-existing metabolic acidosis, hyperkalaemia, and overdosage with tricyclic drugs. It may also be useful in prolonged CPR (eg more than 20 minutes). Bicarbonate treatment is often associated with complications, such as hypernatraemia, hyperosmolality, hypocalcaemia, paradoxical intracellular acidosis, impaired release of oxygen from haemoglobin, and rebound alkalosis.

GUIDELINES   Give sodium bicarbonate at 1 mg/kg IV as a bolus dose, and then use regular arterial blood-gas determinations to guide further treatment. However, during prolonged CPR, arterial blood gases do not necessarily reflect the degree of cellular acidosis.

Calcium chloride

Calcium is no longer routinely recommended during CPR. It may be useful for hyperkalaemia and hypocalcaemia and in cases in which it is suspected that there is toxicity due to calcium-channel blockers.

GUIDELINES   Give 10 ml of calcium chloride (10%).

Lignocaine

Lignocaine is the antiarrhythmic drug of choice for VT when the patient has adequate cardiac output. Patients with VT with no pulse or VF should be immediately defibrillated. Lignocaine may also be useful for cases in which VF remains resistant following the use of adrenaline.

GUIDELINES   Give a 1–1.5-mg/kg bolus, followed by an infusion of 2–4 mg/min.

Bretylium

Bretylium may be useful for resistant VF unresponsive to adrenaline, lignocaine, and electrical countershock. However, there are few data to support its effectiveness.

GUIDELINES

• Give a 5-mg/kg bolus of bretylium.

• Subsequent boluses should be 10 mg/kg, up to a total maximum dose of 30 mg/kg.

• Infuse bretylium at 1–2 mg/min.

FURTHER MANAGEMENT

CONTINUE CPR: WHEN CONDUCTING TESTS, PROCEDURES OR RE-VIEWING AN ELECTROCARDIOGRAM, DO NOT INTERRUPT THE CPR FOR MORE THAN A FEW SECONDS.

A spontaneous palpable pulse is the best evidence that cardiac output has returned. Immediately resume CPR if a pulse is not detected.

Brain resuscitation

The most effective way to maintain cerebral function is to provide efficient CPR. Barbiturates probably are of no use, and calcium-channel blockers and other drugs need further evaluation.

TABLE 10.1   POOR PROGNOSTIC INDICATORS AFTER CPR

No CPR given until 4 minutes or more had elapsed
No defibrillation during the first 8 minutes or more
Age of patient greater than 75 years, and arrest lasting 5 minutes or longer
Severe underlying disease (eg malignancy)
Initial rhythm asystole or PEA
Unwitnessed arrest of unknown duration

WHEN TO STOP

The decision when to stop is largely governed by 'when to start'. The physical conditions of many patients are not suitable for commencement of CPR, and, whenever possible, that should be clarified for each patient before cardiorespiratory arrest occurs. The purpose of CPR is to prevent sudden, unexpected death, not to prolong meaningless life.

Brain-stem signs such as pupil size and reaction to light are unreliable indicators of neurological status during CPR.

If there is a delay of more than 4 minutes before basic CPR is initiated and a delay of more than 8 minutes before defibrillation, the outcomes generally are very poor (Table 10.1).

Prolonging CPR beyond 15 minutes has resulted in a survival rate of less than 5%, and except in exceptional circumstances, such as primary hypothermia or drug overdose, CPR beyond 30 minutes is rarely successful.

POST-CARDIOPULMONARY RESUSCITATION

After resuscitation, a significant amount of organ damage due to ischaemia and/or reperfusion may occur.

It is important to correct as many 'correctables' as possible, in order to optimize tissue perfusion [eg serum potassium and magnesium, blood glucose (hyperglycaemia may exacerbate focal ischaemia), and temperature].

Maintain oxygenation and ventilation. Initially, facilitate carbon dioxide excretion by hyperventilation, in order to correct any accumulated metabolic acidosis. Once that has been achieved, ventilate to normal levels of Pa_{CO_2} (see p. 464).

Obtain a post-resuscitation chest x-ray to exclude pulmonary baro-trauma, rib fractures, aspiration pneumonia, gastric dilatation, and cardiac tamponade, and check the positions of the ETT and invasive monitoring devices in the thorax (eg temporary pacemakers, central venous catheters).

Regarding neurological damage, most studies have shown that if there is to be full neurological recovery, it will occur within the first 48 hours after cardiac arrest. Otherwise there will be varying degrees of permanent damage resulting from the global ischaemia at the time of arrest (see p. 590). There is no evidence that 'cerebral protection' with drugs, such as barbiturates, calcium antagonists, or steroids, can affect the outcome at all.

PREVENTION OF CARDIOPULMONARY ARREST

Up to half of all patients who experience in-hospital cardiac arrest can be shown to have had severe and identifiable abnormalities be-fore arrest. These include tachypnoea, hypotension, oliguria, and de-creased level of consciousness. Because of the increased monitoring and awareness in ICUs, it probably is no coincidence that patients in intensive care rarely experience unexpected cardiorespiratory arrest. It is therefore important that the entire staff of a hospital become better educated in how to recognize patients who are rapidly deteri-orating. Despite considerable advances in our knowledge of cardiac arrest, outcomes have not improved markedly over the past two decades. There is some evidence that the cardiac-arrest team would be more successful being rapidly deployed to patients who were at high risk of having an arrest, rather than to those who had actually arrested.

FURTHER READING

Bass, E. (1985). Cardiopulmonary arrest. Pathophysiology and neurological complications. *Annals of Internal Medicine* 103:920–2.

Emergency Cardiac Care Committee, American Heart Association (1992). Guidelines for cardiopulmonary resuscitation and emergency cardiac care. *Journal of the American Medical Association* 268:2171–298.

Hanashiro, P. K., & Wilson, J. R. (1986). Cardiopulmonary resuscitation. A current perspective. *Medical Clinics of North America* 70:729–47.

Niemann, J. T. (1992). Cardiopulmonary resuscitation. *New England Journal of Medicine* 327:1075–80.

Otto, C. W., Eisenbery, M. S., & Bircher, N. G. (eds.) (1985). Wolf Creek II conference on cardiopulmonary resuscitation. *Critical Care Medicine* 11:881–951 (symposium issue).

11

TEMPERATURE DISORDERS

- A fever has many beneficial effects in the body's fight against infection and should not necessarily be lowered.
- Meticulous supportive care is as important as active measures in the management of hypothermia and hyperthermia.
- Surface cooling for a hyperthermic patient can increase core temperature by encouraging skin vasoconstriction and shivering.

REGULATION OF TEMPERATURE

The body's core temperature remains remarkably stable. This is in spite of the wide range of ambient temperatures to which the body is exposed and the great variations in the metabolic processes that produce heat (thermogenesis) within the body. Heat is normally lost by convection, evaporation, and radiation. Temperature is centrally controlled, probably by the hypothalamus, and the main route for heat control is via the skin. Vasoconstriction is used to cool the skin, diverting blood flow from the superficial circulation to beneath the subcutaneous fat, thus using the skin's insulating properties to conserve body heat (Table 11.1). To lose heat, blood flow is diverted to the skin, facilitating radiant and convective heat losses. However, evaporative loss is the major adaptive mechanism for heat loss. Sweating accounts for heat losses of up to 500 kcal/h.

METHODS FOR TEMPERATURE MEASUREMENT

Temperatures vary considerably throughout the body. The temperatures of different areas of the skin will vary. Similarly, core temperatures measured in the bladder, pulmonary artery, and oesophagus can also vary. A single site for measuring temperature must therefore be chosen for consistency. A record of core temperature, rather than peripheral temperature, is essential in patients with hyper-

155

TABLE 11.1 PHYSIOLOGICAL RESPONSES TO
TEMPERATURE CHANGES

Hypothermia
Skin-vessel vasoconstriction
Muscle-vessel vasodilatation
Tachypnoea
Hypertension
Shivering
Increased metabolic rate
Hyperthermia
Skin vasodilatation
Sweating
Increased minute volume

thermia and hypothermia. Patients who have cardiorespiratory instability, resulting in unpredictable skin blood flow, should also have their core temperatures, rather than peripheral temperatures, recorded.

Simple glass thermometers are suitable for routine measurements of oral or axillary temperature in otherwise stable patients. They usually read 0.4–0.7°C below simultaneously recorded core temperatures. There is little difference in accuracy or ease of use between mercury thermometers and electronic systems for measuring non-core temperatures. Electronic thermistor-type devices are needed for measuring core temperature. It is important to routinely maintain and test these devices for accurate calibration.

HYPOTHERMIA

Hypothermia is said to occur when the body's core temperature is 35°C or less. It is a medical emergency (Table 11.2). Among patients with core temperatures lower than 32°C there is high mortality.

Hypothermia can result from

(a) exposure – when cold stress exceeds the body's maximum heat production

TABLE 11.2   CLINICAL EFFECTS OF CORE HYPOTHERMIA

36°C	Increased metabolic rate, in an attempt to balance heat loss; shivering, vasoconstriction.
32°C	Decreased metabolic activity, consciousness clouded, pupils dilated, shivering ceases, temperature control lost, bradycardia, J waves on ECG.
31°C	Blood pressure difficult to measure; increasing metabolic acidosis.
30°C	Increasing muscular rigidity, slow pulse and respiration, metabolic rate 50% of normal.
28°C	Ventricular fibrillation (VF) may develop if the heart is irritated.
26°C	Unconscious Pupils unreactive Resuscitation may still be No deep-tendon reflexes effective at this stage. Respiratory arrest
24°C	Spontaneous VF, pulmonary oedema, severe coagulopathy.
20°C	Asystole.

Source: The authors are grateful to Dr. R. Lee for permission to use this table.

(b) exhaustion – which results from depletion of the body's available energy sources

(c) failure of central temperature regulation – which is seen mainly in elderly patients and in the newborn

It is important for every intensive care unit (ICU) to have a thermometer capable of measuring core temperatures below 35°C. Arterial blood-gas analysis must allow for body temperature changes.

CAUSES OF HYPOTHERMIA

• Loss of consciousness (eg cerebrovascular events, head trauma).

• Metabolic and endocrine (eg acute diabetic emergencies, myxoedema, pituitary and adrenal failure).

• Accidental hypothermia – in association with low ambient temperature (eg mountaineering and immersion accidents).

• Surgery: Intraoperative hypothermia is common, especially during prolonged procedures involving open body cavities.

• Drugs – especially alcohol and drugs associated with self-poisoning.

Hypothermia is potentiated in

• the elderly (problems with thermogenesis)
• the newborn (problems with thermogenesis)
• the acutely ill (eg patients with pneumonia and renal failure)
• patients with cardiovascular instability (eg congestive heart failure, myocardial infarction, septicaemia)

CLINICAL FEATURES

Adaptive mechanisms such as tachypnoea, tachycardia, and muscle rigidity gradually give way to slowing of respiration, bradycardia, hypotension, and coma (Table 11.2). Electrocardiogram (ECG) changes include QT prolongation, T-wave inversion, J waves, and an increase in the PR interval (Figure 11.1). Ventricular fibrillation (VF) usually occurs when the core temperature drops below 25°C. The VF is often resistant to treatment until the core temperature is increased.

MANAGEMENT

Immediate

Hypothermia is a medical emergency and should be managed in an appropriately monitored area.

AIRWAY   Intubate if the patient is unconscious or has decreased airway reflexes.

BREATHING   All patients require high-flow oxygen, especially if they are shivering. Bradypnoea is usually associated with a core temperature lower than 30°C. Early intubation and artificial ventilation will assist with oxygenation and rewarming.

CIRCULATION   If there is no palpable pulse, perform cardiopulmonary resuscitation (CPR). As a general rule, for every 10°C decrease in body temperature, the time during which there can be hope of recovery from circulatory arrest without CPR can be doubled. This refers only to primary hypothermia (ie people who are instantly cooled to a low temperature). It does not apply to people who have become hy-

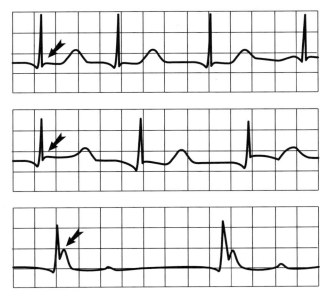

FIGURE 11.1 ECG changes associated with hypothermia. As the temperature decreases (from top to bottom), the heart rate slows, and the QT and PR intervals become more prolonged. J waves (arrows) appear at a temperature of about 35°C (top) and become more prominent at 25°C (bottom). (From Curley & Irwin, 1991, with permission of Little, Brown and Company.)

pothermic secondary to cardiac arrest (secondary hypothermia). Hypotension requires warmed intravenous fluid. Catecholamines are often required (see p. 521). Antiarrhythmics and cardioversion may be ineffective at low temperatures. Treatment of arrhythmias must therefore include aggressive rewarming.

MONITORING Use continuous ECG monitoring, pulse oximetry, vital signs, and other cardiorespiratory monitoring where appropriate.

INVESTIGATIONS Immediate investigations must include arterial blood gases, blood sugar, electrolytes, microbiology, chest x-ray, and 12-lead ECG. Measurement of core temperature with a low-reading thermometer is mandatory.

COAGULOPATHY Hypothermia causes marked disturbances of the enzymes involved in the coagulation cascade, thus predisposing the patient to bleeding. The abnormalities will not be detected if coagulation profiles are constructed at 37°C. The tests must be performed at the patient's core temperature.

Rewarming

CORE TEMPERATURE > 30°C: EXTERNAL WARMING   External rewarming is achieved by covering the patient, conducting the treatment in a warm (>25°C) room, and giving warm intravenous fluids and warmed humidified oxygen. More active techniques, such as immersing a patient in hot water, are unsound and not necessary. A temperature rise of 0.5°C/h should be the target.

CORE TEMPERATURE < 30°C: ACTIVE CORE REWARMING   Surface rewarming is contraindicated when the core temperature is less than 30°C, as it would cause shunting of blood to the dilating skin circulation. The vasodilatation would exacerbate hypotension and cause a further decrease in core temperature, both of which could precipitate VF. Active core rewarming can be achieved in various ways:

• Delivering warmed humidified gases.
• Delivering warmed parenteral fluids.
• Peritoneal dialysis (4–8 L/h at a temperature of 37–42°C).
• Circulating water, heated to 42°C, through a closed irrigation system inserted into the oesophagus or stomach at a rate of about 3 L/h.
• Currently, the technique of choice for several hypothermia probably is haemoperfusion. This procedure employs extracorporeal circulation by a continuous arteriovenous or venovenous technique (see p. 662). The blood is warmed as it flows past a dialysis solution warmed to 40°C.

Active measures can be ceased when the temperature reaches 35°C.

OUTCOME

The mortality among hospitalized patients with core temperatures lower than 30°C can vary from 20% to 85%, depending on the age of the patient, the associated underlying condition, and the severity of hypothermia. **METICULOUS SUPPORTIVE CARE AND THE USE OF**

SOUND RESUSCITATIVE TECHNIQUES ARE JUST AS IMPORTANT AS
THE REWARMING TECHNIQUE.

HYPERTHERMIA

FEVER

Fever in seriously ill patients usually occurs as a result of infection.
The increased temperature is in response to pyrogenic factors that
probably cause a resetting of the central temperature control. Pyrogens are released from leucocytes in response to many types of micro-organisms (bacteria, viruses, and fungi). Trauma and drugs can
also precipitate pyrogen release from leucocytes. Pyrogens are important mediators in cellular activation and antibody production.

EFFECTS OF FEVER

- increased metabolic rate (approximately 10% for each 1°C rise in
temperature)
- increases in oxygen consumption, pulse rate, and cardiac output
- increased protein breakdown
- improved bacteriocidal action
- improved wound healing

MANAGEMENT

Determine the cause of the fever. Exclude infection (see p. 177) and
malfunctioning of the temperature-measuring device; then think of
drug reactions (usually accompanied by an eosinophilia, macu-
lopapular rash, and abnormal liver function tests) and blood-compo-
nent incompatibilities. Fever can also occur as a non-specific reaction
accompanying acute myocardial infarction, pulmonary embolism, or
intracranial abnormalities (eg serious head injuries). In about one-
third of cases, there may not be an obvious explanation for the fever.

Fever can be beneficial for host defenses. If the fever results from
infection, there are good reasons for not lowering the temperature. As
a guideline, if the temperature is below 39°C in an adult or 38.5°C in
a child, it probably should not be specifically treated. If the patient

is intractably hypoxic, the fever may need to be reduced in order to reduce oxygen consumption (see p. 356).

Surface cooling

Ice packs, cooling blankets, and fans have been used to cool patients. However, as a result of peripheral vasoconstriction, secondary to surface cooling by those methods, a paradoxical increase in core temperature can occur. Evaporative techniques (eg fans and tepid sponging) are more efficient than convective techniques (eg ice packs and cooling blankets). Care must be taken that a fan not be directed at the patient's face, as corneal drying and ulceration can occur if the eyes of a semiconscious patient are partially open.

Antipyretic drugs

Paracetamol, non-steroidal anti-inflammatory drugs, and aspirin can all lower body temperature. The drug may have to be given rectally if oral absorption is not possible (eg Indocid, 100 mg per rectum).

HEATSTROKE

Heatstroke can occur as a result of increased heat production by the body or decreased heat loss or a combination of the two. It occurs particularly in certain groups and certain situations:

- the elderly
- athletes participating in endurance sports, particularly in warm temperatures
- people with underlying cardiovascular disease
- hot ambient temperature (eg young children confined in cars)
- infants with febrile illnesses who are wrapped too warmly
- as a result of drugs such as anticholinergics and alcohol

CLINICAL FEATURES

A spectrum of damage will occur as the temperature increases. Heat exhaustion represents failure of the body to maintain a normal core temperature. Heatstroke can then rapidly supervene, and it includes the following features, especially when the core temperature exceeds 42°C:

- tachycardia
- muscle cramps
- hypotension
- hypovolaemia
- weakness

- disorientation
- delirium
- severe vomiting and diarrhoea
- convulsions
- coma

- widespread cellular damage causing rhabdomyolysis, renal failure, hepatic failure, coagulopathy, and thrombocytopenia

THE SEVERITY OF TISSUE DAMAGE WILL BE DETERMINED BY THE DURATION AND DEGREE OF HYPERTHERMIA. RAPID COOLING IS ESSENTIAL.

MANAGEMENT

Heatstroke is a medical emergency. Treatment must be prompt.

AIRWAY AND BREATHING If the patient is unconscious or is having a seizure, or if there is doubt about the airway, intubation and, if necessary, ventilation should be performed.

OXYGEN Initially 100% oxygen should be delivered, and then the inspired oxygen should be adjusted according to the patient's oxygenation.

CIRCULATION Hypovolaemia and hypotension are common. Rapid resuscitation with fluid is required. Cardiac damage may have occurred, necessitating catecholamine infusion in order to support the circulation (see p. 521).

MONITOR CORE TEMPERATURE Use a high-reading thermometer.

CONTINUOUS ECG MONITORING

CONTINUOUS PULSE OXIMETRY

INVESTIGATIONS Conduct baseline measurements: arterial blood gases, electrolytes, renal and liver function tests, blood glucose, haemoglobin, platelet count, coagulation profile, and creatinine kinase.

Cooling

As the severity of tissue damage will be determined by the degree and duration of hyperthermia, rapid cooling is paramount. At the site of injury, this involves removing clothing, moving to a shaded area, wetting the skin, and actively fanning. The temperature must be rapidly dropped to less than 40°C. Core temperatures of more than 39°C may exacerbate the cellular damage.

CONVECTION Although measures such as immersion in cold water or packing the body in ice have been successfully employed, they can precipitate vasoconstriction and shivering, both of which will increase core temperature.

EVAPORATION Evaporation is a more efficient method for cooling. This involves repeated or continuous wetting of the whole body while simultaneously fanning with air. An atomized spray or water spray will make the process even more efficient. Alpha-adrenergic blocking drugs such as chlorpromazine can enhance peripheral dilatation and cooling. However, these drugs should not be given until the cardiovascular system is stable.

CONDUCTION Gastric or bladder lavage with cold fluid will reduce the core temperature.

EXTRACORPOREAL TECHNIQUES Techniques such as continuous haemofiltration (see p. 662) may be suitable for rapid cooling. The lines and filter can be surrounded by cool fluid. The patient may also be dialysed against cooled dialysate.

Other measures

• Monitor urine output.
• Give blood products, as necessary, to correct any coagulopathy.

• Urgent dialysis may be necessary to correct acid–base, potassium, or phosphate disturbances. Intravenous calcium and phosphate replacement can cause widespread precipitation in many tissues, especially muscle, and should be avoided acutely.

• Mannitol at 0.3 g/kg may prevent precipitation of myoglobin in renal tubules.

• Treat convulsions, shivering, and excessive muscle activity in order to limit further temperature increases.

• Dantrolene has been shown to be ineffective for treatment of heat-stroke.

MALIGNANT HYPERTHERMIA

Malignant hyperthermia (MH) is a condition that occurs in association with the use of anaesthesia in genetically susceptible patients. It is an inherited disorder of calcium transport and calcium binding by cell membranes, associated with hyperpyrexia and hypermetabolism.

CLINICAL FEATURES

Malignant hyperthermia typically occurs after induction of anaesthesia, especially with succinylcholine and volatile anaesthetic agents. These patients develop rigidity and hyperpyrexia. Poor relaxation and exaggerated fasciculation can occur after succinylcholine. Other features include tachycardia, fluctuations in blood pressure, arrhythmias, sweating, tachypnoea, cyanosis, skin mottling, and a steady rise in end-tidal CO_2.

Cardiac arrest, secondary to ventricular arrhythmia, can occur, and later complications can include coagulopathy, acute renal failure, rhabdomyolysis, pulmonary oedema, and cerebral oedema.

Non-anaesthetic-related reactions are much less common, but can be triggered by vigorous exercise, hot weather, muscle trauma, infection, shivering, and, perhaps, emotional stress.

Laboratory abnormalities

• marked metabolic acidosis
• respiratory acidosis
• hyperkalaemia

- hypermagnesaemia
- acute renal failure
- massive rise in creatinine phosphokinase (CPK)
- myoglobin in urine and serum
- coagulopathy and thrombocytopenia

Diagnosis

The clinical diagnosis must be made immediately because of the life-threatening nature of this condition. A definitive diagnosis requires eliciting a family history and muscle biopsy studies.

MANAGEMENT

1. An effective treatment protocol and appropriate drugs must be readily available at all sites where anaesthetics are used.

2. Cease the use of suspected anaesthetic agents. Commence narcotics if anaesthesia is still needed. Thiopentone may also be used. Terminate surgery as soon as possible.

3. Give 100% oxygen, and hyperventilate.

4. Change to a vapour-free anaesthetic machine or non-rebreathing circuit.

5. Institute cooling, as described previously (see p. 164). In summary, this may include

- immersion or ice packs
- spraying with water and fanning
- intragastric or intraperitoneal cooling
- an extracorporeal circuit for cooling (eg haemoperfusion circuit with cooled filter or cardiopulmonary bypass)

6. Dantrolene: Initially give $1 \text{ mg} \cdot \text{kg}^{-1} \cdot \text{min}^{-1}$, up to 10 mg/kg, measuring end points such as central temperature, heat rate, and muscle rigidity. Subsequent doses may be required every 15 minutes. A continuous infusion at 1–2 mg/kg, up to 4-hourly, should be continued until all evidence of MH has disappeared.

7. Monitoring

- ECG
- blood pressure

- urinary output
- central temperature
- frequent monitoring of the following:
  arterial blood gases
  electrolytes
  blood sugar
  renal function tests
  coagulation tests
  haematocrit

8. Sodium bicarbonate (1 mmol/kg) may be necessary.

9. Arrhythmias: Procainamide, propranolol, and verapamil have all been used successfully.

10. Avoid cardiac glycosides, calcium, quinidine, and catecholamines, as they can perpetuate MH.

FURTHER MANAGEMENT These patients must have the condition carefully explained to them so that they can avoid the use of the precipitating agents during any future anaesthesia. The families must also be screened and counselled.

NEUROLEPTIC MALIGNANT SYNDROME

Neuroleptic malignant syndrome (NMS) is an idiosyncratic reaction to certain drugs such as the phenothiazines and butyrophenones and is associated with a fever as well as neurological and autonomic dysfunctions. It is probably a central hypothalamic disorder in association with a peripheral muscular mechanism.

CLINICAL FEATURES

- Slow onset (24–72 hours) of increased muscle rigidity and akinesia, involuntary movements, and fluctuating tremor. Extrapyramidal symptoms are features of NMS, especially lead-pipe rigidity.
- Hyperpyrexia, usually more than 39°C.
- Variable levels of consciousness (normal to coma).
- Autonomic dysfunctions (eg tachycardia, tachypnoea, labile blood pressure, diaphoresis, and incontinence).
- Secondary effects such as aspiration and dehydration also occur.

• Differential diagnosis includes any febrile illness superimposed on a neuroleptic-induced dystonic reaction, neuroleptic-related heatstroke, MH, severe dystonic reactions, and acute lethal catatonia.

LABORATORY ABNORMALITIES

• Rhabdomyolysis is almost always present and is associated with an increased CPK concentration. Myoglobin is present in blood and urine.
• Acute renal failure occurs in about half of all cases.
• Leucocytosis is common.
• Abnormal liver function tests.

DRUGS IMPLICATED IN NMS

• phenothiazines
• thioxanthenes
• amantadine
• lithium
• butyrophenones
• tricyclic antidepressants

NMS can occur after first use of the causative drug or at any time during its administration, even years after it has been commenced.

MANAGEMENT

• Cease giving any likely offending drug, and transfer the patient to an ICU.
• Control the airway, breathing, and circulation as for heatstroke.
• Cooling should be instituted as for heatstroke, if necessary (see p. 164).
• Dantrolene sodium has been reported as being successful in NMS, probably because of the similarity between this syndrome and MH. It has been used at dosages of 1–10 mg $\cdot$ kg^{-1} $\cdot$ d^{-1}, either orally or intravenously, as a single dose or for several days.
• Bromocriptine (oral dosage 7.5–30 mg/d for several days) has also been used successfully. There are theoretical synergistic effects when

dantrolene and bromocriptine are used together, and no serious side effects have been reported.

Nifedipine has also been used in NMS.

OUTCOME The mortality has been found to be up to 20–30%.

FURTHER READING

Clarke, D. E., Kimelman, J., & Raffin, T. A. (1991). The evaluation of fever in the intensive care unit. *Chest* 100:213–20.

Curley, F. J., & Irwin, R. S. (1991). Disorders of temperature control. Part I: Hypothermia. In *Intensive Care Medicine,* 2nd ed., ed. J. M. Rippe, R. S. Irwin, J. J. Alpert, & M. P. Fink, pp. 658–73. Boston: Little, Brown.

Editor (1982). Management of heatstroke. *Lancet* 2:910–11.

Ellis, F. R., & Smith, G. (eds.) (1988). Symposium on malignant hyperthermia. *British Journal of Anaesthesiology* 60:251–354.

Gregory, J. S., Bergstein, J. M., Aprahamian, C., Wittmann, D. H., & Quebbeman, E. J. (1991). Comparison of three methods of rewarming from hypothermia: advantages of extracorporeal blood warming. *Journal of Trauma* 31:1247–52.

Ilsley, A. H., Rutten, A. J., & Runciman, W. B. (1985). An evaluation of body temperature measurement. *Anaesthesia and Intensive Care* 11:31–9.

Jolly, B. T., & Ghezzi, K. T. (1992). Accidental hypothermia. *Emergency Medical Clinics of North America* 10:311–27.

Richards, D., Richards, R., Schofield, P. J., Ross, V., & Sutton, J. R. (1979). Management of heat exhaustion in Sydney's The Sun City-to-Surf Fun Runners. *Medical Journal of Australia* 2:457–61.

Schrader, G. B. (1991). The neuroleptic malignant syndrome. *Medical Journal of Australia* 154:301–2.

Tek, D., & Olshaker, J. J. (1992). Heat illness. *Emergency Medical Clinics of North America* 10:299–310.

Yaqub, B. A., Al-Harthi, S. S., Al-Orciney, I. O., Laajam, M. A., & Obeid, M. T. (1986). Heat stroke at the Mekkah pilgrimage: clinical characteristics and course of 30 patients. *Quarterly Journal of Medicine* 59:523–30.

12

TRANSPORT OF THE SERIOUSLY ILL

- Experienced personnel must transport patients.
- Equipment should be simple and robust.
- The level of monitoring during transport must be at least as comprehensive as in the intensive care unit (ICU).

It is crucial to maintain the same high standards of intensive care for seriously ill patients during transport as during their stay in the ICU. This necessitates the following:

1. A high standard of medical and nursing care must be maintained during the transport. The staff not only must be skilled in caring for seriously ill patients but also must have had specific experience in transporting these patients.

2. Equipment and monitoring must be appropriate. The level of monitoring must be at least as comprehensive during transport as when the patient is in the ICU. In determining the equipment and drug supply, one not only must take into account the immediate support for the patient but also must be prepared for the unexpected, such as blocked endotracheal tubes (ETTs), ventilator failure, increased need for sedation, and cardiorespiratory deterioration.

IT IS IN THE INTEREST OF EVERY INTENSIVIST TO ENSURE THE MOST EFFICIENT AND RAPID TRANSFER OF PATIENTS TO AND FROM OTHER SITES OR INSTITUTIONS. SUBOPTIMAL TREATMENT AND DETERIORATION DURING TRANSFER CAN ADVERSELY AFFECT THE PATIENT'S ULTIMATE OUTCOME.

Equally, it is crucial to maintain high standards during transport within the hospital. It is no longer good enough to send the least experienced and most junior members of staff on these journeys. Transport of the seriously ill requires experienced staff.

RETRIEVAL

Primary retrieval

Primary retrieval involves transportation from the site of an incident to a site of definitive medical treatment. It often includes rescue or extraction from difficult terrain or from damaged vehicles. Primary retrieval usually is performed by ambulance personnel or a paramedical service. Depending on the level of sophistication of that service, medical personnel may also be involved.

Secondary retrieval

Secondary retrieval involves transport of a patient from a primary centre to a secondary or referral centre. With increasing rationalization and centralization of expensive resources in the ICU, secondary retrieval is becoming more common.

RETRIEVAL SYSTEM

A retrieval network must be well organized and must have adequate facilities for data collection and peer review in order to monitor the efficiency of the system.

Communications

A comprehensive and integrated communication network is essential. The referring and receiving hospitals need to communicate with each other and with the retrieval team and transport facility. Often there is a co-ordination centre to facilitate communication.

Retrieval teams

It is essential that the retrieval team include medical staff who not only can deliver intensive care medicine equal to the standard of the receiving centre but also are familiar with the problems associated with various modes of retrieval (eg aviation medicine). The team should also include a nurse or assistant with experience in intensive care medicine and retrieval.

Education, data collection, and peer review

There is no point in devoting all effort and resources solely to the medical retrieval system and the receiving centre. The basic principles of initial resuscitation must be implemented at the site of first contact with the patient. This involves a comprehensive education system, data-collection facilities, and peer review in order to locate and correct weak points in the system.

Stabilization

A patient must be resuscitated before transport is undertaken. If, for example, in a patient with multitrauma, the abdomen is expanding and it is difficult to maintain the arterial blood pressure with intravenous fluid, an immediate laparotomy is needed BEFORE transport. If the patient is unconscious and there is doubt about the airway, intubation should be carried out BEFORE transport. Pneumothoraces must be drained, and other life-threatening conditions corrected. Procedures such as these are best attended to before transport. Detection and treatment of such conditions are difficult in the back of an ambulance or during air transport. Once such problems are under control, the attending team can then devote attention to monitoring and maintaining cardiorespiratory stability during transport.

Before transport, the medical team must attend to the following matters:

AIRWAY   Intubate if there is any doubt.

VENTILATION   Institute artificial ventilatory support with an appropriate F_{IO_2}, especially in the presence of head or chest injuries.

CIRCULATION   Ensure adequate fluid resuscitation with blood if necessary. Take adequate reserves of further blood or fluid for use during transport. Arrhythmias should be diagnosed and treated (see p. 531), and the circulation supported with inotropes if necessary (see p. 520).

HISTORY   The history of the event is important, as it may point to potential injuries or other associated injuries (eg high-speed motor-vehicle crash and widened mediastinum).

EXAMINATION The patient must be thoroughly examined from head to foot, noting vital signs (eg arterial blood pressure, respiratory rate, pulse rate, temperature, urine output, peripheral perfusion), assessing stability, and looking for other injuries.

VENOUS ACCESS Short, wide-base cannulae are more appropriate than central lines for use during transport. Measurement of central venous pressure is not necessary during initial resuscitation and transport. If inotropes or other drugs such as concentrated potassium are needed, then a long line from the cubital fossa, rather than a central line placed from the upper chest or neck, should be inserted in order to avoid the possible complication of pneumothorax, especially during flight.

MECHANICS OF FLUID INFUSION Under normal circumstances, a hydrostatic head of more than 75 cm H_2O is sufficient for adequate fluid flow into a peripheral vein. A motorized syringe pump with optional battery pack is the most appropriate method for delivering concentrated drugs such as inotropes, vasodilators, and drugs for sedation and pain relief.

PLEURAL DRAINS A chest x-ray to confirm placement of drain lines must be performed before transport. A flutter valve, such as the Heimlich design, is usually used, rather than an underwater drainage system. Although the Heimlich valve is more convenient and overcomes the problem of having to place the underwater drain below the patient during transport, the lips of the flutter valve can become blocked if it is contaminated by blood or other fluid.

Cardiorespiratory monitoring

Monitoring can be difficult during transport. Outside noise, vibration, and movement can make even simple clinical observations very difficult (eg chest rising with respiration and palpable pulse). Monitoring equipment can be similarly affected. However, there are now robust, portable, battery-operated monitors that work reliably under these conditions. The minimum equipment list should include capabilities for the following:

• continuous ECG monitoring
• invasive/non-invasive determination of blood pressure, adult and paediatric cuffs

- pulse oximetry, with finger and multisite sensors
- end-tidal CO_2 determination, especially for ventilated head-injury patients
- disconnect alarm
- airway-pressure monitoring
- oxygen-failure alarm

Other equipment

Intubating equipment (laryngoscopes, adult and paediatric, Guedel airways, Magill forceps)
Endotracheal tubes (neonatal to adult sizes)
Emergency percutaneous airway set
Chest drains (Heimlich valves, paediatric to adult sizes)
Portable suction equipment and catheters
Manual ventilating system
Oxygen masks
Portable oxygen
Disposable humidifiers
Defibrillator and spare batteries
Syringe pumps, battery-powered
Intravenous fluids, cannulae, giving sets
Syringes, needles, non-return valves
Nasogastric tubes and bags
Urinary catheters and bags

Drugs

The following are the minimum ranges of drugs needed for transport of the seriously ill. The numbers of the various ampoules of the following drugs carried will depend on the length of the journey and the type of patient.

adrenaline	1 : 10,000	10 ml × 5
adrenaline	1 : 1,000	1 ml × 5
atropine	1.2 mg	1 ml
calcium	1 g	10 ml
frusemide	20 mg	2 ml

lignocaine	100 mg	5 ml
dopamine	200 mg	5 ml
isoprenaline	1.0 mg	1 ml
magnesium sulphate	20 mmol	5 ml
propranolol	1 mg	1 ml × 5
verapamil	20 mg	2 ml
bretylium	100 mg	2 ml × 7
NaCl (flushing)	10 ml	
potassium chloride	10 mmol	10 ml
digoxin	1.0 mg	2 ml
thiopentone	500 mg	
water	20 ml	
salbutamol	500 μg	1 ml
dextrose	50%	50 ml
NaHCO$_3$	8.4%	50 ml
neostigmine	2.5 mg	1 ml
morphine	10 mg	1 ml
naloxone	4 mg	10 ml
midazolam	5 mg	1 ml
diazepam	10 mg	2 ml
pancuronium	4 mg	2 ml × 2
vecuronium	4 mg powder × 2	
ketamine	10 g	10 ml
suxamethonium	100 mg	2 ml × 2
(replace weekly in summer and biweekly in cooler weather)		

Mode of transport

The decision to use road transport, fixed-wing aircraft, helicopters, or even water transport depends on many factors. The patient's condition and the urgency for definitive treatment or investigation are the most important factors. However, other factors include the distance between the two points, local geography, weather and visibility, adequacy of roads, facilities for air transport, and comparative costs.

INTRAHOSPITAL TRANSPORT

The principles of transport, whether travelling thousands of kilometres between hospitals or taking a patient from the ICU to the computed tomography (CT) unit, are the same. The patient must be stabilized before transport, and the clinician accompanying the patient must be experienced in the principles of intensive care medicine as well as transport. The list of drugs and equipment to be carried during intrahospital transport is almost the same as for retrieval. Some items, such as nasogastric tubes and urinary catheters, are, of course, unnecessary for intrahospital transport, but appropriate equipment and drugs must accompany the patient in case of an emergency or equipment failure. A standard form of monitoring and a dedicated mobile bed will make intrahospital transport a simple and safe routine, rather than a hazardous venture.

FURTHER READING

Dawson, A. D. G., & Babington, P. C. B. (1987). An intensive care trolley – an economical and versatile alternative to the mobile intensive care unit. *Anaesthesia and Intensive Care* 15:229–33.

Edlin, S. (1989). Physiological changes during transport of the critically ill. *Intensive Care World* 6:131–4.

Ehrenworth, J., Sorbo, S., & Hackel, A. (1986). Transport of critically ill adults. *Critical Care Medicine* 14:543–7.

Gilligan, J. E. (1985). Stabilization, transport, and the critically ill. *Clinics in Anaesthesiology* 3:789–810.

Hageman, J. R., & Fetcho, S. (1992). Transport of the critically ill. *Critical Care Clinics* July:465–661.

Guidelines Committee of the American College of Critical Care Medicine, Society of Critical Care Medicine, and American Association of Critical Care Nurses Transfer Guidelines Task Force. (1993). Guidelines for the transfer of critically ill patients. *Critical Care Medicine* 21:931–7.

Nielson, M. S., & Bacon, R. J. (1989). The transport of critically ill patients within hospital. *Intensive Care World* 6:126–30.

13

INFECTION

- Endogenous sources of nosocomial infections are far more common than exogenous sources.
- The use of antibiotics is only one part of the management of sepsis. The source of the sepsis must be relentlessly sought and treated.
- Avoid broad-spectrum antibiotics and prolonged antimicrobial treatment where possible.

SOURCE OF INFECTION

PRIMARY INFECTIONS

Infections acquired outside the hospital are considered to be primary or community-acquired infections. Such infections include pneumonia, tetanus, acute epiglottitis, urinary-tract infection (UTI), and meningoencephalitis (see p. 610). These usually are well-defined entities, with accepted norms for their diagnoses and treatment.

NOSOCOMIAL INFECTIONS

Nosocomial infections are hospital-acquired infections that represent a major problem, especially in the intensive care unit (ICU). Our current knowledge about the diagnosis and treatment of these disorders is not as extensive as our knowledge of primary infections.

Exogenous infections

Exogenous infections originate in the hospital environment. Patients can acquire such infections either by an airborne route or by direct contact. Apart from sporadic epidemics and problems such as methicillin-resistant *Staphylococcus aureas* (MRSA), exogenous spread is no longer believed to be a major route of infection in intensive care.

ESSENTIAL PRECAUTIONS HAND-WASHING BETWEEN DEALING WITH ANY TWO PATIENTS OR PROCEDURES IS ESSENTIAL. Doctors usually are the worst offenders in regard to failure to wash hands. Strict aseptic conditions for all invasive procedures are also essential.

EQUIVOCAL PRECAUTIONS
- plastic aprons
- isolation rooms
- laminar-flow ventilation
- individual stethoscope for each patient

VERY DOUBTFUL PRECAUTIONS
- shoe covers, sticky or disinfectant mats
- surface disinfectant on floors
- changing clothes before entering the ICU
- routine examinations of environmental cultures
- routine changing of infusion systems every 24 hours
- in-line bacterial filters
- nose and throat cultures from staff, except during epidemics
- routine sterilization of internal ventilatory machinery between patients
- banning of flowers in the ward
- disinfection of sinks and drains

Endogenous infections

These are the most important kinds of nosocomial infections in the ICU, and they account for most episodes of septicaemia. They pose one of the most common and most serious problems among the critically ill.

The normal microbial flora of the human body includes organisms found in the alimentary tract, upper respiratory tract, female genital tract, and skin. The three stages of endogenous infection in the ICU are colonization of normally sterile areas, followed by colonization of

TABLE 13.1 COMMON ORGANISMS CAUSING NOSOCOMIAL
INFECTIONS

Staphylococci
Staphylococcus aureus
MRSA
Coagulase-negative *Staphylococcus* spp.
Streptococcus pyogenes
Enterococcus spp.
Coliforms
Escherichia coli
Klebsiella spp.
Proteus spp.
Enterobacter spp.
Serratia spp.
Acinetobacter spp.
Pseudomonas spp.
Anaerobes
Fungi

major organ systems such as the respiratory tract and bladder, and, finally, overt infection.

A patient's own organisms usually cause nosocomial infections. For example, coliforms colonize the gastro-intestinal tract (GIT), exacerbated by alkalinization of the stomach (Table 13.1).

ANTIBIOTICS, ESPECIALLY BROAD-SPECTRUM ANTIBIOTICS, CHANGE THE MICROBIAL ENVIRONMENT BY SELECTIVELY KILLING SOME ORGANISMS. Thus the original flora is to some extent replaced by a new range of otherwise harmless organisms, such as fungi and *Pseudomonas* species, that often are resistant to antimicrobials. These new micro-organisms are equally as dangerous to a seriously ill patient as the organisms for which the antibiotics were originally prescribed, and often they are markers of unwise use of antibiotics. The host may have been immunocompromised as a result of invasive procedures, malnutrition, and immunosuppressive drugs (Table 13.2), rendering such a patient more susceptible to infection from otherwise benign organisms. The microbiological ecology of the patient should

TABLE 13.2 NOSOCOMIAL INFECTION SITES

Site	Approximate incidence (%)
Urinary tract	30
Generalized septicaemia	20
Pneumonia	20
Skin and subcutaneous tissue	10
Upper respiratory tract (including sinusitis)	10
Wound infection	10

be carefully considered, and empirical treatment with broad-spectrum antibiotics should be avoided wherever possible. Although most clinicians and microbiologists will agree with these principles, in practice they sometimes go astray.

Guidelines for controlling nosocomial infections

• Determine the incidences and types of nosocomial infections in your ICU.

• Rigorously enforce hand-washing after treatment of each patient.

• Limit the number of invasive procedures and the insertion times for intravascular devices.

• Resuscitate early and aggressively. Examine cultures of sputum, urine, and blood routinely, as well as those for wounds, cerebrospinal fluid (CSF), peritoneal fluid, and other sites when necessary.

• Use sucralfate (see p. 32), wherever possible, to prevent stress ulceration, rather than agents that can cause gastric alkalinization and microbial overgrowth (Figure 13.1).

• Make every effort to culture organisms before antibiotics are given.

• Use narrow-spectrum antibiotics where possible.

• If antibiotics are having no obvious effect within 3–5 days, STOP and RECULTURE. Distinguish among normal flora, harmless colonization (particularly *Pseudomonas* species and fungi), and clinically significant infections.

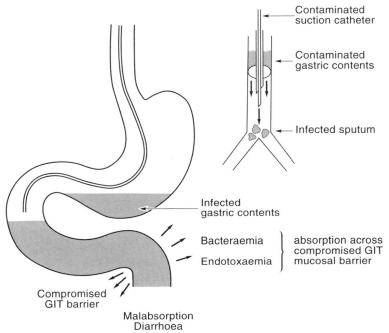

FIGURE 13.1 Potential complications of bacterial overgrowth in the stomach.

• The use of antibiotics will change the microbial ecology and encourage the development of resistance. USE THEM SPARINGLY, FOR SHORT, SHARP BURSTS.

• Review the findings from cultures, and rationalize antibiotic treatment daily.

• Everyone pays lip service to good microbiological practice and wise use of antibiotics. It is crucial to fully incorporate these principles into your own clinical practice.

• Limit peri-operative prophylactic antibiotic regimens to less than 24 hours. Single-dose prophylaxis is appropriate in most cases.

• Avoid routine use of systemic antibiotics for prevention of post-operative pneumonia.

• Improve the immune status of the patient, if possible (eg nutrition, prevention of renal failure, rapid resuscitation, avoidance of drugs that could compromise immune function, such as barbiturates, anaesthetic agents, and corticosteroids).

• Work closely with your microbiology department, and encourage daily ward rounds with a specialist in infectious diseases if possible.

FUTURE PROSPECTS Active and passive immune techniques are currently undergoing evaluation and may be available to decrease nosocomial infections in the near future (see p. 194).

A combined ecological and antibiotic approach is also undergoing investigation – selective decontamination of the digestive tract (SDD). This technique aims to eliminate coliform bacteria and fungi in the GIT by using non-absorbable antibiotics. At the same time, other organisms, particularly the normal gut anaerobes, are allowed to overgrow and help inhibit the growth of more virulent micro-organisms. Clear benefits have not been demonstrated as yet.

SEPTICAEMIA

The term 'septic shock' strikes fear in the heart of even the bravest intensivist. The mortality from septic shock remains around 50%. The terms 'septic shock', 'septic syndrome', 'sepsis', and 'septicaemia' are often used interchangeably. The terms usually refer to evidence of infection accompanied by signs of systemic involvement and altered organ perfusion such as an altered level of consciousness, hypoxia, and oliguria. Positive findings from blood cultures are not necessarily the rule. In fact, sepsis can occur in association with bacteraemia, viraemia, fungaemia, or endotoxaemia, or, indeed, without evidence of any microbes at all. It remains one of the most common and most difficult disorders to treat in intensive care. Cases of sepsis or septicaemia represent inflammatory responses to a variety of insults, including non-infectious insults such as pancreatitis, ischaemia, multitrauma, tissue injury, haemorrhagic shock, and immune-mediated organ injury. It has been suggested that because the host responses are the same, regardless of whether the cause is infective or non-infective, the term should be changed to 'systemic inflammatory response syndrome' (SIRS) (Figure 13.2). The terms 'sepsis' and 'septicaemia' will be used synonymously in this chapter. There are, however, efforts being made to agree on stricter terminology (Table 13.3).

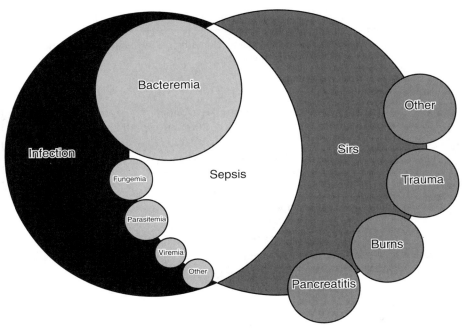

FIGURE 13.2 The interrelationships among systemic inflammatory response syndrome (SIRS), sepsis, and infection. (From Bone, 1992. Reprinted by permission of the ACCP/SCCM Consensus Conference.)

Septicaemia is a disorder of cellular function, but its exact pathophysiology is uncertain. Most of the body's cells probably are affected, but some cells, such as the vascular endothelial cells, appear to be more strongly affected than others.

CLINICAL FEATURES OF SEPTICAEMIA

Because sepsis is primarily a disease involving many types of cells, it usually presents as multiorgan failure (MOF) (see Chapter 9). The initial event in sepsis is peripheral vasodilatation, with a compensatory increase in cardiac output. Other cardiovascular changes will occur before hypotension. These include increases in cardiac output, increases in pulmonary vascular resistance, decreases in systemic vascular resistance, and disturbances in oxygen delivery (Do_2) and oxygen consumption ($\dot{V}o_2$) (see p. 376). These changes continue

TABLE 13.3 SOME SUGGESTED DEFINITIONS RELATING TO SEPSIS

Although there are no universally agreed definitions for clinical syndromes related to sepsis, here are some guidelines:

Bacteraemia: positive blood culture

Sepsis: clinical evidence of infection [eg tachypnoea (respiratory rate > 20 breaths per minute), tachycardia (HR > 90/min), hyperthermia (>39°C), or hypothermia (<35.5°C)]

Sepsis syndrome: sepsis, with evidence of organ dysfunction (eg altered level of consciousness, hypoxia, renal failure, jaundice)

Septic shock: sepsis syndrome with hypotension

Septicaemia: used interchangeably with 'sepsis', 'sepsis syndrome', and 'septic shock'

Refractory septic shock: septic shock unresponsive to fluids and inotropes

Systemic inflammatory response syndrome (SIRS): two or more of the following:
- Temperature > 38.0°C, or temperature < 36°C
- Heart rate > 90 beats per minute
- Respiratory rate > 20 per minute or $Paco_2$ < 32 mm Hg (4.5 kPa)
- White-cell count > 12×10^9 per litre, or more than 10% immature forms

throughout the septic episode (Table 13.4). Low cardiac output in sepsis is rare, even in the latter stages. CONSISTENT CLINICAL SIGNS OF SEPSIS ARE A BOUNDING PRECORDIUM AND A PULSATING NECK, OFTEN VISIBLE FROM THE END OF THE BED.

Patients with sepsis develop abnormalities of cardiac function, even in the early hyperdynamic phase and in the presence of high cardiac output. Manifestations of depressed myocardial function include ventricular dilatation, diminished left and right ejection fractions, and altered diastolic pressure–volume relationships. The mechanism of depressed myocardial function has not yet been fully elucidated, but many of the inflammatory mediators of sepsis may be involved.

Processes other than peripheral vasodilatation that occur in the peripheral circulation include redistribution of blood flow, intravascular pooling, increased microvascular permeability, and microembolization (Table 13.5). Despite elevations in cardiac output and Do_2,

TABLE 13.4   FEATURES OF SEPTICAEMIA

Clinical
Decreased level of consciousness or confusion
Fever or hypothermia
Hypotension
Tachycardia and bounding precordium
Tachypnoea
Oliguria
Jaundice
Ileus
Stress ulceration
Laboratory and monitoring
Manifestations of organ failure (see p. 185):
   Respiratory (eg hypoxia)
   Kidney (eg increased urea and creatinine)
   Cardiac (eg supraventricular tachycardia)
   Liver (eg increased bilirubin)
   Metabolic (eg hyperglycaemia)
   Haematological (eg 'toxic' changes in white cells)

tissues cannot extract adequate oxygen. Cells produce lactate, and other signs of tissue dysfunction begin to appear.

The exact mechanism for ineffective peripheral-tissue metabolism is unknown. The proposed mechanisms have included anatomic shunting, a left shift of the oxygen dissociation curve, and a primary inability of cells to utilize oxygen. Currently, the major dysfunction is thought to be at the microcirculatory level – vasodilatation, microembolization, and endothelial-cell injury. Tissue oedema resulting from cellular injury and inappropriate fluid administration can further impair oxygen diffusion by increasing the diffusion distances and compressing the capillaries. A reduced capacity for peripheral extraction of oxygen is the likely basis for the postulated abnormal dependence of oxygen consumption on the supply. The exact relationship between D_{O_2} and $\dot{V}_{O_2}$ in the presence of sepsis has not yet been determined (see p. 376).

TABLE 13.5 HAEMODYNAMIC RESPONSES TO SEPSIS

Cardiac function
↓ Blood pressure
↑ Cardiac index, ↓ SVR, ↓ LV ejection fraction
↓ Left ventricular end-diastolic volume
↓ ↓ Preload
  Loss of vasomotor tone, splanchnic pooling
    ↑ Microvascular permeability, ↓ circulating blood volume
↓ Contractility
  Myocardial depressant factor
  Often masked by ↓ LV afterload
↓ Coronary blood flow
Regional distribution of blood flow
Loss of vasomotor tone
Vasodilation
Redistribution of blood flow (balance between local tissue mechanisms and
  central mechanisms is disturbed, and local autoregulation malfunctions)
Microcirculation
Vasodilation
Microemboli
Endothelial-cell injury
Tissue O_2 extraction is decreased
Diffusion distance for oxygen is increased
Capillary recruitment

Large numbers of mediators have been suggested as being activated by the presence of micro-organisms. These mediators may be responsible for much of the pathophysiology of sepsis (see p. 186). These include cytokines, eicosanoids, complement, cyclo-oxygenase and lipo-oxygenase products, and effector substances from granulocytes and platelets (Figure 13.3). This area of research is one of the most active in intensive care. However, the clinical implications are, as yet, unclear. For more details, see the publications cited at the end of this chapter.

One of the most promising areas of research involves the free radical nitric oxide (NO). This was formerly called endothelium-derived

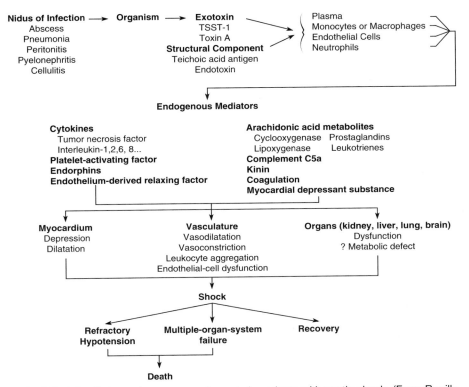

FIGURE 13.3 Pathogenic sequence of events in patients with septic shock. (From Parrillo, 1993, with permission.)

relaxant factor (EDRF). It is produced from arginine and mediates vascular relaxation via cyclic guanosine monophosphate (cGMP). It is suggested that cytokines can induce the enzyme NO synthase (NOS), leading to excess production of NO and hence profound hypotension unresponsive to catecholamines. Trials are under way with NOS inhibitors in an attempt to reverse the vasodilation of sepsis.

OTHER FEATURES

TEMPERATURE DISTURBANCES Fever is common, but it is not an inevitable sign of sepsis. Central temperature should be measured 4-hourly and plotted graphically, so that a swinging fever can be detected – this is a valuable guide to an occult source of sepsis. Fever can also be associated with drugs (including antibiotics), malignancy, or non-infective inflammatory processes (see Chapter 11). However, hypothermia occurs in up to 10% of patients with sepsis and is associated with a worse prognosis.

NAUSEA, VOMITING, DIARRHOEA

CLOUDING OF THE LEVEL OF CONSCIOUSNESS Consciousness is almost always depressed in patients with sepsis. Even before the arterial blood pressure falls, the cerebral blood flow will decrease. The blood–brain barrier is damaged, and the cerebral metabolic rate increases. These changes are reversible.

HYPERVENTILATION AND HYPOXIA The development of adult respiratory distress syndrome (ARDS) is often a marker of infection. It is a common accompaniment of septic shock and MOF (see Chapter 9). Tachypnoea and respiratory alkalosis are among the first signs of systemic sepsis.

SUPRAVENTRICULAR ARRHYTHMIAS Atrial fibrillation (AF) and supraventricular tachycardia (SVT) occur in at least 40% of all patients with septic episodes (see p. 534).

JAUNDICE Jaundice occurs frequently during septic episodes and is related to hepatocellular dysfunction. It is of uncertain aetiology and is reversible, resolving as the sepsis resolves (see p. 674). Biliary obstruction must be considered in the differential diagnosis if the underlying cause of sepsis is not obvious.

GASTRO-INTESTINAL BLEEDING Two of the earliest signs of sepsis are a low gastric pH and mucosal bleeding. Prophylactic treatment should be instituted (see p. 31), and nasogastric (NG) feeding should be commenced whenever possible (see p. 87).

METABOLIC DISTURBANCES

Glucose intolerance Glucose intolerance is very common during sepsis, and insulin usually is not necessary unless the serum glucose is more than 10 mmol/L, when neutrophil function can be compromised. Hyperglycaemia is primarily caused by gluconeogenesis, although there is also a relative insulin resistance.

Catabolism Proteolysis or 'auto-cannibalism' and wasting are universal features of sepsis and cannot be greatly modified by parenteral nutrition (see Chapter 5).

Fat Increasing lipolysis and increasing concentrations of free fatty acids are initial features, followed by decreased triglyceride clearance.

COAGULATION DISORDERS

Thrombocytopenia Thrombocytopenia is common and is due to marrow suppression and increased peripheral consumption. Though often severe ($<30,000/mm^3$), it is reversible, usually is not clinically significant, and does not require transfusion.

Coagulopathy Coagulopathy is very common, but rarely severe, except in specific types of septicaemia such as meningococcal or pneumococcal infection. Fibrin levels are often increased, partial thromboplastin time is increased, and fibrin degradation products (FDPs) or d-dimer levels are equivocal. The associated disseminated intravascular coagulopathy is usually mild, rarely requires active management, and resolves when the sepsis is controlled.

RENAL INSUFFICIENCY

Renal failure is a frequent and dreaded accompaniment of sepsis. The pathophysiology is uncertain. It often presents as oliguria and uraemia, but it can also be non-oliguric (see Chapter 27).

DIAGNOSIS

The diagnosis of sepsis is made on the basis of a cluster of the foregoing features, especially in combination with a defect in the host's defence mechanisms such as occurs in the presence of acute renal failure and granulocytopenia. Immune depression is also a feature of the critically ill or nutritionally depleted patients. The presentation of sepsis is quite variable, with various features being more prominent in various cases. Entities such as 'cold' (vasoconstricted) or 'warm' (vasodilated) sepsis are host-mediated, not organism-mediated. THE DIAGNOSIS OF SEPTICAEMIA IS MADE CLINICALLY. Investigations support the diagnosis.

BLOOD CULTURES Multiple blood cultures should be taken percutaneously. Sterilization of the skin with povidone iodine and alcohol
should be performed prior to taking the specimen, in order to minimize the chances of skin organisms contaminating the culture
medium. Coagulase-negative staphylococci are the commonest skin
contaminants, but their repeated isolation in the culture medium
could implicate these organisms in sepsis, especially if associated with
intravascular devices.

The findings from blood cultures are positive in less than 30% of
patients with septicaemia, either because of concurrent antibiotic
treatment or because the host response is triggered by non-microbial
factors.

WHITE CELLS The whole white-cell count is often elevated in patients
with sepsis, but it can also be reduced. Leucopenia indicates a poor
prognosis. A consistent finding in the presence of sepsis is 'toxic'
changes in the white cells – toxic granulation, vacuolation, Döhle bodies, a disintegrated or 'moth-eaten' appearance of neutrophils.

OTHER INVESTIGATIONS

Identification of a septic source is paramount. Further investigations
are performed in order to identify the septic site.

CHEST X-RAY Pneumonia or lung abscess can be a primary source
of infection. ARDS is a non-specific accompaniment of sepsis from any
site.

RELEVANT CULTURES Take all relevant-culture material (eg sputum,
urine, CSF, wound, dialysate). Specialized techniques may be necessary to isolate lung organisms (see p. 416).

INVASIVE CATHETERS Take a culture from the tip or intradermal section (see p. 199).

IMAGING: ULTRASOUND OR CT SCAN Imaging is especially important if an abdominal source of infection is suspected.

NUCLEAR MEDICINE Leucocyte or gallium scans are non-specific
markers of an inflammatory response.

SINUSITIS Take a lateral skull x-ray or CT scan to exclude sinusitis associated with the NG tube or nasotracheal tube (NTT).

CHEST A CT scan of the chest will sometimes demonstrate an abscess or consolidation not seen on chest x-ray.

SEROLOGY Serology usually involves testing for a rise in antibody titre. The difference between acute-phase and convalescent-phase serology findings usually has to be more than fourfold. An elevated concentration of IgM antibody (an acute-phase specimen) may also be diagnostic. It is important that acute-phase and convalescent-phase sera be titrated together in order to minimize laboratory error. Serology may be important when pneumonia, meningoencephalitis, and myocarditis are thought to be involved in the septic syndrome. Unfortunately, serology is useful only retrospectively.

DIAGNOSTIC SURGERY

EARLY, AGGRESSIVE SURGERY IS OFTEN NECESSARY FOR DIAGNOSIS AND TREATMENT, ESPECIALLY IN THE PRESENCE OF INTRA-ABDOMINAL SEPSIS (see p. 217).

ROUTINE MONITORING

The following are suggested guidelines for monitoring patients with septicaemia:

- Vital signs: blood pressure, pulse rate, respiratory rate, and temperature
- Invasive monitoring [eg central venous pressure (CVP), pulmonary artery wedge pressure (PAWP)]
- Continuous ECG and pulse oximetry
- Urine output, hourly
- Arterial blood gases and pH, twice daily
- Blood sugar, 4-hourly
- Chest x-ray, daily
- ECG, daily
- Platelet count, prothrombin time, fibrinogen, FDPs or d-dimers, daily

- Renal function tests, daily
- Liver function tests, daily

PREVENTIVE MANAGEMENT

- Rapid and efficient resuscitation.
- Aseptic techniques for all procedures.
- Hand-washing between patients.
- Nystatin mouth care, as well as via the NG tube, is useful in preventing fungal colonization.
- Prophylactic antibiotics should be used judiciously.
- Alkalinization of the gastric contents will predispose to bacterial overgrowth and infection. Antacids and H_2-receptor antagonists probably should be avoided, and sucralfate should be used for stress-ulcer prophylaxis (see p. 32).
- Avoid drugs that can depress the immune system (eg certain intravenous anaesthetic induction agents, corticosteroids).
- Support the immune system (eg maintain nutrition).
- Granulocyte infusion in severe neutropenia has proved to be disappointing.
- Passive immunity: Infusions of fresh frozen plasma containing fibronectin and opsonins may improve immunity.
- Active immunization: Recently described antibodies to the lipopolysaccharide walls of bacteria may also be of value in the future.
- Selective bowel decontamination: Like many other conceptually appealing ideas for the treatment of sepsis, this has not yet been shown to reduce mortality (see p. 182).

DEFINITIVE MANAGEMENT (Table 13.6)

Underlying cause

IDENTIFY AND REMOVE THE UNDERLYING CAUSE DRAINAGE OR REMOVAL OF THE SOURCE OF SEPSIS IS CURRENTLY THE MOST IMPORTANT ASPECT OF TREATMENT IN SEPTICAEMIA. No stone can be left unturned in the search for the septic source, even if that means multiple laparotomies or drainage procedures. Necrotic tissue as well as infective tissue must be widely excised.

TABLE 13.6 MANAGEMENT OF SEPTICAEMIA

Preventive
Rapid and efficient resuscitation
Hand-washing between patients
Aseptic techniques
Strict and firmly enforced antibiotic policies
Avoid gastric alkalinization for stress-ulcer prophylaxis
Avoid immunosuppressive drugs, and support immune system

Definitive
DRAINAGE OR REMOVAL OF THE SOURCE OF SEPSIS
Antimicrobials

Supportive
FLUID – OFTEN NEEDED IN LARGE AMOUNTS TO MAINTAIN ADEQUATE CIRCULATING VOLUME
Maintain haemoglobin > 10 g/dl
Maintain Pa_{O_2} to at least 60 mm Hg (8.0 kPa)
  High-flow mask
  CPAP
  Artificial ventilation
Provide catecholamine support once intravascular volume is corrected.
• Adrenaline/noradrenaline ± low-dosage dopamine is a common first-line choice for hypotension
OR
• Dobutamine ± low-dosage dopamine for low-output states
Digoxin and/or verapamil for supraventricular tachyarrhythmias
Prevention of stress ulceration
Nutritional support
Early dialysis if there is renal insufficiency

Antimicrobials (see p. 204)

Antibiotics are discussed in more detail later in this chapter. Although antibiotics have a undisputed role in certain primary or commonly acquired infections, their role in nosocomial infections is less clear. Any antibiotic will have some influence on the flora found in patients, in the hospital, and in the community at large. They lead to the selection of resistant organisms, which in turn demand selective agents with an even broader spectrum. However, coverage with wide-spectrum antibiotics has traditionally been commenced in a blind fashion, after blood and other cultures have been taken. They have proved to be disappointing in the ICU, unless definite bacteria have been isolated. Even then they are valueless unless the source of infection is attended to. If no specific bacteria are found, broad-spectrum antibiotics are worth a trial for a definite and limited period. If there is no response, they should be stopped, and further attempts should be made to isolate the organism. Increasingly the concept of 'non-bacterial septicaemia' is being accepted. In these cases we must question the validity of continuing blind antibiotic treatment.

Corticosteroids

Because of the increasing doubt about the efficacy of steroids in patients with septicaemia, and because of their known complications, their use should be confined to patients with proven adrenal insufficiency and perhaps bacterial meningitis (see p. 765).

Continuous haemofiltration/haemodialysis

These techniques have been demonstrated to improve some aspects of organ function and survival in animal trials. Studies demonstrating efficacy in adults are awaited.

Other drugs

Despite some initial promising trials with drugs such as naloxone and thyroid-releasing hormone, they have little proven benefit in septicaemia.

Several monoclonal antibodies directed against bacterial lipopolysaccharide or endotoxin are currently being developed. So far, two antibodies have been tested: a murine IgM monoclonal antibody raised in mice (E5), and a human IgM monoclonal antibody (HA-1A). Thus far, the evidence for the clinical effectiveness of these antibodies is only suggestive, not conclusive. These drugs are extremely expensive. Other antibodies have been developed against other mediators, such as tumour necrosis factor (TNF). In view of the complexity of sepsis and the fact that a single key mediator has not, as yet, been developed, it is unlikely that a single treatment will be successful in the short term. Treatment along these lines probably will have to be multicomponent treatment, against key mediators and reactions.

SUPPORTIVE MANAGEMENT

There is no guarantee that oxygen and substrates will be delivered through the disordered microcirculation, and even if they are, utilization by damaged cells may be impaired. Nevertheless, the mainstays of supportive treatment, as with other forms of shock, are to optimize arterial oxygen content and tissue perfusion and to match oxygen delivery with consumption (see Chapters 8 and 17).

Arterial oxygen content

OXYGEN DELIVERY = CARDIAC OUTPUT × HAEMOGLOBIN CONCENTRATION × OXYGEN SATURATION × 1.34.

HAEMOGLOBIN   Maintain haemoglobin > 10 g/dl.

OXYGENATION   Adequate tissue concentrations of oxygen are important for the prevention and control of infection. Oxygen transport to the mitochondria from the capillaries is driven by a pressure gradient. The PaO_2 should be kept as close as possible to 'normal'. Although we often accept partial pressures of around 60 mm Hg (8 kPa), pressures closer to the normal of 100 mm Hg (13.3 kPa) are necessary for optimal wound healing and resistance to bacteria.

Monitor oxygen with regular determinations of arterial blood gases and pulse oximetry. Sometimes dual oximetry and determinations of mixed venous oxygen saturation and lactate concentrations may also be useful (see p. 504).

High-flow oxygen delivered via a conventional mask might be sufficient (see p. 365).

Continuous positive airway pressure (CPAP) has many advantages over artificial ventilation (see p. 367). Spontaneous respiration, either with a special mask or via an ETT, should be maintained if possible.

If adequate ventilation is not possible with CPAP, artificial ventilation with positive end-expiratory pressure (PEEP) may be necessary. Where possible, techniques such as 'pressure-limited' ventilation (see p. 466) intermittent mandatory ventilation (IMV) (see p. 472) should be used, rather than intermittent positive-pressure ventilation (IPPV) and PEEP, in order to decrease the effects of intrathoracic pressures (see p. 465).

Patients should be nursed in an upright position, in most cases, in order to achieve optimum oxygenation.

Maintain euvolaemic dehydration: That is, maintain a normal intravascular volume while minimizing interstitial overload in order to minimize tissue oedema and maximize oxygen delivery (see p. 61).

Tissue perfusion

THE KEY TO CARDIOVASCULAR SUPPORT IN PATIENTS WITH SEPTICAEMIA IS FLUID-VOLUME REPLACEMENT, AS THE PRIMARY ABNORMALITY IS VASODILATATION. It is crucial that one aggressively correct cardiovascular impairment, as oxygen utilization is dependent on adequate tissue perfusion.

FLUIDS Giving colloid or blood, depending on the haemoglobin concentration, is the most efficient means of resuscitating the intravascular space, as colloid or blood will correct intravascular-volume deficits more rapidly than can crystalloids, will stay in the circulation longer, and will not cause as much pulmonary and peripheral oedema (see p. 61).

Large amounts (200–800 ml/h) of fluid may be needed to support the circulation in patients with sepsis. Average requirements are about 100–200 ml/h.

The fluid-challenge technique is the most effective means of estimating the intravascular volume (see p. 59). Both before and after a bolus (200–500 ml) of fluid, measure as many indicators of intravascular volume as possible (eg pulse rate, blood pressure, CVP, PAWP, urine output, and peripheral perfusion). The patient's responses will give an indication of the degree of hypovolaemia.

Cardiovascular measurements: Regular or continuous measurements of pulse rate, blood pressure, urine output, and CVP are essential for manipulation of the cardiovascular system in patients with sepsis.

High pulmonary artery pressures can cause misleadingly high CVP readings, even in the presence of significant hypovolaemia.

PAWP does not correlate well with left ventricular filling in patients with sepsis, but like CVP, it is useful to show a trend and as a guide to filling pressures.

Hypovolaemia, vasodilatation, and, more rarely, pump failure may occur simultaneously in the presence of sepsis. Determinations of cardiac output and PAWP may therefore be useful. Determinations of $\dot{V}O_2$ and DO_2 may be of help in optimizing cardiovascular support (see p. 376).

Dual oximetry and continuous measurement of mixed venous oxygen saturation ($S\bar{v}O_2$) may sometimes be useful for determining adequate DO_2 (see p. 504).

INOTROPES AND VASOPRESSORS Cardiac output, even in the advanced stages of sepsis, is usually high, and the peripheral vascular resistance low. In the presence of reduced tissue perfusion, this represents a therapeutic dilemma. Maintaining intravascular volume with fluid in the face of vasodilation is the most important manoeuvre.

Inotropes such as dobutamine and dopexamine cause vasodilation and increased cardiac output, which are already features of sepsis. However, in the presence of demonstrated inadequacies of cardiac output and DO_2, and after correction of hypovolaemia and hypotension, these drugs may have a place. Simultaneous estimations of oxygen delivery and demand (see p. 376) can provide firmer indications for the use of drugs such as dobutamine and dopexamine.

When hypotension is the main cardiovascular problem in a patient with septicaemia, a drug with combined inotropic and vasopressor activities, such as adrenaline or noradrenaline, may be indicated. In moderate dosages, they seem to increase the perfusion pressure for vital organs such as the heart, kidneys, and brain, without causing decreases in peripheral perfusion or renal blood flow.

• adrenaline, 5–20 mg in 500 ml, tritrated against the patient's responses, commencing at 0.5 μg $\cdot$ kg^{-1} $\cdot$ min^{-1}. Very high dosages may be necessary to maintain the blood pressure in patients with severe sepsis.

• noradrenaline, 4–20 mg in 500 ml, titrated against the patient's responses as for adrenaline.

• dobutamine, up to 10 $\mu g \cdot kg^{-1} \cdot min^{-1}$, is usually used to improve cardiac output, in an attempt to match Do_2 with $\dot{V}o_2$ (see p. 376).

Dopamine perhaps should be reserved for its unique dopaminergic actions on the renal and mesenteric circulations at low dosages (1–3 $\mu g \cdot kg^{-1} \cdot min^{-1}$). At higher dosages it has β and α spectra that are simulated by other equally effective and cheaper drugs (eg adrenaline).

After the intravascular volume has been corrected, a combination of these catecholamines may be necessary to maintain perfusion pressure and tissue blood flow.

Even with a satisfactory systemic arterial blood pressure and an adequate blood oxygen content, the tissues at the end of the circulation can still fail (eg gangrenous hands, with palpable radial pulses). Drugs that might seem to be conceptually appealing in this situation have been universally disappointing (eg heparin, aprotinin, vasodilators, prostaglandins, corticosteroids).

Supraventricular arrhythmias

Arrhythmias such as sinus tachycardia, SVT, and AF are very common in patients with sepsis. Each of them cause further cardiovascular compromise. Their management is discussed elsewhere (see p. 540).

Other measures

Use NG feeding if tolerated (see p. 87); otherwise, use intravenous nutrition (see p. 89). Stress-ulcer prophylaxis should be commenced (see p. 31). Sucralfate is probably the drug of choice. Nutritional support, including vitamins, should be given (see p. 91), and early dialysis should be considered if acute renal failure supervenes (see p. 651).

Outcome

Despite the discovery of powerful antimicrobials and the development of sophisticated life-support systems, there continues to be a high incidence of septic shock, with a mortality rate that has remained around 50% for over 20 years.

APPROACH TO UNIDENTIFIED INFECTIONS

Patients in the ICU often have signs of sepsis such as fever, leucocytosis, hyperglycaemia, decreased level of consciousness, hypoxia, hyperventilation, or jaundice. None of these by itself necessarily means that a patient is septic. The diagnosis of septicaemia is based on clinical criteria, and the difficulties associated with that limitation can be compounded by the fact that isolation of an offending microbe often is not possible. There must be a methodical and relentless search for the cause of infection (Table 13.7).

BLOOD CULTURE

If possible, the diagnosis of sepsis should be confirmed by culture of an organism. A search for the organism or site of sepsis must be made, including blood and other routine cultures. Blood cultures should be taken from at least two sites using an aerobic bottle and anaerobic bottle. This will aid interpretation should skin organisms be isolated. There is little value in collecting more than four sets of blood cultures for one infective episode, unless infective endocarditis is suspected, when at least six sets should be taken.

REVIEW OF INVASIVE LINES

The diagnosis of catheter-related sepsis is made on the following basis:

1. Obvious clinical signs of local infection. Clinical signs usually occur late and are more common with peripheral catheters than with central venous catheters. As such, they are not necessarily good indicators of line-related sepsis.

2. Isolation of the same organism from blood cultures and from the removed catheter segment is indicative of line-associated sepsis. The infected catheter segment often is not the tip, but the intracutaneous

TABLE 13.7 APPROACH TO UNIDENTIFIED INFECTIONS

Conduct a physical examination, looking for features of septicaemia (see p. 183). Examine the mouth, wounds, catheter sites, heart sounds, abdomen, pressure areas, and peritoneal fluid if relevant. Examine the chest, and listen for bronchial breath sounds. Examine the patient's back for perianal infections and pressure areas.

Examine for perirectal abscess, decubitus ulcer, or epididymitis associated with prolonged catheterization.

Examine cultures from wounds, blood, sputum, and urine – check Gram stain as well as culture and sensitivity.

Chest x-ray for evidence of pneumonia.

A CT scan of the chest will sometimes demonstrate an abscess or consolidation not seen on chest x-ray.

Viral infections – especially cytomegalovirus and hepatitis B following blood-product transfusion. Examine paired serum cultures and/or use microscopy if suspected.

Leucocyte scanning with indium 111 may be useful for soft-tissue infection or intra-abdominal sepsis, or where there are no localizing signs.

If an intra-abdominal source of sepsis is suspected, nuclear medicine studies, ultrasound, or CT may be helpful.

Exclude acalculous cholecystitis (see p. 221).

Take a lateral skull x-ray or CT scan to exclude sinusitis associated with NG or NTT.

DO NOT HESITATE TO RE-EXPLORE WOUNDS AND PERFORM RE-PEATED LAPAROTOMIES FOR DIAGNOSTIC AND THERAPEUTIC PURPOSES IF THE FINDINGS ON CONVENTIONAL INVESTIGATIONS ARE NEGATIVE.

Strategies such as endobronchial brushing, use of protected catheter cultures, transbronchial biopsy, or open lung biopsy may be necessary for unidentified pulmonary lesions.

Change intravascular lines, and send them for culture studies. Consider other invasive sites.

Consider other causes for fever and leucocytosis (eg drug reactions).

segment. Remember that the catheter itself does not become infected. Biofilms consisting of multilayer thicknesses of bacteria probably are deposited on many inorganic surfaces, such as vascular and urinary catheters. Removing the catheter does not necessarily equate with removing the infection, especially if there is associated skin infection. The intradermal segment or intravenous thrombus will remain contaminated. Another catheter should not, therefore, be inserted in the same site, if it is obviously infected.

Change the catheter, if there is any doubt, and culture the organisms from it. There are, as yet, insufficient data to be dogmatic about the optimum time for routine catheter changes.

Review other invasive sites (eg intraventricular drains, peritoneal dialysate, pacemakers).

Lines should be changed over a guidewire when other venous access is unavailable and ongoing venous access is necessary.

PULMONARY INFECTIONS

Intrapulmonary shadowing seen on a chest x-ray is not specific. It can be related to many different conditions, such as pulmonary oedema, ARDS, and aspiration, and these cannot be specifically differentiated from pneumonia on the basis of a chest x-ray alone. A common dilemma in intensive care is to decide whether or not a patient with chest x-ray shadowing and other signs of infection has pneumonia (see p. 406). Pneumonia, in isolation, rarely causes the clinical picture of systemic sepsis.

Positive findings on sputum cultures are common and usually reflect colonization, rather than infection. This is especially common with Gram-negative rods, including *Pseudomonas* spp., *Candida albicans,* and *Staphylococcus aureus* (including MRSA).

Although sputum cultures from intubated patients are routinely examined, they correlate very poorly with the organisms that cause pneumonia. This is probably because the sputum of intubated patients rapidly becomes colonized.

Transtracheal specimens, bronchial washings, specimens from transbronchial biopsy, and 'guarded' bronchial specimens are more useful (see p. 416), but these secretions still can reflect conditions in the airways, rather than the actual infected lung tissue.

Blood culture is an important way to isolate organisms that cause pneumonia. It is the only common specimen that is specific, but it has low sensitivity.

Biopsy via a bronchoscope or open lung biopsy, thus obtaining tissue from an obviously infected area, may be indicated in severe unresponsive pneumonia of unknown origin. However, other concomitant factors (eg coagulopathy) may make this procedure hazardous.

Common organisms and diseases

COMMUNITY-ACQUIRED PNEUMONIA
- *Streptococcus pneumoniae*
- *Mycoplasma pneumoniae*
- Viral pneumonia
- Legionnaires' disease
- *Haemophilus influenzae*
- Other atypical pneumonias (eg Q fever, psittacosis)

ASPIRATION PNEUMONIA
- Coliforms
- Anaerobic organisms

PNEUMONIA IN IMMUNOSUPPRESSED PATIENTS
- Fungal pneumonia
- *Pneumocystis* pneumonia

NOSOCOMIAL PNEUMONIA
- Coliforms
- *Staphylococcus aureus*

URINARY-TRACT INFECTIONS

Colonization of indwelling catheters invariably occurs, and that predisposes to an increased incidence of urinary-tract infection (UTI). The finding of bacteria and even cells in the urine does not necessarily equate with infection. Treatment should be commenced only if systemic infection is present and the urinary tract is thought to be the source.

Common hospital-acquired UTI organisms include *Escherichia coli, Klebsiella* spp., *Proteus* spp., *Serratia* spp., *Pseudomonas* spp., enterococci, *Staphylococcus aureus,* and *Candida albicans.*

Frequent catheter changes will not reduce the incidence of bacteriuria and infection.

Urinary samples should be obtained by aspirating through prepared tubing, not from the collecting bag.

WOUNDS (see p. 222)

Wounds are often colonized by coliforms, but usually they are not significant. Although orthopaedic wounds can be colonized by coliforms, it is *Staphylococcus aureus* and *Streptococcus pyogenes* that usually cause clinically significant infections. Abdominal wounds associated with bowel perforation can become infected with *S. aureus,* streptococci, coliforms, and anaerobes. Routine wound swabs are very difficult to interpret. Wound aspirates and tissue biopsies will give more accurate information. Findings from blood cultures are rarely positive.

OCCULT INFECTIONS

The search for occult infections includes a thorough physical examination. The following are some causes of occult infections in the ICU:

ABDOMINAL SEPSIS Abdominal sepsis can occur as intra-abdominal abscess or acalculous cholecystitis (see p. 217).

FUNGAL SEPTICAEMIA Long-term patients, especially those on broad-spectrum antibiotics, can develop fungal septicaemia. The use of special blood cultures will allow more rapid diagnosis of fungaemia. However, findings from blood cultures are often negative in patients with systemic fungal infections.

LUNG ABSCESS Especially if associated with aspiration, lung abscess usually can be diagnosed on the basis of chest x-ray or CT scan.

SINUSITIS Sinusitis is especially seen in association with nasotracheal intubation or NG tubes and after facial trauma. This is a common site of infection that often is overlooked. Fluid levels can be seen on routine lateral facial views or CT scan. Sinusitis can cause meningitis, epidural and subdural abscesses, intracranial abscesses, lateral- or cavernous-sinus thrombosis, and osteomyelitis. Orbital cellulitis may indicate infection of the sphenoid or ethmoid sinuses. The causative organisms usually are mixed aerobes and anaerobes, including S. *aureus,* from the upper respiratory tract. Although drainage and tube removal are the most important steps, chloramphenicol, penicillin, and/or metronidazole are suitable antimicrobial agents.

TOOTH ABSCESS   Tooth abscess can occur especially in long-term patients. Routinely inspect the oral cavity.

EPIDIDYMITIS   Epididymitis can occur in association with prolonged catheterization.

BRAIN ABSCESS OR MENINGITIS   These can occur especially in association with head injuries (see p. 599).

PERI-RECTAL ABSCESS   Remember to inspect the patient's back.

DECUBITUS ULCER   Remember to inspect the patient's back.

HEART VALVES   Because of instrumentation of the heart, especially with pulmonary artery catheters, vegetations can grow on the heart valves. Although uncommon, these can become infected. Murmurs are rarely helpful in the diagnosis of right-side endocarditis, which is commonly found in abusers of intravenous drugs, as well as in association with vascular catheterization. If infection is suspected, echocardiography is indicated.

ANTIMICROBIALS

There is little difficulty in choosing the correct antimicrobial agent when the organism has been identified and its sensitivities are known. Unfortunately, that situation is uncommon in the seriously ill. The clinical setting in an ICU often is a microbiological nightmare (eg a septic patient with multiple intravascular lines, an ETT, a urinary catheter, and pre-existing intrapulmonary shadowing of uncertain origin, having recently had an operation and often already on multiple 'blind' antibiotics).

Positive culture of organisms in these circumstances is almost impossible, and even if an organism can be isolated, it will not be for at least 24 hours. This results in the use of 'best-guess' antimicrobials. The guidelines for how long these antibiotics should be used are either non-existent or empirical.

PRINCIPLES OF ANTIMICROBIAL TREATMENT IN INTENSIVE CARE

Community-acquired infections should be treated according to the expected sensitivity of the organism implicated.

Nosocomial or hospital-acquired infections raise complex issues that vary from one hospital to another. Individual ICUs should study their own patterns of organisms and their sensitivities. CLOSE CO-OPERATION WITH SPECIALISTS IN INFECTIOUS DISEASES AND MICROBIOLOGY IS ESSENTIAL.

Most systemic infections in intensive care are caused by the following organisms:

Nosocomial infections	Community-acquired infections
Klebsiella spp.	*Streptococcus pneumoniae*
Proteus spp.	*Haemophilus influenzae*
Enterobacter spp.	*Moraxella catarrhalis*
Citrobacter spp.	*Escherichia coli*
Serratia spp.	*Staphylococcus aureus*
Pseudomonas spp.	*Streptococcus pyogenes*
Acinetobacter spp.	
Candida spp.	
Staphylococcus aureus	

Consider the underlying disease (eg diabetics are often infected with mixed aerobes, and burn patients and patients with leukaemia often have *Pseudomonas* spp.).

The nature of the antimicrobial must be known:

- tissue penetration
- optimum dose
- dosage interval
- toxic effects

- spectrum
- interactions

Use monotherapy where possible. Cost is becoming increasingly important in all facets of medicine. We should no longer feel embarrassed about comparing the costs of antimicrobials and opting for the cheaper one whenever it is appropriate.

Antibiotics will alter the normal flora, encouraging overgrowth by organisms such as *S. aureus, Candida* spp., and *Pseudomonas* spp., especially in the respiratory tract and urinary tract. Broad-spectrum antibiotics encourage this phenomenon to a greater extent than do the more specific antibiotics.

Use empirical antibiotic treatment for 72 hours, and monitor for clinical improvement in those patients from whom no organisms have been isolated. As in many other areas of intensive care, a titrational or challenge approach is most appropriate (ie commence best-guess antimicrobials, and monitor clinical responses). If there has been no improvement, go to the next step:

(a) Consider an occult source of sepsis. Surgery has a more important role than antibiotics in these cases (see p. 192).

(b) Consider that inappropriate antibiotic treatment may have been selected (eg inadequate dose, spectrum, or tissue penetration).

If there has been no improvement after 72 hours and there is no obvious occult infection, cease giving antibiotics, reculture, and empirically commence another antimicrobial combination at a later stage, rather than simply adding one antibiotic after another.

There is no agreement on the duration of treatment or antibiotic 'course' in intensive care. As a guideline, if the antimicrobial has shown an effect within 3 days, cease the drug within 5–7 days. If there has been no effect at all, consider stopping after 3 days.

The original diagnosis of bacterial infection should also be examined (eg fever and leucocytosis do not necessarily mean infection). Consider other possibilities, such as drug reactions, cytomegalovirus infection following transfusion (see p. 708), an occult source of sepsis (see p. 199), pancreatitis, and other non-bacterial infections.

Once-daily intravenous doses of aminoglycosides are less toxic and more bactericidal than are divided daily doses.

PROPHYLACTIC ANTIMICROBIALS WITH SURGERY Prophylactic antibiotics should be used only with a procedure that commonly leads to infection (eg large-bowel resection, contaminated tissue resection) or when an infection could cause devastating results (eg infection of prosthetic heart valve, implantation of foreign materials such as intracranial shunts and joint prostheses).

The antimicrobials selected should have a record of activity against the likely pathogens. Staphylococci should be covered for procedures such as insertion of prostheses. Anaerobes and coliforms need to be covered for gastro-intestinal and genito-urinary surgery.

Antimicrobials should be given about the time of induction of anaesthesia and for no more than 24 hours.

PRACTICAL GUIDELINES TO PRESCRIBING ANTIMICROBIALS

It is beyond the scope of this book to describe detailed antimicrobial guidelines for every infection and to discuss the pharmacology of every drug. Infection is common in intensive care, and antimicrobials are widely used and very expensive. Staff working in ICUs should therefore familiarize themselves with this complex and rapidly changing area and work closely with their own microbiology department.

Clinical, laboratory, and radiological findings will often give some indication of the source of infection.

Patterns of nosocomial infections within a particular ICU will offer further guidelines.

Immunocompromised hosts often require broader coverage against common Gram-positive and Gram-negative bacteria, including *Pseudomonas* spp.

APPROACH TO PATIENTS WITH INFECTIONS OF UNCERTAIN AETIOLOGY

THE FOLLOWING GUIDELINES ARE FOR ONLY THE INITIAL 'BLIND' PHASE OF ANTIMICROBIAL TREATMENT. They must be adjusted according to microbiological findings, sensitivity patterns, and local nosocomial pathogens.

SEPTICAEMIA   Septicaemia of unknown origin can be treated as follows until microbiology findings are available:

• penicillin (eg ampicillin, 1–2 g IV, 6-hourly)
  +
  aminoglycoside (eg gentamicin 5 mg/kg IV as a loading dose, and 3
  mg/kg IV once daily); monitor peak and trough concentrations every
  third day, aiming for a trough < 2 mg/L and a peak of 6–8 mg/L)
  ±
  metronidazole, 500 mg IV, 8-hourly, for abdominal or gynaecological infection
  ±
  flucloxacillin, 1–2 g IV, 6-hourly (especially for community-acquired
  septicaemia)

Pneumonia (see p. 406)

COMMUNITY-ACQUIRED PNEUMONIA

'Typical' lobar pneumonia

• penicillin, 2–3 g IV, 6-hourly, to cover *Streptococcus pneumoniae*
  OR
• ampicillin, 1–2 IV, 6-hourly, if there is underlying chronic lung disease

If the patient is allergic to penicillins, give cephalothin, 1–2 g IV, 6-
hourly, or ceftriazone, 1–2 g IV, daily.
  If the patient has a life-threatening illness, antimicrobials should
initially be extended to cover *S. aureus,* coliforms, and 'atypical' bacteria such as *Legionella.*

'Atypical' pneumonia

'Atypical' pneumonia is becoming a more common form of community-
acquired pneumonia. Legionnaires' disease and *Mycoplasma* pneumonia are the commonest forms, but other forms such as psittacosis
and Q fever need to be excluded.

• erythromycin, 0.5–1 g IV, 6-hourly

Doxycycline is better for psittacosis.

LIFE-THREATENING PNEUMONIA   If the pneumonia is very severe and the diagnosis unsure, often ceftriaxone, penicillin, and erythromycin are commenced simultaneously until a diagnosis is made.

Aspiration pneumonia

Aspiration pneumonia should be suspected in alcoholics, intravenous drug users, and the debilitated. Mixed mouth organisms, mainly anaerobic, need to be covered:

- ampicillin, 1–2 g IV, 6-hourly
  +
  metronidazole, 500 mg IV, 8-hourly (or suppositories, 1 g, 8-hourly)
  OR
  ticarcillin + clavulanate, 3.1 g IV, 6-hourly
  OR
  clindamycin, 300–600 mg IV, 6-hourly

HOSPITAL-ACQUIRED PNEUMONIA

- aminoglycoside (eg gentamicin, 5 mg/kg IV as a loading dose, and 3 mg/kg IV once daily); check concentrations every third day (trough < 2 mg/L; peak, 5–8 mg/L)
  +
  ampicillin, 1–2 g IV, 6-hourly
  OR
  ticarcillin + clavulanate, 3.1 g IV, 6-hourly
  OR
  ceftriaxone, 1–2 g IV, daily

Urinary-tract infection

- ampicillin, 1–2 g IV, 6-hourly
  +
  aminoglycoside (eg gentamicin, 5 mg/kg IV as a loading dose, and 3 mg/kg IV once daily); check concentrations every third day (trough < 2 mg/L; peak, 6–8 mg/L).

If the patient is allergic to penicillins, substitute cephalothin, 1–2 g IV, 6-hourly.

Intra-abdominal infection

• ampicillin, 1–2 g IV, 4-hourly
  +

  aminoglycoside (eg gentamicin, 5 mg/kg IV as a loading dose, and 3 mg/kg IV once daily); check concentrations every third day (trough < 2 mg/L; peak, 6–8 mg/L)
  +

  metronidazole, 500 mg IV, 8-hourly (or suppositories, 1 g, 8-hourly)

Intravascular cannula infection

Remove the cannula and culture its adherent material.

  Possible organisms include *S. aureus, S. epidermidis,* and, more rarely, coliforms or fungi.

• flucloxacillin, 1–2 g IV, 6-hourly
  ±

  aminoglycoside (eg gentamicin, 5 mg/kg IV as a loading dose, and 3 mg/kg IV once daily); check concentrations every third day (trough < 2 mg/L; peak, 6–8 mg/L)

If MRSA is prevalent in the ICU, use vancomycin.

Neutropenic patients

Liaise closely with microbiologists, as the host and invading organisms often will present a challenge. These patients are susceptible to *Pseudomonas* spp., *S. aureus,* fungi, or coliforms, especially from the GIT. The following regimen is for febrile neutropenic patients in whom the source of infection is unknown. These recommendations should be modified as more precise information arrives from culture studies. Initial regimen before culture and sensitivities:

• aminoglycoside (eg tobramycin, 5 mg/kg IV as a loading dose, and 1–1.5 mg/kg IV, 8-hourly); do not use once-daily doses of aminoglycosides in these patients
  +

  ticarcillin + clavulanate, 3.1 g IV, 4-hourly

If there is penicillin allergy, substitute ceftazidime, 2 g IV, 8-hourly. Do not use ceftriaxone or cefotaxime, as their cover for pseudomonads is inadequate.

If the patient remains unresponsive, add

- flucloxacillin, 2 g IV, 6-hourly

If the patient is allergic to penicillins or if MRSA is suspected, use

- vancomycin, according to body weight (BW):
  BW < 70 kg, use 500 mg IV, 8-hourly
  BW > 70 kg, use 1 g IV, 12-hourly

Monitor concentrations every third day (trough < 10 mg/L; peak, 20–40 mg/L). If the patient does not respond after 1 week, use empirical antifungal treatment:

- initial test dose of 1 mg amphotericin B in 20 ml of 5% dextrose solution over 30 minutes
- then 0.3 mg/kg on day 1
- increase to 0.5–0.9 mg/kg for subsequent days

Continue until the neutropenia resolves, and liaise closely with the microbiology department. Do not use fluconazole or other antifungal agents in this situation.

The foregoing drugs for neutropenic febrile patients should be used only initially, followed by a change to specific antimicrobials when an organism has been isolated. The use of antibiotics for empirical treatment should be based on analyses of the sensitivity patterns of the organisms that are causing infections in that particular haematology/oncology unit.

SPECIFIC ORGANISMS

Staphylococcus aureus

If the organism is sensitive to penicillin, use penicillin, $2–3 \times 10^6$ units IV, 4-hourly. It is important to distinguish between a minor side effect and a true allergy.

If the organism is resistant to penicillin, use flucloxacillin, 4–12 g/d, in divided doses. If there is penicillin allergy, use

- cephalothin, 4–12 g IV daily, in 4–6 divided doses
  OR
- cefazolin, 500–1,000 mg, 8-hourly

If the patient is allergic to cephalosporin and penicillin, use vancomycin.

Streptococcus pyogenes

- penicillin, 2–3×10^6 units IV, 6-hourly
  OR alternatively
- first-generation cephalosporin
- vancomycin

Pneococcus

- penicillin, 2–3×10^6 units IV, 6-hourly
  OR, if allergic to penicillins
- cephalothin, 4–8 g IV daily, in 4–6 divided doses
- cefazolin, 2–4 g IV daily, in 4–6 divided doses

MRSA

- vancomycin:
  BW < 70 kg, use 500 mg IV, 8-hourly
  BW > 70 kg, use 1 g IV, 12-hourly

Monitor concentrations every third day (trough < 10 mg/L; peak, 20–40 mg/L).

Vancomycin causes marked thrombophlebitis – use a central line.

Pseudomonas aeruginosa

Liaise closely with the microbiology department in order to determine the hospital sensitivity profiles. Always use an aminoglycoside and an anti-pseudomonal β-lactam, as well as another agent:

- tobramycin, 5 mg/kg IV as a loading dose, and 3 mg/kg IV once daily; check concentrations every third day (trough < 2 mg/L; peak, 6–8 mg/L)

+

ticarcillin + clavulanate, 3.1 g IV, 4-hourly

Alternatively, piperacillin, ceftazidime, or imipenem can be substituted.

Anaerobic infections

Generally speaking, anaerobic infections above the diaphragm have been thought to respond to penicillin, whilst those below the diaphragm have been thought to require metronidazole. However, resistance of oral anaerobes to penicillin is becoming more common.

Anaerobes constitute a common part of the normal flora, especially in the GIT, and they help to prevent overgrowth of coliforms. Antianaerobic drugs should therefore be used only when there is a strong suspicion of anaerobic infection, such as in intra-abdominal infections, infections of the female genital tract, brain abscesses, some cases of aspiration pneumonia, gas gangrene, or soft-tissue infections.

Coliforms

The choice of antibiotic treatment for this, the most common source of nosocomial infection, depends on the sensitivities. Initial therapy:

• gentamicin, 5 mg/kg IV as an initial dose, and 3 mg/kg IV once daily; check concentrations every third day (trough < 2 mg/L; peak, 6–8 mg/L)

+

ampicillin, 1–2 g IV, 6-hourly

Klebsiella spp. are resistant to ampicillin, and ceftriaxone is indicated. Depending on sensitivities, other drugs such as imipenem and ciprofloxacin may have to be used.

SPECIFIC ANTIBIOTICS

Aminoglycosides

Aminoglycosides have narrow therapeutic ranges and need to be monitored closely, as they can cause nephrotoxicity and ototoxicity. Those can be potentiated when aminoglycosides are used with other drugs such as cephalosporins (especially cephalothin) and frusemide. Their main value is their broad-spectrum activity against coliforms. Aminoglycosides usually should be given as once-a-day doses, rather than in divided doses.

Recommended serum concentrations (μg/ml) are as follows:

	Peak	Trough
gentamicin	6–8	<2
tobramycin	6–8	<2
amikacin	20–25	<10

The newer aminoglycosides, such as tobramycin, amikacin, and netilmicin, should be reserved for serious infections that are resistant to gentamicin. Each ICU should determine its prevailing resistance patterns to various aminoglycosides.

Penicillins

PENICILLIN G Penicillin G is still highly active against streptococci, including *Streptococcus pneumoniae, Neisseria meningitidis,* and many anaerobes of the upper respiratory tract.

PENICILLINASE-RESISTANT PENICILLINS Because most strains of *S. aureus* are resistant to penicillin G by virtue of β-lactamase production, treatment requires other agents (eg flucloxacillin or methicillin). Increasingly, resistance to these compounds is being seen, especially in the hospital setting. In some hospitals, up to 50% of the staphylococci isolated are resistant to methicillin.

BROAD-SPECTRUM PENICILLINS Ampicillin and amoxycillin remain useful in intensive care mainly because of their activity against enterococci. They also are usually active against *Haemophilus influenzae,* as well as some strains of *Escherichia coli* and *Proteus mirabilis.* Because about 50% of *E. coli* isolates that cause UTI are resistant to ampicillin, it is inappropriate for empirical treatment of UTI. Widespread use of ampicillin and amoxycillin in intensive care can be associated with the emergence of resistant organisms, such as *Klebsiella* spp.

Ticarcillin, azlocillin, mezlocillin, and piperacillin have wider ranges of activity than do ampicillin and amoxycillin against coliforms, in particular against *Pseudomonas* spp. However, their clinical efficacy may be insufficient when they are used alone to treat *Pseudomonas* spp. infections, and their Gram-negative spectra are not as broad as those of the aminoglycosides. It is recommended, therefore, that they be used with an aminoglycoside. It is thus difficult to assess their true effectiveness in intensive care.

Cephalosporins

It is tempting to resort to the cephalosporins because of their relative safety and because their antibacterial spectra include Gram-positive and Gram-negative activities.

Because the activities of the first- and second-generation cephalosporins are unpredictable against Gram-negative bacteria, they should not be employed for empirical, single-drug treatment. The third-generation cephalosporins feature broad-spectrum, high antimicrobial potencies and excellent tissue penetration. However, several gaps are evident in the overall coverage afforded by all these drugs. For example, some enterococci, *Pseudomonas* spp., and anaerobes are resistant to third-generation cephalosporins. Their activity against *S. aureus* precludes their use as single drugs against this organism. They cannot, therefore, be recommended for single-drug, empirical treatment. Because they are often used in combination with other antibiotics, such as the aminoglycosides, it is difficult to assess their independent usefulness in seriously ill patients.

Cephalosporins are, however, useful in infections caused by sensitive organisms. Specifically, cefotaxime/ceftriaxone are the drugs of choice for most cases of bacterial meningitis, because of their excellent tissue penetration (see p. 610). However, they are not active against *Listeria monocytogenes,* and either penicillin or ampicillin should also be used initially.

Monobactams

Aztreonam is a member of the family of monobactams. It is a highly active compound against the majority of Gram-negative bacteria, and it has no activity against Gram-positive organisms and anaerobes. Its main usefulness is in the treatment of Gram-negative-rod infections for patients who are allergic to β-lactams, as cross-hypersensitivity does not occur.

Carbapenems

The imipenem/cilastatin combination is the major representative of this class. It has activity against Gram-negative bacteria comparable to those of the aminoglycosides. It also has excellent activity against anaerobes and most Gram-positive cocci. However, it may not reliably cover MRSA, and some *Pseudomonas* spp. are resistant.

Vancomycin

Vancomycin is particularly useful in intensive care for treatment of MRSA and infections due to Staphylococcus *epidermidis* or *Corynebacterium* spp. associated with prosthetic heart valves. Oral vancomycin is useful in patients with antibiotic-associated colitis due to *Clostridium difficile.*

Quinolone derivatives

These agents have some theoretical attractions. They are bactericidal, with wide distributions throughtout the body, and have little effect on anaerobic gut flora. The newer agents have wide spectra of activity, including some Gram-positive cocci and many Gram-negative bacteria. However, they are expensive, and their place in the treatment of the seriously ill has not yet been defined. Their greatest usefulness may be in providing an alternative oral treatment for infections with antibiotic-resistant coliforms, thus shortening the duration of hospitalization.

The 'latest' antibiotics

Today there is considerable pressure to use the latest and most expensive antibiotics. Many have been marketed and touted as being broad-spectrum replacements for aminoglycosides, as having stability against β-lactamases, and as being relatively free of serious side effects. However, we need to temper our enthusiasm about their possible roles in the ICU. Some comments about their clinical use in intensive care include:

- There is a danger that if they are over-used, superinfections and resistances will become more common.
- Apart from their use as the first-line treatment for Gram-negative meningitis, third-generation cephalosporins should be used as reserve antibiotics for cases in which there are definite bacteriological indications.
- Often these drugs are prescribed because they are currently fashionable and because of the pressure of product promotion, rather than logic.

Scepticism and caution should be exercised when considering the use of the latest broad-spectrum antibiotics, such as imipenem/cilastatin, aztreonam, and the quinolone derivatives. The mortality from septicaemia remains relatively unchanged, despite the introduction of broader-spectrum antimicrobials. Many other aspects of management (see p. 192) are equally as important as the use of antibiotics, if not more important, especially in the presence of 'non-bacterial' septicaemia (see p. 182). It appears that many of the more recent broad-spectrum antibiotics are expensive and still largely unproven adjuncts to treatment.

INTRA-ABDOMINAL SEPSIS

There is no strict dividing line between generalized intra-abdominal sepsis and an abscess or peritonitis. 'Intra-abdominal sepsis' is a term that loosely refers to a generalized infection and/or localized collections. Intra-abdominal collections or abscesses can be found intraperitoneally, retroperitoneally, or within viscera.

The most important principle in the management of intra-abdominal sepsis is **REMOVAL AND DRAINAGE.** Otherwise, the role of intensive care is to keep the patient alive until the source of the sepsis can be found and evacuated.

The message to reluctant surgeons is this: Rather than viewing patients with intra-abdominal sepsis as being too sick for surgery, they should be viewed as too sick *not* to have surgery.

Intra-abdominal infection remains a common and catastrophic event, entailing high mortality, often associated with MOF (see Chapter 9).

PERITONITIS

Contamination of the peritoneal cavity usually results in abdominal pain, guarding, and rebound tenderness. These signs can become masked or modified in the elderly, in post-operative patients, and in immunocompromised patients.

Diagnosis

The diagnosis of peritonitis is supported by the findings of leucocytosis with toxic changes, fever, and other signs of systemic sepsis (see p. 183). Radiological findings include free abdominal gas and/or fluid. Abdominal ultrasound or a CT scan may demonstrate a source of the peritonitis. Blood cultures and routine investigations should be performed.

Management

SUPPORTIVE CARE   The patient should immediately be prepared for **SURGERY.**

Rapidly restore the intravascular volume, and give blood, if necessary, according to intravascular measurements such as arterial blood pressure, pulse rate, CVP, PAWP, and hourly urine output (see Chapter 21).

Other forms of support, such as low-dose dopamine and inotropes, may be necessary as for generalized sepsis (see p. 195).

SURGERY   **IMMEDIATE SURGERY IS THE MOST IMPORTANT STEP IN THE MANAGEMENT OF PERITONITIS.** The underlying source of contamination must be eliminated.

RADICAL SURGICAL DEBRIDEMENT, as in any other form of infection, is required.

Meticulous inspection and lavage of the intra-abdominal cavity are necessary. Post-operative drainage is essential.

The role of antibiotics in the lavage fluid and the advisability of continuous post-operative lavage have not been established.

Continuing resuscitation and general care of the seriously ill are required until all signs of infection have disappeared. Unfortunately, infection sometimes persists in the form of generalized intra-abdominal sepsis or localized collections, and repeated laparotomies may be necessary.

ANTIBIOTICS

- aminoglycoside (eg gentamicin, 5 mg/kg IV as a loading dose, and 3 mg/kg IV once daily; check concentrations every third day (trough < 2 mg/L; peak, 6–8 mg/L)

  +

  metronidazole, 500 mg IV, 8-hourly, to cover anaerobic bacteria

  +

  ampicillin, 1 g IV, 6-hourly, to cover enterococci

Then tailor antibiotic treatment according to the organisms and sensitivities identified. Continue for 5 days post-operatively, then reassess.

IF FEVER OR SIGNS OF SEPSIS CONTINUE POST-OPERATIVELY, REINVESTIGATION OF THE SOURCE AND FURTHER AGGRESSIVE SURGICAL INTERVENTION ARE REQUIRED – NOT ADDITIONAL ANTIBIOTICS.

INTRA-ABDOMINAL SEPSIS

'Intra-abdominal sepsis' is used here not only to refer to peritonitis but also as a general term encompassing abscesses and generalized infections, as well as possible peritoneal involvement.

Diagnosis

Frequently there are NO ABDOMINAL SIGNS to be found in a patient with an intra-abdominal abscess. Systemic signs and symptoms of generalized sepsis are usually more prominent than local signs. These include the same features seen with septicaemia (see p. 183).

A septic patient may have a classic 'swinging' fever. Also, there may be changes in the patient's mental status, as well as glucose intolerance, a decrease in gastric mucosal pH, cardiovascular decompensation, hypoxia, and ARDS or other signs of MOF (see p. 139).

AN IMMEDIATE, AGGRESSIVE SEARCH MUST BE MADE FOR THE SOURCE OF SEPSIS.

ULTRASOUND The sensitivity and specificity of abdominal ultrasound will vary according to many factors, including the experience of the operator, the quality of the equipment, and the presence of gas, drainage tubes, and dressings, all of which can obscure the image. The use of portable real-time ultrasound and the possibility of fine-needle aspiration for diagnosis and even treatment may prevent unnecessary surgery in some cases. However, extensive debridement at laparotomy is often necessary.

CT SCAN A CT scan may be more suitable than ultrasound for use in the seriously ill and in post-operative patients, because it is not as strongly affected by gas and other artifacts. It can also provide better views of certain areas, such as the retroperitoneal space. Percutaneous drainage in conjunction with CT scanning can also be performed. However, for CT, patients must be transported to an area of the hospital where routine monitoring can be difficult and facilities for continuous supportive care are not ideal (see p. 170).

RADIONUCLIDE IMAGING Although imaging with gallium citrate is unrewarding for investigating collections in the seriously ill, imaging with indium-111-labelled leucocytes can be more useful. However, there can be false-positive findings with indium 111, because the leucocytes are attracted to areas of inflammation and vascularity, as well as definite infective foci. The labelled leucocytes may be taken up by the spleen and liver, but not normally by the kidneys or bowel. There can be false-negative findings when imaging chronic infective sites, such as those involved in osteomyelitis.

SURGERY LAPAROTOMY IN THIS SETTING IS OFTEN AN ESSENTIAL DIAGNOSTIC TOOL. If the patient remains septic and the abdomen is suspected as a continuing source of sepsis, laparotomy is mandatory.

Treatment

DRAINAGE OF THE PUS IS ESSENTIAL. This can sometimes be achieved with fine-needle aspiration, but more often requires surgery, preferably by a surgeon with experience in this area.

Meticulous exploration of the wound and abdominal cavity is mandatory. Extensive debridement and adequate drainage are essential.

If there are any further signs of continuing sepsis (see p. 183), REINVESTIGATION AND RE-EXPLORATION ARE MANDATORY.

Some authors, prompted by the high incidence of recurrence, have proposed

- leaving the abdominal cavity open and packing it, or
- partially closing the abdominal cavity with material such as Marlex mesh.

ANTIBIOTICS Studies of blood cultures and other routine microbiological cultures should be performed in an attempt to isolate the organism.

If there are no positive cultures, empirical antibiotic treatment, as for peritonitis (see p. 219), should be commenced while the source of sepsis is being sought.

OTHER MANAGEMENT PRINCIPLES

- general supportive measures, as for septicaemia (see p. 195)
- general measures for the seriously ill (see Chapter 2)
- cardiovascular support (see Chapter 22)
- fluid therapy (see Chapter 4)
- respiratory support (see Chapter 20)
- nutrition (see Chapter 5)

ACALCULOUS CHOLECYSTITIS

Acalculous cholecystitis is a common disease of the critically ill. There are many predisposing factors, but, as yet, no specific cause has been found. An inflamed gall-bladder often leads to perforation or even gangrene. It leads to high mortality, possibly because of the delay in diagnosis.

Diagnosis

As with other forms of intra-abdominal sepsis, patients usually have systemic manifestations of sepsis (see p. 183), such as decreased levels of consciousness, ARDS, and a hyperdynamic cardiovascular state. The diagnosis is difficult because the signs and symptoms can be masked. Patients are often febrile, but may have concurrent infections. There may be right-upper-quadrant pain or signs of an acute abdomen. Findings on liver function tests, including bilirubin, may be normal or elevated. Ultrasound may show a thickened gall-bladder wall, an enlarged gall-bladder, or a peri-cholecystic collection. CT scanning will often show non-specific dilatation of the gall-bladder or a peri-cholecystic collection. However, sludge formation and non-specific enlargement of the gall-bladder are commonly found as parts of the normal spectrum in seriously ill patients. THE DIAGNOSIS DEPENDS ON A HIGH LEVEL OF AWARENESS, AND LAPAROTOMY OFTEN IS THE ONLY DEFINITIVE WAY TO CONFIRM ACALCULOUS CHOLECYSTITIS.

Management

LAPAROTOMY – Cholecystostomy and drainage of other collections of pus compose the treatment of choice.

WOUNDS

The majority of wound infections involve only the skin and subcutaneous tissues, causing tenderness, swelling, redness, increased warmth, and elevated body temperature. These superficial infections rarely spread to the fascia and muscle.

HOWEVER, AN APPARENTLY BENIGN COLLECTION OF PUS IN A WOUND, WITH LITTLE EXTERNAL EVIDENCE OF INFECTION, CAN, IN SERIOUSLY ILL, IMMUNOCOMPROMISED PATIENTS, CAUSE SYSTEMIC SEPSIS (see p. 183). The incidence of wound infections is increased in patients who have had prolonged surgery.

MANAGEMENT

Prevention

As is true for all other facets of tissue well-being in the critically ill, wounds heal best in ideal homeostatic environments.

BLOOD FLOW TO THE WOUND Rapid healing in areas of good blood flow is demonstrated by the low incidence of infection in well-vascularized areas such as the tongue and heart.

Optimal cardiac output and arterial blood pressure should be maintained.

Take steps to avoid peripheral oedema (see p. 62), which will reduce local blood flow.

OXYGENATION OF THE BLOOD In regard to adjusting the haemoglobin concentration, err on the high side rather than on the lower side.

As for oxygen saturation, maintain higher or 'normal' levels, rather than accepting lower levels.

ADEQUATE TISSUE OXYGENATION AND BLOOD FLOW PROBABLY ARE JUST AS IMPORTANT AS PROPHYLACTIC ANTIBIOTICS IN THE PREVENTION OF WOUND INFECTION.

IMMUNITY White cells have a broader antimicrobial spectrum than do antibiotics:

- antibodies } Active or passive immunization may become
- opsonins } more widespread in intensive care (see p. 194).

NUTRITION The ideal balance of energy and protein needed by patients who are seriously ill is still a matter of contention (see Chapter 5).

Remember that the following are important for optimal healing:

vitamin A	pyridoxine	copper
riboflavin	vitamin D	manganese
niacin	zinc	ascorbic acid

PROPHYLACTIC ANTIBIOTICS

TO BE EFFECTIVE, PROPHYLACTIC ANTIBIOTICS MUST BE GIVEN BEFORE OPERATION OR INJURY.

Definitive treatment

ANTIBIOTICS Following clean operations not involving the gastrointestinal, gynaecological, or respiratory tracts, the organism most commonly found in wound infections is *S. aureus*. The incubation period is 4–6 days. Infection usually is well localized and is characterized by creamy pus. The wound infection is often erythematous, oedematous, and painful. Local drainage procedures are usually effective. Antibiotics usually are not indicated unless there is systemic sepsis or spreading cellulitis.

Following contaminated surgery, there will be a polymicrobial flora resembling the microflora of the resected organ. The incubation period for Gram-negative wound infections is 7–14 days. They produce more diffuse signs than do the staphylococcal infections and more systemic manifestations, such as fever, tachycardia, and bacteraemia. These infections should be treated with local drainage procedures as well as antibiotics.

Infections usually occur beginning on the fourth post-operative day. Wound infections occurring within the first 48 hours characteristically are caused by either clostridial or β-haemolytic streptococci. They rapidly cause systemic symptoms and are associated with high mortality.

SURGERY

WOUND INFECTIONS CAN BE SOURCES OF LIFE-THREATENING, GENERALIZED SEPTICAEMIA (see p. 183). IF THERE IS ANY DOUBT, THE WOUND MUST BE RE-EXPLORED AND DRAINED.

SOME UNUSUAL INFECTIONS

NECROTIZING FASCIITIS

Necrotizing fasciitis is a relatively rare, potentially fatal necrotizing infection of the subcutaneous tissue and superficial fascia, with secondary necrosis of the overlying skin.

The bacteria involved usually are *Streptococcus pyogenes,* staphylococci, or anaerobic bacteria.

The skin rapidly becomes warm, oedematous, painful, and discoloured.

The area of necrotic tissue can eventually be estimated on the basis of the anaesthesia of the overlying skin due to subcutaneous nerve destruction.

The extent of underlying necrosis usually cannot be fully appreciated by simply examining the overlying skin.

THE MOST IMPORTANT ASPECT OF MANAGEMENT IS RADICAL AND REPEATED SURGICAL EXCISION, AS WELL AS AGGRESSIVE DEBRIDEMENT OF THE NECROTIC TISSUE.

High-dosage penicillin should not be commenced until the microbiological findings are available.

LEGIONNAIRES' DISEASE

Legionnaires' disease often occurs as sporadic epidemics caused by inhalation of infected droplets from air conditioning, cooling towers, and similar areas. Although Legionnaires' disease presents primarily as pneumonia, it can also present as a generalized disease with many possible systemic manifestations. *Legionella* spp. pneumonia is discussed elsewhere (see p. 225).

Presentation

These patients present with pulmonary complaints such as coughing and purulent or blood-stained sputum.

Extrapulmonary manifestations can include very high fever, rigors, diarrhoea, myalgia, arthralgia, renal failure, myocarditis, headache, and clouded sensorium.

Diagnosis

Direct fluorescent antibody (DFA) tests on sputum have high numbers of false-negatives and false-positives and may not cover the many different serotypes.

Culture of the organism is the investigation of choice.

Serology is quite sensitive, but can take up to 6 weeks to show positive findings.

Treatment

- erythromycin, 1 g IV, 6-hourly
  ±
  rifampicin, 600 mg orally, 12-hourly

Clarithromycin, 0.25–1.0 g orally, twice daily, is proving an effective alternative to erythromycin.

TOXIC SHOCK SYNDROME

Toxic shock syndrome (TSS) is often associated with the use of tampons by women; it can also follow nasal packing and can accompany influenza episodes and staphylococcal infections, as well as pharyngitis, tracheitis, pneumonitis, and pulmonary abscess. It can also occur in association with streptococcal infections.

Diagnosis

THE DIAGNOSIS IS MADE ON CLINICAL GROUNDS:

- fever exceeding 38.9°C
- diffuse macular, erythrodermal rash, resembling sunburn
- desquamation of superficial epidermis on palms or soles of feet, 7–14 days after onset of symptoms
- hypotension
- multiorgan dysfunction
- vomiting or diarrhoea at onset
- severe myalgia or high concentration of creatinine phosphokinase
- hyperaemia of mucous membranes, involving vagina, oropharynx, or conjunctiva
- renal failure
- abnormal findings on liver function tests
- thrombocytopenia
- altered level of consciousness
- reversible toxic cardiomyopathy

Staphylococcal TSS toxin-1 (TSST-1) and staphylococcal enterotoxin-B are the implicated toxins. Routine cultures for staphylococci and streptococci should be performed, and, if possible, assays for the staphylococcal toxin should be performed.

Treatment

- correction of shock
- anti-staphylococcal antibiotics
- Supportive measures, as for septicaemia (see p. 195)

HUMAN IMMUNODEFICIENCY VIRUS INFECTION

The human immunodeficiency virus (HIV) is a human RNA virus with an enzyme that enables it to make a DNA copy of its RNA genome. The DNA genome then integrates with the genome of the host cell. Consequently, with every replication of the host cell, viral replication is assured. For that reason, infection with HIV is presumed to be life-long.

HIV selectively destroys a subset of T lymphocytes – the helper T lymphocytes. The percentage and absolute number of these cells gradually diminish over months to years, and the infected person becomes susceptible to opportunistic infections and neoplasms, the onset of which defines the diagnosis of acquired immunodeficiency syndrome (AIDS).

AIDS is part of the final stage of a spectrum of infections involving HIV.

AIDS patients may present with Kaposi's sarcoma, pneumonia (usually caused by *Pneumocystis carinii*), fever, lymphadenopathy, malaise, tiredness, loss of weight, diarrhoea, dysphagia, and retrosternal pain. Neurological presentations include meningitis (usually caused by *Cryptococcus neoformans*), facial lesions (*Toxoplasma gondii*, lymphoma, or cryptococcal abscess), and progressive dementia (HIV encephalopathy). The most common neoplasms are Kaposi's sarcoma and non-Hodgkin's lymphoma.

Current evidence indicates that the risk for developing severe HIV disease increases with the duration of infection. In the absence of anti-retroviral intervention, approximately 50% of HIV-infected persons will develop severe HIV disease over a period of 10 years. Accurate figures for any longer period are not yet known.

Diagnosis

Antibodies against HIV usually can be detected within 6 weeks following infection. The antibodies are tested using an enzyme-linked immunosorbent assay (ELISA) or Western immunoblot (WB) test. The ELISA test is currently used for screening because of its excellent specificity and sensitivity, and the WB test is used to confirm anti-HIV status. HIV can be isolated and cultured, but that is time-consuming and requires special expertise.

IMPLICATIONS IN INTENSIVE CARE

HIV can be transmitted by contact with infected blood or blood products and through the transplantation of infected organs, bone grafts, or tissue.

There have been a few cases in which HIV presumably has been transmitted by needle-stick accidents.

Currently there is no evidence to suggest that HIV can be transmitted to hospital staff by contact with the secretions of HIV patients or by aerosol of secretions from patients to staff, but precautions are still mandatory.

At present, there is no cure for AIDS. However, remissions can be achieved, especially of life-threatening *P. carinii* pneumonia. This may involve respiratory support in intensive care or the use of CPAP in a general ward.

Precautions

Every health-care facility must define its policies and address the issues raised by its management of patients with HIV infections and other infectious diseases such as hepatitis.

• Universal precautions: All blood and body fluids should be treated as being potential sources of infection.

• Handling of needles and 'sharps': Work practices that will minimize the handling of sharp instruments and objects should be developed (eg the use of staples or clips instead of sutures during surgery). Used needles should not be re-sheathed by hand. Neither should they be removed from disposable syringes by hand, nor bent or manipulated in any way by hand. Persons handling a sharp must be responsible for its proper disposal. Sharp items should be disposed of in a puncture-resistant container.

• The staff should be educated about the factors associated with transmission of disease and actions to be taken should accidental exposure occur.

• There must be adequate facilities (eg for hand-washing and decontamination).

- Safe systems are needed (eg personal protective equipment and equipment to avoid needle-stick injury).
- There should be a system for the reporting of accidents (eg needle-stick injuries) and follow-up, including counselling.
- Vaccination programmes should be kept current.
- Policies on confidentiality and notification should be clearly stated.

Gloves should be worn for direct or potential contact with blood or body fluids. A combination of mask and protective eyewear or face shield should be worn when aerosolization or splattering of blood is envisaged. Protective apparel (eg gowns, aprons, and overshoes) should be worn during procedures in which blood is likely to be splashed (eg autopsies, trauma, and surgical procedures).

MANAGEMENT OF POTENTIAL HIV EXPOSURE

- Promptly wash away the contaminating fluid.
- Encourage bleeding. Wash with soap and copious amounts of water.
- Report the incident.
- The source patient should be informed, and consent must be gained for serological testing for evidence of HIV antibody and hepatitis.
- If the source patient is positive for HIV antibody or the source is no longer available, baseline HIV serology should be performed.
- Any febrile illness occurring within 12 weeks of exposure should be reported.
- Exposed individuals initially found to be seronegative should be retested after 6 weeks and at periodic intervals thereafter.
- Counselling should be available for exposed individuals.
- If the source patient is seronegative and is not at risk for HIV infection, no further follow-up is necessary.
- Azidothymidine (AZT) prophylaxis may be offered to exposed individuals when the risk of transmission is significant and the exposure is known to involve HIV-positive blood. The suggested dosage is 200 mg orally 5 times per day for 6 weeks.

VIRAL INFECTIONS

IMPORTANCE IN INTENSIVE CARE

Viral infections can sometimes present as primary diseases in patients, such as herpes encephalitis (see Chapter 25) and Guillain-Barré syndrome (see Chapter 26). Secondary infections can occur as a result of reactivations of viruses from a vegetative state, often in immunocompromised hosts.

Though the chances are small, there is always the potential danger that staff members can contract viral diseases after contact with patients, such as hepatitis transmission (see p. 231) and HIV (see p. 227).

DIAGNOSIS OF VIRAL INFECTIONS

Laboratory diagnosis of a viral infection usually comes too late to influence management, and even with more rapid diagnostic techniques, definitive treatment is limited.

The diagnostic techniques available include rapid methods such as DFA, cell culture, serology, and tissue biopsy with electron microscopy. Close co-operation with the microbiologist is needed in this rapidly developing area.

TREATMENT

Because of the parasitic association between viruses and the host cells, drugs that interfere with the viral cycle often are also toxic to the host. However, some recent developments are promising:

ACYCLOVIR   Acyclovir has a high degree of activity against herpes simplex (1 and 2) and somewhat less against varicella zoster viruses. It is available in oral, intravenous (10 mg/kg IV, 8-hourly, for 10 days, for encephalitis or disseminated disease) (see p. 610), and topical preparations. Its toxicity is minimal. Other drugs such as ribavirin, amantadine, and ganciclovir are also used.

INTERFERON   Interferon is a protein with broad-spectrum antiviral activity. Large quantities can be produced using recombinant DNA technology. Current uses include selected cases of hepatitis B and C and genital warts.

VIRAL HEPATITIS

Hepatitis A Virus

Hepatitis A virus (HAV) is transmitted by the orofaecal route and produces the classic short-incubation infectious hepatitis. Several different types of vaccines are being developed for its prevention, but there is no specific treatment.

Hepatitis B virus

Hepatitis B virus (HBV) causes long-incubation serum hepatitis and can be transmitted by chronic carriers who usually are asymptomatic. It has become a major health problem throughout the world and is now responsible for almost half of all cases of hepatitis. The presence of its viral surface antigen (HBsAg) in serum signifies infection, whereas IgG antibody to the surface antigen (anti-HBs) signifies past infection and may indicate immunity. Protection of the staff is particularly important in the ICU, as secretions from patients seropositive for HBsAg are infectious.

The patients who are particularly at risk of being HBsAg-positive are drug addicts, those who have received multiple blood transfusions, homosexually active men, immigrants from areas of high endemicity, and patients on long-term haemodialysis. All staff members who work in intensive care are advised to be actively immunized against hepatitis B infection – 90% will develop antibodies, which will confer almost 100% immunity. An initial course of three intramuscular doses (0, 1, and 6 months) is recommended. All health-care workers are now being encouraged to become immunized.

PRECAUTIONS WHEN TREATING A PATIENT WHO IS HBSAG-POSITIVE
UTMOST CARE MUST BE TAKEN WITH ALL SECRETIONS:

- Handle all needles and sharp instruments with care.
- Wear disposable gloves and gowns.
- Wash hands regularly.

• Bed and linen should be disinfected with suitable chemicals, such as bleach.

• Secretions such as urine, blood, and faeces should be disposed of carefully and labelled prominently for the attention of laboratory staff.

• If a staff member accidentally sustains a needle-stick injury, a standard protocol should be followed, involving testing of the source, if known, vaccination of the staff member, and use of hyperimmune γ-globulin if the staff member has not been vaccinated and the source is HBsAg-positive.

Hepatitis C virus

Hepatitis C virus (HCV) is a recently identified virus that may be responsible for many of the cases of so-called non-A, non-B hepatitis transmitted by blood transfusions, in addition to being associated with chronic active hepatitis, cirrhosis, and hepatocellular carcinoma. All donor blood should be screened for antibodies to HCV. Interferon-α may be useful in patients with chronic hepatitis C.

Non-A, non-B hepatitis

Non-A, non-B (NANB) hepatitis is a diagnosis of exclusion, as no specific test is available. Now that hepatitis C has been separated from the previous NANB classification, it remains to be seen whether or not there will be one or more distinct viruses responsible for NANB hepatitis.

Delta hepatitis (hepatitis D virus)

Delta hepatitis is caused by hepatitis D virus (HDV), which consists of a delta inner core encapsulated by the surface Ag of hepatitis B virus. It can occur only in patients with hepatitis B, either simultaneously or as a superinfection that often makes the primary infection worse. Delta hepatitis infection can be indirectly prevented by vaccinating with hepatitis B vaccine. This is because the HDV is defective and requires active HBV infection in order to survive.

Hepatitis E virus

Hepatitis E virus (HEV) is another recently identified RNA virus responsible for enterically transmitted NANB hepatitis. It is common in developing countries and should be considered a possibility in travellers with a clinical picture of hepatitis A who are negative for HAV IgM.

FUNGAL INFECTIONS

Systemic fungal infections in the ICU usually are associated with prolonged use of broad-spectrum antibiotics or long-term intravenous feeding, or they can occur as complications in immunocompromised hosts. The two most common are caused by *Candida* spp. and *Aspergillus* spp. There are several different species in each genus.

CANDIDA

Candida spp. compose part of the normal human flora. Disseminated infection usually results from an overgrowth of gastro-intestinal *Candida* during antibiotic treatment, particularly with broad-spectrum antibiotics. The body's defence system usually is efficient in dealing with transient systemic candidaemia, but defence is compromised particularly in patients with diabetes or leukaemia, in those receiving corticosteroids, cytotoxic treatment, or parenteral nutrition, and in those with long-term central venous access. Candidaemia can also present as endocarditis, particularly in drug abusers. The clinical picture of systemic *Candida* infection is similar to those for other forms of sepsis (see p. 183).

SYSTEMIC *CANDIDA* INFECTION IS A DIFFICULT DIAGNOSIS TO MAKE, AND AS A RESULT, IT IS OFTEN DELAYED. IT ENTAILS VERY HIGH MORTALITY, AND ITS TREATMENT INVOLVES A HIGH INCIDENCE OF COMPLICATIONS.

Diagnosis

Positive blood cultures are found in only 40–50% of cases, and a positive culture does not necessarily mean generalized infection. An increased yield of positive cultures can be obtained if lysis centrifugation techniques are used. Clinical evidence of generalized infections should be sought, including biopsy and culture of infected tissues. Specific funduscopic signs can be seen in approximately 30% of cases.

Serological tests for antibody and antigen are still experimental.

The diagnosis is usually made clinically, with or without laboratory confirmation.

Treatment

PROPHYLAXIS

• nystatin, 500,000 units, 6-hourly, orally (nasogastrically)

• nystatin mouthwashes may decrease the incidence of fungaemia in patients at risk.

Because the treatment carries its own high risks, it should not be commenced unless there is a strong index of suspicion (eg neutropenic patients or seriously ill patients not responding to multiple antibiotics).

Empirical antifungal treatment is often used in a febrile neutropenic host who has not responded to maximum antibacterial treatment (see p. 210).

AMPHOTERICIN B   Amphotericin B must be given for suspected cases of disseminated *Candida* infection, in spite of its high toxicity.

Dosage: Given an initial test dose of 1 mg in 20 ml of 5% dextrose IV over 30 minutes. Then give 0.3 mg/kg, dissolved in 500 ml of 5% dextrose, given over 2–6 hours on day 1. Increase to 0.5–0.9 mg/kg on subsequent days. Continue until there is clinical improvement. In seriously ill patients, progression to full dosage should be rapid (eg over 24 hours).

Toxic effects: Amphotericin B invariably causes renal toxicity (cease when serum creatinine = 200 μmol/L, and resume after 3–5 days, at same dosage). Alternate-day dosing may decrease renal toxicity. Renal function will gradually return to normal when the drug is reduced or ceased. Amphotericin B also causes thrombophlebitis, anaemia, hypokalaemia, hypomagnesaemia, weight loss, nausea, anorexia, and vomiting. If given rapidly, it can cause anaphylaxis, hypotension, convulsions, and arrhythmias.

Although other antifungal agents might appear to be more attractive, because of their lower toxicities (eg miconazole and ketoconazole), they are not as reliable as amphotericin B for treatment of systemic candidiasis. Combination treatment may be beneficial.

ASPERGILLOSIS

Unlike infections caused by *Candida* spp., aspergillosis is primarily an exogenous infection, and dissemination is usually from a pulmonary source. It is the second most common infection caused by a fungal genus in immunocompromised hosts (apart from patients with AIDS, in whom *Cryptococcus* is more common). Aspergilloma formation and allergic aspergillosis do not usually occur in seriously ill patients.

Diagnosis

Although the growth of *Aspergillus* spp. in tracheal aspirates can be a normal finding, in an immunocompromised patient such a finding should be treated with a high index of suspicion.

Blood cultures are rarely positive for *Aspergillus* spp.

Treatment

Treatment is as for candidiasis (see p. 234).

Itraconazole, a new imidazole derivative, shows greater promise than any other agent. *Aspergillus* spp. are relatively resistant to amphotericin and are unaffected by 5-flucytosine, miconazole, and ketoconazole. For severe cases, amphotericin will also have to be used, as for candidiasis.

TROUBLESHOOTING

IS IT AN AUTOIMMUNE DISEASE?

Occasionally one will see a patient who presents with an acute autoimmune disease. This usually is manifested as single-organ or multiorgan dysfunction and must be differentiated from more common conditions, such as septicaemia.

Autoimmune diseases
Systemic lupus erythematosus (SLE)
Polymyositis
Dermatomyositis
Chronic active hepatitis
Rheumatoid arthritis
Glomerulonephritis
Sjögren's syndrome
Wegeners' granulomatosis
Goodpasture's syndrome

Common presentations of autoimmune diseases
Psychosis, confusion, seizures
Anaemia, pancytopenia
Haemoptysis, dyspnoea
Myocarditis
Jaundice
Cutaneous vasculitis, palpable purpura
Arthralgia, swollen joints
Pain and polymyositis

TROUBLESHOOTING

SCREENING INVESTIGATIONS FOR AUTOIMMUNE DISEASES

Haemoglobin and full blood count

Antinuclear antigen (ANA)   A positive result is suggestive of
SLE
Polymyositis
Dermatomyositis
Sjögren's syndrome
Rheumatoid arthritis

Double-strand DNA   If positive, suggestive of SLE.

Extractable nuclear antigen   Diagnosis depends on which type of antigen is positive.

Rheumatoid factor   Strong indicator of active rheumatoid arthritis.

Complement levels C3, C4, CH$_{50}$ If low, they suggest that a complement-activating disease is present.

Immune complexes   An increase is suggestive of immune-system activation.

Antinuclear cytoplasmic antibody (ANCA)   If positive, indicates Wegener's or crescentic glomerulonephritis.

Anti-glomerular-basement-membrane antibody (anti-GBMAb)   Indicates Goodpasture's syndrome.

Creatinine phosphokinase   If high, consistent with polymyositis.

Antimitochondrial antibody   Indicates primary biliary cirrhosis.

Anti-smooth-muscle antibody   Indicates chronic active hepatitis.

Cryoglobulin   Consistent with essential mixed cryoglobulinaemia.

TROUBLESHOOTING

MICROBIOLOGY: SOME TIPS ON INTERPRETING RESULTS

Microbiology findings, unlike biochemical parameters, are open to interpretation as to their relevance and what, if any, clinical action should be taken. Liaise closely with microbiologists about the relevance of positive findings and the trends in surveillance.

The following should be considered:

1. Does the patient have a clinical infection?

2. Are the microbiology findings relevant to the clinical findings?

3. If the findings are relevant, the most appropriate treatment should be chosen.

Blood cultures   Very useful if positive. About 5% of positive cultures are due to contamination.

Sputum   There is little correlation between the micro-organisms that cause pneumonia and the organisms found in the sputum of seriously ill patients. Positive blood cultures and other techniques are more accurate (see p. 201).

Streptococcus pneumoniae may be present in patients with acute bronchitis or can even be found in the throat of a normal carrier, in addition to being a cause of pneumonia.

Haemophilus influenzae and *Moraxella catarrhalis* are common colonizers in chronic airflow limitation and may not be clinically significant.

Staphylococcus aureus is often associated with the presence of a nasogastric tube and chronic bronchitis.

Mixed growth of non-haemolytic streptococci and *Neisseria* spp. is usual in the normal throat flora.

Coliforms, including *Escherichia coli* and *Klebsiella,* are common colonizers, especially in the seriously ill.

Wounds   *S. aureus* in a pure heavy growth from an inflamed wound is suggestive of wound infection. However, scanty or light growth could represent colonization.

Streptococcus pyogenes, even in small numbers, is probably significant.

Other organisms, even in high numbers, may simply be colonizers of wounds:

Coagulase-negative staphylococci

Gram-negative aerobes, including *Pseudomonas,* diphtheroids, and enterococci

Urine   A count of more than 10^8 viable bacteria per litre in a midstream specimen with red/white cells is suggestive of a UTI if the growth is pure. Catheter samples invariably have red and white cells and colonization, and so a diagnosis of UTI on that basis alone is inappropriate. There must be other signs of systemic infection.

FURTHER READING

General

Bellomo, R. (1992). The cytokine network in the critically ill. *Anaesthesia and Intensive Care* 20:288–302.

Bone, R. C. (ed.) (1992). Definitions for sepsis and organ failure and guidelines for the use of innovative therapies in sepsis. *Chest* 101:1644–55.

Bruining, H. A. (ed.) (1990). Infections in intensive care. *Intensive Care Medicine (Suppl. 3)* 16:181–247 (symposium issue).

Howard, R. J. (1988). Surgical infections. *Surgical Clinics of North America* 68:1–232 (symposium issue).

Parrillo, J. E. (1993). Pathogenetic mechanisms of septic shock. *New England Journal of Medicine* 328:1971–7.

Tibballs, J. (1993). The role of nitric oxide (formerly endothelium-derived relaxant factor, EDRF) in vasodilation and vasodilator therapy. *Anaesthesia and Intensive Care* 21:759–73.

Sources of Infection in the ICU

Daschner, F. D. (1985). Useful and useless hygienic techniques in intensive care units. *Intensive Care Medicine* 11:280–3.

Daschner, F. D., Frey, P., Wolff, G., Baumann, P. C., & Suter, P. (1982). Nosocomial infections in intensive care wards. A multicenter prospective study. *Intensive Care Medicine* 8:5–9.

Levin, S., Goodman, L. J., & Fuhrer, J. (1986). Fulminant community-acquired infectious diseases: diagnostic problems. *Medical Clinics of North America* 70:967–86.

Mackowiak, P. A. (1982). The normal microbial flora. *New England Journal of Medicine* 307:83–93.

Plit, M. L., Lipman, J., Eidelman, J., & Gavavdan, J. (1988). *Intensive Care Medicine* 14:503–9.

Septicaemia

Jacobs, E. R., Bone, R. C. (1986). Clinical indicators in sepsis and septic adult respiratory distress syndrome. *Medical Clinics of North America* 70:921–32.

Karakusis, P. H. (1986). Considerations in the therapy of septic shock. *Medical Clinics of North America* 70:933–44.

Luce, J. M. (1987). Pathogenesis and management of septic shock. *Chest* 9:883–8.

Luce, J. M. (1993). Introduction of new technology into critical care practice: a history of HA-1A human monoclonal antibody against endotoxin. *Critical Care Medicine* 21:1233–41.

Parker, M. M., & Fink, M. P. (1992). Septic shock. *Journal of Intensive Care Medicine* 7:90–100.

Rackow, E. C., Asitz, M. E., Weil, M. H. (1988). Cellular oxygen metabolism during sepsis and shock. *Journal of the American Medical Association* 259:1989–93.

Scott, M. A. J., Norwood, M. C., & Civetta, J. M. (1987). Evaluating sepsis in critically ill patients. *Chest* 92:137–44.

Steele, T. W. (1985). Acute enteric sepsis, bacteriology and antibiotic cover. *Anaesthesia and Intensive Care* 13:241–8.

Thijs, L. G., Schneider, A. J., & Groeneveld, A. B. J. (1990). The haemodynamics of septic shock. *Intensive Care Medicine* 16:S182–6.

Warren, H. S., Danner, R. L., & Munford, R. S. (1992). Anti-endotoxin monoclonal antibodies. *New England Journal of Medicine* 326:1153–7.

Zimmerli, W. (1985). Impaired host defense mechanisms in intensive care patients. *Intensive Care Medicine* 11:174–8.

Approach to Unidentified Infections

Miller, R. T., Kapusnik, J. E., & Sandle, M. A. (1984). The diagnosis and therapy of infections in the intensive care unit. In *Critical Care: State of the Art,* vol. 5, ed. W. C. Shoemaker, pp. 1–58. Fullerton, CA: Society of Critical Care Medicine.

Antimicrobials

Follath, F. (1985). The use of new broad-spectrum antibiotics. *Intensive Care Medicine* 9:277–9.

Hamilton-Miller, J. M. T. (1990). The emergence of antibiotic resistance: myths and facts in clinical practice. *Intensive Care Medicine* 16:S206–11.

Waldvogel, F. A. (1985). Third generation cephalosporins – a panacea for intensive care patients? *Intensive Care Medicine* 11:184–5.

Intra-abdominal Sepsis

Ahrenholz, D. H., & Simmons, R. L. (1983). Peritonitis and intraabdominal abscesses. In *Critical Care: State of the Art,* vol. 4, ed. W. C. Shoemaker & W. L. Thompson, pp. B1–24.

Gerzof, S. G., & Oates, M. E. (1988). Imaging techniques for infections in the surgical patient. *Surgical Clinics of North America* 68:147–66.

Hinsdale, J. G., & Jaffe, B. M. (1984). Reoperation for intraabdominal sepsis. *Annals of Surgery* 199:31–6.

Joseph, A. E. A. (1985). Imaging of abdominal abscesses (editorial). *British Medical Journal* 291:1446–7.

Schein, M., Saddia, R., & Decker, G. A. (1988). The open management of the septic abdomen. *Surgery, Gynecology and Obstetrics* 163:587–92.

Walsh, G. L., Chiasson, P., Hedderich, G., Wexler, M. J., & Meakins, J. L. (1988). The open abdomen. *Surgical Clinics of North America* 68:25–40.

Unusual Infections

Ahrenholz, D. H. (1988). Necrotizing soft tissue infections. *Surgical Clinics of North America* 68:199–214.

Banks, R. A., Lindley, K. J., Pozniak, A. L. (1985). AIDS: a problem for intensive care. *Intensive Care Medicine* 11:169–71.

Chernoff, A. E., & Snydman, D. R. (1993). Viral infections in the intensive care unit. *New Horizons* 1:279–301.

Edwards, J. E. (1991). Invasive *Candida* infections. *New England Journal of Medicine* 324:1060–2.

Franklin, C., & Metry, M. (1992). Life threatening *Candida* infections in the intensive care unit. *Journal of Intensive Care Medicine* 7:127–37.

Gore, M. E., & Selby, P. (1987). Antiviral chemotherapy. *British Journal of Hospital Medicine* 37:22–6.

Hoeprich, P. D. (1992). Clinical use of amphotericin B and derivatives: lore, mystique and fact. *Clinical Infectious Diseases (Suppl.)* 14:114–19.

Jeffries, D. J. (1983). Viruses and intensive care. *Intensive Care Medicine* 9:105–7.

Okrent, D. G., Abraham, E., & Winston, D. (1987). Cardiorespiratory patterns in viral septicaemia. *American Journal of Medicine* 83:681–6.

Shands, K. N., Dan, B. B., & Schmid, G. P. (1981). Toxic shock syndrome: the emerging picture. *Annals of Internal Medicine* 94:264–6.

Stewart, G. J. (ed.) (1993). HIV illnesses. *Medical Journal of Australia* 158:31–3.

Tehrani, M. A., Ledingham, I. M. A. (1977). Necrotizing fasciitis. *Postgraduate Medical Journal* 53:237–42.

14

TRAUMA

- The key to good results in trauma patients is rapid resuscitation.
- A systematic, standardized team approach is required for optimal assessment, resuscitation, management, and definitive treatment of patients.
- Whereas it is common to under-transfuse hypovolaemic patients, it is almost impossible to over-transfuse them.

MULTITRAUMA

THE GOLDEN HOUR

What happens during the first hour or 'golden hour' following severe trauma will largely determine the patient's eventual outcome. Rapid resuscitation is essential. Restoration of the circulation is one of the key goals in managing patients with major trauma. In the presence of significant hypovolaemia, blood is redirected to the so-called vital organs – the brain, heart, and kidneys. The so-called non-vital organs suffer relative ischaemia. This has important implications for the splanchnic circulation. Hypoperfusion of the gastro-intestinal tract (GIT) predisposes to bacterial translocation and endotoxin absorption across a compromised mucosal barrier. This is compounded by ischaemia of the reticuloendothelial system, particularly the liver, which otherwise would filter bacteria and toxins from the portal circulation. It has been proposed that bacterial translocation predisposes to the multiorgan failure (MOF) frequently seen after multitrauma. It seems crucial, therefore, to rapidly restore the circulation. This means not only maintaining a normal blood pressure but also guaranteeing perfusion to the non-vital organs, particularly the GIT.

INITIAL ASSESSMENT AND MANAGEMENT (Table 14.1)

Airway

Initial attempts to establish an airway usually include chin-lift and jaw-thrust manoeuvres. Blood and secretions should be sucked out, foreign bodies removed, and an oropharyngeal airway inserted, if necessary. If there is any doubt about the airway, INTUBATE, especially if the patient is UNCONSCIOUS or has FACIAL INJURIES.

Special attention should be given to the possibility of fracture of the cervical spine. The patient's head should not be hyperextended or hyperflexed when establishing or maintaining an airway. Maintain the cervical spine in a neutral position. This can be facilitated by having an assistant hold the patient's head in the neutral position during intubation. Other ways of immobilizing the cervical spine when damage is suspected or has not been excluded include the use of hard cervical collars or sandbags or taping the head to a spinal board.

Breathing

Ensure adequate ventilation. The patient's breathing may be compromised by a decreased level of consciousness, airway obstruction, pneumothoraces, haemothoraces, diaphragmatic injury, multiple rib fractures, flail chest, cervical spine damage, phrenic nerve damage, or increased intra-abdominal pressure (Figure 14.1).

If there is any doubt about the patient's breathing, INTUBATE and VENTILATE.

If ventilation remains a problem, rule out the possibility of a tension pneumothorax, which would worsen with positive-pressure ventilation.

Rapidly drain any significant collections of air or blood in the pleural cavity.

All patients who are in shock are hypoxic and need OXYGENATION, with as high a concentration of inspired oxygen (F_{IO_2}) as can be administered, until arterial blood-gas tests are performed.

Circulation

RESTORE THE BLOOD VOLUME – hypovolaemia is common in trauma patients (Table 14.2). Blood loss is life-threatening, but it is easily cor-

TABLE 14.1 ASSESSMENT GUIDELINES FOR MULTITRAUMA

Primary survey: assessment of ABCs

1. Airway and cervical spine control:
  • Use chin-lift and jaw-thrust manoeuvres; then oropharyngeal airway, and intubate if in doubt.
  • Protect the cervical spine.

2. Breathing:
  • All patients should be given the maximum inspired O_2 concentration initially.
  • Artificially ventilate if in doubt.
  • Evacuate pneumothoraces and haemopneumothoraces.

3. Circulation, with haemorrhage control:
  • Use at least two large IV cannulae – rapid fluid replacement.
  • Do not hesitate to use group-specific blood.
  • A MAST suit may be used as a temporary measure.
  • Give inotropes, if necessary, and examine for cardiac tamponade.
  • Do not place a patient head-down.

4. Disability: Conduct a brief neurological evaluation.

5. Exposure: Completely undress the patient.

Ensure that the ABC parameters have been stabilized before proceeding to the secondary survey.

RAPIDLY AND SIMULTANEOUSLY ASSESS (history and examination) **AND RESUSCITATE.**

Secondary survey

  1. Head and skull (including ears)
  2. Maxillofacial injuries
  3. Neck
  4. Chest
  5. Abdomen/pelvis
  6. Back, perineum, and rectum – log-roll the patient
  7. Extremities
  8. Complete neurological examination
  9. Appropriate x-rays, laboratory tests, and special studies
  10. 'Tubes and fingers' in every orifice

SUMMARIZE FINDINGS, AND PLAN THE NEXT STAGE OF TREATMENT.

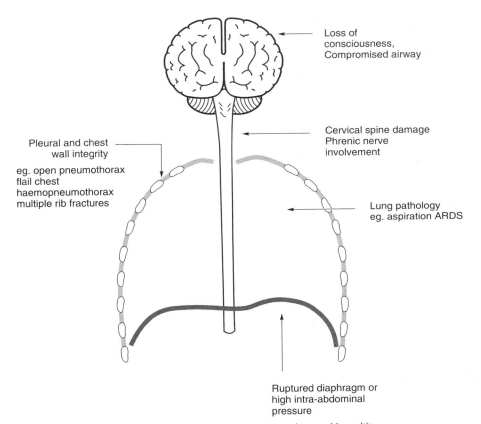

Loss of
consciousness,
Compromised airway

Cervical spine damage
Phrenic nerve
involvement

Pleural and chest
wall integrity

eg. open pneumothorax
flail chest
haemopneumothorax
multiple rib fractures

Lung pathology
eg. aspiration ARDS

Ruptured diaphragm or
high intra-abdominal
pressure

FIGURE 14.1 Factors that can affect ventilation in patients with multitrauma.

rectable. It is difficult to over-transfuse hypovolaemic patients, but it is extremely common to under-transfuse them. Never place a shock patient in the head-down position. Leg elevation is a better temporary measure for hypotension. A MAST suit (medical anti-shock trousers) may also be an advantage in severe hypovolaemia. However, the best treatment for hypovolaemia is rapid fluid replacement. Always use two large (at least 16 gauge) peripheral cannulae. Rule out the possibility of cardiac tamponade (see p. 279).

TYPE OF FLUID FOR INITIAL INTRAVASCULAR-VOLUME REPLACEMENT
There may be advantages in using colloid or even hypertonic saline,

TABLE 14.2 FIVE SITES OF MAJOR BLOOD LOSS

1. External: Conduct an examination, and take a history.
2. Chest: Loss will be obvious on the chest x-ray or as loss from an intercostal catheter.
3. Abdomen: Use lavage or clinical examination.
4. Retroperitoneum: This is a diagnosis of exclusion, if 1–3 are negative. Retroperitoneal losses often are associated with a fractured pelvis.
5. Major fracture: Examine femur, pelvis, and pelvic x-ray.

TABLE 14.3 IMMEDIATE INVESTIGATIONS FOR PATIENTS SUFFERING SEVERE MULTITRAUMA

Get immediate blood cross-match and baseline values for biochemistry, arterial blood gases, and haematology.

Chest x-ray (if there is a widened mediastinum or other signs of ruptured thoracic aorta, an immediate aortogram is necessary).

Lateral x-ray of cervical spine.

Pelvic x-ray.

Diagnostic peritoneal lavage.

Cranial CT scan – for all patients with significant neurological impairments or deteriorating neurological signs.

rather than crystalloid solution, in cases of severe hypovolaemia (see Chapter 8). However, the real challenge is to replenish the circulating volume as rapidly as possible. Because a saline cross-match for ABO compatibility can be performed in less than 10 minutes, rapidly cross-matched (group-specific) blood should be used early in cases of severe bleeding until fully cross-matched blood is available. Fully cross-matched blood (99.9% serologically safe) is only marginally safer than group-specific ABO-compatible blood (99.4% serologically safe).

INITIAL MONITORING (Table 14.3)

As a first step, it is important to simultaneously assess and rapidly resuscitate the patient. **DO NOT SPEND TIME ON COMPLICATED**

MONITORING OR INVESTIGATIONS UNTIL THE PATIENT IS ADE-
QUATELY RESUSCITATED.

Respiration

- adequacy of airway and chest movement
- airway pressure if the patient is ventilated
- color
- respiratory rate
- upright chest x-ray
- pulse oximetry (non-invasive, continuous, easily obtained estimate of oxygenation that can, however, be compromised by poor peripheral perfusion) (see p. 507)

Circulation

- Pulse rate will more accurately 'track' hypovolaemia in the young than in the elderly.
- Blood pressure: Because of well-developed sympatheticoadrenal responses, a young, fit patient often will maintain good arterial blood pressure until just before circulatory collapse, whereas in the elderly, blood pressure tracks the circulation more accurately.
- Urine output: Beware of inappropriate polyuria secondary to use of alcohol, mannitol, or intravenous contrast solution.
- Arterial blood gases, particularly arterial pH, can reflect the status of the circulation.
- Skin perfusion, as estimated by skin temperature, will provide a simple indication of hypovolaemia in multitrauma patients. It may be difficult to estimate when a patient has central hypothermia, when there is a low ambient temperature, or when the local arterial blood supply to a limb is compromised.
- ECG monitoring is easy to perform and can be useful during the early stages of resuscitation, even as a continuous readout of pulse rate.

LATER MONITORING

When a patient is stable, measurement of central venous pressure (CVP) may be useful for estimating fluid replacement. The only value in having a central line initially is to facilitate fluid administration, not to measure intravascular pressures. Even then it is preferable to use large-diameter cannulae. When the patient has been initially resuscitated, measurements such as pulmonary artery wedge pressure (PAWP), cardiac output, oxygen delivery (Do_2), and oxygen consumption ($\dot{V}o_2$) may be useful for fine-tuning the circulation. The place of tonometry (measurement of gastric mucosal pH) (see p. 493) during early resuscitation following major trauma has not been determined. However, early work suggests that it is very promising.

FURTHER ASSESSMENT AND MANAGEMENT

History

A history of the incident should be sought, especially from the first person on the scene, as well as from the patient, if possible, and others who witnessed the incident that caused the trauma.

Examination

A top-to-bottom examination of the patient should be performed: Determine the level of consciousness using the Glasgow coma scale (GCS), and document any lateralizing signs. Look for external scalp lacerations (which can cause significant roadside blood loss), otorrhoea, rhinorrhoea, facial fractures (use palpation), flail segments, and fractured ribs. Examine the neck for tenderness, penetrating wounds, pulses and bruits, venous distension, tracheal position, and evidence of subcutaneous air. Remove all clothing, and carefully examine the abdomen and pelvis. Perform rectal and vaginal examinations. Always examine the patient's back. All this should take only minutes. Finally, assess the limbs. Do not x-ray limbs at this stage; wait until the patient is adequately resuscitated. Radiography is time-consuming. Limb fractures usually are obvious and are not immediately life-threatening.

The next steps

Continue to reassess the **AIRWAY, VENTILATION, OXYGENATION,** and **CIRCULATION** during the initial examination.

TABLE 14.4 FEATURES TO BE NOTED ON A LATERAL VIEW OF THE CERVICAL SPINE

All seven vertebral bodies must be clearly seen, including C7–T1 junction.

Evaluate alignments of the posterior cervical line, the four lordotic curves, the anterior longitudinal ligament line, the posterior longitudinal ligament line, the spinolaminal line, and the tips of the spinous processes.

Evaluate the predental space (<3 mm in adults, 4–5 mm in children).

Evaluate each vertebra for fractures and increased or decreased density (eg compression fracture).

Evaluate the intervertebral and interspinous spaces (an angulation of more than 11° at a single space is abnormal).

Evaluate fanning of the spinous processes, suggestive of posterior ligament disruption.

Evaluate prevertebral soft-tissue distance (<7 mm at C2, and <5 mm at C2–C4).

Evaluate the atlanto-occipital region for possible dislocation.

LABORATORY TESTS Take blood for cross-matching, if necessary, and for other determinations: haemoglobin, haematocrit, white cells, platelets, urea, creatinine, and electrolytes.

CERVICAL SPINE X-RAY Obtain a lateral view of the cervical spine (Table 14.4). If all seven bodies cannot be seen, maintain spinal immobilization until the initial resuscitation is complete, when further views can be contemplated. A lateral film will detect damage in approximately 90% of cervical spine injuries. Conditions that are associated with higher risks for cervical spine damage include neck tenderness, an altered level of consciousness, alcohol intoxication, and other signs and symptoms suggestive of spinal damage; such associated conditions may indicate the need for further spinal views.

UPRIGHT CHEST X-RAY An upright chest x-ray is the next investigation to be performed. Attend to any gas or fluid collections, and check for a widened mediastinum. Further investigation is required in the case of a widened mediastinum. Note fractured ribs, lung contusions, and heart size.

PELVIC X-RAY Following the chest x-ray and a lateral view of the cervical spine, the only other x-ray that should be obtained early in the patient's management is a pelvic x-ray, to exclude fractures that might be sources of substantial blood loss. 'Springing' of the pelvis is a very poor indicator of fractures and probably should no longer be employed. A pelvic x-ray probably is not necessary in a fully conscious patient with no symptoms.

ABDOMINAL EXAMINATION A careful examination of the abdomen should be conducted, including palpation of all four quadrants and a pelvic examination if one has not already been performed. Diagnostic peritoneal lavage should be considered at this stage (see p. 262). If the shock cannot be rapidly corrected, or if the bleeding is obvious and is from such a source that it may be life-threatening, surgery should be performed immediately.

Nasogastric (NG) tubes should be used for intubated patients if there is no contraindication, such as the suspicion of a basilar skull fracture, in which case tubes should be placed orally.

A urinary catheter should be inserted if there is no evidence to suggest urethral disruption (eg blood at the urethral meatus), no perineal, scrotal, or penile injury, and no abnormality on examination of the prostate.

MICROBIOLOGY Tetanus toxoid and tetanus immune globulin, as well as antibiotics, should be administered if they are clinically indicated.

Placement

After resuscitation, patients who have sustained severe trauma should be rapidly placed into other units or sent for further tests:

• Laparotomy, thoracotomy, or decompressive craniotomy in the operating theatre.

• CT scan of the brain.

• Angiography – either aortogram (if there is a widened mediastinum) or pelvic embolization (for uncontrolled bleeding).

• An intensive care environment: All other investigations and x-rays can be performed in an intensive care unit (ICU). In some centres, the initial receiving room or an adjacent area may serve as a site for continuous management, rather than an ICU.

• General ward (if the patient is stable) or discharge (if there was only minor trauma).

As part of the trauma audit process, the time of transfer from the receiving room to another unit should be recorded, and delays should be reviewed.

CONTINUING MANAGEMENT IN INTENSIVE CARE

Continuing management in an ICU has the following goals:

• assessment and continuing resuscitation
• 'fine tuning' during further resuscitation
• monitoring of patients for complications
• co-ordination of all other services, and planning for further definitive care
• secondary examinations for injuries overlooked initially (minor fractures, soft-tissue damage, and nerve injuries can be easily missed during the flurry of initial resuscitation)

Monitoring

A primary, continuing aim during resuscitation is to promote oxygen delivery (Do_2) to the cells (see Chapter 17), with adequate oxygen saturation, haemoglobin, and blood flow. Although continued frequent monitoring of skin perfusion, blood pressure, pulse rate, urine output, chest movement, respiratory rate, and colour is essential in assessing Do_2, further monitoring procedures may be needed (see p. 246):

• arterial blood gases (for assessing oxygenation, ventilation, and adequacy of circulation)
• CVP (may be of help in assessing blood volume)
• pulse oximetry
• PAWP, cardiac output
• optimized Do_2 matched to oxygen consumption ($\dot{V}o_2$)

- frequent chest x-rays and biochemistry and haematology tests
- tonometry

Ventilation and oxygenation

Patients in shock usually are hypoxic. Frequent determinations of blood gases and pulse oximetry are necessary to assess oxygenation. The possible causes of acute respiratory failure in this setting include aspiration, lung contusion, and excessive crystalloid transfusion. Nosocomial pneumonia (see p. 414) or adult respiratory distress syndrome (ARDS) (see p. 400) can develop later.

If the airway is compromised, intubation is necessary. When a patient's ventilation (assessed by clinical appearance and $Paco_2$) is inadequate, artificial ventilation may be needed. If oxygenation is not adequate with an ordinary face mask, continuous positive airway pressure (CPAP) delivered by a special mask, by nasal prongs, or via an endotracheal tube (ETT) may be necessary. Where possible, encourage CPAP or intermittent mandatory ventilation (IMV), rather than mandatory ventilation (with all of its attendant disadvantages) (see Chapter 20).

Fluid replacement

Peripheral perfusion, arterial blood pressure, pulse rate, and urine output remain the most accurate and simple guides to fluid replacement in multitrauma patients. When large amounts of fluid must be used in resuscitation, colloids will cause less peripheral and pulmonary oedema than will crystalloids (see Chapter 4). Maintenance fluids are not necessary during the early stages of resuscitation. Titrate the colloid or blood replenishment against intravascular measurements and serial hematocrit values. FLUID LOSSES OFTEN ARE UNDER-ESTIMATED, BUT RARELY OVER-ESTIMATED.

Haemoglobin is essential for the oxygen-carrying capacity of the blood, and it can be monitored in terms of the haemoglobin concentration (maintain at least 10 g/dl) or haematocrit (more than 30%).

In addition to coagulation studies and ongoing platelet counts, serum potassium and phosphate concentrations should be measured frequently during active resuscitation and replenished as necessary.

Hypothermia can severely impair coagulation and it must be taken into account when performing laboratory investigations.

Pain relief

Adequate pain relief is crucial after multitrauma. Many limb fractures and chest injuries will lend themselves to local or regional anaesthetic techniques when the patient is stable; otherwise, a continuous opiate infusion titrated against pain relief will ensure patient comfort (see Chapter 7).

Other investigations

When trauma patients become relatively stable, other investigations may be necessary. Even if a patient appears stable, it is essential that observation and support by trained staff be continued during any procedure or investigation, especially those involving transport.

CRANIAL CT SCAN   A cranial CT scan is essential for detecting epidural, subdural, and intracerebral haematomas, as well as cerebral oedema and contusions. It is also useful for defining skull and cervical spine fractures. Cranial CT scans should be performed for all patients with neurological impairments or when there are neurological signs of deterioration. This is an essential investigation for all but minor head injuries and is useful for defining the extent of fasciomaxillary injuries.

X-RAYS OF SUSPECT LONG BONES   Rarely is it urgent to x-ray the extremities. That should be delayed until the patient has been fully resuscitated. Exceptions would be fractures causing vascular or acute nerve injury and fractures associated with great loss of blood.

INTRAVENOUS PYELOGRAM   An intravenous pyelogram should be obtained for a patient with significant or sustained haematuria or severe abdominal trauma near a kidney or ureter. A single shot of 100 ml of contrast fluid and a plain abdominal film will give adequate information.

CYSTOGRAM   A cystogram may be necessary for a patient with haematuria in combination with trauma to the lower abdomen or pelvis. Infuse 150–300 ml of contrast fluid into the bladder through a urinary catheter.

URETHROGRAM   For a patient suspected of having a urethral tear, a urethrogram requires injection of 30 ml of contrast material gently through the urethral meatus.

CT OF ABDOMEN, NUCLEAR MEDICINE STUDIES, ABDOMINAL ULTRASOUND   These procedures are used for assessing the liver, spleen, kidneys, pancreas, and retroperitoneal space (see p. 265). Of these, the CT scan is probably the most useful.

THE SPINE   Fractures and dislocations of the spine are uncommon but important complications because of their devastating consequences. After obtaining a lateral cervical x-ray (see p. 249), other views of the cervical and thoracoabdominal spine may be necessary. In these circumstances, anterior–posterior and open-mouth views are probably indicated. If the patient has further unexplained symptoms or signs, or if the films are not satisfactory, then oblique views, flexion–extension views, or a CT scan can also be performed.

THORACIC AORTOGRAM   A thoracic aortogram is necessary if rupture of the thoracic aorta is suspected. Suspicion is aroused by features such as a widened mediastinum, obliteration of the aortic knob, apical capping, pleural effusion, opacification of the angle between the aorta and the left pulmonary artery, and depression of the left main bronchus to an angle of less than 40° with the trachea. Immediate performance of aortography for suspected rupture of the thoracic aorta necessitates a high incidence of investigations whose findings are negative (approximately 80–90%). A thoracic CT scan, even with contrast, is not as accurate as an aortogram in these circumstances. Transoesophageal echocardiography is being increasingly used.

LONG-TERM COMPLICATIONS

THE COMPLICATIONS IN INTENSIVE CARE CAN BE MINIMIZED BY EARLY AND AGGRESSIVE RESUSCITATION.

A patient who has experienced a period of decreased perfusion related to multitrauma will inevitably sustain some cellular injury, and that is the basis for many of the complications that follow severe trauma. The immune system is affected, predisposing to wound infection and sepsis. Decreased visceral perfusion predisposes to acute stress ulceration, renal failure, hepatic insufficiency, pulmonary insufficiency, and MOF (see Chapter 9).

Acute stress ulceration

Preventive measures should be considered in all cases of multitrauma in the ICU (see p. 000). If early enteral feeding is contraindicated, then treatment with either cytoprotective agents (eg sucralfate) or H_2-receptor antagonists should be instituted (see p. 32).

Acute renal failure

Following rapid and efficient resuscitation, low-dosage dopamine should be considered in all patients at risk for acute renal failure, and development of abdominal tamponade should be monitored and treated if renal function is compromised (see p. 699).

Wounds

Meticulous surgical debridement of wounds and removal of foreign bodies are the most important steps in preventing wound infection.

Grossly contaminated wounds will become infected with or without the use of antibiotics. These wounds require debridement and avoidance of primary closure.

Maintaining adequate tissue oxygenation and perfusion is as important as the use of prophylactic antibiotics in preventing infection.

Check the tetanus immunization status of the patient, and give a booster if necessary.

Intra-abdominal complications

Always be alert to an intra-abdominal source of infection. Thorough saline washing at the time of laparotomy is important when there has been gut perforation. Intra-abdominal sepsis is a common and often lethal complication after severe injury. Its management is outlined elsewhere (see p. 217).

It may be inappropriate to use primary closure in the presence of contused and ruptured gut, depending on the extent of damage.

Repeated laparotomies are advisable in patients with mesenteric vascular injuries.

Nutrition (see Chapter 5)

The metabolic responses to trauma are manifested through the neuroendocrine system and include marked protein breakdown. That response can be partially modified by measures such as rapid resuscitation and pain relief. However, the catabolism of trauma is largely obligatory. Enteral feeding should be instituted rapidly if at all possible. The vast majority of patients with severe trauma can tolerate enteral feeding in the early post-operative period. Nasogastric feeding may initially be unsuccessful, and other techniques such as nasoduodenal feeding or a feeding jejunostomy may provide practical and easy alternatives for facilitating enteral feeding. Otherwise, give parenteral nutrition within the limitations of intravenous fluid requirements and only after the patient has been resuscitated (see Chapter 5).

Fat embolism (see Chapter 15)

Fat embolism typically occurs 24–48 hours after trauma. However, most patients are asymptomatic. The fat embolism syndrome (incidence 4–10%) is associated with orthopaedic injuries and results in hypoxia, fever, petechiae, central nervous system deterioration, thrombocytopenia, and anaemia.

Sepsis (see p. 182)

Sepsis is a frequent complication of multitrauma, especially in the presence of renal failure. Rapid resuscitation and surgical debridement will decrease the incidence. Prophylactic antibiotics may sometimes be indicated (eg intra-abdominal soiling). However, continuing awareness of the possibility of a septic focus and an aggressive search for its source (eg intra-abdominal abscess, lung abscess, wound infection) are essential (see p. 217). The use of selective decontamination of the digestive tract (SDD) may decrease the incidence of sepsis among multitrauma patients. Active or passive immune support may play an increasing role in the future (see p. 194).

Rehabilitation

It is important to counsel relatives and friends early during the management of severe trauma and to be honest about the devastating long-term sequelae, especially if there are head injuries. They should be encouraged to accept the possibility that the healing process may take months or even years, and they should pace themselves accordingly. Patients usually need their greatest support from relatives and friends later during the long and frustrating rehabilitation process, not during the first few days of resuscitation.

THE TRAUMA SYSTEM AND SCORING

THE TRAUMA SYSTEM

It is becoming increasingly recognized that severe trauma should be managed by specialized multidisciplinary units. The expertise needed for dealing with trauma is not ensured simply by putting all the components in one place (intensivists, specialist surgeons, accident and emergency specialists, anaesthetists, rehabilitationists, etc). A system must be organized around all that expertise, and adequate numbers of patients must be available for the team to maintain their skills and for the system to work efficiently. As in the case of cardiac surgery, specialist centres are necessary to concentrate the expertise needed to manage severe trauma. Operational protocols, rapid-response multidisciplinary teams, and facilities for education, data collection, and auditing all must be integral parts of this system if trauma is to be managed effectively. The trauma system need not be a specialized stand-alone unit, but can be integrated into existing tertiary referral centres.

TRAUMA SCORING

Measurement of the severity of injury is an essential prerequisite for effective trauma care. The trauma system must be monitored and audited. That requires data collection and analysis, which in turn are based on trauma scoring. Trauma scores are also used for triage, prediction of outcome, epidemiology, research, and planning of trauma services. Systems of scoring fall into two main patterns: physiological and anatomic.

Physiological scoring system

GLASGOW COMA SCALE   The GCS is universally used to classify head injuries (see p. 586).

APACHE II SYSTEM   The APACHE II system is used to classify patients admitted to ICUs and is based on an acute physiological score, age, and chronic health evaluation. This score correlates well with the trauma score and the injury-severity score and complements both.

TRAUMA SCORE   The trauma score is based on a scale of increasing severity from 16 (best prognosis) to 1 (worst prognosis) (Table 14.5). The trauma score can be used as a component of a triage protocol and used together with other scores for predictive purposes. It is based on five parameters: GCS, systolic blood pressure, respiratory rate, respiratory effort, and capillary refill. Scores of 13–16 should be associated with minimal mortality (<1%), scores of 11–12 with less than 20% mortality, and scores of 10 or less with mortality of 70% or more (Table 14.6). Refinements, such as the revised triage score (RTS), are being developed and may be easier to apply, in addition to having greater reliability for predicting outcomes. It uses only three parameters: GCS, systolic blood pressure, and respiratory rate.

Anatomic scoring systems

ABBREVIATED INJURY SCALE   The abbreviated injury scale (AIS) was one of the first anatomic scales developed, and it has been revised several times. The latest is the AIS-90, developed in 1990. The score reflects both the anatomic and pathological results of major trauma. Every injury is coded on the basis of anatomic site, nature, and severity. The AIS correlates well with outcomes.

INJURY-SEVERITY SCORE   The injury-severity score (ISS) was developed specifically to score major injuries, and it expresses a combined score for the most severe injury in each of the three most severely af-

TABLE 14.5 THE TRAUMA SCORE

Parameter	Value	Score	
A. Respiratory rate	10–24	4	
(breaths/minute)	25–35	3	
	$\geq$36	2	
	1–9	1	
	0	0	A ___
B. Respiratory effort	Normal	1	
	Use of accessory muscles or inter- costal retraction	0	B ___
C. Systolic blood pressure	$\geq$90	4	
(mm Hg)	70–89	3	
	50–69	2	
	0–49	1	
	0	0	C ___
D. Capillary refilling time	Normal ($\leq$2)	2	
(seconds)	Delayed ($\geq$2)	1	
	None	0	D ___
E. Glasgow coma scale	14–15	5	
	11–13	4	
	8–10	3	
	5–7	2	
	3–4	1	E ___
Total score (A + B + C + D + E)			___

fected areas of the body. The severity is assigned by the AIS, and the ISS is expressed on a scale of increasing severity (0–75%). The score is calculated by summing the squares of AIS scores. For example, consider this set of injuries:

Abdomen	ruptured spleen	AIS 5
Chest	fractured ribs	AIS 2
Limbs	fractured femur	AIS 3

The ISS score will be $5^2 + 2^2 + 3^2 = 25 + 4 + 9 = 38$.

TABLE 14.6 TRAUMA SCORE AND THE PROBABILITY OF SURVIVAL

Trauma score	Probability of survival (%)
16	99
15	98
14	95
13	91
12	83
11	71
10	55
9	37
8	22
7	12
6	7
5	4
3	1
2	0
1	0

The ISS is used in conjunction with other scores to guide triage and to indicate prognoses, and it has been validated for use with penetrating injuries in adults of all ages and for children over the age of 12 years.

Combined trauma scores

More accurate predictions are often obtained when several scoring techniques are combined. The trauma score (TS) and ISS are often used in combination. The CRAMS scale (Circulation, Respiration, Abdomen, Motor, Speech scale) has attempted to combine features of physiological and anatomic scores, but has been less accurate than the TS. The TS, ISS, and age have been combined to form the TRISS method, which allows comparison of outcome against a baseline rate while controlling for the mix of severities of patients' injuries.

Outcome comparisons

It is becoming increasingly important to measure one's own trauma practice and compare it against other systems, with a view to identifying weaknesses and attempting to achieve better outcomes. Some tools that help us to compare outcomes are as follows:

z statistic The Z statistic is for comparison of outcomes for two population subsets. The Z statistic quantitates the difference between actual and predicted numbers of deaths.

peer review Expert reviewers of trauma deaths (working 'blind') are often used to determine whether or not trauma deaths had any preventable components, based on an arbitrary scale. If this tool is tested for interobserver and intraobserver reliability, it can indicate points of possible weaknesses in the system.

standardized mortality ratio The standardized mortality ratio (SMR) is the ratio between observed deaths and expected deaths. An SMR below unity indicates a decreased risk of mortality in the sample, whereas an SMR greater than unity indicates increased risk.

Paediatric scoring (see p. 312)

BLUNT ABDOMINAL TRAUMA

DIAGNOSIS

Clinical examination

Clinical examination of the abdomen is mandatory and may reveal signs of external trauma, pain on palpation, guarding, rigidity, distension, and so forth. However, such signs sometimes are unreliable in the acute situation, and girth measurements are of no value (see p. 699). Immediate laparotomy should be performed in any case in which there is the suspicion of abdominal trauma and haemodynamic instability.

Upright chest x-ray

This is necessary when looking for features such as fractured ribs over the spleen (ribs 9, 10, and 11) or liver, pneumoperitoneum, or rupture of the diaphragm.

Diagnostic peritoneal lavage

Diagnostic peritoneal lavage (DPL) is a sensitive test for intraperitoneal blood. It is performed as a sterile procedure in the emergency
department by inserting a catheter into the peritoneum just below
the umbilicus, or just above the umbilicus in any patient with a fractured pelvis.

INDICATIONS Indications for DPL are equivocal abdominal findings
(eg where fractured lower ribs or fractured pelvis may obscure findings) or a situation in which there are no clear indications for immediate laparotomy, but the patient

• has unreliable abdominal findings, because of head injury, drugs, or
paraplegia (or because the patient is paralysed and ventilated)
• faces an anticipated lengthy investigation (eg angiography) or
surgery for extra-abdominal injuries
• has unexplained blood loss

TECHNIQUE FOR DPL

1. Decompress the urinary bladder by inserting a urinary catheter.

2. Decompress the stomach by inserting an NG tube.

3. Prepare the abdomen for surgery with antimicrobial solution and
drapes.

4. Inject local anaesthetic down to the peritoneum in the midline,
one-third the distance from the umbilicus to the symphysis pubis
(above the umbilicus where a pelvic fracture is suspected).

5. Vertically incise the skin and subcutaneous tissue down to
fascia.

6. Incise the fascia and peritoneum, and prevent fascial retraction
with a clamp.

7. Direct the dialysis catheter toward the pelvis.

8. Aspirate, and if frank blood or enteric contents appear, there is
urgent need for laparotomy.

9. Infuse warmed isotonic saline at 10 mg/kg (up to 1 litre). Gentle agitation will aid mixing and distribution throughout the abdominal cavity.

10. Wait 5–10 minutes, and then siphon fluid off by placing the isotonic saline container on the floor.

11. A blood clot or heavily bloodstained fluid is unequivocally positive, as is a red-blood-cell count of greater than 100,000/ml. Although such findings are uncommon, the fluid should also be examined for white cells, amylase, and food particles, with a Gram stain used to search for bacteria.

Negative findings at lavage rule out significant haemorrhage in the peritoneal cavity. However, they do not rule out retroperitoneal injuries (eg duodenum and pancreas). Patients with pelvic fractures can have false-positive findings at lavage, as in approximately 15% of cases blood will leak from the retroperitoneal space into the peritoneum. Angiography may help identify the site of bleeding in these circumstances.

RELATIVE CONTRAINDICATIONS
- previous abdominal operations
- morbid obesity
- advanced cirrhosis
- pre-existing coagulopathy
- advanced pregnancy

Laparotomy

If hypovolaemia cannot be rapidly corrected and there is no obvious site of bleeding (eg external, chest, fractures), there is urgent need for laparotomy.

CT scan

CT has an advantage over DPL, because it can detect other intra-abdominal abnormalities, including retroperitoneal haemorrhage. CT scanning is time-consuming and is contraindicated in unstable patients suspected of having uncontrolled intra-abdominal bleeding.

Abdominal ultrasound

In skilled hands, ultrasound is a reliable method for detecting haemoperitoneum, and it offers a valuable non-invasive means for investigating blunt abdominal trauma. Free intraperitoneal fluid is best demonstrated in the hepatorenal pouch. Abdominal ultrasound, scintigraphy, and CT may detect injuries not obvious on DPL, but they cannot substitute for DPL for the detection of intra-abdominal blood.

PRINCIPLES OF MANAGEMENT

Spleen

The spleen is the intra-abdominal organ most commonly affected by blunt trauma. About half of all ruptures are associated with fracture of ribs (9–11) on the left side.

There is no place for drainage: Either totally or partially remove the spleen if active, uncontrollable bleeding is suspected.

It is becoming more common to treat splenic trauma conservatively, especially in children. A CT scan is usually obtained, and the patient is observed for signs of bleeding. Delayed rupture of the spleen occurs in up to 10% of patients with splenic haematomas.

Patients who undergo total splenectomy have a small risk (<1%) of post-splenectomy sepsis. Encapsulated bacteria such as pneumococci and meningococci are the commonest organisms. Vaccination should be carried out in these patients.

Liver

The liver is in second place among the intra-abdominal organs most commonly affected by blunt trauma.

Approximately 70% of all liver injuries can be managed conservatively. Others require resection and, in a small percentage, packing to stop the bleeding. The current approach is to perform the minimum surgery necessary to control bleeding.

Pancreas

Pancreatic injury is relatively rare. However, it is important to mobilize the duodenum and identify the pancreas when performing any laparotomy for trauma. A haematoma around the pancreas at operation should alert the surgeon to the possibility of severe underlying damage.

The amylase concentration is an imprecise diagnostic tool; a CT scan is a much better indicator of pancreatic damage.

With blunt trauma, drainage at laparotomy is often sufficient. Duct damage must be surgically repaired early.

Hollow viscus

The perforation must be repaired early. Liberal peritoneal lavage (10–15 litres of warm isotonic saline) should be used at operation.

Bowel may need to be resected, and the faecal stream diverted.

Adequate drainage and prophylactic antibiotics are necessary for peritoneal soiling.

Repeat laparotomy is advisable after mesenteric-vessel injury, in order to assess gut viability.

Diaphragm

The diaphragm is involved in 4% of all case of multitrauma and must be surgically repaired (see p. 278).

Retroperitoneum and pelvis

PELVIC FRACTURE The diagnosis of a fractured pelvis is made on the basis of an x-ray. 'Springing' of the pelvis is very unreliable. There is increasing interest in surgical fixation of pelvic fractures – either external or internal fixation, with or without traction. Stabilization may be important both for immediate survival (by decreasing the bleeding) and for improvement in long-term functioning. The exact roles of external fixation and internal fixation are not clear at present. Neither is the timing of such procedures. Primary internal fixation may be indicated when laparotomy or bladder repair is being performed in a patient with symphyseal disruption or major-vessel laceration.

RETROPERITONEAL BLEEDING Bleeding into the retroperitoneum is very common, especially in association with a fractured pelvis, and it is best defined by CT scan.

Most retroperitoneal haematomas do not require surgical intervention after blunt trauma, even if discovered at laparotomy. Pelvic retroperitoneal haematoma can result from venous bleeding at fracture sites, disruption of pelvic veins in the posterior pelvic plexus, or disruption of deep pelvic arteries, often distal branches of the internal iliac vessels. Perirenal haematomas and midline haematomas can also occur in the retroperitoneal space.

Although blood loss can be considerable, it usually ceases spontaneously. However, major haemorrhage from this area is frustrating and difficult to treat when it is life-threatening. Pelvic stabilization with a MAST suit or external pelvic fixation can decrease bleeding and is sometimes lifesaving. In the right hands, interventional radiology and, if necessary, embolization can achieve excellent results. It should be performed in all cases of proven retroperitoneal haematomas with uncontrollable bleeding. Continuing bleeding can sometimes be from an arterial source rather than venous plexus bleeding. Arterial bleeding is more amenable to surgery than venous bleeding.

CONTINUING MANAGEMENT IN INTENSIVE CARE

Such patients usually have other injuries and require close monitoring of vital signs, continuing resuscitation, and further investigation of injuries in many cases (see p. 251).

ABDOMINAL TAMPONADE   Patients with abdominal trauma may develop increased intra-abdominal pressure. Such increased pressure will seriously compromise the blood supply to most intra-abdominal organs and can cause renal failure. Girth measurements are of no value in this situation, and all patients should have intravesical pressure measurements (see p. 699).

INTRA-ABDOMINAL SEPSIS   Intra-abdominal sepsis and MOF remain major contributors to mortality following severe trauma. Intra-abdominal sepsis is, in fact, usually characterized by the onset of MOF, rather than by localizing signs. If suspected, it should be aggressively investigated and treated (see Chapter 9).

THORACIC INJURIES

Chest trauma is often associated with trauma at other sites. RESUSCITATE and MONITOR these patients as previously outlined for multitrauma (see p. 243), and maintain a high index of suspicion regarding other injuries.

In particular, closely monitor for signs of blood loss and respiratory distress.

Surgery is seldom indicated for patients who have sustained blunt chest trauma. The major principle of management is to provide support for the patients while their injuries heal. Most chest injuries are adequately treated with chest drains for air and blood collections, as well as adequate pain relief; but do not hesitate to consider surgery for massive air leak or continuing and significant intrathoracic bleeding.

Conservative management depends on **COMPLETE PAIN RELIEF,** often in conjunction with manoeuvres to improve oxygenation (eg CPAP). If that fails, artificial ventilation may be necessary, especially in the presence of associated injuries.

IMMEDIATE RESUSCITATION

The principles of resuscitation are the same as for multitrauma patients (see p. 243).

AIRWAY Establish a reliable airway.

BREATHING Is there respiratory distress? Look for
- tachypnoea
- tachycardia
- decreased movement of one side of the chest (the abnormality will always be on that side)
- low oxygen saturation

Feel for and listen for
- tracheal deviation
- surgical emphysema
- percussion (a large pneumothorax will sound 'hollow')
- air entry

Give all patients 100% oxygen initially.
Rule out the possibility of pneumothorax (simple, tension, or open) and haemothorax.

Restore the mechanics of breathing, if necessary, by artificial ventilation.

CIRCULATION

• Rapidly restore the intravascular volume.

• Hypovolaemic shock is by far the most common cardiovascular problem in trauma patients, but one must exclude the possibility of cardiac tamponade, myocardial contusion, and infarction (see p. 279).

CHEST X-RAY

There is no single investigation that offers more important information than an upright chest film in the presence of chest trauma. Look for

• pneumothoraces and other examples of extra-alveolar air, such as subcutaneous emphysema, mediastinal emphysema, or pneumoperitoneum
• haemothorax
• rib fractures
• lung contusion
• aspiration
• signs associated with a ruptured diaphragm (see p. 278)
• widened mediastinum and, more rarely, cardiac tamponade

IF THERE IS A WIDENED MEDIASTINUM OR OTHER RADIOLOGICAL SIGNS (SEE P. 280), EXCLUDE THE POSSIBILITY OF A RUPTURED THORACIC AORTA BY IMMEDIATE AORTOGRAPHY.

PNEUMOTHORAX

Clinical signs

Decreased entry of air and tracheal deviation usually occur with a significant pneumothorax, together with cardiorespiratory collapse, unless it is drained. If the patient is being ventilated and develops a pneumothorax, the ventilatory pressure can suddenly rise, and the patient can become hypoxic. A high index of suspicion is essential for patients recovering from multitrauma.

Management

OPEN PNEUMOTHORAX   Cover the pneumothorax immediately with an airtight dressing, and insert an intercostal tube, but not through the directly damaged part of the chest.

TENSION PNEUMOTHORAX   If the patient is in severe respiratory distress and a pneumothorax is clinically suspected, insert a 12-gauge catheter in the second intercostal space, mid-clavicular line, in order to decompress the air. Follow this with a chest tube in the fifth–sixth intercostal space.

SIMPLE PNEUMOTHORAX   The rule for all severely injured patients is that a pneumothorax should be drained with a chest tube, no matter how small it is. This is particularly important in the presence of underlying respiratory disease or when a patient is to receive positive-pressure ventilation.

CHEST TUBE   Except in emergency circumstances, insert the chest tube in the fifth or sixth intercostal space, mid-axillary line. It should be a large, straight tube with a blunt plastic tip, rather than a metal trochar tip. Liberal use of local anaesthetic should be followed by an incision of approximately 2 cm, then blunt dissection down to the pleura, and insertion of the tube by directing it posteriorly and superiorly toward the apex. Avoid purse-string sutures; use simple mattress sutures. Confirm the position of the catheter by chest x-ray and by the presence of bubbling and swinging of the fluid level in the underwater seal. Check the chest x-ray for correct siting of the distal holes within the pleural cavity. Place the underwater seal under the bed during transport. Never clamp an intercostal tube. Suction is often necessary to drain blood, and sometimes to drain air. However, suction may exacerbate the air leak. A single tube is usually adequate for air and fluid drainage. Multiple tubes in appropriate positions may be necessary for loculated collections. If a single-chamber drainage bottle is used to drain chest fluid, it should be changed frequently; otherwise, as the level of fluid rose, the efficiency of drainage would decrease.

OTHER MANIFESTATIONS OF EXTRA-ALVEOLAR AIR

Whereas a pneumothorax and localized subcutaneous emphysema resulting from a punctured lung are the most common manifestations of extra-alveolar air, gas can also collect in other sites, leading to conditions such as mediastinal emphysema, pneumoretroperitoneum, and pneumoperitoneum. These can occur in association with blunt chest injuries. The mechanism is not necessarily related to puncture of the lung by fractured ribs. It usually involves severe blunt injury against a closed glottis. That causes simultaneous rupture of alveoli at the time of trauma, in a manner similar to a massive Valsalva manoeuvre. Air moves in the adventitia of pulmonary vessels as pulmonary interstitial emphysema to the mediastinum to cause mediastinal emphysema, then up into the neck and over the anterior chest wall to produce subcutaneous emphysema. It can break through the thin mediastinal pleura to cause a pneumothorax, or alongside the oesophagus and aorta to yield pneumoretroperitoneum and pneumoperitoneum. The clinical importance of such phenomena is as follows:

(a) Subcutaneous emphysema in the neck, rather than at the site of fractured ribs, may indicate extra-alveolar air formation by this mechanism, rather than by lung puncture. Subcutaneous emphysema and mediastinal emphysema can also occur in combination with a pneumothorax associated with rupture of the tracheobronchial tree. Rarely, subcutaneous emphysema and mediastinal emphysema can occur after a ruptured oesophagus.

(b) The presence of subcutaneous emphysema and mediastinal emphysema, simultaneously, without a pneumothorax, points to massive pulmonary interstitial emphysema as the mechanism rather than a punctured lung.

(c) Positive-pressure ventilation can predispose to further extra-alveolar air.

(d) Pneumoperitoneum and pneumoretroperitoneum must be differentiated from a ruptured abdominal viscus.

(e) Management of extra-alveolar air formation involves reducing the level of positive-pressure support. For example, use CPAP rather than intermittent positive-pressure ventilation (IPPV) where possible. Use techniques such as pressure support in order to reduce the level of positive pressure (see p. 473).

RUPTURE OF THE TRACHEOBRONCHIAL TREE

A bronchopleural fistula (BPF) is a communication between the bronchial tree and pleural space, resulting in a massive air leak. Simultaneous rupture of many alveoli (see p. 270) can also cause a large air leak.

Diagnosis

- presence of a large, continuous leak from the chest tube
- persistent pneumothorax, despite chest drains
- bronchoscopy – most rupture 1–2 cm from the carina

Management

1. Use a large-diameter intercostal catheter (see p. 269).

2. Drainage: The catheter either can be attached to an underwater drain or can be connected to suction. Usually a suction level of no more than 20 cm H_2O is sufficient to facilitate flow.

3. Ventilatory strategies:

(a) Lowest effective tidal volumes, peak inspiratory pressures, and positive end-expiratory pressures (PEEP) should be employed to encourage healing of the BPF.

(b) High-frequency ventilation (see p. 475) can encourage decreased ventilatory pressure and healing of the BPF.

(c) Independent lung ventilation (see p. 437), using either CPAP or low tidal volumes on the affected side, and normal tidal volumes and pressures on the other side, can reduce the leak in a BPF.

4. Sealing or sclerosing agents given via the intercostal catheter can be used to occlude the fistula site (eg tetracycline).

Surgery (eg bronchial-stump stapling or decortication) is sometimes necessary when the leak will not respond to the foregoing measures.

HAEMOPNEUMOTHORAX

The bleeding from a haemopneumothorax usually stops without surgical intervention. Any significant haemothorax (ie visible on chest x-ray) should be drained via a large intercostal tube. The same tube can be used to drain both air and blood if a pneumothorax is also present. Blood loss is accurately reflected by the loss from the intercostal tube. Continued bleeding usually indicates arterial loss from an intercostal artery, rather than from the low-pressure pulmonary circuit.

Thoracotomy should be considered when the total blood loss is more than 1,500 ml or when drainage of blood exceeds 300 ml/h for more than 4 hours.

LUNG CONTUSION

Lung contusion or 'bruised' lung is usually associated with rib fractures, especially a flail chest. In children, contused lung occurs commonly without rib fractures, because a child's rib cage is more flexible.

Lung contusion usually is seen on initial chest x-ray as a patchy infiltrate that typically progresses over the next 24–48 hours before it begins to clear. Lung contusion is invariably associated with hypoxia, which can be very severe. The spectrum of severity ranges from mild to life-threatening pulmonary oedema. There can be simultaneous alveolar rupture, necessitating a ventilatory technique that employs relatively low intrathoracic pressures, such as CPAP (see p. 367), in order to avoid further lung damage and extra-alveolar air formation. Some patients with severe hypoxia and contusion can develop long-term changes in respiratory function and exercise tolerance. The long-term changes probably result from underlying lung damage in combination with high ventilatory pressures.

Treatment (see the general principles of treating respiratory failure, p. 360)

The principles of management are as follows:

• Use a face mask with a high concentration of inspired oxygen.

• Use CPAP via a mask or tube if it can be tolerated, provided there are no contraindications such as a fracture of the base of the skull, and provided adequate ventilation is possible.

• Maintain the cardiovascular system with colloid or blood, avoiding excessive amounts of crystalloid.

• Use positive-pressure ventilatory techniques, such as IMV, pressure-support ventilation, or IPPV, if ventilation is inadequate (see Chapter 20).

• Pain relief: Epidural, intrapleural, or intercostal nerve blocks will provide excellent pain relief when there are associated rib fractures (see p. 120).

Monitor progress with

• serial chest x-rays (at least daily)
• serial determinations of arterial blood gases or pulse oximetry

FRACTURED RIBS

• Fractured ribs are usually associated with severe pain. Pain restricts coughing and breathing, predisposing to sputum retention, atelectasis, pneumonia, and respiratory failure.

• Fractured ribs are often associated with underlying lung contusion.

• Fractured ribs can puncture underlying structures.

• Fractured ribs are often difficult to diagnose on initial chest x-ray. As an empirical rule, the actual number of fractured ribs will be double the number seen on chest x-ray.

• The fractures may be simple or multiple or part of a flail chest.

• Fractures of the first and second ribs are associated with higher incidences of damage to the myocardium, major vessels, and bronchi.

• Even a small number of simple rib fractures in an elderly patient or in a patient with underlying lung disease can cause life-threatening complications such as hypoventilation, collapse, and pneumonia. IT IS EASY TO UNDER-ESTIMATE THE SERIOUSNESS OF FRACTURED RIBS AND FLAIL CHEST. They should be aggressively treated with pain relief, with or without CPAP. These patients tend to look best at admission and to slowly deteriorate, especially those who are old or obese or have underlying lung disease.

• There is little, if any, place for surgical repair of fractured ribs.

FLAIL CHEST   Flail chest is caused by fractures in two or more locations on each of three or more adjacent ribs. Whereas the paradoxical movement of the flail segment can interfere with ventilation, the flail segment is more important as a marker of underlying severe lung contusion.

TREATMENT   The thrust of treatment has moved away from stabilization of rib fractures and mechanical ventilation.

The cornerstone of conservative treatment is **COMPLETE PAIN RELIEF.** Pain relief can be provided by intermittent or continuous dosages of narcotics or by regional local anaesthetic techniques such as intercostal nerve block (see p. 27), thoracic epidurals (see p. 120), and intrapleural catheters (see p. 123). The choice of a technique will depend on the extent of the rib fractures, the severity of pain and associated injuries, and the expertise of the operator.

COMPLETE PAIN RELIEF often allows adequate **SPONTANEOUS VENTILATION.** Assisted ventilation usually is not necessary, even in the presence of multiple rib fractures or severe flail chest. However, **OXYGENATION** is often a problem. Adequate oxygenation can be achieved by delivering oxygen through a simple face mask or by using CPAP (delivered either nasally, with a face mask, or via an ETT). CPAP masks should not be used for patients who have depressed levels of consciousness, facial fractures, or base-of-skull fractures.

INTUBATION and **ARTIFICIAL VENTILATION** are sometimes necessary, especially if there are associated injuries such as head trauma or spinal injuries, or when a patient is obese or has grossly unstable rib fractures. Where possible, mask CPAP and complete pain relief should be used, rather than intubation, ventilation, and systemic narcotics, as the former are associated with fewer complications. **EARLY TRACHEOSTOMY** should be considered in patients with fractured ribs who need intubation, as they usually require at least 2–3 weeks of respiratory support.

PLEURAL DRAINAGE

Drainage of air or fluid from the pleural space requires an airtight system to maintain the subatmospheric intrapleural pressure. To drain air or fluid, a low-resistance tube is needed, with a one-way valve (usually underwater). The amount of suction generated is determined by the distance between the pleural cavity and the collection chamber. The lower the chamber, the more suction. However, when air pockets break the continuity of the fluid column, less suction is generated. Thus, in addition to lowering the collection chamber, negative pressure may be necessary to facilitate air and fluid removal. The collection chamber should always be more than 100 cm below the chest, in order to prevent fluid from being sucked up into the chest when large subatmospheric pressures are generated (eg during obstructed inspiration). Unless precise flow measurements are used, the amount of suction needed is empirical. Excessive suction can potentiate air leaks. A small amount of suction (less than -20 cm H_2O) can help overcome resistance to airflow within the system.

A large-diameter chamber (about 20 cm in diameter) will maintain the underwater seal, with minimum resistance to drainage. The catheter should be placed about 2 cm under the water. If a one-bottle system is used, there is increasing resistance as the chamber fills, as well as difficulty in measuring in the presence of bubbling and foaming. Two-, three-, and four-bottle systems will increase safety and efficiency, but they are more cumbersome and expensive. Commercial devices that are compact and disposable, using two, three, or four bottles, are beginning to be used in many ICUs (Figures 14.2 and 14.3).

The system is monitored by observing synchronous oscillations. If blockage is suspected, gentle milking of the tube can be performed. The pleural tube should never be clamped, and the collection chamber should always be kept below the level of the chest during transport. Consideration should be given to removing the intercostal catheter after bubbling has ceased for more than 12 hours. A chest x-ray is needed after removal of the catheter to exclude re-collections of air or fluid.

ASPIRATION

Aspiration should always be considered a possibility, especially in association with coma, intoxication, and facial fractures.

Aspiration can be distinguished from contusion on the basis of its distribution on a chest x-ray, as well as on the basis of the appearance and smell of the tracheal aspirate. Look for radiopaque foreign bodies (eg teeth). Consider bronchoscopy if obstruction by a foreign

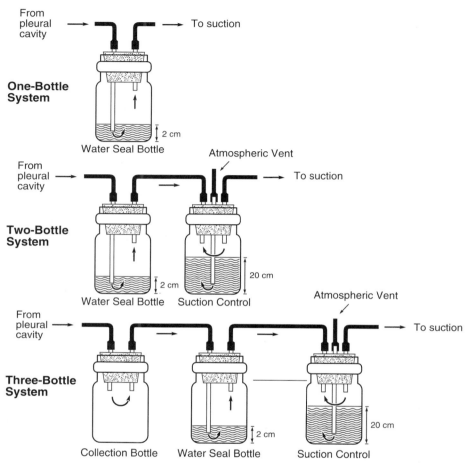

FIGURES 14.2, 14.3 Pleural drainage systems. The drainage system consists of a water seal, drainage trap, pressure-control chamber, and connecting tubes. In the case of a single bottle, the water seal also acts as the drainage trap for fluid and air (above). The bottle either is vented to air or has suction attached to it. A two-bottle system contains a bottle that acts as a drainage trap as well as a water seal, and a separate bottle for suction control. A three-bottle system has one bottle for drainage, one as a water seal, and the third for suction control. Commercially available systems can combine the three-bottle setup into one disposable lightweight and transportable package that allows a separate drainage area, underwater seal compartment, and suction-control compartment (right). (From Gilbert et al., 1993, with permission of Blackwell Scientific Publications Inc.)

Underwater Seal Drainage System

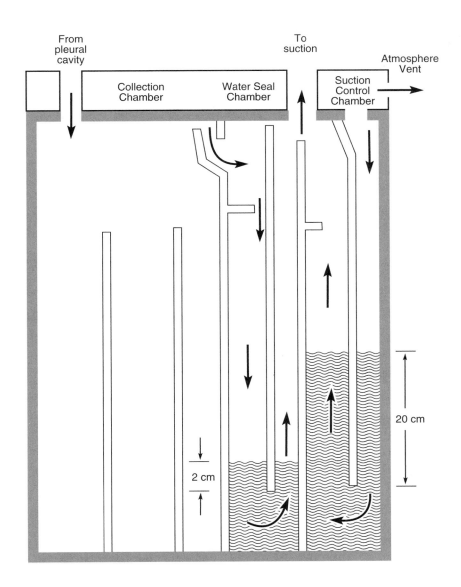

body is suspected. Respiratory support for aspiration involves the same general principles as for contusion (see p. 272).

TRAUMATIC RUPTURE OF THE DIAPHRAGM

Rupture of the diaphragm occurs in approximately 5% of cases of blunt trauma to the trunk. The left side is more commonly ruptured than the right, which is protected by the liver.

Presentation

• A ruptured diaphragm is very difficult to detect clinically, particularly if the patient is on positive-pressure ventilation.
• Diminished chest expansion and air entry.
• Tracheal deviation, with underlying mediastinal shift.
• Bowel sounds in the chest.

Investigations

Chest x-ray is by far the most important investigation, but it can be difficult to interpret. Abnormalities can include
   • elevated left hemidiaphragm
   • herniation of abdominal organs
   • mediastinal shift
   • haemothorax
   • atelectasis
   • abnormal position of NG tube
Liver scintigraphy
Ultrasound
CT scan
Laparoscopy

Management

All diaphragmatic lacerations should be surgically repaired at an early stage because of the risk of herniation of an abdominal viscus.

OESOPHAGEAL TRAUMA

Oesophageal trauma usually is a result of a penetrating injury. Symptoms include pain and dysphagia. Signs include mediastinal air and gastric contents draining from the chest tube. Treatment is surgical. Oesophageal rupture after blunt trauma is rare and usually fatal.

CARDIAC INJURIES

MYOCARDIAL CONTUSION

Myocardial contusion is associated with blunt anterior chest injuries, especially involving a fractured sternum. The contusion can be diagnosed on the basis of serial ECGs, creatine phosphokinase (CPK) MB-fraction levels, technetium-99m scanning, ECG-gated scintigraphy, or two-dimensional echocardiography. None of these is entirely satisfactory, either for diagnosis or for demonstrating the extent of the contusion or prognosis. The most promising method for assessment is echocardiography.

Cardiac contusion usually responds to conservative measures and is rarely associated with significant heart failure or arrhythmias. Patients with normal ECGs and normal clinical findings on admission usually do not require monitoring.

PENETRATING CARDIAC INJURIES

CHEST INJURIES ASSOCIATED WITH CARDIAC INJURIES

• Penetrating wounds that are unlikely, judging from site and direction, to be associated with cardiac injury, occurring in patients with no evidence of shock. This grouping comprises approximately 80% of such cases. Treatment includes observation with or without drainage.

• Suspicious chest wounds, usually over the cardiac area, in patients who are hypotensive but who respond well to fluid replacement. Approximately 50% of these patients will deteriorate and need surgical exploration. Monitoring and resuscitation must be carried out while transport is quickly arranged to an institution where facilities for immediate cardiac surgery are available. Echocardiography should be performed. These account for approximately 15% of all such cases.

• Highly suspicious chest wounds in a small group (approximately 5%) of moribund patients who require immediate thoracotomy to relieve tamponade, rapid fluid resuscitation, and internal cardiac massage. Many of these will achieve full recovery if treatment is rapid.

PERICARDIAL TAMPONADE

Pericardial tamponade usually is associated with penetrating injuries, but it can result from severe blunt trauma.

Initially the tamponade is lifesaving, because it prevents massive blood loss, but it soon becomes life-threatening by interfering with cardiac function.

Patients with cardiac tamponade classically present with hypotension, distended neck veins, and muffled heart sounds. If a patient is also hypovolaemic, the neck veins may not be raised. If the neck veins are raised, consider tension pneumothorax, myocardial contusion, and myocardial infarct as alternative diagnoses.

Emergency thoracotomy, rather than pericardiocentesis, is usually needed, even if the patient appears moribund, as the blood within the pericardium is often clotted. Further bleeding into the pericardium usually occurs after aspiration, and lacerations of the heart and coronary vessels can occur during aspiration by inexperienced operators.

CARDIOGENIC SHOCK

Hypovolaemic shock is by far the most common type of shock associated with trauma. However, cardiogenic shock can occur in some patients (eg the elderly) who have myocardial infarcts, either as precipitating causes of their accidents or coincidentally (see p. 555).

GREAT-VESSEL INJURY

Great-vessel injury is relatively rare after blunt trauma. The diagnosis should be considered in all cases of severe deceleration injuries (eg a head-on collision, being thrown from a car, or a fall of more than 10 metres). Usually a high index of suspicion is required for this diagnosis, and these injuries have serious consequences if they are overlooked.

Most patients with ruptures of the great thoracic vessels die instantly. A survivor will have a contained haematoma and will need rapid management, as half of the surviving patients will die each day if left untreated.

A ruptured thoracic aorta usually is suspected when an upright chest x-ray shows a widened mediastinum and blurring of the aortic knob. Other associated radiological signs (Figure 14.4) include fractures of the first and second ribs, deviation of the trachea to the right, and a pleural cap. However, these signs are inconsistent and difficult to interpret on an anterior–posterior x-ray made with the patient supine.

If the mediastinum is seen to be widened on upright chest x-ray, aortography, rather than thoracic CT, is the investigation of choice.

Transesophageal echocardiography has also been shown to be useful in the diagnosis of thoracic aortic rupture.

Surgical repair is best performed in specialized centres with cardiopulmonary bypass facilities.

SPINAL INJURIES

INJURIES OF THE CERVICAL SPINE

Any patient who has suffered trauma and who has a compromised level of consciousness should be assumed to have injuries of the cervical spine, until proved otherwise. Although a high index of suspicion should always be maintained, resuscitation procedures should not be compromised or delayed. Compared with airway obstruction, hypovolaemia, and respiratory impairment, spinal injuries are uncommon. If the airway is compromised, intubation has the highest priority, and it can almost always be safely achieved by holding the head and neck in a neutral position during the procedure.

Injuries of the cervical spine often are associated with certain activities (eg sporting injuries, diving into a shallow pool) or with severe multitrauma, especially in association with head injuries. Injuries of the cervical spine are found in 5–10% of patients who are unconscious after a fall or a vehicle crash.

One should suspect spinal injury in the presence of the following:

- flaccid areflexia
- localized pain, or sensory and motor deficits

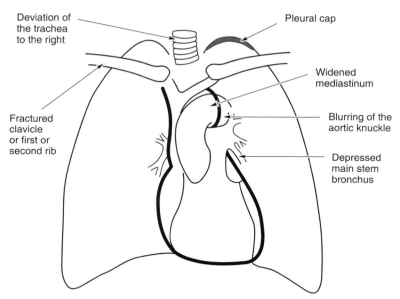

FIGURE 14.4 Radiological signs of a ruptured thoracic aorta.

- unexplained hypotension, normal pulse rate, and peripheral vasodilatation
- diaphragmatic breathing
- absence of anal and bulbocavernous reflexes
- priapism

Lateral x-rays of the cervical spine should be obtained for any patient who has sustained severe multitrauma, as soon as the patient is adequately resuscitated (see p. 249). All seven vertebrae must be visualized. Simple anteroposterior and lateral cervical views will exclude most fractures. More sophisticated views may be necessary after resuscitation. When cervical spine damage is suspected in a patient with head injuries, CT views of the cervical spine area in question should be obtained at the same time as CT views of the head. Subluxation will not be demonstrated on a CT scan.

MANAGEMENT

SPINAL IMMOBILIZATION IS THE MAINSTAY OF TREATMENT:

• hard collar (soft collars are of little value)
• sandbags on each side of the head, and the head taped to a spine board
• manual in-line immobilization, with the head in a neutral position

Immobilization helps to reduce fractures and dislocations, correct spinal misalignments, and decompress the cord and nerve roots. Definitive treatment usually involves traction. Surgery is sometimes indicated for patients with unstable fractures, in order to facilitate nursing care and reduce delays in mobilization.

Intubation and ventilation may be required if the cord lesion involves the phrenic nerve at C3, C4, C5, or above. Intubation usually can be safely achieved by an experienced operator with an assistant performing manual in-line immobilization. Atropine (0.4 mg IV) should be given for persistent bradycardia, and inotropic support (eg adrenaline infusion, see p. 523) is sometimes necessary to correct persistent hypotension. It is important to maintain an adequate perfusion pressure in these patients. Over-zealous administration of fluids can cause pulmonary oedema.

A urinary catheter and NG tube should be inserted.

Methylprednisolone, 30 mg/kg stat, and $5.4 \text{ mg} \cdot \text{kg}^{-1} \cdot \text{h}^{-1}$ for 23 hours, given within 8 hours of injury, may in the long term help to preserve sensory and motor functions, although more research data are needed on this point.

Selective hypothermia, naloxone, hyperosmotic agents, and coma treatment have shown equivocal results.

All patients with significant spinal injuries should be transferred to a specialized spinal unit as soon as they have been resuscitated.

FRACTURES OF THE THORACIC AND LUMBAR SPINE

If a thoracic or lumbar spinal injury is suspected, immobilization must be achieved above and below the site (ie head and neck, chest, pelvis, and extremities may all need to be immobilized on a spine board).

Once resuscitation has been achieved, log-roll the patient and assess for pain and a palpable deformity.

Thoracic spine

The commonest fracture in this region is a wedge fracture from hyperflexion. This fracture is usually stable.

Lumbar spine

Fractures of the thoracolumbar and lumbar spine are more likely to be unstable than are injuries of the thoracic spine. As the spinal cord terminates at L1–L2, cord lesions at this site can cause a mixture of spinal cord signs (bladder and bowel signs) and cauda equina signs (sensory deficits in lower limbs).

GENITO-URINARY TRAUMA

• Genito-urinary trauma is commonly associated with pelvic fractures.

• Trauma to the urethra, bladder, and kidneys is relatively common, whereas trauma to the ureters is rare.

• A rectal examination should be performed before a urinary catheter is passed.

• Haematuria is a common non-specific sign. Only when the haematuria is significant and prolonged should investigation of the urinary tract be undertaken. An intravenous pyelogram (IVP) probably is worthwhile only if there are more than 30 red blood cells per high-power field. The only exception may be haematuria in a patient with severe abdominal trauma, in order to determine the state of renal blood flow.

• Urological investigations are time-consuming, and only rarely are the injuries immediately life-threatening. They should be delayed until the patient is fully resuscitated.

• An IVP can be obtained with 30% contrast material at 1–2 ml/kg (up to 100 ml), followed by a plain abdominal film within 5–10 minutes. This will show most major abnormalities in the kidney and collecting system. If a kidney is not visualized, selective renal angiography may be indicated. Delayed films and tomography may be needed to further evaluate the renal parenchyma and ureters. In the presence of abnormal IVP findings, CT is often the next diagnostic step, as it is highly sensitive and accurate.

Kidney trauma

Trauma to the kidneys usually results in contusions or lacerations, which often will heal with conservative management. Persistent haemorrhage or extravasation of urine will require surgery.

Bladder trauma

Among patients who sustain blunt trauma, bladder rupture is rare when the bladder is empty, usually occurring only when it is full (eg after prior alcohol intake), especially in association with fractured pelvic rami or a separated pubic symphysis. Rupture can present as haematuria, positive findings on peritoneal lavage, anuria, or even peritonitis.

A retrograde cystogram may be indicated in the presence of haematuria and a fractured pelvis. It can be readily performed by gravity infusion of 150–300 ml of water-soluble contrast material. Anteroposterior, oblique, and post-drainage views are necessary to exclude injury. The priority of IVP over cystography hinges on whether upper- or lower-tract injury is more likely. CT with IV contrast is increasingly being used to evaluate the urinary tract in the presence of pelvic fractures.

Urethral trauma

Urethral trauma is a rare problem. When it does occur, it is usually in association with severe blunt trauma to the pelvis and perineum. A high-riding prostate, blood at the urethral meatus, and a scrotal haematoma are contraindications for placing an indwelling bladder catheter. Either a suprapubic cystostomy, if the bladder can be palpated, or a urethrogram should be considered.

If the patency of the urethra is in doubt, a urethrogram should be obtained before catheterization, by gentle injection 30 ml of water-soluble contrast through the urethra via a urinary catheter secured in the meatal fossa by balloon inflation to about 3 ml.

PENETRATING TRAUMA

The early management of a patient who has suffered penetrating trauma is the same as for those with other injuries (see p. 243). The patient should be managed with the same systematic approach in the primary and secondary surveys, as well as for definitive treatment. Much of this is discussed under specific sections in this chapter (eg abdomen, chest, extremities). However, there are specific aspects of penetrating trauma that one should remember during assessment and treatment.

PENETRATING CHEST INJURIES

• Lacerations of intrathoracic organs can cause catastrophic blood loss. Rapid fluid replacement and even emergency thoracotomy may be necessary. The indications for emergency thoracotomy are discussed elsewhere (see p. 272).

• When the positioning of a penetrating foreign object or the entry and exit wounds suggest that the mediastinum has been traversed, exploratory thoracotomy is mandatory, even if the patient is initially stable, as the probability of damage to vital structures is high.

• Pulmonary lacerations are associated with pneumothorax or haemothorax (see p. 268). Major, life-threatening lacerations are uncommon, representing about 4% of thoracic trauma cases, usually accompanied by haemoptysis or haemopneumothorax with parenchymal haematoma. These patients usually require thoracotomy.

• Cardiac lacerations can result in rapid exsanguination into the pleural space, cardiac tamponade (see p. 279), and other injuries, depending on the site of penetration.

• Large-vessel penetration presents as massive bleeding in more than 50% of cases. If the damage is intrapericardial, pericardial tamponade can result (see p. 279). Less serious injuries can result in false aneurysms or arteriovenous fistulae. Rapid volume replacement and early surgery are required.

• A lacerated diaphragm, like rupture of the diaphragm from blunt trauma (see p. 278), is a difficult diagnosis to make. Exploratory laparotomy may be necessary, especially when the site of penetration raises suspicion that a knife or bullet may have gone through the diaphragm.

PENETRATING ABDOMINAL TRAUMA

• Blood loss can be severe. Rapid replacement through large-bore cannulae and early cross-matching are essential.

• Every entry wound must be noted, particularly when they are multiple. If there are exit wounds in the back, bear in mind the possibility of penetration of abdominal viscera.

• Radiographs may demonstrate missiles or foreign objects within the body.

• Penetration of the peritoneal cavity may be evident from the locations of the entry or exit sites or from radiographic visualization.

• Stable patients with stab wounds may require only local wound exploration or peritoneal lavage (see p. 262).

• Laparotomy is mandatory if the lavage fluid contains blood (see p. 263) or increased amylase.

• Early administration of prophylactic antibiotics with a wide spectrum, covering anaerobes and Gram-negative bacteria, and tetanus prophylaxis should be commenced if laparotomy is to be performed.

BURNS

The initial assessment, management, and investigations should be carried out simultaneously, according to the priorities for the particular patient.

HISTORY

It is important to determine the circumstances of the burn:

• Explosions (liquid, steam, fire): Look for other features, such as fractures and intra-abdominal bleeding.

• Burning wood, chemicals, plastic: Think of cyanide poisoning and water-soluble gases causing pneumonitis.

• Burns in an enclosed space: Consider carbon monoxide poisoning.

INITIAL MANAGEMENT

ENSURE A PATENT AIRWAY.

ASSESS AND TREAT RESPIRATORY DYSFUNCTION.

REPLACE LOST FLUIDS.

RELIEVE THE PATIENT'S PAIN.

CONSIDER ESCHAROTOMY OR FASCIOTOMY.

TRANSFER TO A BURN CENTRE AS SOON AS THE PATIENT IS RE-SUSCITATED.

AIRWAY AND PULMONARY INHALATION INJURIES

Tracheobronchial and pulmonary parenchymal injuries are due to direct effects of heat or chemicals.

Inhalation injuries are seen in about 20% of burn patients and are associated with various factors:

- fire in an enclosed space
- a period of unconsciousness before rescue (especially in association with drugs, alcohol, or head injuries)
- facial burns/singed facial hair
- hoarseness/stridor
- carbonaceous sputum
- dyspnoea, wheezing

The diagnosis is usually obvious on the basis of history and clinical presentation.

The key to management of these patients is close observation in an environment in which intubation can be achieved rapidly by skilled personnel. Early intubation is recommended when facial and airway oedema is becoming a problem.

Acute upper-airway obstruction can develop **SUDDENLY,** in which case one should intubate and then either artificially ventilate or deliver CPAP (see p. 367). Tracheostomy can be performed safely in burn victims.

All patients suspected of having inhalational injuries should have maximum concentrations of inspired oxygen. Chest x-ray and arterial blood-gas determinations should be used to assess the severity of the damage. The initial chest x-ray may show nothing abnormal.

Parenchymal lung injury or ARDS can be related to the primary injury or, less commonly, can result from overly aggressive fluid resuscitation. Treatment is outlined in Chapter 19.

Carbon monoxide poisoning should always be considered a possibility in burn patients (see p. 338). Determine carboxyhaemoglobin levels if in doubt. Symptoms can occur if these levels are higher than 15%. Myocardial ischaemia can occur when levels are higher than 25%. A cherry-red skin colour is an uncommon and unreliable sign.

FLUID REPLACEMENT

The goal of fluid resuscitation is to maintain adequate tissue perfusion without exacerbating the burn oedema. The composition of the resuscitation fluid is less important than is titration of the correct amount for the individual patient's need.

Estimate the percentage of the body burned and the thickness of the burn injury (Figure 14.5). Fluid loss is directly related to the fluid sequestered as a result of thermal injury. Little further sequestration of fluid will occur 18–30 hours post burn.

Intravenous fluid is required if more than 15% of the body is burned.

The choice between colloid and crystalloid solutions is still controversial. Although some of the colloid particles will leak out of the intravascular space in the affected area, colloids may be more efficient in terms of restoring plasma volume and causing less pulmonary and peripheral oedema in the unaffected areas.

Despite the myriad formulae for fluid replacement, the aim is to MAINTAIN ORGAN PERFUSION. This is best assured by maintaining urine output of at least $0.5 \ \mathrm{ml \cdot kg^{-1} \cdot h^{-1}}$ for adults and 1 $\mathrm{ml \cdot kg^{-1} \cdot h^{-1}}$ for children. This will mean giving intravenous fluid at a rate of 3 ml/kg × percentage of body burned (% burn) per day for adults.

Guidelines

Following are two suggested fluid regimens, assuming that all times are calculated from the moment of injury. Alterations will have to be made according to the patient's clinical status.

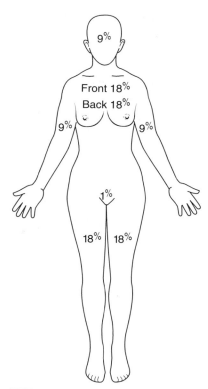

FIGURE 14.5 The 'rule of nines' for rapid assessment of percentage body burned. Do not include simple erythema.

1. Give Ringer's lactate at 2 ml/kg × (% burn) per day.

Give colloid at 1 ml/kg × (% burn) per day.

Give half of each over 8 hours, and the remainder over 16 hours.

Then give only the colloid after the initial 24 hours – titrate against intravascular measurements (see p. 55).

GIVE BLOOD AS NECESSARY (usually required if more than 30% of body is burned).

Intravenous water in the form of dextrose and water may be necessary, in addition to the foregoing requirements, as maintenance fluid, in order to prevent hypernatraemia. The amount of water can be empirically titrated against the serum sodium concentration (usually 1–3 L/d).

2. Give a balanced salt solution (Ringer's lactate or Hartmann's solution) at 2–4 ml/kg × (% burn) per day. Administer half of the amount in the first 8 hours. Then give colloid or blood and maintenance fluid as necessary.

Remember that the volume necessary to resuscitate patients with burns is dependent on the severity of the burn, age, physiological status, and other associated injuries. Resuscitation formulae are only guidelines.

IMMEDIATE INVESTIGATIONS

Arterial blood gases
Urea and electrolytes
Haemoglobin, blood grouping, and cross-matching
Chest x-ray
Carbon monoxide levels
12-lead ECG

IMMEDIATE MONITORING

Pulse rate and continuous ECG
Respiratory rate
Pulse oximetry
Arterial blood pressure
Urine output
Level of consciousness

ANALGESIA

INTRAVENOUS OPIATES SHOULD BE GIVEN IN LIBERAL QUANTITIES FOR THIS DISTRESSING INJURY. An opiate is best given as a continuous intravenous infusion, titrated against its pain-relieving effects (see p. 115).

ESCHAROTOMY

Immediate escharotomy or fasciotomy is occasionally indicated. Rapid excision of devitalized tissue, combined with early and continuous wound closure with autograft or artificial skin, is essential.

NUTRITIONAL SUPPORT

Patients with burns have markedly increased metabolic rates, increased rates of glucose production and utilization, decreased rates of lipid metabolism, and increased rates of protein catabolism and anabolism. The principles of nutritional support are the same as outlined for other seriously ill patients (see Chapter 5). Enteral feeding is preferred, where possible, to intravenous nutrition. Enteral feeding should be initiated within 48 hours of burn injury, utilizing feeding tubes until the patient is capable of taking adequate amounts orally. The diet should provide approximately 50% of calories as carbohydrate, 25% as protein, and 25% as fat.

PROPHYLACTIC ANTIBIOTICS AND CORTICOSTEROIDS SHOULD NOT BE USED.

TRANSFER THE PATIENT TO A SPECIALIZED BURN UNIT AS SOON AS ADEQUATE RESUSCITATION HAS BEEN ACHIEVED.

OVERALL COURSE OF BURNS

Days 1–2
Resuscitation:
- airway
- breathing
- fluids and support of the circulation

Days 2–5
Oedema reabsorption
Increase in urine output, with potassium losses

Day 6
Marked increase in metabolic rate

ELECTRICAL INJURIES

The damages sustained during electrical injuries are related to various factors:

- type of current
- duration of current flow – the longer the contact, the greater the damage (AC worse than DC because of tetanic effect on muscles)
- surface area contacted (greater current density in a small area)
- resistance (more severe damage occurs in areas of high resistance)
- amperage (the higher the amperage, the greater the damage)
- voltage (anything greater than 40 volts is potentially dangerous)
- current pathway (related to resistance and voltage)

PATHOPHYSIOLOGY

Electrical injuries are related to primary electrical trauma and electrothermal burns that result from electrical energy being converted to heat as it passes through tissues. Flame burns can also occur if the current ignites clothing or other material.

CLINICAL FEATURES

COAGULATION NECROSIS This is the major feature of electrical injuries, and it occurs as a result of vessel thrombosis and heat damage. It can result in extensive tissue necrosis, similar to that seen with a crush injury.

CUTANEOUS WOUNDS Usually there is a charred entry wound, with multiple exit sites.

Cardiac

- conduction defects, including ventricular fibrillation (VF), ventricular tachycardia (VT), supraventricular tachycardia (SVT), bundle branch blocks and heart block
- myocardial rupture
- coronary ischaemia

Respiratory

- upper-airway burns
- haemopneumothorax

Neurological

- confusion, seizures, and loss of consciousness
- cerebral haemorrhage, oedema, and focal damage
- peripheral nerve damage
- spinal-cord damage
- long-term memory and behavioural problems

Musculoskeletal

- tetanic contractions
- disruption of muscle cells (release of potassium and CPK)
- fractures of vertebral bodies and other bones
- dislocations

Gastro-intestinal

- nausea, vomiting
- bleeding
- paralytic ileus
- perforated bowel
- parenchymatous injury (eg pancreas, spleen, gall-bladder)

Renal

- renal failure (albuminuria, haemoglobinuria, myoglobinuria)

Vascular

- arterial and venous thromboses and rupture
- haemolysis

- microcirculation thrombosis
- aneurysm formation

Infection
Cataracts

MANAGEMENT

Initial measures

Remove the patient from the source of the current and ensure ABC:

AIRWAY: Secure the airway, and, if necessary, intubate.
BREATHING: Assist breathing, if necessary.
CIRCULATION: Give external cardiac massage. Defibrillate, if necessary. Begin aggressive fluid replacement.

Renal function

Renal function deteriorates secondary to hypovolaemia and myoglobinuria. The treatment for the latter is outlined elsewhere (see p. 298).

Initial investigation and monitoring

Continuous ECG monitoring and pulse oximetry
Regular monitoring of vital signs (blood pressure, pulse rate, respiratory rate, and urine output)
Haemoglobin and haematocrit
Urea and electrolytes
Arterial blood gases
Renal function tests
Examine for spinal fractures (see p. 281)
Chest x-ray (upright if possible)

Further management

Assessment, debridement, and fasciotomy, if necessary.
Avoid correcting the serum calcium concentration, because of the possibility of ectopic calcification.

Tetanus toxoid prophylaxis and intravenous penicillin as prophylaxis against clostridial infections of open wounds.

LIGHTNING INJURIES

Lightning injuries are more than simply high-voltage electrical injuries. Although the amount of energy in a lightning bolt is enormous, it is in contact with the body for only a brief period. Thus, skin damage is usually minimal. Moreover, because of the 'flashover' effect, the energy tends to travel around the body, rather than through it, causing rapid dissipation of energy.

Mechanisms of injury from lightning strikes

• direct strike: cutaneous entry and exit wounds relatively rare
• contact voltage: when the victim is touching an object struck by lightning
• sideflash: from another object hit by the strike
• ground current: when the strike spreads along the ground
• blunt injury: from being thrown as a result of the strike

Clinical features

CARDIOVASCULAR

• cardiac arrest (the most common cause of death)
• arrhythmias
• ischaemia

NEUROLOGICAL

• seizures or loss of consciousness
• paralysis paraesthesias (usually transient)
• intracranial haemorrhage
• long-term neuropsychiatric problems
• spinal-cord damage

RESPIRATORY

• respiratory arrest
• ARDS (rarely)

MUSCULOSKELETAL, CUTANEOUS, AND RENAL COMPLICATIONS
• relatively rare

Management

Conduct initial resuscitation, management, and investigations as for other electrical injuries (see p. 293. Victims who are still alive after lightning strikes usually have uneventful recoveries.

CRUSH INJURIES AND ACUTE COMPARTMENT SYNDROME

CRUSH INJURIES

Although the term 'crush injury' is sometimes used to cover a wide range of pathological changes, from very minor to severe, it is usually reserved for cases at the more severe end of the spectrum. The clinical signs are determined by the extent of the compressed area and the depth and duration of the compression. Such injuries involve both ischaemia and muscle destruction.

AETIOLOGY

PATIENT'S OWN WEIGHT (eg unconsciousness related to poisoning or long operations) The heavier the patient, the more severe the damage.

EXTERNAL FORCE (eg use of antishock garments, limbs caught in machinery, injuries resulting from collapse of a building, other traumatic events causing compression and crushing).

CLINICAL FEATURES

If an injury is severe enough, a crush syndrome will result, caused by disintegration of muscle tissue and rhabdomyolysis, with influxes of myoglobin, potassium, uric acid, and phosphorus into the circulation. All of that results in two main categories of complications:

• Local: There will be variable degrees of pain, swelling, and sensory changes.

• Systemic: In more severe cases, hypovolaemia, acute renal failure, severe coagulopathies (including disseminated intravascular coagulation), ARDS, and shock can all occur.

ASSESSMENT

The extent of both local and systemic damages will require careful monitoring, including regular testing of sensory and motor nerves and assessment of peripheral pulses. Detection of peripheral pulses does not exclude severe crush injury. Direct pressure measurements of muscle compartments may be necessary (see p. 300).

Treatment

RESUSCITATION

• Administer fluids aggressively – hypovolaemia must be rapidly corrected.

• Regular measurements of arterial blood gases and serum sodium, potassium, magnesium, phosphate, creatinine, urea, uric acid, and calcium are necessary.

• Serum creatine kinase activities greater than five times normal are diagnostic of muscle damage in the absence of other injuries.

• Regular coagulation studies and haemoglobin and platelet counts are necessary.

• Renal function, respiratory function, and cardiovascular function should be closely monitored.

• A CT scan of the affected area may demonstrate myonecrosis.

RESPIRATORY FAILURE ARDS should be treated early (see p. 400).

RENAL FAILURE Correction of hypovolaemia is the most important step in the prevention of renal failure. Renal-dosage dopamine (1–3 $\mu g \cdot kg^{-1} \cdot min^{-1}$) may be given to at-risk patients. Alkalinization of the urine may also help to prevent renal failure. Aim to keep the urine pH above 6.5 by infusion of sodium bicarbonate (10–20 mmol/h).

Diuresis: Induction of diuresis with mannitol (0.3 mg/kg IV initially, followed by a continuous IV infusion) may also help to prevent renal failure. Discontinue the infusion if the patient becomes oliguric or anuric. Beware of the exacerbation of hypovolaemia that can occur with the use of diuretics. Dialysis may be necessary if these measures fail (see p. 652).

LOCAL INJURY Excision of dead muscle is not necessarily essential if the wound is closed. Open crush injuries require fasciotomy and immediate radical debridement of dead muscle. Major bleeding is a common complication.

Dead muscle is an excellent medium for infection and sepsis. Amputation should be considered early, especially for a severely injured limb with skin lacerations.

Fasciotomy should be considered when there is a high compartment pressure or when distal pulses and capillary filling are absent. Because this will convert the wound into an open wound, radical debridement should accompany the fasciotomy. Amputation should be strongly considered in all patients who have sepsis or open wounds in the presence of severe crush injuries. This is because the muscle tissue is already dead in true crush syndrome, as opposed to a simple compartment syndrome.

ACUTE COMPARTMENT SYNDROME

A compartment syndrome is a condition in which high pressure within a closed fascial space (muscle compartment) reduces capillary blood perfusion below the level necessary for tissue viability. Permanent loss of function and limb contracture can occur, and therefore capillary perfusion should be restored as soon as possible.

Aetiology

- fractures (especially of the tibia)
- contusions
- bleeding disorders
- burns
- trauma

- venous obstruction
- post-ischaemic swelling after arterial injury or thrombosis
- strenuous exercise
- prolonged limb compression (eg drug or alcohol overdose)
- tight plaster cast

Clinical features: the five P's

PAIN Pain is the most important symptom. It is described as deep and throbbing, with a feeling of unrelenting pressure. The pain is said to be worse on stretching.

PRESSURE The compartment is swollen and palpably tense, although palpation offers only a crude indication of pressure.

PARAESTHESIAS Paraesthesias may also be found.

PARESIS Paresis may also occur independently as a result of nerve and muscle damage.

PERIPHERAL PULSES Capillary refilling and peripheral pulses usually can be detected in compartment syndrome, even in the presence of severe muscle ischaemia. This should not lead to a false sense of security.

All of these signs and symptoms can occur independently as a result of trauma, and they are difficult to assess in an unconscious patient.

Measurement of tissue pressure

Because palpation offers only a crude estimation of tissue pressure, and the presence or absence of capillary refilling and peripheral pulses is no guide to the extent of muscle ischaemia, direct measurement of tissue pressure is a more accurate guide to the need for surgical intervention. The principle of such a measurement is a continuous column of fluid from the compartment to a pressure-measuring device. Flushing is necessary to guarantee accurate measurements. Devices that can be inserted into the compartment to measure pressure include needles, wicks, and slit catheters.

It is suggested that fasciotomies should be performed when the pressure is more than 30 mm Hg. In the absence of a pressure measurement, the symptoms and signs previously mentioned can be used as guidelines.

Treatment

Fasciotomy is the treatment of choice for compartment syndrome. If the muscle appears necrotic, debridement should be carried out, and skin incisions not closed. Partial skin closure (if possible, with further debridement) should occur after 3 or 4 days. Other procedures that can reduce pressure, such as fracture reduction or escharotomy, should also be performed.

NEAR-DROWNING

The aim of treatment is to re-establish cardiorespiratory function before neurological damage occurs. This is more a function of first-aid, rather than intensive care. Rapid initial resuscitation will significantly influence outcome in the ICU.

PRECIPITATING EVENT

Near-drowning incidents often are associated with precipitating causes:

- epilepsy – Obtain a history, and determine anticonvulsant levels.
- alcohol intake – Obtain a history, and determine the blood alcohol level.
- spinal-cord or head injury – especially in association with diving or surfboard accidents.
- child abuse – Do a skeletal survey.
- cardiac causes – arrhythmias, acute myocardial infarction.

AIRWAY

If the patient is unconscious, or if there is doubt about the patency of the airway, INTUBATE.

RESPIRATORY FUNCTION

People who drown or nearly drown rarely aspirate large amounts of water. At least 10% aspirate no water and probably develop laryngeal spasm – the so-called dry drowning. However, hypoxia is universal in near-drowning incidents. In drowning without aspiration, hypoxia results simply from apnoea. When the victim aspirates, the volume and composition of the fluid contribute to the hypoxia. Stomach contents and contaminated water, even in small amounts, can cause severe hypoxia. Pulmonary oedema occurs in both fresh-water and salt-water drowning and frequently occurs acutely.

ARDS and bronchopneumonia can occur later, usually in association with aspiration.

Management

The standard approach to hypoxia should be used (see Chapter 17).

PRINCIPLES

• Use a face mask with a high concentration of inspired oxygen.
• Use CPAP via a mask or tube if it can be tolerated and if ventilation is not a problem.
• Maintain the cardiovascular system with colloid or blood, and limit the use of crystalloid fluids.
• Use IMV or IPPV/PEEP if ventilation is inadequate.
• Monitor progress:

serial chest x-rays (at least daily)
serial blood-gas determinations or pulse oximetry

BLOOD VOLUME AND ELECTROLYTES

Animal models have shown that fresh water is absorbed into the blood volume, causing dilution, haemolysis, and electrolyte disturbances,

whereas salt water simultaneously decreases the blood volume by os-
mosis and is absorbed in excessive amounts. However, in clinical practice there is little difference between salt-water and fresh-water near-
drowning episodes. Many near-drowning victims are **HYPOVOLAEMIC**
as a result of pulmonary oedema. Colloid should be used for resuscitation. Major electrolyte disturbances are not common. Nevertheless,
serum osmolality determinations and serum biochemistry tests should
be regularly performed.

The cardiovascular system should be monitored by routine measurements of parameters such as arterial blood pressure, pulse rate,
peripheral perfusion, arterial pH, serum lactate, and urine output,
and, if necessary, CVP and pulmonary artery catheterization should
be used.

HYPOTHERMIA

These patients often are hypothermic. If a patient's temperature is
above 30°C, allow passive, slow rewarming. Many need catecholamine
infusions to maintain the cardiovascular system if the body's core temperature is below 30°C. Low temperature alone does not indicate improved chances for good survival. Patients who become hypothermic
in water that is near 0°C before they go into arrest (primary hypothermia) have a better prognosis than do patients who arrest early
in non-icy waters and then become hypothermic (secondary hypothermia). Treatment of hypothermia is described elsewhere (see
Chapter 11).

Deliberate induction of hypothermia as part of treatment is controversial.

NEUROLOGICAL MANAGEMENT

The most important aspect in the management of near-drowning victims is maintenance of neurological functions. Cerebral oedema and
increased intracranial pressure usually become evident after 24
hours. Active management of the neurological sequelae (eg corticosteroids, barbiturate coma, induced hypothermia) has largely been
abandoned. Nevertheless, the basic principles of treating cerebral
oedema should be applied if the patient is unconscious (see Chapter 24):

PRINCIPLES

• Sit the patient head-up (>30° inclination to facilitate venous drainage); however, maintain arterial blood pressure and cerebral perfusion pressure (CPP).

• Keep the head straight, and do not tie the ETT with constricting tapes, which could prevent adequate cerebral venous drainage.

• Avoid stimulating procedures, or use prior sedation, to prevent hypertensive surges in the presence of an increased intracranial pressure (ICP) and damage to the blood–brain barrier.

• Maintain adequate oxygenation; avoid hypercarbia and acidosis.

• Minimize the use of crystalloid solutions – maintain 'euvolaemic dehydration'.

• ICP monitoring can help to increase awareness of the factors that can exacerbate an already elevated ICP. However, it has not, as yet, been shown to influence survival. Sustained intracranial hypertension is a poor prognostic sign.

MISCELLANEOUS CONSIDERATIONS

Coagulopathy: Severe coagulopathy can sometimes occur. Management is described elsewhere (see p. 715).

Renal function: Acute renal failure can occur after near-drowning incidents (see Chapter 27).

GIVE NO STEROIDS.

GIVE NO PROPHYLACTIC ANTIBIOTICS.

USE ROUTINE INTENSIVE CARE:

  prevention of acute stress ulceration (see p. 31)

  nutrition (see Chapter 5)

  sedation (see Chapter 7)

  prevention of septicaemia (see Chapter 13)

PROGNOSIS

These patients are classified on the basis of their status on admission to hospital following their rescue:

A AWAKE, 100% survival

B BLUNTED LEVEL of consciousness (ie obtunded, but can be roused), at least 90% survival. Most deaths are due to cardiorespiratory causes. Patients in this group should recover full neurological functions.

C COMATOSE

Adults: More than 50% survive, with variable percentages having some degree of neurological damage, and the remainder die. Children: Fewer than 50% survive neurologically intact; variable percentages of survivors will have some degree of brain damage.

The occurrence of a FIRST GASP within 30 minutes of the initiation of the resuscitation effort and an early resumption of SPONTANEOUS RESPIRATION are good prognostic indicators, as is neurological responsiveness at the scene of the incident. Very poor prognostic indicators are a submersion duration greater than 10 minutes and unproductive resuscitation efforts lasting longer than 25 minutes.

Each patient must be assessed individually, especially with regard to body temperature, whether or not neurological improvement occurs, and at what rate it occurs (see p. 590).

TRAUMA IN OBSTETRIC PATIENTS

The treatment priorities are the same as for multitrauma (see p. 243). However, management of obstetric patients involves special considerations, because pregnancy alters the maternal physiology, and the fetus is a second potential victim. An obstetrician and paediatric surgeon should be enlisted in most cases.

The uterus is initially protected by the pelvic ring, but it becomes more prone to injury as it enlarges. In the latter part of pregnancy, the uterus is vulnerable to injury and offers little protection to the fetus. Fetal death is much more common than maternal death. Even minor injuries can result in death of the fetus.

There are many physiological changes during pregnancy (see p. 775) that can affect the mother's reaction to blood loss and injury. Cardiac output, tidal volume, blood volume, and pulse rate are all increased. The gravid uterus can compress the inferior vena cava and severely reduce venous return when the patient is in the supine position – the supine hypotension syndrome.

The uterus is prone to rupture as a result of blunt trauma. Placental abruption occurs in 1–5% of minor injuries and in up to 50% of major injuries, and it can occur up to 3 days after the initial trauma. Labour can be precipitated, and direct fetal injury can also occur. The fetus must be carefully monitored during this period, for in addition to the danger of abruption, shock and hypoxia in the mother can cause fetal distress. Immediate delivery is required in the event of fetal distress if the gestation is past 26 weeks.

FETAL ASSESSMENT

• Monitor fetal movements.

• Time the uterine contractions.

• Monitor the fetal heart rate (normal, 120–160/min).

• Cardiotocographic monitoring should be commenced as soon as possible. Continuous monitoring, rather than intermittent auscultation, is preferable.

• Doppler ultrasound may be useful to determine gestational age and assess fetal well-being if the findings from cardiac monitoring are equivocal, as well as to estimate the volume of amniotic fluid if rupture of the amniotic membrane is suspected. However, cardiotocographic monitoring usually is a superior means for assessment.

MANAGEMENT

The general principles of management are the same as for other patients with multitrauma (see p. 243).

Airway and breathing

In the latter stages of pregnancy, intubation can be difficult. There may be laryngeal oedema. These patients can rapidly become hypoxic because of decreased functional residual capacity and increased oxygen consumption.

Secure the airway, by intubating if necessary. Always give a high concentration of inspired oxygen, and immobilize the neck with a rigid collar if there is doubt about the cervical spine.

Circulation

The fetal circulation is not self-regulating. Uterine blood flow is largely dependent on systemic blood pressure. Hypovolaemia must be aggressively corrected.

TABLE 14.7 NORMAL PAEDIATRIC VITAL SIGNS (APPROXIMATE)

	Pulse (beats/min)	Arterial blood pressure (mm Hg)	Respiration (breaths/min)
Infant	150	80	40
Pre-schooler	130	90	30
Adolescent	110	100	20

Systolic blood pressure (mm Hg): $2 \times$ age + 70

Weight (kg): $2 \times$ age + 8

Blood volume (ml/kg): 80

Endotracheal-tube size: (age/4) + 4

Establish intravenous access with large cannulae, and aggressively infuse fluids in order to reverse any hypovolaemia. Do not hesitate to infuse rapidly cross-matched blood (Rh-negative) (see p. 706). Patients should remain in the left lateral decubitus position if possible.

DPL can be performed using a supraumbilical minilaparotomy.

DO NOT HESITATE TO PERFORM EMERGENCY INVESTIGATIONS AND TREATMENT (EG LAPAROTOMY) AS FOR ANY OTHER PATIENT.

PAEDIATRIC TRAUMA

The general principles of resuscitation and management of children who have suffered trauma are the same as for adults. However, there are some important specific differences between children and adults (Table 14.7). It is mainly these that will be emphasized in this section.

AIRWAY AND CERVICAL SPINE

If there is any doubt about the airway, endotracheal intubation with an uncuffed tube is recommended (Table 14.8). There should always be provision for a small leak at approximately 20 cm H_2O airway pressure. The size of the tube should roughly correspond to the diameter of the child's fifth finger or external nares (see p. 752). The

TABLE 14.8 APPROXIMATE SIZES OF PAEDIATRIC EQUIPMENT ACCORDING TO AGE (APPROXIMATE WEIGHT)

Equipment	0–6 months (1–6 kg)	6–12 months (4–9 kg)	1–3 years (10–15 kg)	4–7 years (16–20 kg)	8–11 years (22–33 kg)
Airway/breathing					
Oxygen mask	0	0/1	1	1/2	2/3 (adult)
Oral airways	000/00	0/1	0/1	1/2	2
Resuscitator	Baby	Baby	Baby/adult	Adult	Adult
Breathing system	T-piece	T-piece	T-piece	T-piece	Coaxial
Laryngoscope	Straight blade	Straight blade	Child Macintosh	Child Macintosh	Adult Macintosh
Tracheal tubes (uncuffed)	2.5–3.5	3.5–4.0	4.0–5.0	5.0–6.0	5.5–7.0
Suction catheter (French gauge)	6	8	8–10	10	12
Circulation					
Intravenous cannula (gauge)	24/22	22	22/18	20/16	18/14
Central venous pressure cannula (gauge)	20	20	18	18	16
Arterial cannula (gauge)	24/22	22	22	22	20
Ancillary equipment					
Nasogastric tube (French gauge)	8	10	10–12	12	12–14
Chest drain (French gauge)	10–14	12–18	14–20	14–24	16–30
Urinary catheter (French gauge)	5-gauge feeding tube	5-gauge feeding tube	Foley (8)	Foley (10) (10–12)	Foley

relative shortness of the trachea will increase the risk of endo-bronchial intubation or accidental extubation. Although injuries of the cervical spine are uncommon in children who survive accidents, the neck should be immobilized in any seriously injured child until spinal damage is excluded.

Failure to maintain the airway is the commonest cause of pre-ventable death in children with trauma.

BREATHING

Assess the following:

- chest expansion
- tracheal position
- respiratory rate
- neck-vein distension
- breath and heart sounds

As with adults, an early chest x-ray is mandatory.
Examine for pneumothorax and haemothorax.

CIRCULATION

Assessment

Tachycardia is a primary response to hypovolaemia.

Children, as a rule, have greater physiological reserves than adults and compensate better during hypovolaemia. However, that can be dangerous, because hypotension is a late sign indicating severe hy-povolaemia. (The systolic blood pressure should be 70 mm Hg plus twice the child's age in years.)

Hypotension, altered mental status, and absence of peripheral pulses in the presence of hypvolaemia signal imminent cardiorespi-ratory arrest.

Fluid replacement

The principles of fluid replacement are the same as for adults (see Chapter 4).

Among children, the body weight (in kilograms) is approximately twice the age (in years) plus 8. Blood volume is approximately 80 ml/kg body weight. Tibial interosseous infusion of fluids and drugs is easy and effective in children up to the age of 6 years.

INITIAL CHALLENGE Give colloid or crystalloid solution at 20 ml/kg as an initial fluid challenge. This represents approximately 25% of the normal blood volume (80 ml/kg).

FURTHER FLUID Rapidly restore the circulating volume by giving further 10–20-ml/kg boluses of fluid, according to the physiological responses, until rapidly cross-matched blood is ready.

BLOOD Blood must be given early, as for adults (see p. 246). Blood transfusion is essential after the total of infused crystalloid or colloid has reached 40 ml/kg.

Group-specific blood usually can be obtained within 15 minutes. Any child who is in shock or is hypovolaemic should receive warmed blood as soon as possible.

Blood can be given in amounts 20 ml/kg as soon as rapid cross-matching is complete, with the infusion rate titrated against the physiological responses. Surgery should be considered if the circulation remains unstable despite aggressive resuscitation.

THERMOREGULATION

The high ratio of body surface to body mass in children, their thin skin, and their relative lack of subcutaneous tissue predispose them to hypothermia, especially smaller children. Blood should be warmed, and humidifiers should be used, and overhead heaters or thermal blankets may also be necessary.

CHEST TRAUMA

Because a child's chest wall is compliant, allowing efficient energy transfer, pulmonary contusions and haemorrhages are common, but fractured ribs are uncommon. Pneumothorax is a common cause of preventable deaths in children. Diaphragmatic ruptures and great-vessel injuries are rare, compared with their rates in adults. The approach to diagnosis and management is the same as for adults (see p. 266). Almost all these injuries will resolve with supportive treatment, and thoracotomy is rarely required.

ABDOMINAL TRAUMA

Non-operative management of patients with blunt abdominal trauma is becoming increasingly accepted for solid visceral injuries in children, especially when the vital signs and haematocrit are stable. The most common injuries are to the spleen, liver, and kidneys.

Blunt abdominal injuries compose the second most common cause of preventable death in children.

Guidelines for laparotomy in children
• persistent bleeding, as indicated by failure to respond to aggressive fluid replacement (eg blood totalling more than 40 ml/kg)
• suspicion of injury to hollow viscera
• severe concomitant head injury and an unstable circulation due to unexplained hypovolaemia that may be compromising cerebral perfusion

The need for DPL in children probably is restricted to multiply injured children with severe head injuries in whom intra-abdominal injuries are suspected and in whom there is unexplained hypovolaemia. Children who are haemodynamically stable should have abdominal CT.

EXTREMITY TRAUMA

Blood loss associated with pelvic and long-bone fractures is proportionately greater in children (eg up to 500 ml can be lost into the thigh from a fractured femur).

Because the bones are less well mineralized, interpretation of x-rays, especially around the joint, is difficult. Comparison with the opposite side is useful.

There should be a careful examination for growth-plate fractures after the patient has been resuscitated.

TABLE 14.9 PAEDIATRIC TRAUMA SCORE[a]

Parameter	+2	+1	−1
		Score	
Weight	>20 kg	10–20 kg	<10 kg
Airway	Normal	Oral/nasal airway	Intubated/ tracheostomy
Systolic blood pressure	>90 mm Hg	50–90 mm Hg	<50 mm Hg
Central nervous system	Awake	Obtunded	Coma/ decerebrate
Open wound	None	Minor	Major/penetrating
Skeletal	None	Closed fracture	Open/ multiple fractures

[a]Possible range −6 to +12. A score of 8 or less indicates potentially serious trauma.

Supracondylar fractures of the elbow are associated with a high incidence of vascular injuries and growth deformity.

HEAD INJURY

An elevated ICP is more common in children, and focal mass lesions are less common.

Head injuries should be assessed and treated as for adults (see p. 599).

Children tend to recover better than adults.

Seizures early after injury are more likely in children.

Children under 6 months of age can become hypovolaemic from intracranial blood loss.

Vomiting is common after head injuries in children and does not necessarily mean an elevated ICP.

The severity of a head injury is usually measured by depth and duration of coma. Coma lasting less than 20 minutes is usually considered mild; up to 6 hours, moderate; 6–48 hours, severe; over 48 hours, very severe. However, at 1 week after injury, prediction of outcome category with respect to disability is accurate in only 70% of cases.

Even so-called mild injuries can result in some permanent brain damage.

PSYCHOLOGICAL ASPECTS

Psychological sequelae in children are common after severe trauma. They need to be continually comforted and reassured. In many cases, children's close relatives will also be involved, especially in traffic accidents, and may be unable to offer the necessary reassurance and comfort.

PAEDIATRIC TRAUMA SCORE

Increasingly, trauma scoring is being used for comparison and prediction. A simple, widely accepted score is outlined in Table 14.9.

TROUBLESHOOTING

TRAUMA PATIENTS: THE NEXT DAY

Once patients who have suffered serious multitrauma have been resuscitated and investigated and perhaps have undergone surgery, they are usually managed in the ICU. It is then time for a careful review of each case.

Airway An early decision may have to be made regarding whether or not a tracheostomy is indicated. This will largely depend on the anticipated length of ventilatory support. As a general rule, if intubation is anticipated for more than 2 weeks, early tracheostomy should be considered.

Hypoxia There are many possible causes of hypoxia at this stage, but the most common are post-traumatic ARDS (see p. 400), lung contusion (see p. 272), aspiration (see p. 423), and fat emboli (see p. 320).

Fractured ribs and flail chest If there are significant fractures of ribs or there is a large flail segment, early tracheostomy should be performed, particularly if the patient is age 50 years or older or has significant chronic underlying lung disease, especially related to smoking. Epidural analgesia should also be considered (see p. 120).

Hypotension and oliguria In the early stages of recovery from multitrauma, hypotension must be considered to be related to continued bleeding, until proved otherwise. Transfuse the patient, and look for the cause – pelvis, chest, abdomen, and long bones are the most likely.

Fever and tachycardia Nosocomial infection is unusual within the first 48 hours. However, fever and tachycardia are non-specific and relatively common accompaniments of severe trauma. Consider the possibility of fat emboli. Early fever and sepsis can also be related to aspiration, a ruptured abdominal viscus, or contaminated wounds.

Delayed abdominal injuries An overlooked abnormality or its delayed onset can cause features such as an acute abdomen or sepsis (eg ruptured viscus) or bleeding and haemoglobin reduction (eg ruptured spleen).

Feeding A decision must be made whether the patient can tolerate enteral nutrition (see p. 87) or whether intravenous nutrition must be commenced (see p. 89).

Pain It is important to provide adequate pain relief for patients who have suffered multitrauma (see p. 116).

Major fractures and plastic repair Major fractures and dislocations should be treated early rather than late (see p. 265). Similarly, definite times should be arranged for plastic repair of injuries (eg faciomaxillary injury).

Overlooked bone and soft-tissue injuries It is common to discover previously overlooked small-bone fractures and soft-tissue injuries (eg torn ligaments) up to many weeks after severe multitrauma. If a patient is unconscious, the only hint may be swelling or instability during passive movement. Although such indications may seem minor at the time, they can lead to severe disability.

Fat emboli These can cause hypoxia and confusion within 24 hours of fractures (see p. 320).

Prophylaxis against pulmonary embolism Low-dosage heparin probably should be commenced once active bleeding has ceased.

Continuing haematuria Investigate.

Relatives and friends It is never too soon to explain to relatives and friends that the patient may be in the hospital for weeks or even months, with the possibility of a lengthy rehabilitation period.

TROUBLESHOOTING

ACUTE LIMB CONDITIONS

TIME IS OF THE ESSENCE IN ASSESSING AND
TREATING AN ACUTE LIMB CONDITION

Important history and signs

- pain
- numbness
- temperature changes
- abnormal pulses
- slow capillary return
- crepitus
- cellulitis
- weakness

The examiner must inquire as to the state of the muscles, nerves,
and distal organs – not simply how the skin appears.

Major adverse outcomes

Focal death leading to loss of function
Global death leading to limb loss
Inflammation and infection that can lead to distant organ dysfunc-
  tion and even loss of the patient's life

Three main entities to consider

Ischaemia (eg arterial or graft thrombosis)
Infection (eg gas gangrene, diabetic foot)
Compartment compression (eg trauma)

Ischaemia

If it looks ischaemic, it must be considered ischaemic until proved oth-
  erwise.
This is a medical emergency, needing rapid restoration of blood flow.
The initial surgery should be definitive.

Infection

Rapidly spreading necrosis and gas formation may not be obvious simply from skin appearance.
Superficial cellulitis often is a marker of deep suppuration tracking
  along tendons and fascial planes.
Rapid diagnosis is essential, and definitive surgical debridement or
  amputation may be needed.
Debridement often must be repeated.

Compartment syndrome (see p. 299)

The term refers to increased pressure within one or more encapsulated compartments of a limb.

The causes can include crush syndrome, ischaemia, reperfusion, closed fracture, haematoma, and electrical burns.

Unrelieved pressure will result in impaired venous return, impaired arterial inflow, nerve and muscle ischaemia, and necrosis.

Decompress rapidly with a fasciotomy.

FURTHER READING

General Aspects of Multitrauma

Trunkey, D. D. (ed.) (1983). Symposium on trauma. *Surgical Clinics of North America* 62:1–195 (symposium issue).

Trunkey, D. D., & Lewis, F. (eds.) (1984). *Current Therapy of Trauma*. Philadelphia: BC Decker.

Wilson, R. F. (1980). Trauma. In *Critical Care: State of the Art*, vol. 1, ed. W. C. Shoemaker & W. L. Thompson, pp. T1–87. Fullerton, CA: Society of Critical Care Medicine.

The Trauma System and Scoring

Deane, S. A., Gaudry, P. L., Pearson, I., Misra, S., McNeil, J., & Read, C. (1990). The hospital trauma team: a model for trauma management. *Journal of Trauma* 30:806–11.

Smith, E. J., Ward, A. J., & Smith, D. (1990). Trauma scoring methods. *British Journal of Hospital Medicine* 44:114–18.

Blunt Abdominal Trauma

David, J. J., Cohn, I., & Nance, F. (1979). Diagnosis and management of blunt abdominal trauma. *Annals of Surgery* 183:672–8.

Feliciano, D. V. (1990). Management of traumatic retroperitoneal haematoma. *Annals of Surgery* 211:109–22.

Kellarn, J. F., McMurry, R. Y., Paleg, D., & Tile, M. (1987). The unstable pelvic fracture. *Orthopedic Clinics of North America* 18:25–41.

Thoracic Injuries

Baumann, M. H., & Sahn, S. A. (1990). Medical management and therapy of bronchopleural fistulas in the mechanically ventilated patient. *Chest* 97:721–8.

Besson, A., & Saegesser, F. (eds.) (1982). *A Colour Atlas of Chest Trauma and Associated Injuries*. London: Wolfe Medical.

Bolliger, C. T., & Van Eeden, S. F. (1990). Treatment of rib fractures. Randomized controlled trial comparing ventilatory and non ventilatory management. *Chest* 97:943–8.

Demling, R. H., & Pomfret, E. A. (1993). Blunt chest trauma. *New Horizons* 1:402–21.

Gilbert, T. B., McGrath, B. J., & Soberman, M. (1993). Chest tubes: indications, placement and complications. *Journal of Intensive Care Medicine* 8:73–86.

Hillman, K. (1985). Pulmonary barotrauma. *Clinics in Anaesthesiology* 3:877–98.

Worthley, L. I. G. (1985). Thoracic epidural in the management of chest trauma. *Intensive Care Medicine* 11:312–15.

Cardiac Injuries

Anonymous (1986). Blunt trauma to the heart. *Lancet* 2:724.

Hiatt, J. R., Yeatman, L. A., & Child, J. S. (1988). The value of echocardiography in blunt chest trauma. *Journal of Trauma* 28:914–18.

Kron, I. L., & Cox, P. M. (1983). Cardiac injury after chest trauma. *Critical Care Medicine* 11:524–6.

Taggart, D. P., & Reece, I. J. (1987). Penetrating cardiac injuries. *British Medical Journal* 294:1630–1.

Spinal injuries

Fraser, A., & Edmonds-Seal, J. (1982). Spinal cord injuries. *Anaesthesia* 37:1084–98.

Gilbert, J. (1987). Critical care management of the patient with acute spinal cord injury. *Critical Care Clinics* 3:549–67.

Green, B. A., Eismont, F. J., O'Heir, J. T. (1987). Spinal cord injury – a systems approach: prevention, emergency medical services and emergency room management. *Critical Care Clinics* 3:471–93.

Burns

Boswick, J. S. (ed.) (1987). Symposium on burns. *Surgical Clinics of North America* 67:1–195 (symposium issue).

Deitch, E. A. (1990). The management of burns. *New England Journal of Medicine* 323:1249–53.

Demling, R. H. (1993). Smoke inhalation injury. *New Horizons* 1:422–34.

Pruitt, B. A. (1992). Progress in burn care. *World Journal of Surgery* 16:1–96 (symposium issue).

Tompkins, R. G., & Burke, J. K. (1985). Burn therapy. Acute management. *Intensive Care Medicine* 12:289–95.

Crush Injuries and Acute Compartment Syndrome

Better, O., & Stein, J. H. (1990). Early management of shock and prophylaxis of acute renal failure in traumatic rhabdomyolysis. *New England Journal of Medicine* 322:825–9.

Mubarak, S. J., & Hargens, A. R. (1983). Acute compartment syndromes. *Surgical Clinics of North America* 63:539–65.

Mubarak, S. J., & Owen, C. A. (1975). Compartment syndrome and its relation to the crush syndrome. A spectrum of disease. *Clinical Orthopaedics and Related Research* 113:277–80.

Reis, N. D., & Michaelson, M. (1986). Crush injury to the lower limbs. *Journal of Bone and Joint Surgery* 68:414–18.

Rorabeck, C. H., Castle, G. S. P., & Hardie, R. (1989). Compartment pressure measurements. An experimental investigation using the slit catheter. *Journal of Trauma* 21:446–51.

Stewart, I. P. (1987). Major crush injury. *British Medical Journal* 294:854–5.

Electrical Injuries

Dixon, G. F. (1983). The evaluation and management of electrical injuries. *Critical Care Medicine* 11:384–6.

Hiestand, D., & Colice, G. G. (1988). Lightning-strike injury. *Journal of Intensive Care* 3:303–14.

Lee, R. C., Craralho, E. G., & Burke, J. F. (1993). *Electrical Trauma: The Pathophysiology, Manifestations and Clinical Management.* Cambridge University Press.

Near-Drowning Episodes

Modell, J. H. (1993). Drowning. *New England Journal of Medicine* 328:253–6.

Pearn, J. The management of near drowning. *British Medical Journal* 291:1447–50.

Trauma in Obstetric Patients

Pearlman, M. D., Tintinalli, J. E., & Lorenz, R. P. (1990). Blunt trauma during pregnancy. *New England Journal of Medicine* 323:1609–13.

Paediatric Trauma

Jaffe, D., & Wesson, D. (1990). Emergency management of blunt trauma in children. *New England Journal of Medicine* 324:1477–82.

Lloyd-Thomas, A. R. (1990). Paediatric trauma. *British Medical Journal* 301:334–6, 380–2.

Mackway-Jones, K., Molyneux, E., Phillips, B., & Wieteska, S. (eds.) (1993). *Advanced Paediatric Life Support: The Practical Approach*. London: BMJ Publishing Group.

Mayer, T. A. (1985). *Emergency Management of Pediatric Trauma*. Philadelphia: Saunders.

Yaster, M., & Haller, A. (1987). Multiple trauma in the pediatric patient. In *Textbook of Pediatric Intensive Care*, vol. 2; ed. M. C. Roger, pp. 1265–322. Baltimore: Williams & Wilkins.

15

FAT EMBOLISM SYNDROME

- Suspect fat embolism in all patients with long-bone fractures.
- Early fixation of fractures will decrease the incidence of respiratory complications.
- Aggressive initial resuscitation may prevent development of the fat embolism syndrome.

Fat embolism occurs in approximately 90% of patients with long-bone fractures. Only 3–4% of those will go on to develop the florid fat embolism syndrome (FES) – severe hypoxia, decreased level of consciousness, and petechiae.

THEORIES OF FAT EMBOLISM

Fat embolism is most common in patients who have suffered trauma, but it can also occur in the presence of non-traumatic conditions (eg burns, liposuction, pancreatitis, diabetes, renal transplantation). There are two main theories:

1. Mechanical theory Trauma to the long bones releases fat droplets from the marrow or adipose tissue. These travel to the lung and either are trapped as emboli or reach the systemic circulation to cause embolization in the kidney, retina, and brain.

2. Biochemical theory There are two possible explanations: Either circulating free fatty acids released at the time of trauma adversely affect the lung pneumocytes, or a factor released from the fracture site affects the solubility of lipids in the blood, which then coalesce and embolize.

There appears to be good evidence for each of these theories. What is not yet explained is why some patients get full-blown FES, whereas others who have suffered similar trauma develop only fat emboli, not

TABLE 15.1   CLINICAL FEATURES OF FAT EMBOLISM

Major
1. Petechial rash
2. Respiratory symptoms plus bilateral signs, with positive radiographic changes
3. Cerebral signs unrelated to head injury or any other condition

Minor
1. Tachycardia
2. Pyrexia
3. Retinal changes (fat or petechiae)
4. Urinary changes (anuria, oliguria, fat globules)
5. Sudden drop in haemoglobin
6. Sudden thrombocytopenia
7. High erythrocyte sedimentation rate
8. Fat globules in the sputum

Source: From Gurd (1970), with permission.

the full-blown syndrome. It is suggested that shock, hypovolaemia, or sepsis may be required to convert embolized fat into the FES.

CLINICAL PRESENTATION

There is a wide spectrum of presentations, ranging from mild hypoxia to full-blown FES.

Ninety percent of patients will develop symptoms within 24 hours of injury, but some can have a latent period up to 72 hours post injury.

The diagnosis is normally made using Gurd's criteria (Table 15.1). One major sign and four minor signs are necessary for a diagnosis of FES. Bronchoalveolar lavage may be useful in intubated patients. Cells from the lavage may show fat droplets. However, this is not specific for FES.

In examining any trauma patient, maintain a high index of suspicion for fat emboli.

Respiratory failure

Dyspnoea, tachypnoea, and hypoxia are the initial signs. Bilateral infiltrates can be seen on the chest x-ray. Adult respiratory distress syndrome (ARDS) and pulmonary hypertension can develop rapidly in patients with severe FES.

Central nervous system

Signs can range from anxiety, irritation, and confusion to convulsions and coma (a score of 9 or less on the Glasgow coma scale). Exclude other causes (eg head injury in trauma). A CT scan may show cerebral oedema. Petechial haemorrhage is common; larger haemorrhages are rare.

Skin and other areas

A petechial rash (axillae, anterior chest, or conjunctivae) will appear in 25–50% of patients.
Retinal findings include exudate, haemorrhage, and cotton-wool spots.
Tachycardia and fever (>38°C) are common.

LABORATORY FINDINGS

• hypoxaemia, often with a large alveolar–arterial oxygen gradient (see Chapter 17)
• hypocarbia
• decreased haemoglobin
• thrombocytopenia
• coagulopathy
• hypocalcaemia
• chest x-ray – bilateral infiltrates

MANAGEMENT

Prophylactic

• Keep a high index of suspicion in trauma patients; use frequent determinations of arterial blood gases and Sao_2 monitoring.

- Rapid, expert resuscitation is needed.
- Early fixation of fractures will decrease the risk of FES and decrease the respiratory and septic complications in multitrauma patients. The 'horizontal crucifix position' (patient in traction, lying flat in bed) makes nursing care, mobilization, and respiratory care very difficult. These patients will need prolonged ventilatory support and larger dosages of antibiotics, and they will have a higher incidence of sepsis.

THE MAINSTAY OF TREATMENT IS SUPPORTIVE – THERE IS NO DE-FINITIVE TREATMENT.

Respiratory

The principles of treatment are as for any other form of acute respiratory failure and ARDS (see p. 400):

- Oxygen treatment to maintain $Sa_{O_2} > 95\%$.
- Use continuous positive airway pressure (CPAP) or ventilatory support.
- Maintain the intravascular volume with blood and colloid, and restrict clear fluids.

Cardiovascular

- Maintain oxygen delivery – adequate haemoglobin, cardiac output, and Sa_{O_2}.
- Right-side pressure may be high secondary to pulmonary hypertension.
- Inotropes with or without vasopressors may be required.
- Diuretics can decrease the extravascular water in the lungs.

Central nervous system

Coma in patients with FES usually is completely reversible.

Specific drugs

There is no role for aspirin, dextran, ethyl alcohol, or heparin. The place of corticosteroids is not yet clear. Several studies have suggested that prophylactic steroids can benefit high-risk patients, but others have maintained that outcomes are just as good with supportive care only.

Prognosis

The pathophysiology in patients with fat emboli is completely reversible, and survival should be 100%. The mortality rate for FES can approach 10%, mainly because of respiratory failure.

FURTHER READING

Fabian, T. C., Hoots, A. V., Stanford, D. S., Patterson, C. R., & Mangiante, E. C. (1990). Fat embolism syndrome: prospective evaluation in 92 fracture patients. *Critical Care Medicine* 18:42–6.

Gurd, A. R. (1970). Fat embolism: an aid to diagnosis. *Journal of Bone and Joint Surgery* 52:732.

Levy, D. (1989). The fat embolism syndrome. A review. *Clinical Orthopaedics and Related Research* 261:281–6.

Schein, M., & Saadia, R. (1990). Early operative fracture management of patients with multiple injuries. *British Journal of Surgery* 77:361–2.

16

POISONING

- The first priority in the management of poisoning is the initial resuscitation – airway, breathing, and circulation.
- Supportive care is the cornerstone of management in the intensive care unit (ICU).
- The use of specific antidotes is only rarely lifesaving.
- Self-poisoning often involves multiple drugs, commonly including alcohol.

INITIAL ASSESSMENT

The possibility of poisoning should be considered in all unconscious patients. First-line treatment involves securing the airway, giving high-flow oxygen, and supporting the patient's breathing and circulation. Examine the patient's entire body carefully for signs of intravenous drug abuse, trauma, and pressure areas (Table 16.1). Perform a thorough neurological examination. Smell the patient's breath. The possibility of hypoglycaemia must be considered. Elicit a history from the patient, ambulance officers, friends, or relatives. Thiamine (100 mg IM or IV) should be given to all known alcoholic patients in order to treat or prevent Wernicke's encephalopathy.

Although active intervention, such as the use of antidotes, forced alkaline diuresis, and dialysis, can sometimes play a crucial role, basic resuscitation measures usually are more important. OUR CONCERN IN POISONING IS TO SAVE THE PATIENT, NOT THE POISON!

AIRWAY

If there is doubt about the patency of the airway, rapidly intubate the patient with pre-oxygenation and cricoid pressure. As a guideline, patients with Glasgow coma scale scores of 9 or less should be intubated. It is dangerous to attempt to elicit a gag reflex, as the patient

325

TABLE 16.1 THE MOST COMMON TOXIC SYNDROMES

Anticholinergic syndromes	
Common signs	Delirium, with mumbling speech, tachycardia, dry and flushed skin, dilated pupils, myoclonus, slightly elevated temperature, urinary retention, and decreased bowel sounds. Seizures and dysrhythmias can occur in severe cases.
Common causes	Antihistamines, antiparkinsonism medication, atropine, scopolamine, antispasmodic agents, mydriatic agents, skeletal-muscle relaxants, and many plants (notably jimsonweed and *Amanita muscaria*).
Sympathomimetic syndromes	
Common signs	Delusions, paranoia, tachycardia (or bradycardia if the drug is a pure α-adrenergic agonist), hypertension, hyperpyrexia, diaphoresis, piloerection, mydriasis, and hyperreflexia. Seizures, hypotension, and dysrhythmias can occur in severe cases.
Common causes	Cocaine, amphetamines, methamphetamine and its derivatives, and over-the-counter decongestants (eg phenylpropanolamine, ephedrine, and pseudoephedrine). In caffeine and theophylline overdoses, similar findings can occur.
Opiate, sedative, or ethanol intoxication	
Common signs	Coma, respiratory depression, miosis, hypotension, bradycardia, hypothermia, pulmonary oedema, decreased bowel sounds, hyporeflexia, and needle marks. Seizures can occur after overdoses of some narcotics, notably propoxyphene.
Common causes	Narcotics, barbiturates, benzodiazepines, ethchlorvynol, glutethimide, methyprylon, methaqualone, meprobamate, ethanol, clonidine, and guanabenz.
Cholinergic syndromes	
Common signs	Confusion, central nervous system depression, weakness, salivation, lacrimation, urinary and faecal incontinence, gastro-intestinal cramping, emesis, diaphoresis, muscle fasciculations, pulmonary oedema, miosis, bradycardia or tachycardia, and seizures.
Common causes	Organophosphate and carbamate insecticides, physostigmine, edrophonium, and some mushrooms.

Source: From Kulig (1992), with permission of the *New England Journal of Medicine*.

may aspirate stomach contents. Paradoxically, further sedation may be needed if the patient is restless or is having a seizure. The patient's level of consciousness and airway patency must be constantly monitored, and intubation must be carried out if there is any doubt. Slow-release preparations can cause delayed effects.

BREATHING

Oxygen (at least 30–40%, via a face mask) should be administered to any patient with a compromised level of consciousness. Many drugs (eg narcotics, sedatives, tricyclic antidepressants) can cause hypoventilation, hypercarbia, and respiratory acidosis.

Monitor the patient's respiratory rate, check arterial blood gases frequently, and use pulse oximetry and clinical assessment to determine the need for artificial ventilation with intermittent positive-pressure ventilation (IPPV). Whereas all intubated patients should initially be ventilated, those who are making some spontaneous respiratory effort may be suitable for a change to some partial mode of ventilatory support, such as mandatory minute volume (MMV) or intermittent mandatory ventilation (IMV) (see p. 472).

CIRCULATION

Many of these patients are hypotensive on admission. This can be related to several factors:

• vasodilatory actions of many drugs (**MOST COMMON**)
• direct cardiac toxicity
• hypovolaemia due to decreased fluid intake or fluid loss (eg vomiting)

Hypotension

Hypotension can almost always be reversed with replenishment of intravascular fluid. The fluid must be titrated against cardiovascular measurements – particularly blood pressure and peripheral perfusion. Occasionally, large volumes are required. Inotropic support is sometimes needed for resistant hypotension (see p. 520).

Cardiac problems

Correct hypoxia, acidosis, and hypokalaemia, as they predispose to arrhythmias and depress cardiac function. The poison itself can have a direct cardiodepressant effect on the heart (eg β-blockers).

INVESTIGATIONS AND MONITORING

Most patients need only monitoring and the basic investigations. Initially, frequent (every 15 minutes) monitoring of vital signs, such as pulse rate, blood pressure, respiratory rate, and level of consciousness, may be required.

CHEST X-RAY An x-ray may show signs of aspiration or atelectasis.

ECG Use initial 12-lead ECG and continuous monitoring if indicated.

OXIMETRY Continuous monitoring for hypoxia is necessary.

ROUTINE HAEMATOLOGY AND BIOCHEMISTRY Creatinine phosphokinase (CPK), for instance, may be increased because of rhabdomyolysis; theophylline and tricyclic antidepressants can cause hypokalaemia.

ARTERIAL BLOOD GASES Their determination may reveal, for instance, persistent unexplained acidosis due to salicylates, carbon monoxide, methanol, and ethylene glycol.

SERUM OSMOLALITY When compared with calculated osmolality, the serum osmolality may be helpful in diagnosing poisoning due to methanol or ethylene glycol.

DRUG ASSAYS Urine, blood, and gastric contents can be used for drug screening. Early samples of gastric contents (50 ml) and urine (50 ml) should be used for diagnostic and medico-legal purposes. Specific, rapid screening tests are available for drugs such as paracetamol, salicylates, benzodiazepines, opiates, and barbiturates. There is also a screening test, based on thin-layer chromatography (TLC), that covers about 200 substances. Although blood cannot be used for the TLC screening test, blood samples should be taken to test specifically for other substances, including alcohol. Specific serum or plasma concentrations are useful for dealing with the following drugs: paracetamol, iron, salicylates, theophylline, digoxin, anticonvulsant agents, lithium, ethanol, methanol, and ethylene glycol.

SPECIAL PROBLEMS

HYPOTHERMIA

Hypothermia is common after poisoning, but it rarely requires active measures (see p. 156). Always measure the central temperature (eg rectal or oesophageal). Hypothermia is a marker of increased risk for rhabdomyolysis and aspiration as a result of coma.

Treatment for hypothermia begins with covering the patient with metallic foil to reduce heat loss. Warm the intravenous fluids and humidified gas to 37°C. More active measures are sometimes needed (see p. 156).

HYPERTHERMIA

Hyperthermia is uncommon and sometimes is associated with tricyclic antidepressants, antipsychotics, antihistamines, amphetamine, cocaine, phencyclidine, and salicylates. Hyperthermia must be controlled by aggressive means, in order to prevent complications (see p. 161). Fever as a result of infection can, of course, occur (eg aspiration).

SEIZURES

Seizures can occur as direct results of the poison and may be difficult to control. Seizures can occur in association with anticonvulsants, phenothiazines, antihistamines, theophylline, and tricyclic antidepressants. Seizures can also occur as indirect results of the poison (eg hypoglycaemia or hypoxia). Drug or alcohol withdrawal can also precipitate seizures.

Seizures are medical emergencies, as they can cause cerebral oedema, hyperthermia, hypoxia, and aspiration. The principles of management are listed here, but they are discussed in detail elsewhere (see p. 613):

• Intubate and assist ventilation if in doubt about the airway. Initially give intravenous benzodiazepines. If the seizures are not controlled with benzodiazepines, use intravenous barbiturates (see p. 616).

• Concurrently given phenytoin (15 mg/kg IV over 1 hour as a loading dose, then 5 mg/kg IV daily as a single dose over 1 hour).

• If muscle relaxants are given, EEG monitoring should be used to assess electrical seizure activity.

RHABDOMYOLYSIS

Rhabdomyolysis usually occurs in association with pressure necrosis. It can complicate narcotic and cocaine abuse without coma. ALWAYS SUSPECT RHABDOMYOLYSIS IN A PATIENT WHO IS IN A PROLONGED COMA. Rhabdomyolysis can cause hypovolaemia, shock, hyperkalaemia, hypocalcaemia, acidosis, and renal failure (see p. 298). Early, aggressive correction of hypovolaemia and acidosis is essential. Active treatment of hyperkalaemia (see p. 76) and renal failure (see p. 640) may be necessary. Fasciotomy is sometimes required to relieve compartment pressure and prevent further tissue ischaemia (see p. 301).

ATELECTASIS AND ASPIRATION

A chest x-ray should be obtained as soon as possible after admission to detect features such as atelectasis and collapse (see p. 391) due to hypoventilation, or aspiration (see p. 423) as a result of coma and depressed reflexes.

OTHER GENERAL SUPPORTIVE MEASURES

The key to effective management of a patient who has been poisoned, whether accidentally or deliberately, is METICULOUS SUPPORTIVE CARE. Supportive measures are based on the principles essential for management of all critically ill patients (see p. 10):

- regular assessment of airway, breathing, and circulation
- regular turning and pressure care
- nasogastric tube
- catheterization of the bladder
- mouth, eye, and limb care
- prophylactic measures for stress ulceration (see p. 31)

FOLLOW-UP

It is often helpful to obtain psychiatric and/or social-worker opinions before a poisoning patient is transferred from the ICU. It is important that the ICU staff present a positive attitude toward these patients. Because self-poisoning presents a situation in which it is difficult and frustrating to have to be supportive of the patient in the long term, these patients often are not managed in the acute situation with the dignity and sensitivity that they deserve.

ACTIVE MEASURES

DECREASED DRUG ABSORPTION

The exact role of gastric emptying, gastric lavage, and whole-gut irrigation, as well as the use of ipecac and charcoal, remain controversial.

Any active attempt to empty the stomach is accompanied by the danger of aspiration. The patient must have an intact cough reflex or have a cuffed endotracheal tube (ETT) in place before an attempt is made to aspirate stomach contents.

For patients poisoned by drugs that cause coma and respiratory depression, aggressive removal of the drugs is not warranted. Active gastric emptying of such drugs might give the attending medical staff a sense that they were doing something positive (or punitive, regarding these drugs), but good supportive care usually is all that is required.

Active measures to empty the gut should be considered for toxic drugs such as aspirin, colchicine, paraquat, organophosphates, iron, tricyclic antidepressants, and paracetamol. Active measures should be avoided in cases involving corrosive chemicals and petroleum products.

Induced emesis

This technique has been used primarily for small children soon after ingestion of the toxin. However, it seems to be falling out of favour, even for that group. Emesis should not be induced if

- the child is not fully alert, with intact laryngeal reflexes
- acid, alkali, or petroleum distillates have been ingested
- more than 3 hours have passed since ingestion

Ipecac syrup has traditionally been recommended for young children, but not for adults, in whom sedation and poor drug recovery are problems. Its effectiveness is largely unproven. Paediatric ipecacuanha mixture (0.12% alkaloids) is usually used: 5 ml for children up to 1 year of age; 10–20 ml for those age 1–5 years.

Gastric lavage

The exact role and usefulness of gastric lavage have not been fully established. It should always be CONSIDERED, but not done simply as a routine.

It is probably useful within 4 hours of ingestion, and also when one suspects that potentially lethal quantities of a drug have been taken. It can also be useful if slow-release preparations of drugs have been taken. Gastric lavage can be successful for up to 12 hours after ingestion for salicylates, quinidine, tricyclic antidepressants, and paracetamol.

Lavage should not be attempted when ingestion of corrosives, caustics, acids, or petroleum derivatives is suspected.

TECHNIQUE Place the patient in the semiprone position, with the head dependent. Insert a special large-bore gastric tube to aspirate the stomach. Instil water (1 ml/kg) at body temperature, and recover that amount before instilling more. Repeat the cycle until the return water is clear.

Charcoal

If given early enough, activated charcoal can reduce the gastro-intestinal absorption of many drugs, including aspirin, paracetamol, phenobarbitone, digoxin, carbamazepine, theophylline, and phenytoin. It is of little value for highly charged molecules, such as iron, lithium, and cyanide, and other compounds such as alcohol. There may be the added benefit of clearance from the systemic circulation by 'gastro-intestinal dialysis': A concentration gradient for the drug is established between the systemic circulation and the lumen of the gastro-intestinal tract (GIT). Clearance is thus encouraged from the circulation into the GIT lumen, where it is adsorbed onto the charcoal.

The efficiency of charcoal absorption may be reduced in the presence of shock or impaired gastro-intestinal motility. Just as we remain uncertain about many aspects of management after poisoning, the exact role of charcoal has not been established. In practical terms, repeated doses of charcoal do not tend to transit rapidly through the gut.

TECHNIQUE Administer activated charcoal at 1 g/kg, either orally or through a nasogastric (NG) tube. Its action can be enhanced by repeating that dose every 4 hours, especially for drugs that rely on the enterohepatic circulation. Alternatively, continuous NG infusion of charcoal (30–50 g/h) can be used (for paediatric patients, 0.25 $g \cdot kg^{-1} \cdot h^{-1}$). As with adults, there is little evidence for the effectiveness of charcoal in paediatric poisoning. Metoclopramide may speed the gastric emptying of charcoal. Charcoal can be used for long periods after drug ingestion, as it can enhance the clearance of drugs already absorbed. Repeated doses of activated charcoal may decrease the half-lives and increase the clearances of a wide range of drugs, including the following:

- dapsone
- theophylline
- glutethimide
- digoxin
- phenylbutazone
- barbiturates
- quinine
- tricyclic antidepressants
- salicylates
- carbamazepine

Whole-bowel irrigation

Some agents, such as polyethylene glycol electrolyte solutions, can decrease drug absorption by decreasing the time for the drug to transit the gut. Such agents do not act by means of an osmolar effect within the gut. They can be useful for purging intact tablets from the gut (eg in cases of iron poisoning). It is a technique suitable for conscious patients who have ingested tablets that do not bind well to charcoal and can be identified on a plain radiograph. Because polyethylene glycol will bind to charcoal, the two probably should not be used together.

TECHNIQUE   These compounds come as commercially available water-soluble powders (eg Go-lytely or Colyte) to be dissolved in about 4 litres of water. They can be taken orally or delivered via NG tube. For adults, give the solution at a rate of 1–4 L/h (children 0.5 L/h), and continue until the patient passes clear fluid from the bowel (usually after about 3– 5L) or until the tablets are cleared from the gut.

INCREASED DRUG EXCRETION

These techniques are employed only in specific circumstances.

Forced alkaline diuresis

Forced alkaline diuresis is a dangerous and unproven technique that is now largely discouraged. It was considered theoretically attractive because it encourages ion trapping in the renal tubules. However, it can result in dehydration, hypokalaemia, and pulmonary oedema. Even in acute and severe salicylate poisoning, it has not been shown to improve outcome.

Faecuresis

Just as we are uncertain about many of the active measures used in the management of poisoning, the effectiveness of giving an osmolar agent is uncertain. Mannitol is sometimes given together with charcoal. Apart from its uncertain effectiveness, mannitol can lead to hypovolaemia, as a result of its osmolar effect in the gut, as well as hypokalaemia and hypomagnesaemia.

Haemodialysis

Haemodialysis is effective mainly for low-molecular-weight drugs that are not effectively bound to plasma proteins and have small volumes of distribution and low rates of spontaneous clearance. It has a limited role, but it can be useful for potentially lethal doses of specific drugs, such as lithium, ethylene glycol, and salicylates.

Haemodialysis should be CONSIDERED when these drugs are present at certain high concentrations:

- salicylates (>1.2 g/L initially; >1.0 g/L at 6 hours)
- methanol, ethylene glycol (>0.5 g/L)
- lithium (>4 mmol/L)

Haemodialysis can also be useful for the acute acid–base or electrolyte disturbances that accompany poisoning. It is of no benefit for drugs that have large volumes of distribution, such as tricyclic antidepressants.

Haemoperfusion

Haemoperfusion involves passing the patient's blood through a device containing charcoal or adsorbent particles, such as resin columns. The technique has anecdotally been reported to be successful for many drugs, but it should be CONSIDERED only when their concentrations are high:

- salicylates (>1.2 g/L initially; >1.0 g/L at 6 hours)
- theophylline (>600 μmol/L)

Haemoperfusion can also be considered for patients with paraquat poisoning, mushroom poisoning, and late-presentation paracetamol poisoning. The technique for haemoperfusion is described in the chapter on renal failure (see p. 651).

ANTIDOTES

Some drugs and conditions require immediate antidotal treatment:

Drug	*Antidote*
carbon monoxide	oxygen
paracetamol	N-acetylcysteine
anticholinergics	physostigmine
insulin	glucose
β-blockers	glucagon/adrenaline
organophosphates	atropine and pralidoxime
benzodiazepines	flumazenil
ethylene glycol	ethanol
bromide	sodium chloride
calcium-channel blockers	calcium
cyanide	amyl nitrate, sodium nitrite, sodium thiosulphate
heavy metals	chelating agents
isoniazid, hydrazine	pyridoxine
iron	desferrioxamine
methaemoglobinaemia	methylene blue
narcotics	naloxone
warfarin	vitamin K
digoxin	digoxin antibody fragments

For more details, see the specific poisons discussed in the next section.

Immunotherapy

In the future, antibodies to a given drug that can result in inhibition of that drug's action may play an important role. Thus far, immunotherapy has been used for severe digoxin poisoning (see p. 340).

SOME SPECIFIC POISONS
β-BLOCKERS

FEATURES

• Common effects include bradycardia, hypotension, peripheral vasospasm, bronchospasm, coma, convulsions, and respiratory depression.

MANAGEMENT

- Supportive management is recommended.
- Atropine, isoprenaline, adrenaline, or glucagon infusions may be necessary. Transvenous pacing may also be required. Glucagon can be given as a bolus at 50 μg/kg IV, up to 10 mg; a maintenance dosage of 2–10 mg/h can be used.

CARBAMAZEPINE

CARBAMAZEPINE CAN BE A PARTICULARLY DANGEROUS DRUG.

FEATURES

- Mild ataxia to profound coma
- Marked depression of brain-stem reflexes (see p. 587)
- Convulsions or myoclonic activity
- Cerebellar dysfunction
- Marked cardiovascular toxicity, including
    Tachyarrhythmias and bradyarrhythmias
    ECG: prolonged PR intervals, QRS complex, and QT interval
    Conduction disturbances
    Severe hypotension
- Thrombocytopenia and leucopenia
- Pulmonary oedema
- Anticholinergic effects

MANAGEMENT

- The drug has extensive protein-binding capacity (75–85%) and a large volume of distribution (1.5 L/kg), making it relatively inaccessible to active measures for drug elimination.
- Management is mainly supportive:

    Intubation.
    Artificial ventilation.
    Fluid resuscitation (see p. 61).
    Inotropes are often necessary (see p. 520).
    Cardiac pacing may be necessary.
    Seizures must be controlled with aggressive measures (see p. 616).

Drug removal can be facilitated by multiple doses or even continuous infusion of activated charcoal via NG tube. Haemoperfusion with a charcoal column has also been used.

CARBON MONOXIDE

FEATURES

• Carbon monoxide displaces oxygen from haemoglobin, myoglobin, and the cytochrome system. This causes widespread cellular damage because of decreased oxygen delivery and utilization.

• A pink colour of the skin is uncommon; cyanosis and skin pallor are more common.

• Carbon monoxide poisoning should be considered a possibility in all patients who have been trapped in a fire.

MANAGEMENT

• General supportive measures are recommended (see p. 10).

• Give as high a concentration of inspired oxygen as possible (100%, if possible) by a tight-fitting mask or ETT (if necessary) until the carboxyhaemoglobin concentration is less than 5%. Remember that pulse oximeters will be misleading, because they measure carbon monoxide as well as oxygen.

• Many patients have had long-term neuropsychiatric deficits after carbon monoxide poisoning. For that reason, hyperbaric oxygen is now used earlier and more aggressively. Some units use hyperbaric oxygen when the carboxyhaemoglobin concentration is more than 20–30% or when the patient either has lost consciousness at any stage or has neurological deficits or cardiac abnormalities.

COCAINE

FEATURES

• Stimulation of both peripheral and central nervous systems.

• Clinical features include euphoria, agitation, hyperthermia, seizures, confusion, tachycardia, and hypertension.

• Cardiac arrhythmias, cerebral haemorrhage, coagulopathy, cerebral oedema, and rhabdomyolysis can also occur.

MANAGEMENT

- It is important to reduce the psychomotor agitation, using diazepam intravenously, as required.
- Close monitoring and aggressive resuscitation are essential.
- Neuroleptic agents should be avoided.
- β-blockers can result in excessive α activity and hypertension.
- Severe hypertension may require the use of labetalol or sodium nitroprusside.
- A CT scan may be necessary to exclude cerebral haemorrhage.

CYANIDE

FEATURES

- Cyanide toxicity can occur as a result of ingestion or inhalation, as well as secondary to the use of sodium nitroprusside.
- Cyanide inhalation during a fire can bring an onset of symptoms within seconds, and death can occur within minutes.
- When cyanide is ingested or absorbed through the skin, symptoms appear in minutes, and death can occur within hours.
- Cyanide is a cellular poison that prevents the utilization of oxygen, leading to metabolic acidosis.
- Symptoms reflect cellular hypoxia: drowsiness, convulsions, coma, tachypnoea, and dyspnoea, followed by bradypnoea, initially hypertension then hypotension, and cardiovascular collapse.

MANAGEMENT

- General supportive measures are recommended (see p. 10). Assess and support the airway, breathing, and circulation. Give high-flow oxygen. Gastric lavage should follow antidotes, not precede them.
- If cyanide is inhaled as a result of a fire, then carbon monoxide and other gases should also be considered.
- Mouth-to-mouth breathing can lead to cyanide toxicity in the rescuer.
- Antidotes:

    Sodium thiosulphate will convert cyanide to thiocyanate. Initial dose 150 mg/kg IV, followed by an infusion of $30\text{--}60 \text{ mg} \cdot \text{kg}^{-1} \cdot \text{h}^{-1}$.

Nitrates will cause methaemoglobinaemia and will complex with cyanide to form cyanomethaemoglobin, thereby restoring cytochrome oxidase. Amyl nitrate can be administered by inhalation, or sodium nitrite can be given as an intravenous infusion (for adults, give 10 ml of 3% solution at 2.5–5 ml/min).

Cobalt EDTA will complex with cyanide. Give 600 mg IV over 1 minute. A further 200 mg can be given if there is no response.

Hydroxycobalamin will form cyanocobalamin. The dose is empirical; 100 μg/kg has been suggested.

DIGOXIN

FEATURES

• Nausea, vomiting, drowsiness, and mental confusion.

• ECG: Almost any change is possible, including sinus bradycardia, atrioventricular block, ventricular and atrial ectopics, and asystole.

MANAGEMENT

• Gastric lavage and support.

• Temporary cardiac pacing and specific treatment of individual arrhythmias may be necessary.

• Treatment is mainly supportive.

• Serum digoxin concentrations will not give a good indication of the severity of digoxin toxicity.

• Digoxin-specific antibody fragments are becoming increasingly available. They bind digoxin and hasten its elimination. They should be used for cardiovascular instability secondary to arrhythmias.

• A recommended regimen is 160 mg as a loading dose, followed by 160 mg as an intravenous infusion over 7 hours. Alternatively, 6–8 mg/kg, repeated over 30–60 minutes, can be given. A further dose can be given in cases of incomplete reversal or recurrence of toxicity. Digoxin antibody fragments interfere with digoxin measurements that employ immunoassay techniques.

IRON SALTS

FEATURES   Iron-salt poisoning is most severe in young children:

Stage I: Acute gastric disturbances: epigastric pain, nausea, vomiting, and haematemesis, leading sometimes to necrosis and perforation of the stomach. Rapid pulse and respiratory rate. There may be a symptom-free period for up to 24 hours.

Stage II: Acute encephalopathy: headache, confusion, delirium, convulsions, coma. Respirations deep and rapid. Cardiovascular collapse may supervene. Hyperglycaemia and leucocytosis.

Stage III: If the patient survives to this stage, acute liver failure may develop, with jaundice, hepatic coma, and death.

MANAGEMENT

• **TREATMENT MUST BE RAPID.**

• A plain abdominal x-ray usually will demonstrate the number of tablets. Gastric lavage with a **LARGE-BORE TUBE** may facilitate removal of tablets.

• There is little or no place here for activated charcoal, as it does not bind iron. Lavage with desferrioxamine, 2 g in 1 litre of warm water, then leave 10 g in 50 ml in the stomach to chelate the remaining iron in the GIT.

• Whole-bowel irrigation with polyethylene glycol electrolyte solution, especially in children, may be useful (see p. 334).

• Desferrioxamine can be given by intravenous and intramuscular routes. The dosage is the same for both routes and the same for adults and children: a 1-g loading dose, then 500 mg 4-hourly for two doses. Thereafter, 500 mg between 4-hourly and 12-hourly, depending on the severity of poisoning. The total dose should not exceed 6 g in 24 hours. The intravenous rate should not exceed 15 mg $\cdot$ kg^{-1} $\cdot$ h^{-1}.

• Treatment should be continued until serum levels and clinical status are improved.

• If anuria or oliguria supervenes, dialysis should be commenced immediately.

LITHIUM

FEATURES

• Polyuria, thirst, vomiting, diarrhoea, and agitation.

• With larger doses, coma, hypertonia, involuntary movements, and convulsions can occur.

MANAGEMENT

• General supportive measures are recommended (see p. 10).

• Correct hypertonicity with 5% dextrose solution.

• Haemodialysis should be considered if there are severe complications or high concentrations of lithium (eg >4 mmol/L).

MONOAMINE OXIDASE INHIBITORS

FEATURES

• Drug and food interactions can cause headache, fever, and hypertensive crises.

• Overdoses usually cause coma, hypotension, and, more rarely, convulsions and hyperthermia.

MANAGEMENT

• With drug and food interactions, severe hypertension is the main problem (see p. 544).

• With overdosage, airway control and intravascular fluids to correct the hypotension usually are sufficient.

NARCOTICS

FEATURES

• Coma and respiratory depression are the most common presenting signs.

• Look for needle marks, miosis, hypotension, bradycardia, hypothermia, pulmonary oedema, hyporeflexia, and decreased bowel sounds.

• Seizures can occur after overdoses of some narcotics (eg pethidine and propoxyphene).

MANAGEMENT

• Precautions should be taken against transmission of hepatitis B and C and HIV virus.

• General supportive measures are recommended (see p. 10).

• Intravenous naloxone is a specific antagonist. However, it has a short half-life, and coma can recur. Give naloxone, 0.8 mg IM, followed by naloxone at 0.5–2 mg IV. The IM dose has a longer duration of action, and coma is less likely to recur, especially if the patient absconds after the IV dose! More may be needed, and sometimes an infusion (1–4 mg/h). Less can be used for addicts, in whom acute withdrawal can be precipitated. The paediatric dose is 0.1 mg/kg, and infusion at 0.01 mg · kg^{-1} · h^{-1}.

- There may also be concurrent infection, rhabdomyolysis, tricuspid valve abnormalities, subacute bacterial endocarditis, pulmonary oedema, and problems associated with narcotic withdrawal.

ORGANOPHOSPHATES

FEATURES

- Symptoms usually appear within 2 hours of exposure.
- Usually there is a distinctive smell about the patient.
- Cholinesterase inhibition causes parasympathetic over-activity, as well as sympathetic, neuromuscular, and central neurological abnormalities.
- Signs and symptoms include

salivation	bronchorrhoea
bronchospasm	sweating
lacrimation	headache
restlessness	muscle weakness
confusion/convulsions	nausea
vomiting	abdominal cramps
diarrhoea	bradycardia
hypotension	shock

MANAGEMENT

- Gastric aspiration and supportive measures.
- Staff should exercise care in handling the aspirate – the odour of the organophosphate usually will be evident in the ICU for many days during management of the patient, and it has been implicated in feelings of malaise and headache amongst the staff. Staff should wear gloves, gowns, masks, and glasses during the initial management of these patients, in order to decrease absorption.
- Atropine should be titrated against signs and symptoms. Aim to

maintain the heart rate and reduce pulmonary secretions with a continuous intravenous infusion or intravenous increments. Commence with an intravenous infusion of 5 mg/h, and increase as necessary. Very high infusion rates, up to 30 mg/h may be required initially. Glycopyrrolate could be used instead of atropine.

• Pralidoxime will result in specific reactivation of cholinesterase, but it needs to be given early (within 24 hours). The dose is 1–2 g IV within 2 minutes. Repeat after 30 minutes if necessary, and then give 1–2 g 4-hourly when indicated. Monitor plasma cholinesterase levels until recovery.

• Direct cardiotoxicity has been reported, and often inotropic support is necessary.

PARACETAMOL

FEATURES

• No symptoms initially
• Then anorexia, nausea, vomiting.
• Severe vomiting, abdominal pain, and hepatic tenderness on the second day.
• Hepatic toxicity is maximum on days 2–4 and can lead to fulminant liver failure (see p. 666).

MANAGEMENT

• The outcome will be determined by the amount taken and by the time elapsed before effective treatment is provided.

• Use gastric lavage and activated charcoal (see p. 332) for patients who present within 4 hours; these may be useful up to 12 hours.

• Intravenous *N*-acetylcysteine is the treatment of choice for paracetamol poisoning and should be used if

more than 10 g has been ingested

there is doubt about the amount ingested

the plasma concentration of paracetamol, plotted on a semilogarithmic graph against time (Figure 16.1), falls above a line drawn between 1.32 mmol/L (200 mg/L) at 4 hours and 0.33 mmol/L (50 mg/L) at 12 hours after the overdose. A copy of this chart should be in every ICU and emergency department. *N*-acetylcysteine is

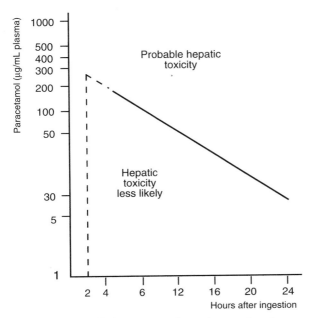

FIGURE 16.1 Toxic concentrations of paracetamol.

very effective up to 8 hours. There is now evidence to suggest that the antidote should be given to all patients, regardless of presentation, even if they have developed fulminant hepatic failure.

• Give *N*-acetylcysteine, 20% solution, 150 mg/kg in 200 ml of 5% dextrose over 15 minutes initially; then 50 mg/kg in 500 ml of 5% dextrose over 4 hours; finally, 200 mg/kg in 1 litre of 5% dextrose over the next 16 hours (total dose 400 mg/kg in 20 hours). Urticaria, bronchospasm, or anaphylaxis can occur in up to 10% of patients given *N*-acetylcysteine, especially asthmatics.

• Patients who ingest large amounts of paracetamol or who present late may develop renal failure (see Chapter 27) or acute hepatic failure (see Chapter 28). Monitoring the prothrombin time (PTT) and its 12-hourly rate of rise is the best marker of hepatic necrosis: Peak elevation occurs at 72–96 hours. Treat hypoglycaemia, as indicated, with dextrose infusion.

• Patients should be transferred to a specialist centre if fulminant hepatic failure is suspected.

PARAQUAT

FEATURES

• This potent herbicide causes ulceration of the mucous membranes, nausea, sweating, vomiting, tremors and convulsions, and severe pulmonary oedema. Lung fibrosis can occur up to a week after ingestion.

• Cardiovascular collapse and renal failure can also occur.

MANAGEMENT

• General supportive measures (see p. 10).

• Fuller's earth helps adsorb paraquat in the gut. A suspension of 30%, 200–250 ml every 4 hours, should be used until the stools contain Fuller's earth. Activated charcoal can also be given (see p. 333).

• Avoid a high oxygen concentration unless it is absolutely necessary, as it can potentiate pulmonary fibrosis. Immediate plasma exchange or haemofiltration may be effective, but this remains unproven.

QUININE, QUINIDINE, AND CHLOROQUINE

FEATURES

• vomiting
• tinnitus
• deafness
• blurred vision
• headache
• hypotension
• cardiac arrhythmias
• tachypnoea
• renal failure
• coma

• ECG changes: prolonged QT interval, widened QRS complex, and T-wave flattening.

MANAGEMENT
- Support of the cardiorespiratory system is the key to management.

SALICYLATES

FEATURES
- The toxic effects are complex and are related to acid–base disturbances, uncoupling of oxidative phosphorylation, and disordered glucose metabolism.
- Initially there will be nausea, vomiting, abdominal pain, and tinnitus, which can progress to deafness.
- Next will come hyperventilation, flushed skin, sweating, and hyperthermia.
- Salicylates have two separate, independent effects on acid–base balance. The first is respiratory alkalosis, as a result of central respiratory stimulation. The second is metabolic acidosis, resulting from accumulation of organic acid metabolites and lactate.
- Arterial blood pH is initially normal or raised because of the respiratory alkalosis, but metabolic acidosis usually supervenes. This pattern is more common in children.
- Respiratory complications include aspiration pneumonia, pulmonary oedema, and adult respiratory distress syndrome (ARDS).
- Cardiovascular abnormalities: Mortality is often due to cardiovascular depression, which can be unresponsive to treatment. ECG changes include a widened QRS complex. Atrioventricular block and ventricular arrhythmias can occur.
- Metabolic disturbances can include hypoglycaemia or hyperglycaemia and hypokalaemia.
- Coagulation disturbances: hypoprothrombinaemia, prolonged bleeding time, thrombocytopenia, and disseminated intravascular coagulopathy (DIC), often causing GIT bleeding.
- More rarely, there may be hyperpyrexia, renal failure, and hypoglycaemia.

MANAGEMENT
- Gastric lavage – within 24 hours of ingestion.
- Administer gastric charcoal.

- Maintain intravascular volume aggressively (see p. 61).
- Glucose infusion if hypoglycaemic.
- Monitor and correct electrolyte disorders.
- Vitamin K may be necessary for hypoprothrombinaemia.
- Marked metabolic acidosis should be corrected with sodium bicarbonate.
- Early determination of the plasma salicylate level is essential:

  mild toxicity, <500 mg/L
  moderate toxicity, 500–750 mg/L
  severe toxicity, >750 mg/L
  in CHILDREN, toxicity can occur at 300 mg/L

- Although forced alkaline diuresis has largely been abandoned, it is important to give enough fluid to maintain a brisk diuresis.
- Haemodialysis should be considered in cases of moderate or severe toxicity where the levels have not decreased after 2 hours. Dialysis is also indicated for acute renal failure or pulmonary oedema unresponsive to diuretics.
- Other anti-inflammatory agents, such as indomethacin, do not have the same toxic effects as salicylates, and treatment is largely supportive.

SEDATIVES AND NEUROLEPTIC DRUGS

- Barbiturates
- Benzodiazepines
- Glutethimide
- Methaqualone
- Phenothiazines

FEATURES
- Mainly coma and cardiorespiratory depression.

MANAGEMENT
- General supportive measures (see p. 10).
- INTUBATE if there is doubt about the airway.
- VENTILATE if there is doubt about breathing.

• INTRAVENOUS FLUIDS are commonly needed in large amounts in order to support the circulation (see Chapter 4).

• Benzodiazepine antagonists such as flumazenil (at a dosage of no more than 0.1–0.2 mg/min; 1–2 mg is usually sufficient; the paediatric dose is 5 μg/kg IV stat, to a total of 40 μg/kg) can reverse the effects of benzodiazepines and may play a limited role in the management of benzodiazepine poisoning. However, not all the effects of the benzodiazepines are reversed, and the relationship between the amount of benzodiazepine ingested and the amount of flumazenil needed to offset the effect is not linear. The half-life of flumazenil is about 1 hour. It can induce acute withdrawal syndromes in patients on long-term benzodiazepines. Flumazenil should not be given to patients who are suspected of having taken tricyclic antidepressants or to patients who are having seizures.

THEOPHYLLINE

FEATURES

• Nausea, vomiting, abdominal pain.

• Haematemesis, hypotension, tachyarrhythmias.

• Renal failure and rhabdomyolysis.

• Central nervous system excitability and convulsions.

• Hypokalaemia, hyperglycaemia, hypophosphataemia, hypomagnesaemia, hypocalcaemia.

• Acid–base disturbances.

• Leucocytosis.

MANAGEMENT

• ECG monitoring

• Gastric lavage, with activated charcoal (see p. 332).

• Correction of hypotension with fluid and inotropes if necessary.

• Aggressive measures to control seizures (see p. 613).

• Correction of electrolyte disorders: RAPIDLY CORRECT HYPOKALAEMIA, as well as phosphate and magnesium levels.

• Determination of electrolyte concentrations at least 4-hourly.

• For serious arrhythmias, propranolol may be useful.

• The plasma concentrations do not correlate well with the clinical severity, and therefore the concentrations can serve only as guidelines. Therapeutic concentrations are 80–120 μmol/L.

• Haemoperfusion using a charcoal column should be considered if the serum concentration is high (>600 μmol/L) or if serious complications occur (eg seizures, intractable vomiting, severe metabolic acidoses, renal failure, arrhythmias).

TRICYCLIC ANTIDEPRESSANTS

FEATURES   Remember the three C's: coma, convulsions, and cardiac arrhythmias.

• Arrhythmias (tachycardia, atrioventricular block, intraventricular conduction disturbances)
• Hypotension
• Respiratory depression
• Anticholinergic effects (dry mouth, dilated pupils, urinary retention)

MANAGEMENT
• Secure the airway, and ventilate if necessary.
• Treat seizures aggressively.
• Give intravascular fluids to correct hypotension.
• Correct electrolyte and acid–base disorders.
• Avoid physostigmine, as it can worsen convulsions and cardiac effects.
• Arrhythmias:
   Most occur within the first 12 hours.
   May need adrenaline, atropine, or temporary pacing for brady-arrhythmias. β-blockers or lignocaine may be useful for tachy-arrhythmias and intraventricular conduction disturbances.
   Bicarbonate (1–2 mmol/kg IV) may be useful for conduction delay or ventricular arrhythmias. Titrate to response and arterial pH. Hyperventilation may also be useful.

TROUBLESHOOTING

POISONING

Establish control of the airway, breathing, and circulation before concentrating on drug removal. Supportive care is all that is required for most patients.

Airway Intubate and ventilate if the score on the Glasgow coma scale (GCS) is less than 9.

Breathing Give high-flow oxygen, via mask if not intubated. Artificially ventilate if still hypoxic.

Circulation Fluid will correct most cases of hypotension. Inotropes are rarely needed.

Monitoring and investigation Vital signs such as blood pressure, respiratory rate, temperature, pulse rate, and GCS should be measured frequently (eg every 15–30 minutes) on admission, and then according to progress. Also monitor

- blood sugar/electrolytes
- arterial blood gases
- ECG
- pulse oximetry

Corrections Correct hypoxia, acidosis, and electrolyte disorders.

Drugs Identify by direct observations of aspirated tablets. Get a history from witnesses. Conduct a drug screen (see p. 328).

To decrease absorption (see p. 331)

- Use NG aspiration.
- Use lavage if ingestion occurred less than 1 hour earlier.
- Give charcoal, 1 g/kg via NG tube; repeated doses may be indicated (see p. 331).
- Induced vomiting should be considered only for children (see p. 332).

To increase excretion Procedures such as faecuresis and haemodialysis are indicated only for specific drugs above certain concentrations (see p. 335).

Antidotes Antidotes are available for some drugs (see p. 336).

Sequelae The sequelae of poisoning, such as hypothermia, hyperthermia, rhabdomyolysis, and seizures, must be recognized early and treated aggressively.

FURTHER READING

Dreisbach, R. H. (ed.) (1980). *Handbook of Poisoning: Prevention, Diagnosis and Treatment*, 10th ed. Los Altos, CA: Lange Medical.

Goldfrank, L. R., Flomenbaum, N. E., Lewin, N. A., Weisman, R. S., & Howland, M. A. (1990). *Goldfrank's Toxicologic Emergencies*, 4th ed. Englewood Cliffs, NJ: Prentice-Hall.

Kulig, K. (1992). Initial management of ingestions of toxic substances. *New England Journal of Medicine* 326:1677–81.

Levy, G. (1982). Gastrointestinal clearance of drugs with activated charcoal. *New England Journal of Medicine* 307:676–8.

Pond, S. M. (1991). Extracorporeal techniques in the treatment of poisoned patients. *Medical Journal of Australia* 154:617–22.

Thompson, W. L. (1980). Poisoning: the twentieth century black death. In *Critical Care: State of the Art*, vol. 1, ed. W. C. Shoemaker & W. L. Thompson, pp. N1–94. Fullerton, CA: Society of Critical Care Medicine.

Todd, J. W. (1984). Do measures to enhance drug removal save life? *Lancet* 1:331.

Vale, A., Meredith, T., & Buckley, B. (1984). Eliminating poisons. *British Medical Journal* 289:366–9.

Wright, R. C. (1974). A simple plan for the management of drug overdose. *Anaesthesia and Intensive Care* 4:288–302.

17

ACUTE RESPIRATORY FAILURE

- Oxygen is the first-line drug for acute respiratory failure.
- High concentrations of inspired oxygen almost never depress ventilation in patients with acute respiratory failure.
- Artificial ventilation will improve hypercarbia, but may not improve hypoxia.

This chapter will cover the pathophysiology and general principles of treatment for acute respiratory failure. Specific respiratory conditions will be discussed in Chapter 19.

The respiratory system can be seen as being divided into a gas-exchange system (the lungs) and a pump to ventilate that system (the diaphragm). The main functions of the lungs are to take up oxygen and eliminate carbon dioxide. Oxygen is needed for basic metabolism, and carbon dioxide is produced as a result of that metabolism. Respiratory failure occurs when either gas exchange fails or the pump fails. The classic definitions for the onset of acute respiratory failure that cited exact levels of oxygen and carbon dioxide were inflexible and misleading.

Acute respiratory failure can be divided into failure of oxygenation and/or failure of ventilation leading to hypercarbia (Table 17.1). Although hypoxia and hypercarbia can coexist, it is helpful, for an understanding of acute respiratory failure, to look at them separately.

FAILURE OF OXYGENATION

There are four types of hypoxia that can lead to decreased oxygen supply to the tissues. They are described in the equation for oxygen-carrying capacity:

oxygen-carrying capacity = cardiac output
× haemoglobin concentration
× saturation of haemoglobin
× 1.34

353

TABLE 17.1 CAUSES OF ACUTE RESPIRATORY FAILURE

Ventilatory problems

AIRWAY (eg obstruction)

NEUROMUSCULAR PATHWAY

- brain (eg coma from any cause)
- spinal cord (eg poliomyelitis, trauma)
- nerve (eg neuropathies)
- neuromuscular (eg myasthenia gravis)
- muscular disease (eg dystrophies)

MECHANICAL SYSTEM: interference with the bellows action of the ventilatory system (eg kyphoscoliosis, obesity, pneumothorax, pain, flail chest). Exhaustion as a result of lung abnormalities (increased airway resistance and
decreased compliance) also represents a failure of the mechanical system.

Gas-exchange problems

DECREASED F_{IO_2}

DECREASED VENTILATION (will also cause hypercarbia and hypoxia)

DIFFUSION DEFECT

$\dot{V}/\dot{Q}$ MISMATCH (usually, critically ill patients will have a spectrum of $\dot{V}/\dot{Q}$ mismatch and shunting)

SHUNTING

- stagnant hypoxia – decreased cardiac output
- anaemic hypoxia – decreased haemoglobin
- hypoxic hypoxia – decreased saturation
- histotoxic hypoxia – decreased oxygen-binding capacity (1.34 ml of
oxygen normally bind to every 1 g of haemoglobin)

Although oxygen delivery to the tissues can be compromised at all
levels, including inadequate cardiac output, anaemia, and decreased
oxygen-binding capacity, this chapter will concentrate on the principles of oxygen exchange in the lungs, where 'hypoxic hypoxia' occurs.

Hypoxic hypoxia

Acute respiratory failure is generally associated with hypoxic hypoxia
(ie there is a problem in getting the oxygen from the inspired gas

The oxygen cascade

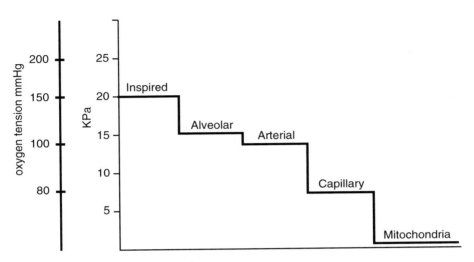

FIGURE 17.1   The oxygen cascade.

through the lungs into the capillaries). All causes of hypoxic hypoxia can be related to the oxygen-cascade concept (Figure 17.1).

DECREASE IN INSPIRED OXYGEN   Usually, a decrease in inspired oxygen (FIO_2) is a problem only at high altitudes or where there is a fault in the gas-supply system.

ALVEOLAR HYPOVENTILATION   If the lungs are otherwise normal, hypoxia will occur only with severe hypoventilation. An increase in FIO_2 will correct hypoxia in most cases of moderate hypoventilation.

DIFFUSION   The term 'diffusion' describes the movement of molecules down a concentration gradient. Diffusion disorders of the lung can occur in diseases such as emphysema. However, diffusion abnormalities play only minor roles in most cases of acute respiratory failure.

VENTILATION/PERFUSION MISMATCH   Ventilation/perfusion ($\dot{V}/\dot{Q}$) mismatch is the commonest cause of hypoxia in patients with acute respiratory failure. Ventilation and perfusion are well matched in the

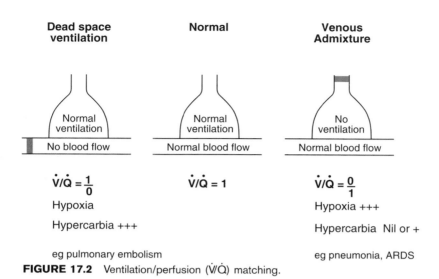

FIGURE 17.2 Ventilation/perfusion ($\dot{V}/\dot{Q}$) matching.

normal lung. Mismatching affects the exchange of oxygen and carbon dioxide, resulting in hypoxia and, to a lesser extent, hypercarbia, as carbon dioxide is a more diffusible gas.

SHUNT There is some variable degree of true shunting in the presence of acute respiratory failure (ie blood and gas do not match at all) (Figure 17.2). Most shunting occurs as a result of venous admixture, where capillary blood and alveolar gas do not equilibrate. The larger the shunt, the less responsive it is to added oxygen.

Other factors

INCREASED OXYGEN CONSUMPTION Increased consumption of oxygen can contribute to arterial hypoxia. For example, as a result of hypercatabolism, or in patients with excessive fever, the existing hypoxia can be exacerbated. An increase in peripheral oxygen consumption will decrease the mixed venous levels of oxygen, which, after becoming involved in defective gas exchange in the lungs, will result in arterial hypoxia.

OXYGEN EXTRACTION In order to ensure optimal oxygen extraction, the oxyhaemoglobin curve can be manipulated by encouraging peripheral oxygen unloading. However, the ultimate benefit of such manipulation has not been proved. Some of the manoeuvres include encouraging mild acidosis, avoiding alkalosis, correcting hypophosphataemia, and maintaining a normal or slightly elevated $Paco_2$.

HYPOXIC PULMONARY VASOCONSTRICTION Alveolar hypoxia causes pulmonary vasoconstriction, which can diminish the $\dot{V}/\dot{Q}$ mismatch (ie a decreased amount of blood will perfuse partially ventilated alveoli). Although the sensors for hypoxic pulmonary vasoconstriction are unknown, mediators may be released from cells, or hypoxia may act directly on pulmonary vessels. Vasodilating drugs such as glyceryl trinitrate and calcium-channel blockers can inhibit the hypoxic pulmonary vasoconstriction and worsen the hypoxia.

Effects of hypoxia

Hypoxia causes severe disruptions of cellular function so central cyanosis is not a reliable sign of hypoxia, and more accurate monitoring or measurement is needed in the critically ill. Similarly, signs and symptoms of hypoxia often are late and unpredictable. They can include confusion, irritability, tachypnoea and tachycardia, hypertension eventually leading to bradycardia, and hypotension.

The degree of hypoxia can be measured by comparing Pao_2 to Fio_2, by determining the difference between alveolar oxygen and arterial oxygen, or by measuring the degree of shunting (see p. 506). Oxygen saturation is continuously monitored in the intensive care unit (ICU) with a pulse oximeter. This is described in more detail in the section on cardiorespiratory monitoring (see p. 507).

FAILURE OF VENTILATION

The commonest cause of hypercarbia is alveolar hypoventilation. Its causes in the ICU include coma and exhaustion secondary to respiratory failure (Table 17.2).

$$Paco_2 \propto \frac{\text{CO}_2 \text{ production}}{\text{alveolar ventilation}}$$

$$\text{alveolar ventilation} = \text{total ventilation} - \text{dead-space ventilation}$$

TABLE 17.2   MAJOR CAUSES OF HYPERCARBIA IN INTENSIVE CARE

Decreased CO_2 elimination

• There are many causes of hypoventilation (eg airway obstruction, drugs, central and peripheral nervous disorders) (see p. 426).

• Decreased minute volume (eg end-stage acute respiratory failure because of exhaustion).

• Ventilation–perfusion inequality is the commonest cause of hypercarbia in patients with chronic lung disease and acute respiratory failure. It is often seen in association with destruction of lung architecture, either chronically (largely as a result of smoking-related diseases) or acutely (as a result of pulmonary barotrauma in acute respiratory failure).

Excess CO_2 production

• This is an uncommon cause of hypercarbia and usually is important only when CO_2 elimination is impaired.

• Hyperpyrexia.

• Inappropriate carbohydrate load (see p. 90).

• Hypercatabolism.

• Thyrotoxicosis.

Increased dead space

• In the setting of an ICU, increased dead space usually is due to increased equipment dead space or decreased pulmonary artery blood flow.

An increase in dead space will decrease alveolar ventilation. Increases in anatomic dead space usually result from the use of artificial airways and ventilatory circuits in the setting of intensive care. Increased physiological dead space usually occurs as a result of a $\dot{V}/\dot{Q}$ mismatch.

Hypercarbia usually is associated with hypoventilation (Table 17.3), but it can also result from under-perfused alveoli consequent to hypovolaemia, from lung destruction as a result of barotrauma (see p. 466), or from increased CO_2 production (eg as with fever, excessive carbohydrate intake, or increased activity).

Effects of hypercarbia

• increased respiratory drive
• anxiety, restlessness, tachycardia, hypertension

TABLE 17.3 MAJOR CAUSES OF HYPOVENTILATION IN INTENSIVE CARE

Brain
    Drug overdose
    Neurotrauma
    Post-operative anaesthetic depression
    Cardiovascular accident

Spinal cord
    Poliomyelitis
    Spinal-cord trauma

Neuromuscular system
    Myasthenia gravis
    Tetanus
    Organophosphate poisoning
    Neuromuscular blocking drugs
    Peripheral neuritis
    Guillain-Barré syndrome
    Muscular dystrophies

Thorax
    Massive obesity
    Kyphoscoliosis
    Chest trauma and flail chest
    Pneumothorax and pleural effusion

Upper-airway obstruction

Exhaustion
Especially in the latter stages of acute respiratory failure, as a result of low lung compliance or increased resistance

- peripheral vasodilation
- increases in cerebral blood flow and intracranial pressure (ICP)
- decreased level of consciousness, and coma
- acute rise in endogenous catecholamines, causing increases in cardiac output and blood pressure
- decreased oxygenation, by displacing alveolar oxygen

Carbon dioxide usually is monitored by intermittent sampling of arterial blood gases in the ICU. Capnography can also be used. Monitoring of carbon dioxide is described in the section on cardiorespiratory monitoring (see p. 493).

PRINCIPLES OF TREATMENT

FAILURE OF VENTILATION

Obviously the airway is crucial for respiratory function, and it must always be the first consideration in dealing with any respiratory problem. Gas cannot move in and out of the lungs, no matter how efficient they are, if the airway is blocked. Always consider the possibility of a compromised airway, and replace the endotracheal tube or tracheostomy tube if there is any doubt about its patency (see p. 29).

Treatment and diagnosis of hypoventilation go hand in hand (Table 17.3). If necessary, the airway must be secured, and artificial ventilation commenced, while the cause of the ventilatory failure is being determined and treatment selected.

HYPOXIC PATIENTS NEED OXYGENATION, NOT NECESSARILY MORE VENTILATION. Indeed, acute respiratory failure is usually marked by hyperventilation and hypocarbia in the face of hypoxia. In other words, the patient's existing ventilation usually is more than adequate, especially in the earlier stages. Oxygen uptake is affected more than carbon dioxide excretion. As the lungs become heavier and less compliant, the patient has to work harder, and eventually the increased work will lead to respiratory-muscle exhaustion and hypoventilation. The oxygen consumption related to respiratory work may also be unacceptably high. In the event of hypoventilation or an unacceptable increase in respiratory work, artificial ventilation may eventually be necessary.

If ventilation is impaired and the carbon dioxide concentration rises, the possible reversible causes should be examined and ruled out; then, if necessary, artificial ventilation should be commenced or increased. Unless the ICP is elevated, hypercarbia is not as dangerous as hypoxia; this is particularly relevant when ventilating patients with asthma (see p. 443) or chronic airway limitations (see p. 451). There is an increasing tendency to accept Pa_{CO_2} values higher than 'normal', so long as the arterial pH remains acceptable. Achieving 'normal' Pa_{CO_2} values in patients with acute respiratory failure can result in an unacceptably high peak inspiratory pressure and a high incidence of complications, such as pulmonary barotrauma (see p. 466).

Ventilation should be commenced with a tidal volume of no more than 10 ml/kg at a respiratory rate consistent with adequate lung emptying at the end of expiration. Carbon dioxide levels should be reduced slowly, especially if there is evidence of subacute or chronic hypercarbia. The aim of artificial ventilation is to maintain oxygenation at the lowest level of positive intrathoracic pressure. It is not necessary, and may even be detrimental, to achieve 'normal' Pa_{CO_2} values.

FAILURE OF OXYGENATION (Table 17.4)

Treating hypoventilation with artificial ventilation is relatively straightforward, as compared with managing hypoxia. THE REAL CHALLENGE IN PATIENTS WITH ACUTE RESPIRATORY FAILURE IS TO MAINTAIN ADEQUATE OXYGENATION.

Management of patients with acute respiratory failure involves the right balance of FI_{O_2}, positive end-expiratory pressure (PEEP), sedation, fluid treatment, drugs, and positive intrathoracic pressure – all of which involve potential dangers. TREATMENT OF PATIENTS WITH ACUTE RESPIRATORY FAILURE IS USUALLY A HOLDING OPERATION WHILE THE LUNGS HEAL THEMSELVES. Avoidance of any iatrogenic complications of the ventilatory therapy is paramount.

The primary aim in treating acute respiratory failure is to provide more oxygen to the cells, and sometimes to reduce their consumption. Oxygen delivery depends on the following relationship:

oxygen delivery = cardiac output
  × haemoglobin concentration
  × oxygen saturation × 1.34

The following sections will take up each aspect of oxygen delivery in turn, but in clinical practice they must, of course, be considered as complementing and interacting with each other.

For example, more oxygen might be available on each haemoglobin molecule if PEEP were applied to the lungs, but the cardiac output might be depressed, and therefore oxygen transport would be decreased. Capillary flow might be encouraged because of the fewer numbers of haemoglobin molecules that would result from decreasing the viscosity. However, the oxygen content in the blood would then be decreased. Oxygen delivery requires a balance of many factors, and

TABLE 17.4   PRINCIPLES OF TREATMENT FOR ACUTE RESPIRATORY
FAILURE

Treat underlying cause
Increase oxygen delivery
- Oxygen
- PEEP
- CPAP
- Fluid treatment
- Artificial ventilation
- Nursing and physiotherapy
- Haemoglobin
- Perfusion

Decrease oxygen consumption
Improve oxygen extraction
Miscellaneous (eg bronchoscopy, antibiotics)
Match oxygen delivery to oxygen consumption

the oxygen-delivery equation is one of the most important tools in intensive care.

OXYGEN DELIVERY

INCREASED OXYGEN SATURATION OF HAEMOGLOBIN (Table 17.5)

oxygen delivery = cardiac output
× haemoglobin concentration
× oxygen saturation × 1.34

OXYGEN IS THE FIRST-LINE DRUG FOR HYPOXIA. It may have to be delivered via an endotracheal tube (ETT) with artificial ventilation, but in many cases that is not necessary. Many patients with acute respiratory failure are hyperventilating and do not need increased ventilation.

TABLE 17.5 PRINCIPLES OF OXYGENATION

The following guidelines are listed in order of increasing escalation of measures needed to maintain oxygenation in patients with acute respiratory failure:

1. **Oxygen**

   Increase F_{IO_2}, but aim to keep below 0.5 with face mask.

2. **CPAP**

   CPAP mask or intubation with CPAP at 5–20 cm H_2O initially, using efficient circuit $\pm$ IMV with pressure assist.

3. **Ventilation**

   IPPV + PEEP – preferably with a technique to maintain spontaneous respiration, such as IMV with pressure support, or APRV.

   Use low tidal volumes (eg 7 ml/kg) in order to reduce PIP and a respiratory rate consistent with adequate carbon dioxide excretion.

   Use sedation only if necessary and with continuous narcotic $\pm$ muscle relaxant to reduce excessive movement and fighting of the ventilator.

   Use conventional IPPV and PEEP if reverse I:E ratio is not available.

   Aim to keep peak inspiratory pressures below 35 cm H_2O when using positive-pressure ventilation, even if it is at the expense of a high Pa_{CO_2}.

4. **Fluid treatment**

   Use minimal crystalloids, while maintaining intravascular volume with colloid or blood, in all hypoxic patients.

5. **Diuretic**

   Give diuretic in frequent small doses (eg 5–10 mg frusemide initially 4-hourly, or continuous intravenous infusion may help to reduce lung water). The circulation must simultaneously be maintained with colloid or blood.

6. **Position**

   Position the affected lung up in the presence of a unilateral abnormality. Otherwise, sit the patient up at an angle of 40° or more.

7. Give 100% oxygen during endotracheal suctioning.

8. Actively cool the patient to reduce severe hyperpyrexia, in combination with sedation and/or paralysis to prevent shivering.

9. LFPPV + ECCO$_2$R or extracorporeal oxygenation if available (see p. 376).

Note: See the sections on ventilatory techniques (Chapter 20) for IPPV, PEEP, CPAP, APRV, IMV, MMV, HFPPV, LFPPV + ECCO$_2$R, reversed I:E ratios, and weaning.

Complications of oxygen treatment

CARBON DIOXIDE NARCOSIS Apart from the fact that it can sometimes explode and can support combustion, oxygen is a very safe drug. For some inexplicable reason, medical students are taught, and seem to remember forever, that oxygen is a dangerous drug. One almost expects to see it counted out, molecule by molecule, like pills. Many hypoxic patients, with or without chronic respiratory components in their illnesses, are found behind their masks inhaling 24% oxygen – 3% more than in room air! Oxygen **NEVER** inhibits breathing in **ACUTE** respiratory failure and **RARELY** inhibits breathing in **ACUTE OR CHRONIC** respiratory failure. When it does, the onset is slow enough to allow monitoring with pulse oximetry, blood-gas analysis, and clinical status.

OXYGEN TOXICITY In the past, fear of oxygen toxicity had been another reason for depriving hypoxic patients of oxygen. High levels of inspired oxygen can cause atelectasis, decreased alveolar macrophage activity, decreased ciliary action, and, in the long term, lung fibrosis. Oxygen has never been shown to cause lung damage if the F_{IO_2} has been less than 0.5. If at all possible, it should be kept below that level. However, if oxygen is essential for preventing hypoxia, it should not be withheld because of fear of toxicity. Oxygenation should be carefully monitored (eg arterial blood gases, pulse oximetry), with the F_{IO_2} reduced to a safe level as soon as possible. Because the shunt fraction in the lung is constant, increasing the F_{IO_2} may not have much effect on Pa_{O_2}. In that situation, an excessive F_{IO_2} may be unnecessary and dangerous. On the other hand, hypoxia is definitely dangerous!

CONCENTRATION OF INSPIRED OXYGEN In view of the conflict between the potential dangers of oxygen and its essential nature, the amount given will depend on the amount needed. In acute respiratory failure, keep the Pa_{O_2} above 60 mm Hg (8 kPa), or 90% saturation. That is the critical point at the top of the oxyhaemoglobin dissociation curve. Below that, the curve becomes closer to vertical, and saturation of the haemoglobin molecule diminishes rapidly.

TABLE 17.6 APPROXIMATE O_2 CONCENTRATIONS RELATED TO FLOW RATES

Oxygen flow rate (L/min)	Approximate F_{IO_2}
4	0.25–0.35
6	0.30–0.50
8	0.35–0.55
10	0.4–0.60
12	0.45–0.65

Delivery systems (Table 17.6)

No mask or catheter device can deliver 100% oxygen unless it can provide a peak inspiratory flow rate (PIFR) of at least 40 L/min. There are two main types of systems for delivering oxygen:

(a) inspired oxygen independent of patient factors (fixed-performance masks, eg Venturi masks)

(b) inspired oxygen dependent on the patient's respiratory pattern (variable-performance masks)

NASAL CATHETERS F_{IO_2} is dependent on respiratory rate and tidal volume. As the respiratory rate and tidal volume increase, F_{IO_2} decreases. The nasal catheter (2–6 L/min) functions by filling the nasopharyngeal reservoirs with oxygen, which is entrained as the patient inspires. Flow rates higher than 6 L/min offer no advantage for oxygenation and can cause patient discomfort.

SIMPLE OXYGEN MASKS The oxygen flow must be more than 5 L/min in order to avoid carbon dioxide retention. F_{IO_2} is dependent on respiratory rate and tidal volume. As the respiratory rate and tidal volume increase, F_{IO_2} decreases. F_{IO_2} varies between 0.35 and 0.50 as the oxygen flow is increased from 5 to 8 L/min.

VENTURI OXYGEN MASK
The F_{IO_2} value depends on the degree of entrainment. A variety of entrainment valves can provide F_{IO_2} values between 0.24 and some-

thing approaching 1.0. F_{IO_2} may not be independent of respiratory pattern in patients with very high PIFRs.

RESERVOIR OXYGEN MASK This mask potentially can provide an F_{IO_2} of 1.0. For efficient operation, the oxygen reservoir should be fully expanded.

If a patient is unable to protect and maintain the airway, or if the patient becomes exhausted, an ETT should be inserted. This will allow efficient delivery of oxygen and maintenance of PEEP and continuous positive airway pressure (CPAP), as well as artificial ventilation, if required.

PEEP (Table 17.7)

Positive end-expiratory pressure occurs when, instead of allowing airway pressure to return to atmospheric pressure between ventilator breaths, an end-expiratory pressure is applied. Just how PEEP improves oxygenation is not fully understood. The end-expiratory pressure probably prevents collapse of the alveoli, in addition to recruiting non-ventilated alveoli, thus enabling greater numbers to participate in gas exchange and thereby lessening $\dot{V}/\dot{Q}$ mismatch.

OPTIMAL PEEP Although PEEP will improve oxygenation, it may decrease overall oxygen transport by decreasing cardiac output. The increased intrathoracic pressure causes a decrease in venous return, which is usually reversed by the use of intravenous fluids and/or inotropes. Extrathoracic oxygen blood flow is also compromised by PEEP. A combination of decreased cardiac output (blood flow to the organ) and decreased venous return (blood flow from the organ) can markedly reduce blood flow to extrathoracic organs such as the brain, liver, and kidneys. The optimal PEEP is the best match between improving the oxygenation and decreasing the oxygen transport due to decreased cardiac output. Another way of expressing the idea of optimal PEEP is that it is the minimal PEEP at which adequate oxygenation is maintained.

TABLE 17.7 POSITIVE END-EXPIRATORY PRESSURE

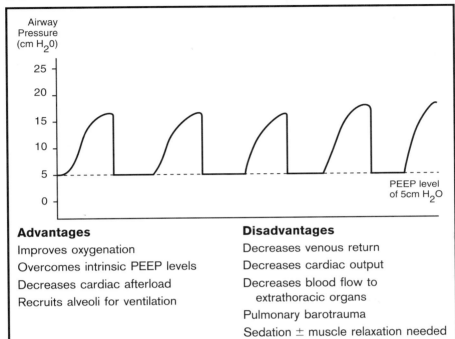

Advantages	Disadvantages
Improves oxygenation	Decreases venous return
Overcomes intrinsic PEEP levels	Decreases cardiac output
Decreases cardiac afterload	Decreases blood flow to extrathoracic organs
Recruits alveoli for ventilation	Pulmonary barotrauma
	Sedation $\pm$ muscle relaxation needed

Uses

Patients with hypoxia who are artificially ventilated (eg atelectasis, pneumonia, ARDS)

Practical aspects

Start at 5 cm H_2O, and do not exceed 20 cm H_2O. Give a fluid bolus (200–400 ml) before commencing IPPV + PEEP, in order to prevent hypotension as a result of decreased venous return.

DISADVANTAGES OF PEEP The complications of PEEP are the same as those for the increased intrathoracic pressure achieved with artificial ventilation. Barotrauma and decreased cardiac output occur. These are described in more detail elsewhere (see p. 466).

CPAP (Table 17.8)

Continuous positive airway pressure is a technique whereby gas is delivered to the airways at a constant pressure, facilitating sponta-

TABLE 17.8 CONTINUOUS POSITIVE AIRWAY PRESSURE

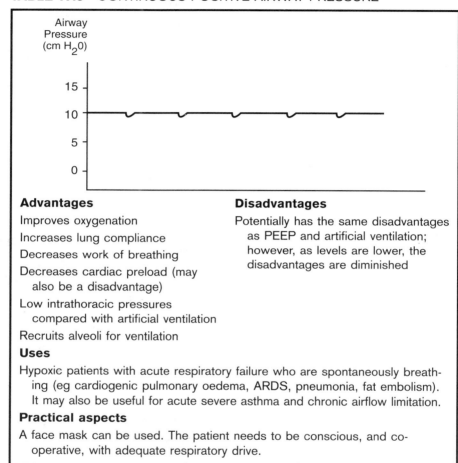

Advantages

Improves oxygenation

Increases lung compliance

Decreases work of breathing

Decreases cardiac preload (may also be a disadvantage)

Low intrathoracic pressures compared with artificial ventilation

Recruits alveoli for ventilation

Disadvantages

Potentially has the same disadvantages as PEEP and artificial ventilation; however, as levels are lower, the disadvantages are diminished

Uses

Hypoxic patients with acute respiratory failure who are spontaneously breathing (eg cardiogenic pulmonary oedema, ARDS, pneumonia, fat embolism). It may also be useful for acute severe asthma and chronic airflow limitation.

Practical aspects

A face mask can be used. The patient needs to be conscious, and co-operative, with adequate respiratory drive.

neous inspiratory effort, as well as providing PEEP. It is a technique used to support SPONTANEOUS respiration and to correct hypoxia, not hypoventilation. In many cases of acute respiratory failure, CPAP will increase lung compliance and decrease the work of breathing and thus may eliminate the need for assisted ventilation. It can be delivered by lightweight plastic masks, nasal prongs, ETTs, or tracheostomies. A CPAP mask or nasal prongs can be used in any patient who is

TABLE 17.9 ADVANTAGES OF CPAP AS COMPARED WITH IPPV + PEEP

Less sedation needed

Lower peak inspiratory pressure needed

Better oxygenation during spontaneous respiration

Less barotrauma

Better blood flow to extrathoracic organs

Better venous return and cardiac output

Better lung lymph drainage

- conscious and co-operative, with an intact airway
- hypoxic, with consistent respiratory drive

Some masks have an adjustable head strap to prevent leaks. After adequate explanation to the patient, they are usually well tolerated. An efficient circuit must be employed (see p. 472). Inefficient CPAP, which occurs in many demand systems incorporated into sophisticated intensive care ventilators (see p. 472), can cause increased work of breathing and impairment of gas exchange. The increased work of breathing in these systems can be counteracted by use of the inspiratory 'assist' mode. However, it is probably cheaper and more efficient to use a continuous-flow device (see p. 472).

Table 17.9 compares PEEP and CPAP.

Artificial ventilation

Artificial ventilation will not necessarily improve oxygenation. In some patients it will decrease oxygen delivery by altering the $\dot{V}/\dot{Q}$ matching. Matching of ventilation and perfusion is more efficient in spontaneously breathing patients than in those on artificial ventilation. Patients should not necessarily be ventilated for hypoxia, unless they are becoming exhausted or unless there is a concurrent abnormality, such as a head injury. Other modalities should be explored first, such as increasing the F_{IO_2} with appropriate oxygen masks or applying CPAP by mask. If ventilation is required, the following guidelines should be used (see Chapter 20 for more details).

Aim to keep the lung expanded with a minimum peak inspiratory pressure (PIP), using low tidal volumes, even in the presence of higher rather than 'normal' carbon dioxide levels. This concept has been called 'elective hypoventilation' or 'permissive hypercarbia'. The aim is to achieve oxygenation, with a minimum of complications resulting from the use of positive pressure. Some of the techniques that can facilitate positive-pressure ventilation with minimal complications include intermittent mandatory ventilation (IMV), pressure-support ventilation (PSV), airway-pressure-relief ventilation (APRV), and pressure-limited, reverse-I : E ratio ventilation (see Chapter 20). Conventional intermittent positive-pressure ventilation (IPPV) with PEEP should be avoided in favour of these other modes, where possible.

Fluid treatment

Poor fluid treatment in intensive care can impair gas exchange: DRY LUNGS ARE MORE EFFECTIVE THAN WET ONES.

THE AIM OF FLUID TREATMENT IS TO KEEP THE INTERSTITIAL SPACE AS DRY AS POSSIBLE, WHILE MAINTAINING A NORMAL INTRAVASCULAR VOLUME – SO-CALLED EUVOLAEMIC DEHYDRATION (see Chapter 4). Thus, the lungs should be kept as dry as possible while not compromising organ perfusion.

There are quite enough causes of increased lung water and adult respiratory distress syndrome (ARDS) in the ICU without us contributing to the list by giving excessive salt and water. Irrespective of the colloid osmotic pressure (COP), at least three-quarters of any crystalloid solution is distributed to the interstitial space. Excessive use of crystalloids should be avoided, if possible, in patients with acute respiratory failure (see p. 62).

The pulmonary artery wedge pressure (PAWP) at which lung water will accumulate is lower in patients with acute respiratory failure than in normal patients. Therefore, excessive use of intravascular fluid should also be avoided.

Assessment of lung water is difficult. Currently, the chest x-ray is the best clinical guide to the volume of lung water. There is good correlation between the extent of lung water and the degree of chest x-ray opacification. Peripheral oedema may also be a clinical indicator of increased lung water.

RESTRICT INTAKE OF SALT AND WATER If possible, limit the intake of 'clear' fluids to less than 2,000 ml over 24 hours in normal-size adults with severe respiratory failure. Use non-sodium-containing fluids (eg 5% dextrose) if the serum sodium concentration is normal, especially if fluids such as colloid (with a high sodium concentration) or blood are being used concurrently. Maintain the intravascular volume and cardiovascular stability with colloids or blood products and inotropes, according to the available cardiovascular measurements (see p. 55).

Reduction of the lung's interstitial-space fluid

DIURETIC Small doses of a loop diuretic (eg fursemide, 5–10 mg IV, 4-hourly, or the equivalent amount in a continuous intravenous infusion) may reduce lung water. However, colloid or blood usually will have to be given simultaneously in order to maintain the intravascular volume while depleting the interstitial space with the diuretic. Cations such as potassium, magnesium, and hydrogen will become depleted during aggressive diuretic treatment. Their serum levels need to be measured at least once each day (more often for potassium). Meticulous replacement is necessary.

DIALYTIC MODES Patients on dialysis or haemofiltration can readily have their fluid status altered by increasing or decreasing the ultrafiltration. The fluid removed is the ultrafiltrate of blood – almost the same constituents as interstitial-space fluid. Ultrafiltration is a very efficient and convenient way of selectively decreasing the volume of the interstitial fluid. As with diuretic treatment, the intravascular space must be maintained simultaneously with colloid or blood products.

Nursing and physiotherapy

POSITIONING OF PATIENTS The dependent part of the lung is perfused best. Generally speaking, patients with respiratory failure should be sat up, at least 40°, so that perfusion will be directed to the bulk of alveoli at the base of the lung. The head-down position can cause hypoxia. However, depending on where the pulmonary abnormality is, the patient should be positioned to maximize the matching of ventilation and perfusion (eg if the abnormality is more in the left lung, it may help to turn the patient so that the right lung is down).

PROCEDURES Nursing procedures can contribute to hypoxia, especially tracheal suctioning. Intratracheal negative pressure can exacerbate pulmonary oedema and will always cause hypoxia. The hypoxia can sometimes be severe and can lead to bradycardia. Intratracheal suctioning should always be preceded by 100% oxygen for 3–5 minutes; its use should be minimized for patients with acute respiratory failure and avoided in those with active pulmonary oedema. With the use of special devices on endotracheal connectors, PEEP and ventilation can be maintained during suction.

CHEST PHYSIOTHERAPY Physiotherapy is aimed mainly at clearing the sputum confined to the central airways, in addition to preventing collapse and atelectasis. It cannot modify the course of acute respiratory failure, as the abnormality is parenchymatous, rather than in the airways. Care must be exercised in positioning and suctioning patients during physiotherapy, as hypoxia can be exacerbated.

HAEMOGLOBIN

oxygen delivery = **cardiac output**

$\times$ $\boxed{\textbf{haemoglobin concentration}}$

$\times$ **oxygen saturation** $\times$ **1.34**

Oxygen is carried on haemoglobin in red blood cells. Each gram of haemoglobin carries 1.34 ml of oxygen. Anaemia is common in the seriously ill, often as a result of coagulopathy and multiple blood tests. The haemoglobin concentration should be kept to at least 10 g/dl in hypoxic patients in order to maintain their oxygen-carrying capacity. There is an increasing tendency to keep the haemoglobin concentration around normal during acute respiratory failure.

PERFUSION

oxygen delivery = $\boxed{\textbf{cardiac output}}$

$\times$ **haemoglobin concentration**
$\times$ **oxygen saturation** $\times$ **1.34**

Optimizing the saturation on the haemoglobin molecule and ensuring an adequate haemoglobin concentration are of no avail unless there is sufficient blood flow to take the oxygen to the cells. To improve cardiac output, the following need to be optimum (see also Chapter 22):

• Preload: Titrate the fluid against cardiovascular responses.
• Use of inotropes: Increase the cardiac output and peripheral perfusion with inotropes.
• Afterload: Decreasing the afterload is a manoeuvre used more in patients with primary heart disease than in the seriously ill with multiorgan failure (see p. 525).

Regional blood flow is a function of the perfusing pressure and the resistance to flow. At the tissue level, the factors determining oxygenation are the number of capillaries and the diffusing distance for the gas between the capillary and the cell. Whereas cardiac output and global oxygen delivery are relatively easy to measure and alter, tissue blood flow and oxygen delivery are not amenable to accurate measurement, nor are they easily manipulated.

COMBINING POWER OF HAEMOGLOBIN AND OXYGEN

> **oxygen delivery** = **cardiac output**
> × **haemoglobin concentration**
> × **oxygen saturation** × $\boxed{\textbf{1.34}}$

The factor 1.34 is mentioned for completeness. It is of minor relevance in acute respiratory failure. For each 1 g of haemoglobin, 1.34 ml of oxygen are attached. Occasionally, and in the presence of a normal Pa_{O_2}, the combining ability is compromised (eg carbon monoxide toxicity and cyanide poisoning). Such poisons also affect the ability of the cells to utilize oxygen. The combining power of haemoglobin and oxygen is described by the oxyhaemoglobin dissociation curve (Figure 17.3).

OXYGEN CONSUMPTION

On the other side of the oxygen equation is consumption. A decrease in the consumption of oxygen should be considered a possibility in se-

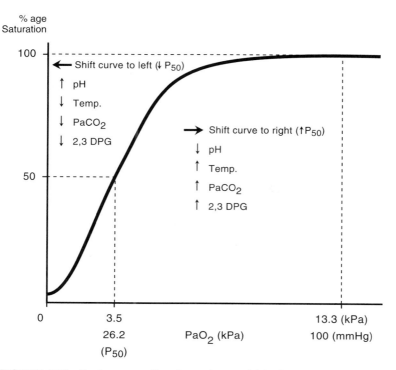

FIGURE 17.3 Factors controlling the oxyhaemoglobin dissociation curve.

verely hypoxic patients when the factors determining oxygen delivery have been optimized and the patient remains hypoxic.

TEMPERATURE   Oxygen consumption will increase markedly with increasing fever. If a patient's oxygenation is marginal, aggressive measures should be taken to treat the cause of the fever (eg infection,
heatstroke, malignant hyperthermia, drugs) and to reduce the fever
(see p. 161).

Surface cooling is an efficient method for lowering temperature so
it can be facilitated by creating a wind-tunnel effect, with a fan blow-
ing from the end of the bed, and a sheet tightly attached to the upper part of the chest, to avoid corneal drying and ulceration.

Tepid sponging can increase the efficiency of this form of cooling.
Sedation with or without muscle relaxation may also have to be employed to reduce the shivering response. Paracetamol should be used

with caution in patients with liver dysfunction. Avoid the use of ice packs for febrile patients, as that would simply decrease the skin circulation.

Aim for moderate temperature reduction (eg to 38.0°C), rather than hypothermia. A fever may be necessary for an optimal immune response in the presence of infection (see p. 161).

MINIMIZING MOVEMENT Except for the diaphragm, movement should be discouraged for hypoxic patients. Hypoxic confusion sometimes leads to excessive movement, at a high oxygen cost. Reassurance and sedation often are the only measures needed. For intractable cases, sedation and induction of paralysis may be necessary. This, of course, means mandatory ventilation, with its own costs. Epilepsy and excessive muscle movements must be aggressively treated in hypoxic patients (see p. 613).

HYPERCATABOLISM Hypercatabolism is often a feature of the seriously ill and is refractory to manipulation, apart from treating the underlying cause. Avoidance of high-carbohydrate feeds may help to reduce excessive carbon dioxide production.

MISCELLANEOUS CONSIDERATIONS

The principles of management for patients with acute respiratory failure are based on physiological considerations. Drugs have limited but well-defined roles.

DRUGS

BRONCHODILATORS Use bronchodilators if there is any evidence of bronchoconstriction (see p. 441).

ANTIBIOTICS Use antibiotics for infections (see p. 207).

NITRIC OXIDE Nitric oxide was previously known as 'endothelium-derived relaxant factor', and it is both an endogenous vasodilator and a cellular messenger for the vasodilating actions of nitrates. Inhaled nitric oxide is a selective pulmonary vasodilator, reducing pulmonary vascular resistance without affecting systemic vascular resistance, and improving cardiac output and oxygen delivery. Nitric oxide requires a special delivery system and gas analysis, as metabolites of nitric oxide, such as nitrogen dioxide (NO_2), cause toxicity secondary to their oxidising effects.

Small trials in adults with ARDS, CAL, and idiopathic pulmonary hypertension have shown significant reductions in pulmonary vascular resistance. The place of nitric oxide in the management of ARDS is not certain; large randomised trials are awaited.

OTHER DRUGS   Steroids, prostacyclin, aprotinin, artificial surfactant, heparin, thrombolytic agents, indomethacin, imidazole, meclofenamate, antioxidants, and anti-inflammatory prostanoids have all been tried or are being tested for treatment of acute respiratory failure, with, as yet, equivocal results.

EXTRACORPOREAL GAS EXCHANGE

If all else fails, some form of extracorporeal support can be considered. Although extracorporeal membrane oxygenation (ECMO) is rarely used today, more recent variations, combining low-frequency positive-pressure ventilation (LFPPV) and extracorporeal CO_2 removal ($ECCO_2R$), have proved to be successful in some cases of severe acute respiratory failure: Carbon dioxide is eliminated through an extracorporeal circuit, while oxygenation is achieved using oxygen insufflated directly into the trachea. Two to three artificial breaths each minute are delivered, with pressures limited to less than 35 cm H_2O.

MATCHING OXYGEN DELIVERY AND CONSUMPTION

Oxygen delivery (DO_2) is the amount of oxygen delivered to body tissues, and usually it is well matched to metabolic requirements. Under basal conditions, oxygen consumption ($\dot{V}O_2$) is about 25% of DO_2, yielding an oxygen extraction ratio of 0.25. Decreases in DO_2 are usually matched by increases in the oxygen extraction ratio, allowing $\dot{V}O_2$ to remain constant. However, once oxygen extraction is maximum, further decreases in DO_2 will be matched by parallel decreases in $\dot{V}O_2$ – the so-called supply dependence (Figure 17.4). This critical point is reached when tissue extraction cannot increase enough to compen-

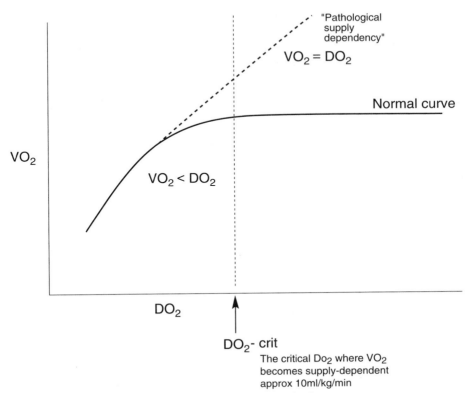

FIGURE 17.4 Relationship between oxygen consumption ($\dot{V}O_2$) and oxygen supply (DO_2).

sate for the reduction in oxygen delivery. The critical value is the same whether the reduced DO_2 results from lowering the haemoglobin concentration or decreasing the oxygen concentration in inspired air. The critical level at which this occurs in animal models is about 8–$10 \; ml \cdot kg^{-1} \cdot min^{-1}$. When an oxygen debt occurs, anaerobic metabolism produces lactic acid. If the condition goes uncorrected, tissue hypoxia will occur, eventually leading to cellular damage and death.

In the presence of certain conditions, such as septic shock, adult respiratory distress syndrome (ARDS), and multiple trauma, there will be increases in oxygen consumption. As oxygen delivery is increased, so is oxygen consumption. The amount of oxygen consumed is dependent on the amount delivered, the so-called pathological supply dependence.

This phenomenon is characterized not so much by the absence of a plateau phase in the relationship between DO_2 and $\dot{V}O_2$ as by an impairment in oxygen extraction. This can result from arteriovenous shunting, capillary obstruction due to microemboli or localized disseminated intravascular coagulation, capillary compression due to excessive peripheral oedema, primary cellular dysfunction, or maldistribution of perfusion, with over-supply of oxygen to some tissues and under-supply to others. Vasomotor reactivity could also be impaired by the release of vasoactive agents in precapillary sphincters and arterioles.

In patients in whom supply dependence is suspected (especially in cases of sepsis or ARDS), an 'oxygen-challenge' test can be considered. To achieve this, the DO_2 is increased (eg by fluid-volume loading or adding an inotrope), and the response in $\dot{V}O_2$ is measured. If the increase is significant (eg more than 10–20 ml/m^2), that confirms a pathological supply dependence, and delivery should be maintained at a higher level. The ideal rate of oxygen delivery is difficult to define for the seriously ill. Whereas it is easy to recommend that we provide oxygen delivery adequate to meet the demand, measurements of demand usually require intensive and time-consuming monitoring, with all of its disadvantages. Moreover, it is difficult to draw conclusions about cellular oxygen supply from $\dot{V}O_2$, as $\dot{V}O_2$ reflects only cellular oxygen consumption, which is not necessarily the same as actual cellular requirements. In addition, interpretation of absolute whole-body $\dot{V}O_2$ values is complicated by the fluctuations that can occur with the patient's activities, such as positioning, independent of real changes in consumption. It has been suggested that a pathological $\dot{V}O_2/DO_2$ relationship does not occur in the absence of lactic acidosis. Thus, normal blood levels of lactate can reasonably rule out the existence of tissue hypoxia. On the other hand, elevated blood levels of lactate do not always imply $\dot{V}O_2/DO_2$ dependence.

Recently, the concept of supply dependence has been questioned. It has been suggested that if the components of delivery and consumption are all measured or calculated via a pulmonary artery catheter, then the relationship observed – oxygen consumption ($\dot{V}O_2$) depends on oxygen delivery (DO_2) – is the result of a mathematical linkage, not a real phenomenon. In studies where $\dot{V}O_2$ has been measured using respired-gas analysis, a clear dependence of $\dot{V}O_2$ on DO_2 has not been demonstrated. One recent study (Hayes et al., 1994) suggested increased mortality among patients who had undergone aggressive efforts to increase oxygen consumption.

Allowing for accurate and continuous measurements, how do we interpret DO_2 and $\dot{V}O_2$? This remains a challenge for intensivists. $\dot{V}O_2$ represents the oxygen consumed, not the metabolic need. Part of the problem is related to the global representation of oxygen flow by measuring DO_2 and $\dot{V}O_2$. We must also take into account regional variations and the barriers to oxygen delivery at the tissue level as delivered oxygen passes from the erythrocytes to the mitochondria. Tissue damage may be occurring in certain organs, despite an adequate global DO_2. Conversely, other tissues may have adequate regional DO_2 despite inadequate global DO_2 levels.

UNTIL THESE DILEMMAS ARE RESOLVED, WE PROBABLY SHOULD AIM FOR AT LEAST NORMAL OXYGEN DELIVERY, AS THIS HAS BEEN DEMONSTRATED TO REDUCE THE INCIDENCE OF ORGAN FAILURE AND TO IMPROVE OUTCOMES. Thus, a patient should have adequate fluid resuscitation, an oxygen saturation of at least 90%, and a haemoglobin level of at least 10 g/dl. Inotropes and vasopressors may also be necessary. Thus, the emphasis probably should be more on oxygen delivery, and away from consumption, which currently is beset by many problems of interpretation.

TROUBLESHOOTING

SUDDEN ONSET OF HYPOXIA

Observe for chest movement.

Hand-ventilate the patient on 100% oxygen.

Check the oxygen delivery system (ventilator/circuit/artificial airway).

Listen for air entry and pathological breath sounds (eg pneumothorax, bronchospasm, acute lung collapse, or aspiration).

Ensure that any chest drains are not blocked.

If hypoxia does not resolve quickly with 100% oxygen, then intubate the patient if that has not already been done.

Immediately obtain a chest x-ray.

> Treat according to the underlying abnormality (eg titrate PEEP for pulmonary oedema, drain pneumothorax).

TROUBLESHOOTING

HYPOXIA: WHERE TO GO WHEN THE PATIENT IS ALREADY ON 100% OXYGEN

Often there is little more that one can do for these patients, but here are some suggestions for fine tuning:

Check oxygen delivery   Check ventilator, gas delivery, lines, etc.

Review   Reassess the chest x-ray and physical examination in order to exclude the possibility of a reversible component (eg collapse, effusion, or loculated pneumothorax).

Position   Change the patient's position in order to match ventilation with perfusion more effectively. This may involve placing the more heavily affected lung uppermost, or sitting the patient up at an angle of 40° or more if the abnormality is equally distributed.

PEEP   The PEEP should be adjusted to optimize oxygen delivery (see p. 366).

Decrease oxygen consumption   One should consider decreasing the patient's oxygen consumption (eg cooling or sedation).

Use of paralysis   Coughing and 'fighting' the ventilator can exacerbate hypoxia. Muscle relaxants can help to reduce oxygen consumption in these patients.

Fluids   Fluids should be used carefully. The intravascular volume should be maintained with colloid or blood, and excessive use of crystalloid infusion avoided. Small amounts of diuretic may help to reduce lung water. Similarly, increased water removal during dialysis may improve oxygenation.

Ventilator techniques   Trial and error with different ventilatory techniques (see p. 470) may improve oxygenation. For example:
• Increased spontaneous breathing will sometimes improve oxygenation.
• Reverse the I : E ratio to 3 : 1 or 4 : 1 with PEEP at 5 cm H_2O and pressure limited to less than 40 cm H_2O.

> • Decrease inspiratory flow rates to avoid excessive peak inspiratory pressure and pulmonary barotrauma.
> • Use differential ventilation in cases of unilateral lung disease (see p. 437).
> **Extracorporeal oxygenation techniques** Extracorporeal techniques (see p. 376) may benefit some patients in this group.

FURTHER READING

Demling, R. H., & Knox, J. B. (1993). Basic concepts of lung function and dysfunction: oxygenation, ventilation and mechanics. *New Horizons* 1:362–70.

Edwards, J. D. (ed.) (1990). Practical applications of oxygen transport. *Intensive Care Medicine* 16:S133–80.

Hayes, M. A., Timmins, A. C., Yau, E. H. S., Palazzo, M., Hinds, C. J., & Watson, D. (1994). Elevation of systemic oxygen delivery in the treatment of critically ill patients. *New England Journal of Medicine* 330:1717–22.

Hickling, K. G. (1990). Ventilatory management of ARDS. Can it affect outcome? *Intensive Care Medicine* 16:219–26.

Nunn, J. F. (ed.) (1987). *Applied Respiratory Physiology*, 3rd ed. London: Butterworth.

Pontoppidan, H., Geffin, B., & Lowenstein, E. (1972). Acute respiratory failure in the adult. *New England Journal of Medicine* 287:680–98, 743–52, 799–806.

Robin, E. D., Cross, C. E., & Zelis, R. (1973). Pulmonary edema. *New England Journal of Medicine* 288:239–46, 292–304.

Shoemaker, W. C., Appel, P. L., Kram, H. B., Waxman, K., & Lee, T. (1988). Prospective trial of supranormal values of survivors as therapeutic goals in high-risk surgical patients. *Chest* 94:1176–86.

Tibballs, J. (1993). The role of nitric oxide (formerly endothelium-derived relaxing factor, EDRF) in vasodilation and vasodilator therapy. *Anaesthesia and Intensive Care* 21:759–73.

Tobin, M. J. (1992). Breathing pattern analysis. *Intensive Care Medicine* 18:193–201.

Tuman, K. J. (1990). Tissue oxygen delivery. *Anesthesiology Clinics of North America* 8:451–69.

West, J. B. (1987). Assessing pulmonary gas exchange. *New England Journal of Medicine* 316:336–8.

18

INTERPRETATION OF CHEST FILMS

- The chest x-ray is one of the most useful tools for assessing seriously ill patients, and x-rays should be taken at least once daily for all patients.
- A routine for assessing radiographs should be developed and followed in every case so that nothing will be missed.
- All plain chest radiographs should be taken with the patient sitting erect, unless there is an absolute contraindication.

An anteroposterior (AP) chest film is one of the most useful tools in critical care medicine. It is a mandatory supplement to the examination of the respiratory system. A chest x-ray should be obtained at least daily, in addition to x-rays following intubation or placement of an intrathoracic line and in response to sudden changes in the patient's clinical state, such as fever, hypoxia, or increased ventilatory pressure.

There is an art to interpreting chest x-rays in the ICU. These patients often are unconscious and difficult to position, they usually cannot co-operate in breath-holding, and they can move during the exposure, causing blurring. Also, the AP projection magnifies the heart and mediastinum, making interpretation of those regions difficult.

Although it may be tempting to take a chest x-ray with the patient supine, it is crucial that one gain the co-operation of both nursing and radiology staff so that the film can be exposed with the patient sitting erect. Air–fluid interfaces can be visualized accurately only with the patient erect. Moreover, pneumothoraces, the distribution of pulmonary vessels, and lung oedema can be interpreted more accurately when the patient is erect.

Computed tomography (CT) is sometimes useful, especially for abnormalities around the lung bases, for differentiating between effusions and intrapulmonary abnormalities, for localizing loculated pneumothoraces, and for documenting chronic changes following an acute insult case such as adult respiratory distress syndrome (ARDS).

A ROUTINE FOR INTERPRETATION

A routine should be established and followed assiduously in every case in order to avoid overlooking anything. With practice, a chest film can be rapidly interpreted. The nursing staff and others involved in the care of patients, such as physiotherapists, should also be trained in interpretation and should be made aware of the most important findings on each patient's chest x-ray. The following is a suggested routine:

1. Determine the patient's name and the date.

2. Check whether the patient was erect or supine, anteroposterior (AP) or posteroanterior (PA).

The next four steps involve assessing the quality of the film, in order to distinguish between real abnormalities and artifacts. Features that must be assessed include position, exposure, movement, and expansion:

3. Position: Check that the film is centered. The spinous processes of the thoracic vertebrae should be midway between the heads of the clavicles. If the film is not centered, the mediastinal anatomy can be distorted.

4. Exposure: The fourth thoracic vertebral body should just be visible behind the mediastinum. Over-exposure can cause under-estimation of pulmonary abnormalities, whereas under-exposure can result in over-estimation of pulmonary abnormalities. Sometimes over-exposure is necessary (eg to detect fractured ribs).

5. Movement: Check for sharpness. If respiratory motion occurs during the exposure, or if exposure times are long, blurring can occur. This can simulate early pulmonary oedema. The thicker the chest wall, the greater the chances of movement artifact, because of the longer exposure time needed to penetrate the tissue.

6. Expansion: This must be assessed in comparison with previous radiographs. If expansion is not taken into account, an abnormality can falsely appear to be improving or worsening. Expansion should be to the fifth anterior rib or the ninth rib posteriorly.

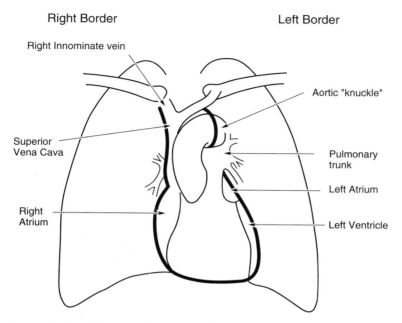

FIGURE 18.1   Diagrammatic representation of the chest, showing the left and right mediastinal borders. (From Ellis & Feldman, 1993, with permission of Blackwell Scientific Publications, Inc.)

The next four steps involve looking at the abnormality:

7. Tubes and lines (see p. 385): Check the positioning of the hardware and any complications associated with its insertion.

8. Lung fields: Check the trachea, and compare one lung to the other. Inspect around the hilum and apex, then laterally, and then over the diaphragm.

9. Heart and mediastinum: Check for features such as the size and shape of the cardiac silhouette, hilar lymphadenopathy, and signs of pulmonary hypertension (Figure 18.1).

10. Soft tissues and bones: Soft-tissue features such as subcutaneous emphysema, peripheral oedema, and obesity can be seen on chest films. Sometimes fractures outside the thoracic cage, such as the jaw and humerus, can also be detected on a chest film. Even more subtle features, such as the superimposition of the head in the mediastinum, indicating a semiconscious patient, can offer clues useful to a trained observer.

Any interpretation of a film will be limited without clinical data and previous radiographs.

TUBES AND CATHETERS

Endotracheal tube, nasotracheal tube, and tracheostomies

• Correct placement of every tracheal intubation should be checked by a chest film. The tip of the tube should be at least 2 cm above the carina, and the cuff should be at least 2 cm distal to the vocal cords to allow for the considerable movement (up to 2 cm) that can occur during flexion and extension of the head.

Nasogastric tube

• Check to see that the tube is below the diaphragm and within the stomach and is not curled in the pharynx or oesophagus.

Central venous catheters

• A chest film should be obtained immediately after placement to confirm correct positioning and to check for iatrogenic complications, such as bleeding or pneumothorax.
• The tip should be located beyond all peripheral valves, and in the superior vena cava, not within the right atrium. This corresponds to the aortic knuckle or T4 on an upright chest x-ray. Bleeding, as a result of puncturing large central veins during insertion, characteristically produces an opacity over the apex of the lung or widening of the upper mediastinum.
• The catheter tip can perforate a vessel and move extravascularly over time. Evidence for this will be seen on a chest x-ray as a pleural effusion due to misplaced intravenous fluid. If misplacement is suspected, aspirate from the distal limb for confirmation.

Pulmonary artery catheters

• These catheters are associated with the same complications described for central lines, as well as potentially more dangerous developments such as pulmonary embolism, infarction, or even haemorrhage as a result of vessel rupture.

• The position of the tip of the catheter may help in interpreting readings of wedge pressure. Ideally, it should be directed toward the base of the lung in the so-called West zones (3 or 4) and should be no more than 2–3 cm beyond the heart border. Excessive coiling of the catheter in the heart can predispose to migration and wedging of the catheter.

Transvenous pacemakers

• Depending on where the catheter is inserted, there can be complications similar to those seen with central-line placement.

• The tip of the pacemaker should be positioned at the apex of the right ventricle, wedged between the trabeculae carneae to ensure stability as well as direct contact with the endocardium.

Pleural drains (see p. 274)

• Assess the effectiveness of air and/or fluid drainage after insertion.

• A radiopaque strip demonstrating the commencement of side holes can help to guarantee that the catheter is placed within the pleural cavity, not in the soft tissues of the chest wall. Check that all the side holes are within the pleural cavity.

• The chest film should allow one to rule out the possibility of complications such as local lung damage.

DIFFERENTIATING INTRAPULMONARY ABNORMALITIES

The lung appears to react in much the same fashion to many different insults, at least from a radiological point of view. There are no absolute radiological patterns that would allow one to distinguish among pathological processes such as cardiogenic pulmonary oedema, aspiration, ARDS, pneumonia, and fat embolism. The reading of the chest film must be tempered by clinical findings, together with knowledge of the time periods for onset and disappearance of shadows resulting from the natural history of the disease process and treatment.

Moreover, accurate assessment of pulmonary abnormalities is dependent on the volume of air in the lungs. For example, a large tidal volume, or a high positive end-expiratory pressure (PEEP), may make the abnormality appear less severe.

PULMONARY OEDEMA

Chest radiography is, at present, the best technique, in terms of availability, reproducibility, non-invasiveness, practicality, and cost, for assessing the presence and extent of pulmonary oedema. The technique is as sensitive as the double-indicator dilution technique for measuring extravascular lung water (EVLW) and can detect EVLW increases as small as 10%.

CARDIOGENIC PULMONARY OEDEMA

- Classic findings (Figure 18.2) include the following:
  Spectrum of changes from pulmonary venous congestion to widespread alveolar shadowing
  Blurring of hilar vessels
  Upper-lobe blood diversion
  Diffuse micronoduli
  Central or bat-wing distribution of lung water
  Interstitial oedema (fluid in fissure, Kerley B lines, and peribronchial cuffing)
  Alveolar oedema (homogeneous opacification with air bronchograms)
  Cardiomegaly
  Pleural effusions
- The pulmonary artery wedge pressure (PAWP) correlates well with changes:
  PAWP < 12 mm Hg: normal appearance
  PAWP = 12–22 mm Hg: dilatation of peripheral vessels, and interstitial oedema
  PAWP > 22 mm Hg: alveolar oedema
- Movement by the patient can cause blurring on the film, which can simulate early pulmonary oedema.

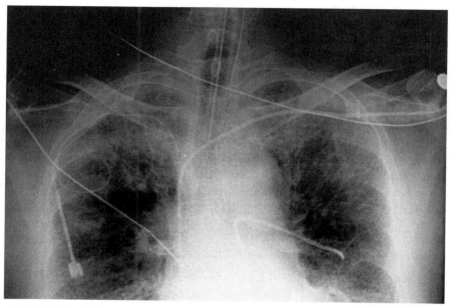

FIGURE 18.2   Patient with cardiogenic pulmonary oedema and bilateral basal collapse, with right-side subclavian central venous catheter, left-side subclavian pulmonary artery catheter, and endotracheal tube. Note that the intrapulmonary opacity is difficult to distinguish from other pulmonary abnormalities, such as ARDS (Figure 18.3).

• A patient with normal lungs may have radiographic signs that mimic pulmonary oedema if a supine AP film is taken (eg upper-lobe blood diversion and peribronchial cuffing). Chest films should be taken upright if at all possible.

• Abnormalities of lung parenchyma and the integrity of the vascular bed will affect the distribution of pulmonary oedema. It is very common, for example, to see atypical patterns of pulmonary oedema in the presence of chronic lung disease.

ADULT RESPIRATORY DISTRESS SYNDROME (ARDS)

• ARDS is a form of pulmonary oedema. It may be difficult to distinguish radiologically from other intrapulmonary abnormalities, such

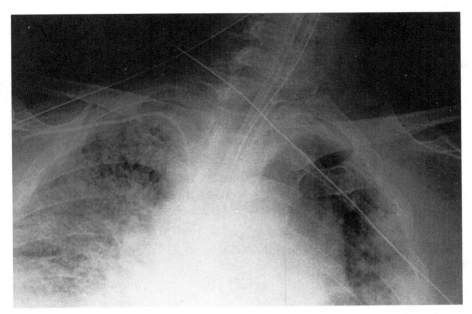

FIGURE 18.3 Patient with severe ARDS, with right-side central venous subclavian catheter, endotracheal tube, nasogastric tube, and ECG leads. Note that the intrapulmonary opacities are difficult to distinguish from those in Figure 18.2.

as aspiration, cardiogenic pulmonary oedema, and pneumonia (Figure 18.3). It must therefore be differentiated on clinical grounds (see Chapter 19).

• The radiographic findings can vary from mild changes to a 'white-out' of both lung fields.

• Radiological signs usually can be detected within 24–36 hours of the precipitating insult and include a perihilar haze, interstitial oedema, and alveolar filling.

• Classic findings include

Air bronchograms.

Increased lung opacification distributed relatively equally over central and peripheral regions.

Enlargement of right ventricle and main pulmonary arteries is sometimes seen.

• Changes that occur later, and possibly as a result of ventilatory pressures, rather than the disease process (see p. 406), include cavitation and fibrosis. These changes can take many months to resolve.

PNEUMONIA

• Pneumonia is a clinical pathological condition with no definite radiological appearance to distinguish it from other intrapulmonary abnormalities. The radiograph is a helpful adjunct to the diagnosis.

• Lung opacification may be lobar or widespread. The so-called atypical pneumonias are usually associated with widespread and discrete opacifications that can become confluent as the disease progresses.

• Often air bronchograms will be associated with the opacification.

• Although the opacification associated with cardiogenic and non-cardiogenic pulmonary oedema can be difficult to distinguish from that seen with pneumonia, bronchial breathing is more commonly associated with pneumonia, presumably because consolidation leads to a more dense area around the airways than does oedema.

• Radiological changes classically do not become detectable until after the first clinical signs and symptoms, and there is a similar delay before radiological signs of improvement can be seen in the recovery stage.

• Apart from showing lobar consolidation, a chest film is more a tool to follow the course of treatment, rather than a specific diagnostic indicator.

ASPIRATION

The sequelae of aspiration will depend on the type of material aspirated, its volume and distribution, and the host's reactions to the aspirated material. The radiological features can vary from localized shadowing to a bilateral whiteout.

FOREIGN BODY, PARTICULATE MATTER

• The distribution will depend on the position of the patient at the time of aspiration. It is common to aspirate into the right main bronchus.

- Radiopaque material can be directly visualized.
- Atelectasis, air trapping, or mediastinal shift may be seen.

INFECTED MATERIAL
- Consolidation occurs slowly over 5–7 days, often accompanied by pleural exudate, and it may take weeks to clear.
- Cavitation may occur at a later stage.

LIQUID ASPIRATION
- A wide spectrum of radiological changes can be seen, depending on the nature and volume of the aspirated liquid.
- The distribution is usually bilateral.
- Severe damage can occur; for example, aspiration of gastric acid can result in ARDS.

SMOKE INHALATION AND TOXIC GASES
- A wide range of damages is possible.
- Focal or patchy alveolar filling can occur within a few hours.

ATELECTASIS AND COLLAPSE

- 'Collapse' usually refers to a lobe or lung, whereas atelectasis affects a smaller subunit (Figure 18.4).
- Radiological signs include the shadow of the collapsed portion of lung and displacement of other structures to take up the space normally occupied by that collapsed lung, including crowding of lung markings in the collapsed area, separation of lung markings in the non-involved area, elevation of a hemidiaphragm, and mediastinal shift.

PULMONARY EMBOLISM

- Radiography is not an accurate method for diagnosing pulmonary emboli.
- Non-specific signs include focal redistribution of blood flow, pulmonary infarction, atelectasis, pleural effusion, and an elevated hemidiaphragm.

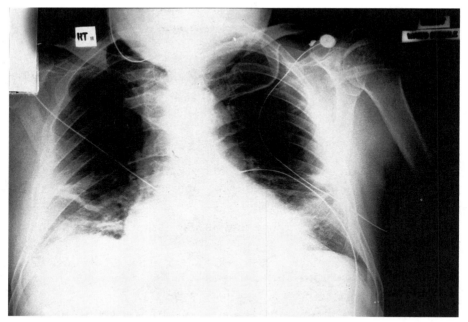

FIGURE 18.4 Patient with severe pancreatitis, with bilateral basal collapse and reduced lung volumes. Note that the head is dipping onto the mediastinum. This is usually an indication of exhaustion or a decreased level of consciousness and is a strong predictor of imminent intubation.

PLEURAL EFFUSION

• Blunting of the costophrenic angle is commonly seen when the effusion is small.

• On an upright film, the effusion classically forms a homogeneous density at the base of the lung, with a meniscus extending laterally through which lung markings can sometimes be seen.

• On a supine film, the fluid usually is seen to be distributed evenly over the whole pleural space, causing a 'veiling' effect through which lung markings can be seen.

• Effusions can also become loculated anywhere in the pleural space.

• More accurate definition of the effusion can be obtained by the use of ultrasound or CT scanning.

ABDOMINAL ABNORMALITIES AFFECTING CHEST X-RAY

• A chest x-ray can be an excellent reflection of intra-abdominal abnormalities in intensive care (eg intra-abdominal sepsis causing ARDS).

• An intra-abdominal mass effect can cause elevation of the diaphragms and atelectasis. Abdominal pain can also cause atelectasis. Basal effusions can occur post-operatively or as a result of sub-diaphragmatic infection.

• Gastric dilatation commonly accompanies resuscitation efforts involving the use of a mask.

• Pneumoperitoneum can result from recent laparotomy, from a ruptured intra-abdominal viscus, or from pulmonary barotrauma (see p. 466).

EXTRA-ALVEOLAR AIR (see p. 466)

• Excessive alveolar pressure can cause distension and rupture: The air will travel from the ruptured alveoli along the vascular sheaths toward the mediastinum as pulmonary interstitial emphysema (PIE). This is difficult to detect radiologically, but it can be seen as a generalized, irregular, radiolucent mottling, especially in the perihilar region, and sometimes as cysts.

• Under continuing pressure, the extra-alveolar air (EAA) can then produce mediastinal emphysema. The gas can then move into the tissue planes of the neck, and possibly elsewhere over the chest, as subcutaneous emphysema.

• Under further pressure, the EAA can burst through the thin mediastinal pleura, causing pneumothorax, and even into the abdomen, causing pneumoretroperitoneum and pneumoperitoneum.

CHEST TRAUMA

For both blunt trauma and penetrating trauma, an upright chest x-ray should be among the first investigations ordered. The features to be looked for include the following:

PNEUMOTHORAX EAA   These often are due to penetration of lung tissue by fractured ribs, but they can also occur as a result of blunt injury (see p. 266).

HAEMOTHORAX   Haemothorax often accompanies other abnormalities, such as pneumothoraces, lung contusion, and rib fractures. If it can be seen on the chest radiograph, then there will be at least 500 ml in the pleural cavity, and it should be actively drained.

CONTUSION   Contusion represents oedema or haemorrhage into alveoli, as a result of blunt trauma. It is usually obvious within the first 24 hours and begins clearing after 2–3 days, with total resolution by 1–2 weeks. However, with severe contusion, it may be several weeks before resolution begins.

FRACTURED RIBS   Rib fractures often are seen together with lung contusion and should be documented, especially for purposes of pain relief. Remember that it is difficult to image all rib fractures, and often there are more than can be seen on the chest x-ray: As a general rule, there are approximately twice as many fractured ribs as can be seen on the chest film.

OTHER POSSIBLE FEATURES   Diaphragmatic rupture, signs of oesophageal trauma, pericardial tamponade, a widened mediastinum suggesting large-vessel injury, and tracheobronchial tears are all rarer, but serious, complications. Further investigations, such as angiography, CT scan, bronchoscopy, or oesophagoscopy, may also be necessary.

TROUBLESHOOTING

HYPOXIA WITHOUT SIGNIFICANT CHEST X-RAY SHADOWING

Non-respiratory problems
- Compromised airway (consider the possibility of a blocked airway)
- Problems with the oxygen delivery system or ventilatory malfunction

- High oxygen consumption (eg hyperthermia)
- Intracardiac shunt

Respiratory problems
- Pulmonary emboli
- Asthma
- Chronic lung disease
- Early stage of abnormality, such that radiological changes are not yet obvious (eg pneumonia)

TROUBLESHOOTING

INTERPRETING NON-SPECIFIC OPACITIES ON THE CHEST X-RAY

Determine that the opacity is genuine (ie not a result of movement, under-exposure, or rotation).

Rule out the possibility of other opacities, such as pleural abnormalities and soft-tissue abnormalities (usually extend outside the chest wall).

Parenchymal or intrapulmonary opacities in ICU patients usually are due to **BLOOD**, **OEDEMA**, or **INFECTION**. Other causes, such as carcinoma, are rare.

Oedema   There can be cardiogenic and non-cardiogenic (ARDS) pulmonary oedema, as well as fluid overload.

Features of Oedema on Chest X-Ray

- Interstitial oedema
  Fluid in fissures
  Pleural effusions
  Kerley B lines
  Peribronchial cuffing
- Alveolar oedema
  Confluent homogeneous opacities that are usually bilateral
  Air bronchograms
- Cardiogenic pulmonary oedema
  Large heart, and increases in size and density of hilar vessels
  PAWP > 20 mm Hg
  Perihilar distribution and upper-lobe diversion

- Non-cardiogenic pulmonary oedema
  Small heart (normal)
  Peripheral and generalized distribution
  PAWP < 20 mm Hg

The patient's history and clinical signs are essential for distinguishing between cardiogenic and non-cardiogenic pulmonary oedema, and the chest x-ray is a helpful adjunct to the diagnosis.

Blood Pulmonary haemorrhage can, for example, occur as a result of
- Trauma (contusion)
- Ruptured pulmonary vessel, as a complication of using a pulmonary artery catheter

Features

- Sudden onset
- No air bronchograms
- Confluent and discrete opacity

Infection Pneumonia

Features

- Air bronchograms, with bronchial breathing
- Slowed radiological indications of onset and resolution
- Spectrum from lobar pneumonia to bronchopneumonia (see p. 406)
- Usually accompanied by clinical signs of infection

FURTHER READING

Ellis, H., & Feldman, S. (1993). *Anatomy for Anaesthetists*, 6th ed. London: Blackwell.

Goodman, L. P., Putman, C. E. (eds.) (1983). Imaging of the critically ill. Philadelphia: Saunders.

Kox, W., Boultbee, J., & Hillman, K. (1988). The interpretation of the portable chest film and the role of complementary imaging techniques. In *Imaging and Labelling Techniques in the Critically Ill. Current Concepts in Critical Care,* ed. W. Kox, J. Boultbee, & J. Donaldson. Berlin: Springer-Verlag.

Winer-Muram, H. T., Rubin, S. A., Miniati, M., & Ellis, J. V. (1992). Guidelines for reading and interpreting chest radiographs in patients receiving mechanical ventilation. *Chest* 102:565S–70S.

19

SPECIFIC RESPIRATORY PROBLEMS

CARDIOGENIC PULMONARY OEDEMA

Cardiogenic pulmonary oedema is usually seen in the setting of acute left ventricular failure (LVF) in association with ischaemic heart disease (IHD).

Cardiogenic pulmonary oedema as an accompaniment to LVF can result from conditions such as acute myocardial infarction (AMI), arrhythmias, cardiac tamponade, and valvular abnormalities. However, no specific cause is obvious in the majority of cases. This is especially true with paroxysmal nocturnal dyspnoea or 'flash' pulmonary oedema. The oedema presents acutely, often at night, with the patient suddenly waking up breathless. These patients typically are old, with histories of IHD and hypertension. Many of these patients have normal systolic function, and it is thought that the cause of the pulmonary oedema is left ventricular diastolic dysfunction. The precipitating event may be silent myocardial ischaemia. Patients with acute cardiogenic pulmonary oedema often have accompanying tachycardia, hypertension, and hypoxia, which in turn will increase left ventricular dysfunction and exacerbate the pulmonary oedema. Moreover, the increased work of breathing and the increased inspiratory effort can, in themselves, further exacerbate the oedema (Figure 19.1).

INVESTIGATIONS, DIAGNOSIS, AND MONITORING

• The history and examination should strongly suggest the diagnosis.
• Chest x-ray will demonstrate Kerley B lines, thickened fissures, peribronchial cuffing, increased vessel diameter and upper-lobe diversion, a perihilar bat-wing appearance, and intrapulmonary shadowing, often with cardiomegaly.
• Examine 12-lead ECG to exclude the possibility of ischaemia, AMI, etc.

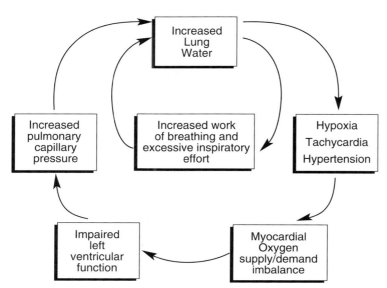

FIGURE 19.1   Factors exacerbating cardiogenic pulmonary oedema.

• Measure arterial blood gases to determine the extent of the gas-exchange abnormality and the acidosis.

• Monitor vital signs (eg arterial blood pressure, pulse rate, respiratory rate, urine output).

• Continue ECG monitoring.

• Monitor with pulse oximetry.

FEATURES

• a history of dyspnoea and orthopnoea, usually when sitting upright, and tachypnoea, with an obvious increase in the work of breathing

• often sweaty, with increased pulse rate and blood pressure

• crepitations, wheeze, and, in severe cases, pink frothy sputum

• signs of cardiac failure, such as cardiomegaly, third heart sound, and elevated jugular venous pressure

MANAGEMENT

RESUSCITATION   Control the airway, maintain a high F_{IO_2}, and support the breathing and circulation where necessary.

REVERSIBLE CAUSES Reverse any contributing cause (eg arrhythmia, hypertension, cardiac tamponade).

POSITION Sit the patient up, if possible.

CONTINUOUS POSITIVE AIRWAY PRESSURE (CPAP) CPAP has revolutionized the management of cardiogenic pulmonary oedema. It can be delivered by a face mask or a cuffed endotracheal tube (ETT) and is a very effective and easily applied measure for controlling pulmonary oedema. **FOR SUCCESS, HOWEVER, ONE MUST ENSURE ABSOLUTE INTEGRITY OF ALL PARTS OF THE CPAP CIRCUIT** (see p. 472). CPAP improves oxygenation, decreases hypercarbia, and increases lung compliance, thus making it easier for the patient to breathe. The increased intrathoracic pressure as a result of CPAP also decreases the preload and afterload, improving left ventricular function, increasing cardiac output, and relieving the pulmonary oedema. By improving the efficiency of the work of breathing and decreasing inspiratory effort, CPAP can limit the formation of further oedema. CPAP has been shown to correct hypoxia rapidly and to reduce tachypnoea and hypertension, all of which can adversely affect left ventricular diastolic dysfunction.

DIURETIC A diuretic (eg frusemide, 20 mg IV, if not already on a diuretic, or 40 mg IV otherwise) will cause immediate venodilation and eventually will reduce lung water. More diuretic may be necessary, but use it judiciously, as excessive diuresis can cause hypovolaemia and cardiovascular impairment.

VASODILATION Use vasodilating drugs **SLOWLY** and **CAREFULLY** and only if the arterial blood pressure is normal or high for that patient. Use a drug such as nitroglycerin, with mainly venodilating effects, in order to decrease preload (see p. 526). Where hypertension is of prime concern, a drug with both venous and arterial effects, such as sodium nitroprusside, can be used (see p. 525).

NARCOTIC Give morphine, in increments of 2 mg IV, titrated slowly over 2 minutes, to reduce dyspnoea, to decrease anxiety, and to contribute to vasodilation.

INOTROPIC AGENTS An intravenous inotropic agent such as dobutamine may also be beneficial in cases of severe pulmonary oedema (see p. 522). However, beware of increases in pulse rate and arterial blood pressure, both of which will increase myocardial oxygen demand and adversely affect left ventricular function.

INTUBATION AND VENTILATION Intubation and ventilation with positive end-expiratory pressure (PEEP) can be a last resort, but usually that can be avoided by the use of CPAP.

INTRAVASCULAR VOLUME Hypovolaemia, paradoxically, can be a problem in the management of pulmonary oedema. It is related to fluid losses from the lung capillaries and aggressive use of diuretics, and it can be exacerbated by inappropriate use of vasodilators. Because these patients often need higher preload than usual for optimum ventricular function, they can become hypotensive and oliguric, requiring fluid resuscitation in order to correct the hypovolaemia. Because of the delicate balance between pulmonary oedema and hypovolaemia in these patients, more invasive monitoring, with a pulmonary artery catheter, may sometimes be necessary in order to measure pulmonary artery wedge pressure (PAWP), as a guide to volume replacement (see p. 55).

ADULT RESPIRATORY DISTRESS SYNDROME (ARDS)

Since its initial description in 1967, there probably has been more written about this particular syndrome than about any other in intensive care medicine. Precise definitions are difficult because of the huge spectrum of the syndrome. It is loosely defined as hypoxia in the right clinical circumstances, with a normal or low left atrial pressure – or so-called non-cardiogenic pulmonary oedema. It is characterized by diffuse alveolar infiltrates seen on chest x-ray, dyspnoea, tachypnoea, decreased compliance, increased shunting, severe hypoxia, and an increase in lung water. ARDS is not so much a specific disease, but rather the sum of the lung's general responses to critical illness.

AETIOLOGY

There probably are several distinct ARDS states, each with its own initiating cause, but all ending in a common pulmonary response.

The term 'ARDS' is often used synonymously with 'acute respiratory failure' (see Chapter 17) and is usually a complication of another disease process, such as sepsis or multiorgan failure (MOF). In fact, ARDS probably represents one manifestation of a generalized inflammatory process leading to endothelial-cell injury and eventually MOF, rather than being a disease in its own right. It has many causes, which are usually divided according to the origin of the insult (Figure 19.2). These insults are believed to lead to a final common pathway by damaging the alveolus–capillary interface, which damage, in turn, causes fluid to leak into the interstitial space and/or causes flooding of alveoli with protein-rich fluid:

Insults via the airway (eg aspiration of acidic gastric contents, smoke inhalation, near-drowning incidents)

Insults via the circulation (eg septicaemia, shock, MOF, fat embolism, amniotic fluid embolism and pancreatitis)

Direct insults (eg pulmonary contusion)

Combination insults (eg pneumonitis, such as bacterial or viral pneumonia)

Despite extensive research, the exact cause of the alveolus–capillary membrane damage is uncertain. Leucocytes, platelets, microemboli, neurogenic influences and mediators such as prostaglandins, oxygen radicals, complement, leukotrienes, activated neutrophils, and alveolar macrophages have all been implicated (Table 19.1). The process usually is widespread and often affects capillary beds other than the lungs. Whether the lungs initiate this process or are simply among the organs involved as part of MOF is unknown. Conclusions in this area are difficult, because animal models do not necessarily reflect what happens clinically.

MEASUREMENT OF PULMONARY OEDEMA

CHEST X-RAY The chest x-ray remains the reference point for estimating lung water, and its indications usually correlate very well with

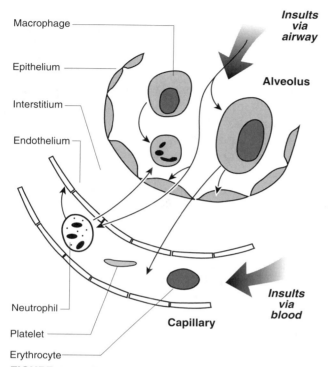

FIGURE 19.2 Factors that influence the progression to ARDS. (From Repine, 1992, with permission.)

TABLE 19.1 POSSIBLE CONTRIBUTORY FACTORS IN ARDS

Complement
Oxygen radicals
Proteases (elastase)
Endotoxin
Eicosanoids (eg thromboxanes, prostaglandins, leukotrienes)
Platelet-activating factor
Cytokines (eg tumour necrosis factor, endothelin)
Growth factors
Kallikreins (kinins)
Fragment D

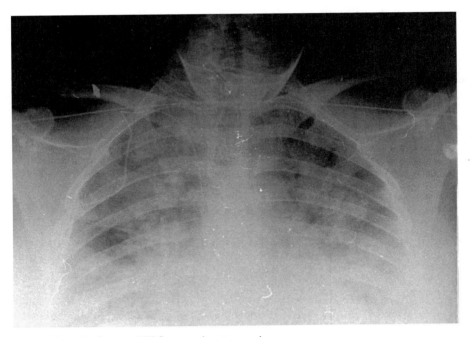

FIGURE 19.3 Severe ARDS secondary to sepsis.

those from more sophisticated and expensive techniques, such as double-indicator dilution.

There are characteristic chest x-ray findings in patients with ARDS (Figure 19.3).

- normal pulmonary vascular pattern
- absence of septal (Kerley's) lines
- air bronchograms
- infrequent perivascular cuffing
- normal heart size

COMPUTED TOMOGRAPHY (CT) A CT scan offers a more accurate way of quantifying lung water than does a chest x-ray. However, it is limited by its expense and the difficulties of transporting critically ill patients.

MAGNETIC-RESONANCE IMAGING Nuclear magnetic-resonance imaging of protons in water permits quantification of lung water. The problem of motion during breathing can be overcome by 'gating'. However, the technique is still expensive and cumbersome in its application.

DOUBLE-INDICATOR DILUTION   The correlation between lung-water measurement with the indicator technique and autopsy-measured lung water is good. The double-indicator dilution technique relies on heat as the diffusible indicator and uses a pulmonary artery catheter. It is more expensive and more complex than the method of chest x-ray, and thus far it has not been demonstrated to be more accurate.

FEATURES AND MANAGEMENT

Only the main features of ARDS will be discussed here. The principles of management for this syndrome are summarized in tables (see p. 363) and are discussed in detail in Chapter 17.

1. Gas-exchange abnormalities   Hypoxia is due to a mismatch between perfusion and ventilation, mainly because of perfusion of non-ventilated or under-ventilated alveoli, which is in turn is caused by atelectasis or alveolar flooding.

Failure of carbon dioxide exchange is also due to a mismatch between perfusion and ventilation, mainly as a result of ventilation of unperfused alveoli, which in turn is a consequence of vascular obstruction. Hypercarbia occurs only during end-stage ARDS. Initially a patient will compensate by hyperventilation.

2. Pulmonary hypertension   Pulmonary hypertension develops early in ARDS and is a result of vasoconstriction and vascular occlusion. Nitric oxide, a selective pulmonary vasodilator, may be useful (see p. 375).

3. Decreased pulmonary compliance   An increase in lung water results in increased lung stiffness, tachypnoea, diffuse intrapulmonary shadowing seen on chest x-ray, decreased airway calibre, and a marked increase in the work of breathing.

ARDS often accompanies MOF of various causes (see p. 137). Often it is impossible to distinguish between pneumonia (see p. 390) and ARDS on clinical grounds and chest x-ray. The features of the two entities overlap.

Although cardiac function is usually normal in patients with ARDS, the amount of fluid that collects in the lungs in ARDS patients is a function of the pulmonary hydrostatic pressure, which is related to left atrial filling pressure and the degree of capillary leak. Thus, intravascular volume replacement should not be excessive. Crystalloids will be distributed mainly to the interstitial space (ISS), independent of the left atrial filling pressure, and so the use of large amounts of crystalloids should be avoided in ARDS patients (see Chapter 4).

The rate of accumulation of extravascular fluid in ARDS patients is related to gravity, structural compression from within the lung, and the underlying alveolus–capillary membrane leak. The improvement in gas exchange with the use of artificial ventilatory techniques probably is related to the number of recruitable alveoli that initially were not involved in gas exchange because of oedema or atelectasis. Alveoli that are involved in a consolidation process, such as pneumonia, are less amenable to recruitment. Thus, intermittent positive-pressure ventilation (IPPV), PEEP, and CPAP are less effective in patients with pneumonia than in those with ARDS and cardiogenic pulmonary oedema.

There is usually a peripheral defect in oxygen utilization associated with ARDS. This may be due to the widespread nature of microvascular permeability, as a result of the primary disease process or as a result of inappropriate fluid replacement causing interstitial oedema (see p. 62).

The pathophysiological changes seen with ARDS can vary over time. Initially there will be hypoxia, dyspnoea, and tachypnoea, with little in the way of changes visible on chest x-ray. That will be followed by the classic changes seen on chest x-ray, with worsening hypoxia. That state can worsen, with more dense and more extensive changes appearing on the chest x-ray, accompanied by clinical deterioration. After approximately 10 days, long-term changes, such as fibrosis, can supervene and cause long-term respiratory disability.

There is active research in a number of areas having to do with modifying the mediators of lung damage. Possible mediators include neutrophil proteases, oxygen radicals, lipid peroxides, plasma proteolytic enzymes, lipoxygenase products, platelet-activating factor, free fatty acids, and cytokines. Although that research is to be encouraged, the final common pathway (if there is one in ARDS) has not been found. The use of a single drug that acts via one mediator may be of little benefit. If there is to be a pharmacological cure for ARDS, the answer may be in finding a 'cocktail' of modulators, rather than a single one. The principles of management for ARDS are the same no matter what the cause, and they are discussed in detail elsewhere (see Chapter 17). The principal challenge is to address the underlying problem.

OUTCOME

The outcome for a patient with ARDS will depend on its cause (eg when ARDS is associated with prolonged MOF, the mortality is high). Abnormal pulmonary function is found in approximately 40% of survivors 6 months after recovery from ARDS, but by 1 year, lung function usually will return to normal. Thoracic CT scans will reveal extensive fibrosis in many of these patients. Those changes will slowly resolve with time.

PNEUMONIA

Pneumonia can be defined as an inflammatory process in which the host reacts to uncontrolled multiplication of pathogenic organisms in the distal airways and alveoli of the lung.

Pneumonia does not encompass inflammation of the large airways – a condition that results in production of sputum and bronchitis. Most intubated and many non-intubated patients in an ICU will have bronchitis or colonization of the airways. This is important when interpreting sputum cultures, because detection of organisms in sputum is very common in an ICU. However, that does not signify pneumonia, and even if pneumonia coincidentally exists, the organisms grown in the sputum usually bear no relationship to the organisms causing the pneumonia, especially in the case of nosocomial pneumonia.

FEATURES

Lung consolidation: Air in the alveoli is replaced by exudate and cellular material, leading to the following manifestations:

• radiological opacities – presenting either a picture typical of consolidation or an interstitial pattern, or a combination of the two (Figure 19.4)

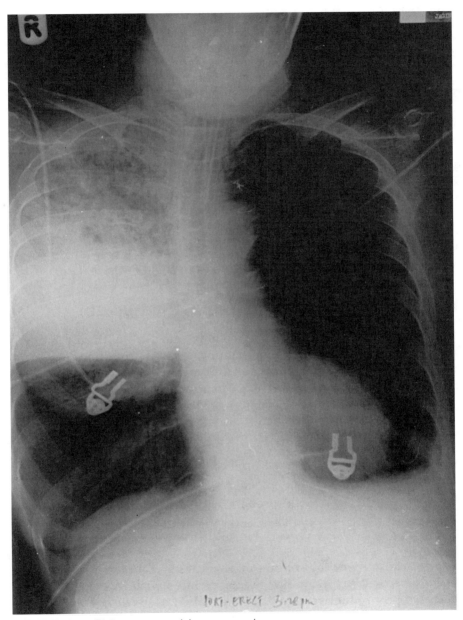

FIGURE 19.4 Right-upper-zone lobar pneumonia.

- bronchial breath sounds on auscultation
- non-compliant lungs
- impaired gas exchange – hypoxia, hyperventilation, and hypocarbia, until exhaustion supervenes, at which time hypercarbia will occur.

Classically, primary pneumonia is associated with one or more of these features:

- fever
- cough
- sputum production (increases in colour and viscosity)
- dyspnoea
- pleuritic pain
- tachypnoea
- malaise

PRIMARY PNEUMONIA (COMMUNITY-ACQUIRED)

Pneumonia remains a leading infectious cause of death in the developed world. Patients with pneumonia who require admission to intensive care have a very high mortality rate.

Infection of lung tissue results in intrapulmonary shunting, impaired distribution of ventilation, and decreased lung compliance, in addition to the systemic effects that result from the infection. The features include

- fever
- leucocytosis
- cough
- dyspnoea
- tachycardia

- sputum production
- tachypnoea
- widespread rales and bronchial breath sounds
- cyanosis and other features of hypoxia

The typical history for community-acquired pneumonia is acute onset of fever, with chills and rigors, associated with dyspnoea, tachypnoea, and a productive cough. The so-called atypical pneumonias include those caused by *Mycoplasma pneumoniae, Legionella* spp., *Chlamydia* spp., *Coxiella burnetii, Pneumocystis carinii*, and viruses.

The pneumonias in this group are typified by extrapulmonary features, diagnoses made primarily by serologic methods, and failure to respond to conventional antibiotics. For that reason, in patients with severe pneumonias of unknown origin, erythromycin is usually included in the first-line treatment.

INVESTIGATIONS AND DIAGNOSIS

The history and examination should strongly suggest a diagnosis of pneumonia:

Chest x-ray: demonstrates the distribution, extent, and complications (eg abscess, effusion) associated with the pneumonia
Blood count: leucocytosis
Arterial blood gases: demonstrate extent of impaired gas exchange

Isolation of the organism

This can be difficult, and often no organism can be isolated, especially if antibiotics have been commenced. Common organisms that cause primary pneumonia include

Streptococcus pneumoniae
Mycoplasma pneumoniae
Legionella spp.
Staphylococcus aureus
Haemophilus influenzae
viruses (particularly influenza A)

Less common organisms include

Chlamydia psittaci
Streptococcus (other species)
Coxiella burnetii
coliforms
Pneumocystis carinii
Chlamydia pneumoniae

Despite thorough screening, in almost one-third of cases no organism can be found.

SPUTUM

• Obtain a good sputum specimen. Salivary specimens are useless and will be discarded by the microbiology laboratory.

• Gram stain: Look for polymorphonucleocytes (PMN) and a heavy and pure population of bacteria as evidence of microbiological pathogenicity.

• Culture for bacteria (eg pneumococcus and *Haemophilus*).

• Special tests are required only in certain situations, such as special stains and cultures for fungi and acid-fast bacilli (AFB), and cultures to exclude tuberculosis (TB) or direct-fluorescence antibodies (DFA) for *Pneumocystis* and *Legionella*.

Bacteria in the sputum do not necessarily equate with infection of the lower respiratory tract, even in patients with pneumonias such as the more typical pneumococcal pneumonia. If the sputum has an abundance of PMN and a pure growth of bacteria, it is more likely to be pathogenic.

BLOOD CULTURES   Blood cultures are mandatory, because pneumonia is an infection of the lung parenchyma, and organisms are isolated from blood in about 30% of cases of pneumococcal pneumonia and at much lower rates for other types of pneumonia. Positive findings from blood cultures are strongly predictive of infection with the isolated bacteria.

SEROLOGY   Paired sera must be tested for antibodies to

Mycoplasma pneumoniae
Legionella spp. (Legionnaires' disease) – may take up to 6 weeks to seroconvert
Coxiella burnetii
viruses
Chlamydia psittaci (psittacosis)

Legionella: The laboratory diagnosis of legionnellosis is based on isolation of the organisms, seroconversion, and direct detection by fluorescent-antibody techniques or DNA probes. Direct immunofluorescence of the sputum, bronchial washings, or pleural fluid has a sensitivity of less than 80%. Although serum or indirect fluorescent antibody is commonly employed, some patients never seroconvert.

Mycoplasma: The laboratory diagnosis of *Mycoplasma* pneumonia is generally retrospective, based on serologic evidence of infection. It is a slowly growing and fastidious organism that is difficult to culture. A DNA-probe test for *M. pneumoniae* is now available. Cold agglutinins can be demonstrated in over 50% of cases, but that is not a specific test. Positive tests for IgM are reported in up to 90% of patients at presentation.

Chlamydia pneumoniae: Although the diagnosis can be made serologically and by isolation from respiratory samples in cell culture, specific confirmation reagents are not yet commercially available.

More invasive techniques for isolation and culture of micro-organisms are discussed in the section on nosocomial pneumonia (see p. 414).

TREATMENT

TREATMENT IS USUALLY COMMENCED ON CLINICAL GROUNDS BEFORE AN ORGANISM IS ISOLATED. Even after extensive investigation, up to 60% of micro-organisms remain undetected. These cases are often called 'viral pneumonia', without any evidence to support the diagnosis. The term 'viral pneumonia' should be reserved for cases where a viral cause is actually demonstrated.

OXYGEN The F_{IO_2} should be adjusted according to frequent assessments of oxygenation via arterial blood gases or pulse oximetry.

FLUIDS The intravascular volume must be aggressively resuscitated (see p. 61), while not overloading the ISS with excessive crystalloids (see p. 62).

VENTILATORY SUPPORT Ventilatory support (see p. 470) may be necessary, but it is not as effective in patients with pneumonia as in those with pulmonary oedema, probably because there are fewer recruitable alveoli (see p. 366). Because of the dangers of positive-pressure ventilation (see p. 466), spontaneous respiration with CPAP should be encouraged before mandatory ventilation is utilized. The most appropriate ventilatory techniques are discussed in detail elsewhere (see p. 470).

PHYSIOTHERAPY   Physiotherapy is of little value in the acute stage of pneumonia.

Features and specific antimicrobials

Streptococcus pneumoniae: This is the most common causative organism, accounting for more than 70% of all community-acquired pneumonias. These patients usually are systemically ill and present early. Approximately half of them will have positive sputum cultures.

Treatment
- benzylpenicillin, $2–3 \times 10^6$ units, 6-hourly
  OR
- for those with true penicillin allergy, ceftriaxone, 1–2 g IV, once daily

Haemophilus influenzae: This is relatively uncommon and often is associated with bronchitis in patients with chronic airflow limitation (CAL).

Treatment
- ampicillin, 1–2 g IV, 6-hourly
  +
  ceftriaxone, 1–2 g IV, daily

Legionella species: Legionnaires' disease often presents as severe progressive pneumonia, and it can be associated with a wide variety of other manifestations that often precede pulmonary involvement. The presence of several of the following features should suggest the diagnosis:

- prodromal flu-like illness, with dry cough, myalgia, rigors, watery diarrhoea, dyspnoea, malaise, or headache
- renal failure, myoglobinuria, and a high level of creatinine phosphokinase (CPK)
- hyponatraemia and hypophosphataemia
- central nervous system involvement (headache, confusion, disorientation, stupor, seizures, coma)

- myocarditis (tachycardia and bradycardia)
- very high fever (>39°C)

Isolation of this organism is very difficult. The diagnosis can be confirmed by detection of an antibody rise in paired sera or by a rapid DFA test on sputum or bronchial washings. Some patients never seroconvert. If in doubt, commence treatment on clinical grounds. There are more than 30 species of *Legionella*, and therefore it may not be detected even with the use of paired sera, which can test only the more common varieties. *Legionella* is discussed in more detail elsewhere (see p. 225).

Treatment
- erythromycin, 4 g IV, daily, in divided doses, for 3 weeks (because of the danger of thrombophlebitis, use a central line)

±

rifampicin, up to 600 mg IV, daily, in divided doses, for severe cases

Mycoplasma pneumoniae: General symptoms such as fever, malaise, and headache precede the chest symptoms by 1–5 days. A chest x-ray will show patchy opacities, often in only one lobe. Cough and radiographic changes can persist for weeks if there is no treatment. Death is rare.

Extrapulmonary manifestations include erythema multiforme, Stevens-Johnson syndrome, myocarditis, anorexia, nausea, vomiting, hepatitis, thrombocytopenia, coagulopathy, and meningoencephalitis.

Treatment
- erythromycin, 1 g IV, 6-hourly (a 2-week course may be needed for eradication and should be recommenced in cases of relapse)

OTHER ORGANISMS THAT SHOULD BE CONSIDERED IN CASES OF PRIMARY PNEUMONIA:

Viruses
Klebsiella pneumoniae (in older or alcoholic patients)
miliary tuberculosis (in debilitated or alcoholic patients)
Coxiella burnetii (Q fever, in abattoir workers or people working on farms)
Pneumocystis carinii (in patients suspected of having AIDS, or in other immunocompromised patients) (see p. 421)

Chlamydia psittaci (associated with exposure to pet birds, especially if the pets are ill or have died)

No definite organism

USUALLY, NO DEFINITE CAUSE IS DETERMINED. A regimen that will cover most cases of primary pneumonia is as follows:

- penicillin, $2–3 \times 10^6$ units IV, 6-hourly
  OR
- ampicillin, 1 g IV, 6-hourly
  +
  erythromycin, 1 g IV, 6-hourly
  ±
  third-generation cephalosporin: ceftriaxone, 1–2 g IV, once daily

If psittacosis is suspected, add

- rolitetracycline, 275 mg, daily

NOSOCOMIAL PNEUMONIA

Dealing with nosocomial or hospital-acquired pneumonia is not as straightforward as treating primary pneumonia:

- The diagnosis is very difficult to make.
- There are many possible causative organisms.
- The causative organisms are difficult to isolate.

While there is a lack of general agreement on such fundamental issues as how to define nosocomial pneumonia, it is even more difficult, perhaps even impossible, to reach consensus on basic information such as incidence, treatment, and outcome.

DIAGNOSIS

The diagnosis of pneumonia is usually made on the basis of a combination of some of the following criteria. However, in the setting of the seriously ill, each of these criteria has inadequacies.

• Fever or hypothermia: Fever is common in patients in an ICU, for a great variety of reasons.

• Leucocytosis or leucopenia: These are both very common features in seriously ill patients and may not even indicate infection.

• Purulent secretions: These are almost universal findings in seriously ill patients, especially intubated patients, and often they indicate bronchitis or colonization, rather than pneumonia.

• New or progressive infiltrations seen on chest x-ray: Progressive infiltrates seen on chest x-ray are common in the seriously ill and often are related to other lung abnormalities, such as ARDS or aspiration. The onset and persistence (for at least 24 hours) of a new infiltrate seen on a good-quality chest x-ray are suggestive of nosocomial infection. A CT scan of the thorax often can help to define intrapulmonary abnormalities.

The diagnosis is likely if all four of these criteria are met, and probable if three are met. Nosocomial pneumonia by itself often is not accompanied by the systemic features of sepsis (eg hypotension, decreased level of consciousness, jaundice, renal failure) (see p. 183).

Pathogenic organism

Because of the difficulty in making a clinical diagnosis of nosocomial pneumonia, the key to making the diagnosis is to find a definite pathogenic organism.

COLONIZATION OF THE AIRWAYS, ESPECIALLY WITH GRAM-NEGATIVE ORGANISMS, IS A FEATURE OF MANY PATIENTS IN AN ICU. THIS USUALLY DOES NOT INDICATE PNEUMONIA. IN FACT, IN THE SETTING OF THE SERIOUSLY ILL, THERE IS LITTLE CORRELATION BETWEEN THE ORGANISMS ISOLATED FROM SPUTUM AND THE PRESENCE OR ABSENCE OF PNEUMONIA. Organisms such as pseudomonads, *Acinetobacter*, fungi, and methicillin-resistant staphylococci are common colonizers in intubated patients. Their continuing presence is facilitated by indiscriminate use of antimicrobials.

The source of such an organism may be related to aspiration of oropharyngeal secretions. Gastric contents made alkaline in order to prevent stress ulceration will encourage bacterial overgrowth and may be a source of oropharyngeal organisms, which are then aspirated.

Isolation of organisms

TRACHEOBRONCHIAL SECRETIONS There are great discrepancies between the organisms in the sputum and the pathogens in the lower respiratory tract. Concurrent antibiotic treatment further complicates this picture. Conventional sputum cultures are very unreliable for intubated patients. To be of any use, the sputum must be induced and must not be contaminated with saliva. If there is a pure growth accompanied by polymorphonucleocytes, the significance of the pathogenicity is increased.

BLOOD CULTURES Positive findings from blood cultures offer the only real proof of pneumonia, but the findings are positive in fewer than 20% of patients with nosocomial pneumonia.

IMMUNOLOGICAL METHODS The delay inherent in obtaining positive results from paired sera makes that method unsuitable for assisting in rapid therapeutic decisions. Immediate antigen or antibody tests seem to offer a lot of promise for the future, but thus far they are of limited use for nosocomial pneumonia.

BRONCHOSCOPY Samples obtained by suction through a fibre-optic bronchoscope (FOB) are usually contaminated by upper-airway organisms. Techniques that use protected specimen brushes (PSB) are expensive and complicated, but provide more accurate results (Table 19.2). In order to get the ideal specimen that will allow one to distinguish between colonization and infection, the bronchoscope must be guided to the appropriate area, and the specimen must be protected from contamination if it is to yield quantitative cultures that can meet validated diagnostic thresholds. Both the sensitivity and specificity of PSB techniques have ranged between 60% and 100%. Some of the limitations of PSB techniques are unreliability when a patient is already being treated with antibiotics, the limited area of the lung that can be sampled, and the delay in processing the microbial cultures. The use of bronchoalveolar lavage combined with PSB techniques may add diagnostic accuracy.

BRONCHOALVEOLAR LAVAGE Bronchoalveolar lavage (BAL) is lavage of a lung subsegment using 100–200 ml of physiological solution

TABLE 19.2 PSB TECHNIQUE

1. High-dosage nebulized lignocaine, 10–15 ml of 4% solution, until gag reflex is abolished in non-intubated patients.
2. In intubated patients, sedation and a short-acting paralytic agent are recommended.
3. Do not inject lignocaine through the suction channel of the FOB or the ETT.
4. Position the FOB close to the orifice of the study area with new or increased infiltrate seen on chest x-ray.
5. Advance the PSB catheter 3 cm out of the FOB to avoid collection of pooled secretions on the catheter's tip.
6. Advance the inner cannula to eject the distal carbon-wax plug into a large airway.
7. Advance the catheter into the desired subsegment.
8. Advance the brush, and wedge it into a peripheral position; gently rotate it several times. If purulent secretions are visualized, rotate the brush into them.
9. Retract the brush into the inner cannula, and the inner cannula into the outer cannula, and remove them from the bronchoscope.
10. The distal portions of the outer and inner cannulae must be separately and sequentially wiped clean with 70% alcohol, cut with sterile scissors, and discarded.
11. Advance the brush out, and sever it with a sterile wire clipper into a container with 1 ml of saline solution or Ringer's lactate solution to avoid drying and rapid loss of bacteria.
12. Submit for quantitative culture within 15 minutes.

Source: From Meduri (1990), with permission.

through an FOB wedged in an airway. BAL provides sampling of a larger amount of lung tissue than does the PSB technique, but it is subject to the same risk of contamination. BAL is an accurate technique for diagnosing pneumonia caused by organisms that do not colonize the upper airway, and it has largely replaced open lung biopsy for diagnosis of opportunistic infections in immunocompromised patients. The main complication of BAL is hypoxia during the procedure, and also there is the possibility of translocating toxins or organisms during the procedure. The best results are obtained when patients are not already receiving antimicrobials.

PROTECTED BAL   Protected BAL involves selection of a sampling area using an FOB, based on the chest x-ray appearance: A transbroncho-scopic balloon-tipped catheter is advanced into the segment, the balloon is inflated with 1.5 ml of air to occlude the bronchial lumen, and aspiration is performed with 30-ml aliquots of sterile saline solution. The specimen obtained is then centrifuged, cultured, and examined with Gram and Giemsa stains. Protected BAL has higher specificity and sensitivity than other current techniques.

TRANSBRONCHIAL BIOPSY   Biopsy not only is helpful for isolating bacteria but also is useful for viruses and fungi and for differentiating between non-infective lesions (eg carcinoma, Wegener's granulomatosis) and infective lung lesions. The complications of biopsy can include pneumothorax.

TRANSTHORACIC NEEDLE ASPIRATION   Aspiration offers the advantage of allowing one to identify parenchymal infections that are solid, but it is associated with high incidences of pulmonary bleeding and pneumothorax, especially in artificially ventilated patients.

OPEN LUNG BIOPSY   Open lung biopsy is the most accurate method for achieving a definite histological or microbiological diagnosis. It is crucial that any obviously affected lung be biopsied for isolation of microbes. This technique is very invasive and entails a far higher risk of complications than do the other procedures.

The false-negative rates and the overall success for any of these diagnostic techniques cannot be assessed yet, as there is no gold-standard technique for diagnosing nosocomial pneumonia, and even post-mortem examination involves potential sources of error.

The simple techniques are unreliable, and the more reliable techniques are complicated.

Organisms

The most common isolates are Gram-negative organisms such as

Pseudomonas aeruginosa
Enterobacter spp.
Klebsiella spp.

Escherichia coli
Serratia spp.
Proteus spp.
Acinetobacter spp.
Haemophilus influenzae

Less common organisms include

Staphylococcus aureus
Streptococcus pneumoniae
anaerobic bacteria
fungi

IMMUNOSUPPRESSED HOSTS   In patients with cellular and humoral immunosuppression, one also must consider

Pneumocystis carinii (especially in association with AIDS and after organ transplantation)
cytomegalovirus (CMV) (especially after organ transplantation)
Aspergillus spp. (especially in patients with leukaemia)
Cryptococcus neoformans (especially in patients with lymphomas)

ARDS and pneumonia

Pneumonia and ARDS overlap considerably in the seriously ill. They are impossible to distinguish without isolation of a specific organism. Patients with ARDS can develop a superimposed pneumonia, and patients with pneumonia can develop features of ARDS. The diagnostic criteria for ARDS (see p. 400) and nosocomial pneumonia (see p. 414) are so non-specific that they are often considered together. This causes confusion, especially when considering antimicrobial treatment.

TREATMENT

Preventive treatment

• Prevent airway colonization by judicious use of parenteral antibiotics (for sound indications and for limited periods).
• Use of local antibiotics in the oropharynx and stomach may decrease the incidence of nosocomial pneumonia (see p. 182).

• The use of sucralfate, rather than H_2-receptor antagonists or antacids, to prevent stress ulceration may decrease the incidence of colonization and nosocomial pneumonia (see p. 32).

• Minimize instrumentation and intubation of the upper airways.

• Attempt to preserve the cough reflex, where possible, and limit the time a patient is intubated and ventilated.

• Prevent aspiration past ETT cuffs by clearing pharyngeal secretions and maintaining cuff pressure.

• Use meticulously sterile technique for endotracheal suction.

• Strictly enforce hand-washing between any two procedures.

• Maintain the integrity of the gastro-intestinal-tract (GIT) mucosa (see p. 31).

Definitive treatment

TREATMENT IS LARGELY BASED ON EMPIRICAL USE OF ANTIBIOTICS – A BEST-GUESS APPROACH. The choice of the appropriate antibiotic combination must be based on the bacteria isolated. However, it is uncommon to isolate a definite microbe. One of the most difficult decisions in intensive care is to choose the initial antibiotic treatment for suspected cases of nosocomial pneumonia – not only which antibiotics, but whether or not any antibiotic at all should be commenced. The diagnosis is almost impossible to make with certainty, and the organism, if any, is rarely found. It is further complicated by the fact that Gram-negative pneumonia does not respond rapidly to antibiotic treatment, and therefore it is difficult to judge the success of the selected antibiotic on clinical grounds. On the other hand, the mortality remains high, and it is a bold intensivist who can resist the temptation to use antibiotics. The incidence of nosocomial pneumonia and survival patterns have not been in any way affected by the influx of the latest and most expensive broad-spectrum antibiotics. The following combinations of antibiotics are given as guidelines. Close microbiological surveillance and liaison with the microbiology department are essential in order to define the particular spectrum of organisms in an individual ICU.

Initial treatment

- aminoglycoside
  +
  a penicillin (eg benzylpenicillin or a penicillinase-resistant synthetic penicillin)
  OR
- aminoglycoside
  +
  a third-generation cephalosporin
  OR
- a cephalosporin (eg cefotaxime, cefuroxime, or cefamandole) for suspected coliform infections

When *Pseudomonas aeruginosa* is suspected, a combination of an aminoglycoside and piperacillin or ciprofloxacin is usually selected. Imipenem is also used as a broad-spectrum alternative when an organism has not been isolated. If aspiration is suspected, clindamycin plus an aminoglycoside can be used. If *Staphylococcus aureus* is suspected, vancomycin should be used. *Legionella* spp. can also cause nosocomial pneumonia.

Further antibiotic strategy will depend on clinical response and isolation of organisms. If there is no improvement within 3 days, consideration should be given to reinvestigation and either ceasing the antibiotics or changing them.

OUTCOME

The outcome figures for nosocomial pneumonia depend on the difficult issue of the accuracy of the initial diagnosis, and as there currently is no gold standard for diagnosis, outcome figures must be viewed with caution. Various studies have cited mortality figures ranging from 40% to 90%.

STRATEGY IN IMMUNOCOMPROMISED PATIENTS WITH PULMONARY INFILTRATES (Table 19.3)

ROUTINE TESTS Conduct a full examination and routine investigations, including extensive sputum and blood cultures.

TABLE 19.3 SOME CAUSES OF PULMONARY INFILTRATES IN IMMUNOSUPPRESSED PATIENTS

Infection
Bacteria
Staphylococcus aureus
coliforms
Legionella spp.
Nocardia
Protozoans
Pneumocystis carinii
Fungi
Aspergillus
Cryptococcus
Candida
Viruses
CMV
Herpes simplex
Herpes zoster
Non-infectious causes
Pulmonary oedema
ARDS
Cytotoxic drug injury
Radiation infiltration
Pulmonary haemorrhage

DRUGS   Exclude the possibility of drug-related causes (eg bleomycin).

TRANSTRACHEAL ASPIRATION   This procedure may be useful for bacterial isolation.

BRONCHOALVEOLAR LAVAGE   Use 150–200 ml of normal saline in 30-ml aliquots, with the FOB wedged in an appropriate subsegmental bronchus. Conduct a microscopic examination of the centrifuged sample for bacteria, fungi, mycobacteria, and *Pneumocystis carinii*. Use direct immunofluorescent-antibody staining for *Legionella* and CMV. As BAL can cause hypoxia, close monitoring during the procedure is necessary.

ENDOBRONCHIAL BRUSHING

- The incidence of barotrauma is significant.
- Sensitivity is approximately 75% for fungi and *P. carinii*.
- The use of a PSB culture will facilitate the diagnosis in cases of bacterial pneumonia.

TRANSBRONCHIAL BIOPSY

- With fluoroscopic guidance, taking three specimens will yield tissue in up to 95% of cases.
- There are risks for pneumothorax (about 10%) and haemorrhage (about 20%).
- Examine the tissue as in open lung biopsy.

OPEN LUNG BIOPSY

- The diagnostic yield is at least 90%.
- Yields will largely depend on the quality of the laboratory technique, not the size of the specimen.
- Pleural leak for more than 3 days occurs in 10–25% of cases.
- Use direct examination for bacteria, mycobacteria, fungi, *P. carinii*, and CMV. Use direct immunofluorescent-antibody staining for *Legionella* and CMV. Examine cultures for bacteria, mycobacteria, fungi, and viruses.

EMPIRICAL APPROACH   A broad-spectrum, best-guess antibiotic regimen is usually undertaken where adequate examination facilities are not available or when treatment cannot be delayed.

ASPIRATION

Aspiration occurs most often in patients with decreased levels of consciousness (eg head injury, epilepsy, recent operation) who have impaired cough and gag reflexes. The sequelae of aspiration into the lungs will depend on the type of material aspirated, its volume, its distribution within the lungs, and the patient's reactions to the aspirated material.

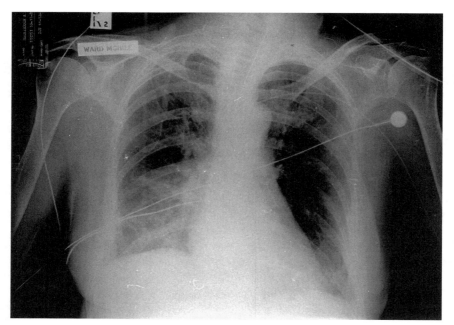

FIGURE 19.5   Right-side aspiration.

Foreign body or particulate matter

A foreign body often will lodge in the right main bronchus. Such material often can be visualized radiologically if it is radiopaque (eg a tooth). Otherwise, the sequelae from the aspirated material can be visualized (eg atelectasis, air trapping, mediastinal shift, local hyperinflation) (Figure 19.5).

TREATMENT   In order to prevent long-term complications, such as chronic infection, the obstructing material should be removed under direct vision or by lavage.

Infected material

Apical segments of the right upper and lower lobes often are involved if the patient was recumbent at the time of aspiration. Otherwise, the right lower zone of the lung is most commonly involved. Consolidation occurs slowly over at least 5 days and may take weeks to clear. It should be noted that infection after aspiration is rare, and antibiotics should not be commenced as a routine.

TREATMENT If infection is suspected, antibiotic treatment should include cover for anaerobes (eg clindamycin, cefoxitin, or benzylpenicillin). Abscess formation and cavitation, with or without fluid levels and empyema, may occur as late complications.

Non-toxic material (eg blood)

Depending on the volume and distribution, there can be a wide spectrum of radiological changes, sometimes with atelectasis and pleural effusion, as well as parenchymal involvement. Radiographic evidence of clearing usually can be seen rapidly if the case is uncomplicated by infection.

TREATMENT The treatment for this type of aspiration is non-specific and is the same as for other forms of acute respiratory failure, as outlined in Chapter 17. Usually there will be complete and uncomplicated resolution.

Toxic-liquid aspiration (eg acid aspiration from stomach)

Toxic liquid from acidic stomach contents can cause severe and extensive parenchymal damage, with alveolus–capillary membrane leak and pulmonary oedema. This pathologic condition is often classified as ARDS. Radiographic changes will develop within 24–36 hours.

TREATMENT The treatment is non-specific and is outlined in Chapter 17. There is a relatively high indicence of infection if the stomach contents have been aspirated, and antibiotics should be considered (eg benzylpenicillin, 1 g IV, 4-hourly). Because of the increasing resistance of oral anaerobes to penicillin, metronidazole (500 mg IV, 8-hourly) is often added to penicillin or used instead of it. Clindamycin (600 mg IV, 6-hourly) can be used alone. There is no indication for the use of steroids.

Mixed forms

Many cases of aspiration can include most or all of the previously mentioned manifestations in seemingly infinite combinations. Each case must be individually evaluated.

PRINCIPLES OF TREATMENT

• Prevention: ensure adequate airway protection, and encourage the patient to cough.
• Use bronchoscopy if particulate matter or a foreign body is suspected.
• Use antibiotics if infected material is suspected.
• Treat as for acute respiratory failure (see p. 360).
• Beware of late abscess formation (usually anaerobic).

HYPOVENTILATION

The causes of hypoventilation are shown in Figure 19.6, and the specific disorders of neuromuscular function that can affect the respiratory system are listed in Table 19.4.

The most common cause of hypoventilation and hypercarbia is their deliberate induction, related to the current approach to artificial ventilation: In order to avoid over-inflation of alveoli and pulmonary barotrauma (see p. 466), tidal volumes are reduced, and the peak inspiratory pressures are limited to less than 30–40 cm H_2O. This strategy is called elective hypoventilation or permissive hypercarbia (see p. 471). Hypoventilation in these circumstances is an acceptable trade-off in order to limit lung damage.

MANAGEMENT

Treatment and diagnosis go hand in hand. The specific treatment for hypoventilation will depend on the cause, as discussed in Chapter 17.

The AIRWAY must be secured, and ventilation commenced (if necessary), while the cause of the ventilatory failure is being determined. VENTILATION should be commenced with a tidal volume of no more than 10 ml/kg, at a respiratory rate designed to reduce CO_2 levels slowly, especially if there is evidence of subacute or chronic hyper-

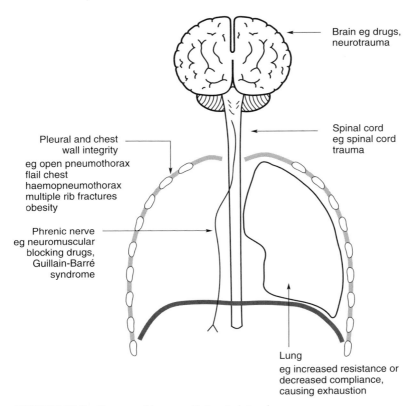

Brain eg drugs, neurotrauma

Spinal cord eg spinal cord trauma

Pleural and chest wall integrity
eg open pneumothorax
flail chest
haemopneumothorax
multiple rib fractures
obesity

Phrenic nerve
eg neuromuscular
blocking drugs,
Guillain-Barré
syndrome

Lung
eg increased resistance or
decreased compliance,
causing exhaustion

FIGURE 19.6 Causes of hypoventilation in intensive care.

carbia. The aim of ventilation is to maintain oxygenation at the lowest level of positive intrathoracic pressure, keeping the Pa_{CO_2} and arterial pH within reasonable limits – it is not necessary to achieve a so-called normal Pa_{CO_2} (see p. 471).

UPPER-AIRWAY OBSTRUCTION IN ADULTS

Acute upper-airway obstruction is a medical emergency. The common causes are outlined in Table 19.5.

MANAGEMENT

The specific management will depend on the cause, but in general terms, the principles are as follows:

TABLE 19.4 DISORDERS OF RESPIRATORY NEUROMUSCULAR FUNCTION

Level	Examples	Clinical characteristics
Upper motor neuron	Hemiplegia	Weakness
	Quadriplegia	Hyperreflexia
	Extrapyramidal disorders	Increased muscle tone
		Perhaps sensory and autonomic changes
Lower motor neuron	Poliomyelitis	Weakness
		Atrophy
		Flaccidity
		Hyper-reflexia
		Fasciculations
		Bulbar involvement
		No sensory changes
Peripheral neuron	Guillain-Barré syndrome	Weakness
	Acute intermittent porphyria	Flaccidity
		Hyporeflexia
	Diphtheria	Bulbar involvement
	Lyme disease	Sensory and autonomic changes
	Toxins (eg lead)	
	Critical illness polyneuropathy	
Myoneural junction	Myasthenia gravis	Fluctuating weakness
	Botulism	Fatigability
	Organophosphate poisoning	Ocular and bulbar involvements
		Normal reflexes
		No sensory changes
Muscle	Muscular dystrophies	Weakness
	Polymyositis	Normal reflexes
		No sensory or autonomic changes

Source: From Kelly and Luce (1991), with permission.

TABLE 19.5 COMMON CAUSES OF UPPER-AIRWAY OBSTRUCTION IN ADULTS

Compromised airway secondary to decreased level of consciousness

Obstructed ETT or tracheostomy tube

Post-operative obstruction secondary to neck surgery or haematoma (eg carotid artery surgery, thyroidectomy)

Trauma

Foreign body

Inhalation injury and oedema

Complications of artificial airways (eg post-extubation oedema)

Adult epiglottitis

Severe tonsillitis or pharyngitis

Acute on chronic obstruction (eg laryngeal tumour)

Anaphylaxis and laryngeal oedema

BASIC AIRWAY MANOEUVRES For non-intubated patients, the following should be employed:

- head tilt
- chin lift
- jaw thrust
- suction
- oxygen

OBSTRUCTED ARTIFICIAL AIRWAY Ensure that the artificial airway is not obstructed: Pass a suction catheter, or, if there is any doubt, **IMMEDIATELY REMOVE THE TUBE AND REPLACE IT WITH ANOTHER.** With very viscous secretions, the suction catheter may pass through with relative ease and totally occlude on withdrawal.

UNDERLYING ABNORMALITY Where possible, correct the underlying abnormality (eg remove foreign body, drain haematoma, treat infection).

ENDOTRACHEAL INTUBATION If necessary, endotracheal intubation should be performed. This can be achieved by a variety of techniques, according to the clinical circumstances and the skills of the operator: direct laryngoscopy with intravenous or gaseous anaesthetic induction, fibre-optic laryngoscopy, rigid bronchoscopy, or blind nasal intubation. If those measures fail, emergency cricothyroidotomy, tracheostomy, or insertion of a minitracheostomy tube may have to be performed.

POST-OPERATIVE CHEST COMPLICATIONS

Many patients are admitted to the ICU for post-operative management, including ventilation. These patients often have chest complications:

- microatelectasis and infection
- collapse secondary to hypoventilation, sputum retention, and intra-abdominal abnormalities
- interstitial oedema because of excessive peri-operative fluid
- hypoventilation
- aspiration
- pleural effusion
- pulmonary emboli
- acute or chronic lung problems

Pre-existing lung disease, age, body status, and the site of operation will all affect the incidence and severity of complications.

SOME ASPECTS OF MANAGEMENT

It is assumed that appropriate oxygen treatment (see p. 365) and monitoring (see p. 21) will be undertaken.

Pre-operative assessment and preparation

Careful assessment of cardiorespiratory function is essential. Physiotherapy, especially for patients with pre-existing chronic lung disease, may be required as part of the preparation for surgery.

Patient position and mobilization

Where possible, the patient should be sat up, in order to improve oxygenation and minimize basal collapse. As soon as possible, the patient should be sat up, out of bed, and mobilized at the earliest stage.

Physiotherapy

Incentive spirometry, encouragement of coughing, and aggressive physiotherapy are useful for clearing secretions and preventing atelectasis. These manoeuvres, combined with adequate pain relief to facilitate breathing, are particularly valuable in patients with chronic airflow limitation (CAL).

Continuous positive airway pressure

CPAP, via a mask or nasal prongs, is excellent treatment for post-operative hypoxia and may prevent atelectasis. It can be used either continuously or intermittently (eg 10 minutes every hour). It may be necessary to deliver continuous CPAP through an ETT or tracheostomy tube when a prolonged post-operative course is anticipated (eg obese patients with CAL and upper-abdominal wounds).

Fluid replacement

Rational fluid treatment is necessary – excessive amounts of crystalloid fluid should be avoided (see Chapter 17).

Pain relief

Pain relief is of paramount importance, particularly after abdominal and thoracic procedures. This is most efficiently achieved with regional or local analgesia. Otherwise, liberal and efficient use of narcotics should be employed. Paradoxically, adequate pain relief with an appropriate dosage of narcotic may enhance ventilation, rather than depress it. The right dosage of narcotic must be achieved – a fine line balancing the advantages of achieving pain relief and facilitating coughing and breathing against the disadvantages of respiratory depression. Use of horizontal, rather than vertical, abdominal surgical incisions and injection of the wound with local anaesthetics at the end of the operation can reduce pain and improve respiratory function.

For the analgesic regimen, see Chapter 7.

Minitracheostomy

Temporary use of a 'minitracheostomy' tube inserted through the cricothyroid membrane, with frequent tracheal suction, may be helpful in patients with sputum retention, lung collapse, and failure to cough adequately. It can be particularly useful in patients with CAL.

Artificial ventilation

The indications for post-operative ventilation have not been precisely defined. However, it is common practice to ventilate patients overnight or for several hours after major or prolonged surgery (eg cardiothoracic surgery, major vascular surgery, emergency abdominal surgery). It has the advantages of providing adequate ventilation in the face of post-anaesthetic drug effects, ensuring adequate pain relief without compromising ventilation, and facilitating tracheal toilet. However, positive-pressure ventilation also has disadvantages (see p. 466), and spontaneous ventilation, with adequate pain relief and oxygenation, should be established as soon as possible.

ATELECTASIS AND COLLAPSE

Atelectasis can vary from microatelectasis of a small part of the lung to collapse of a lobe or even a whole lung. It is a common occurrence in intensive care. Atelectasis should be looked for each day on routine chest radiography in all seriously ill patients, whether ventilated or spontaneously breathing (Figure 19.7).

RADIOLOGICAL FEATURES

These features include opacification of lung parenchyma distal to the occluded airway, as well as displacement of structures such as the diaphragm, trachea, and mediastinum and other structures within the affected lung.

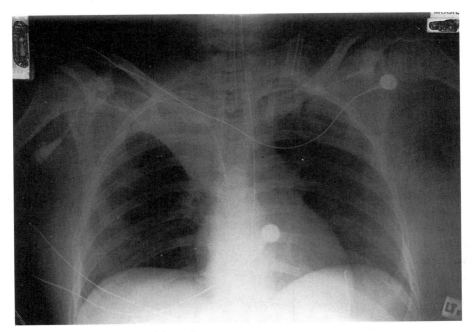

FIGURE 19.7 Right-upper-lobe collapse.

AETIOLOGY

The cause of atelectasis in intensive care is related to regional hypoventilation and retention of viscous sputum as a result of poor diaphragmatic movement. It is often secondary hypoventilation resulting from a decreased level of consciousness or pain. Despite reflex hypoxic vasoconstriction within the collapsed area of lung, some hypoxia will result, and secondary infection can occur within the atelectatic area.

MANAGEMENT

Preventive management

Aggressive physiotherapy is necessary for all at-risk patients. Meticulous regular care for the airway, with regular tracheal suction, is required, especially in intubated patients. Early mobilization and total pain relief are also useful in preventing lung collapse.

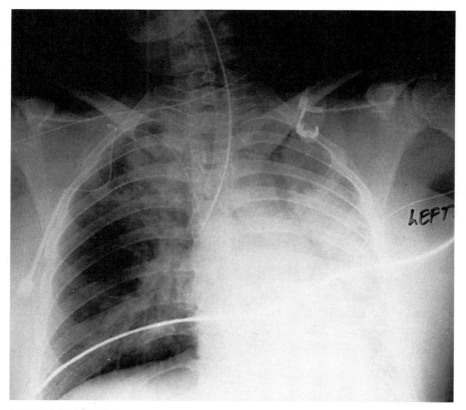

FIGURE 19.8   Left-lung collapse following intubation of the right main bronchus.

Definitive management

MICROATELECTASIS   Physiotherapy, adequate pain relief and deep breathing, incentive spirometry, and minitracheostomy are useful.

COLLAPSED LUNG LOBE   Collapse of a lung lobe or a major lung unit usually is the result of sputum retention. This should respond either to appropriate physiotherapy manoeuvres or to bronchoscopic intervention. Occasionally, selective reinflation with a bronchoscope fitted with an inflatable balloon is useful (Figures 19.8 and 19.9).

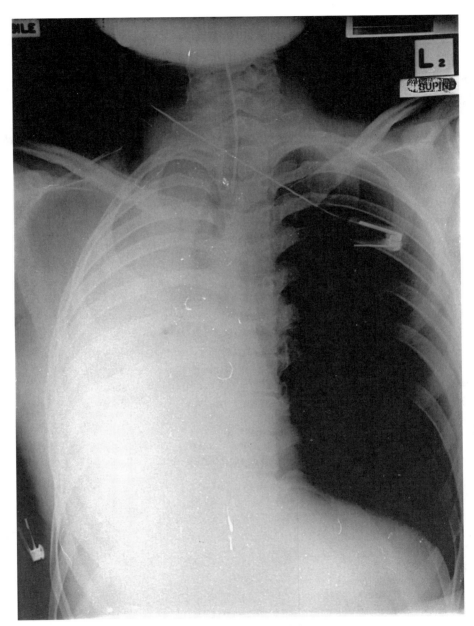

FIGURE 19.9   Right-lung collapse. Note mediastinal shift.

FIBRE-OPTIC BRONCHOSCOPY IN INTENSIVE CARE

In addition to being used for diagnostic purposes, such as tumour biopsy and sputum collection, the FOB is useful for visualizing and removing airway obstructions, such as sputum plugs.

A special membrane in the ETT connector, through which the FOB is inserted, is available for use with intubated patients.

PRECAUTIONS

• It is advisable to have an additional clinician solely to monitor the patient during bronchoscopy, especially if the patient is intubated and ventilated.

• Pre-oxygenate with 100% oxygen for 5 minutes, and use 100% oxygen during the procedure, as patients often are hypoxic to begin with.

• Use 4% lignocaine solution to anaesthetize the airway, in order to avoid paralysing the patient.

• Cease the use of positive end-expiratory pressure (PEEP), as the FOB creates a PEEP effect within the lumen of the artificial airway.

• Monitor the inspiratory ventilator pressures closely.

• Aspirate for short periods, monitor the patient's oxygenation and vital signs (eg pulse rate, blood pressure, pulse oximetry), and observe for signs of pulmonary barotrauma. A post-bronchoscopy chest x-ray is necessary, both to look for complications and to observe the benefits of the procedure.

UNILATERAL LUNG ABNORMALITIES

Severe, predominantly unilateral lung abnormalities are rare, but they can cause hypoxia resistant to conventional respiratory support (Figure 19.10). If positive pressure is applied to these patients, it will cause over-inflation of the unaffected lung and diversion of pulmonary blood flow to the affected lung. Increasing the PEEP in these circumstances can paradoxically worsen the hypoxia.

MANAGEMENT

Correct any reversible abnormalities in the affected lung by means of physiotherapy or bronchoscopy if collapse is suspected.

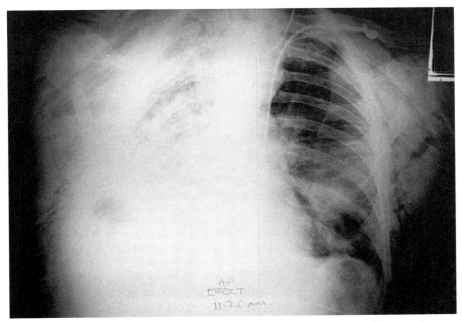

FIGURE 19.10 Predominantly unilateral lung abnormalities with right-side consolidation. Note the evidence of pulmonary barotrauma, probably as a result of excessive total volume into the remaining normal lung tissue.

These patients can be nursed laterally, with the affected lung uppermost to maximize pulmonary blood flow to the unaffected lung. This can, of course, be done only for limited periods of time and may cause infected contents from the uppermost lung to drain into the lower (normal) lung.

If these measures fail and the hypoxia is severe, independent lung ventilation may be indicated.

TECHNIQUE OF INDEPENDENT LUNG VENTILATION

Intubate using a plastic endobronchial tube (EBT) with suitable cuffs for long-term use. These patients can be very hypoxic, and a meticulous intubation technique is necessary. These patients must be heavily sedated to allow adequate controlled ventilation in cases of selective lung ventilation.

The unaffected lung should be ventilated with a normal tidal volume for one lung (250–350 ml), minimal PEEP, and appropriate F_{IO_2}.

The affected lung can be connected either to CPAP or a separate source of ventilation. It is not necessary to synchronize the two ventilators. Higher levels of PEEP should be applied to the affected lung, and a tidal volume and rate should be used to minimize the peak inspiratory pressure and maintain oxygenation. Alternatively, a constant pressure (CPAP) can be applied to the affected lung in order to improve oxygenation without the danger of high peak pressures. High-frequency ventilation (see p. 475) has also been applied to the affected lung using an EBT.

INDICATIONS FOR SELECTIVE LUNG VENTILATION

This technique should be restricted to patients with severe intrapulmonary abnormalities such as aspiration, pulmonary oedema, ARDS, or pneumonia that is predominantly unilateral and unresponsive to conventional treatment. It can also be used for unilateral air leaks and bronchopulmonary fistulae, as well as for cases of unilateral collapse resistant to normal manoeuvres.

ACUTE SEVERE ASTHMA

'Acute severe asthma' is now preferred to the term 'status asthmaticus', and it describes asthma that over a short period of time becomes increasingly severe and does not respond to the usual treatments. The pathogenesis is uncertain.

CLINICAL FEATURES AND ASSESSMENT

- History of asthma.
- Altered level of consciousness.
- Silent chest on auscultation.
- Difficulty in completing sentences without a pause for breath.
- Tachypnoea.
- Serial measurements demonstrating a decrease in peak expiratory flow rate (PEFR) or forced expiratory volume in 1 second (FEV_1).

- Pulse rate > 110 beats per minute, and bradycardia as hypoxia supervenes.
- Arterial blood pressure is usually raised.
- Pulsus paradoxus > 10 mm Hg.
- Use a chest x-ray to determine the degree of hyperinflation and to rule out infection and pneumothoraces.
- Cyanosis or severe hypoxia. Hypoxaemia is invariable and may paradoxically worsen with the use of bronchodilators.
- Pa_{CO_2}: Hypocarbia occurs initially, and as the patient's condition worsens, the Pa_{CO_2} rises.
- Low arterial pH.
- Subjective impressions: increased work of breathing, sweating, and distress, with exhaustion eventually supervening.
- No single index has yet been developed that could accurately predict the severity of asthma.

MANAGEMENT (Table 19.6)

It is not surprising, given that the pathophysiology of acute asthma is poorly understood, that there are many controversies about its management.

Preventive management

Certain asthmatic patients are particularly at risk for sudden deterioration and death:

- those with childhood-onset asthma that has continued for over 20 years
- women over 45 years of age
- those with chronic persistent asthma with remission periods of less than 3 months.
- those with a history of previous life-threatening asthmatic episodes
- those with night attacks and early morning deterioration in lung function
- those recently discharged from hospital after an episode of acute asthma

TABLE 19.6 MANAGEMENT OF ACUTE SEVERE ASTHMA

Reassurance

Oxygen

Initially give 100% oxygen, and then as according to oximetry.

Bronchodilators

- Nebulized β_2-agonist: Give continuous nebulized drug if necessary.
- Intravenous β_2-agonist: Give if nebulized drug is unsuccessful

  $\pm$

  adrenaline

  $\pm$

  aminophylline

Corticosteroids

Fluids

CPAP

Artificial ventilation

Preload with intravascular fluid.

100% oxygen initially.

Monitor cardiorespiratory system closely.

Avoid cardiovascular depression with drug.

Elective hypoventilation.

Keep PIP < 50 cm H_2O.

Other measures

Chest compression

Extracorporeal oxygenation

Other drugs, such as

    ketamine

    halothane

    ether

    magnesium

The ICU staff must carefully instruct these patients (as well as their relatives and attending physicians) regarding the particular regimen suitable for the individual patient. These patients need to understand how to monitor the disease, preferably each with an individual peak-flow metre, and how to avert attacks. In severe cases, and after lack of success with conventional nebulized bronchodilators, the relatives can be instructed in how to deliver 0.5 mg of adrenaline subcutaneously (SC). There must be a sound plan, already in place, for rapid referral to a specialist centre with advanced facilities for intensive care.

Definitive management

OXYGEN All patients should receive the maximum F_{IO_2} that can be delivered by face mask if there is no element of chronic obstructive lung disease. Oxygen does not depress ventilation in patients with acute severe asthma.

FLUIDS If a patient is unable to tolerate oral fluids, give 2–3 litres of intravenous fluids over 24 hours for adults. There is no firm evidence that excess intravenous fluid will decrease the incidence of viscous sputum.

STEROIDS Hydrocortisone (100 mg IV, 6-hourly) or methylprednisolone (40–125 mg IV, 6-hourly) is recommended. Because the effectiveness of steroids becomes maximum after 6–8 hours, their role in immediate resuscitation is limited. Nevertheless, asthma is primarily an inflammatory disease of the airways, rather than a bronchoconstrictive disease, and therefore anti-inflammatory drugs such as steroids are essential to reverse the underlying problem.

β_2-AGONISTS Controversy surrounds the use of bronchodilators for patients with acute severe asthma: the choice of drug, the dosage, the route of administration, and the timing. β_2-agonists such as salbutamol (2.5–10 mg, nebulized) are the first-line drugs and are effective for reducing life-threatening bronchoconstriction for most patients. Other β_2-agonists, such as terbutaline, rimiterol, fenoterol, and reproterol, can also be used. Increasingly, higher doses of nebulized β_2-agonists are being recommended for acute episodes, in order to preclude the need for intubation and ventilation. Under controlled circumstances, continuous administration of nebulized β_2-agonists should be used, when necessary, or until unacceptable side effects occur (eg serious tachycardia or arrhythmias). Although intravenous administration of β_2-agonists may be no more effective than the nebulized form, the intravenous route should be used for acute severe asthma when the patient has difficulty in breathing and adequate delivery cannot be ensured. Aerosol delivery is particularly unpredictable in intubated patients, as much of it becomes deposited on the ETT. The intravenous dosage for salbutamol is 5–10 μg/kg, slowly over 15 minutes, as a loading dose, if there has been no previous salbutamol, then 5–20 μg/min for adults, titrated against the severity of the asthma.

ANTICHOLINERGIC BRONCHODILATORS Ipratropium bromide (500 μg, nebulized) may provide a small additional benefit when used with β_2-agonists.

AMINOPHYLLINE Intravenous aminophylline is usually used when high dosages of β_2-agonists have not been effective. There is little evidence, however, that it improves bronchodilatation, and it has toxic side effects, such as arrhythmias, agitation, and seizures. Patients must be monitored with a continuous ECG display, and potassium levels must be checked regularly. Many facilities no longer recommend the use of aminophylline for acute severe asthma. One must question patients about prior use of slow-release oral theophylline and decrease the initial aminophylline intravenous dose accordingly. Serum potassium concentrations must be determined immediately, as chronic theophylline use will decrease serum and total-body potassium levels, and acute intravenous use will decrease the serum potassium further. Hypokalaemia predisposes to arrhythmias.

The aminophylline dosage is initially 6 mg/kg, as a loading dose, over 30 minutes, then 0.2–0.9 mg $\cdot$ kg^{-1} $\cdot$ h^{-1} if the patient is not already on theophylline. Otherwise, use 2–3 mg/kg as a loading dose. The pharmacodynamics of aminophylline are complicated. Aim to keep plasma concentrations at 10–20 mg/L.

ADRENALINE Adrenaline has been used successfully for many years in the form of a subcutaneous injection. The action of intravenous adrenaline, however, is more rapid and more reliable. As is the case for most drugs, the role of intravenous adrenaline in treating patients with acute severe asthma is as yet unclear, but a trial of adrenaline may allow one to avoid the use of intubation and ventilation. It can be used immediately after a nebulized β_2-agonist has been determined a failure.

The dosage of adrenaline should be 5–10 ml of a 1:10,000 solution IV over 5–10 minutes, repeated as necessary.

All patients should be monitored with continuous ECG display.

If a patient is stable after the initial dose of adrenaline, a continuous infusion at 1–20 μg/min should be commenced and titrated against the patient's symptoms. This can be achieved by diluting 5 mg of adrenaline in 100 ml of isotonic saline and empirically titrating it against a clinical effect.

Paradoxically, blood pressure and pulse rate usually will decrease with the use of adrenaline, as the patient's condition improves. If the blood pressure rises, if serious arrhythmias occur, or if the patient's condition is rapidly deteriorating, alternative treatment must be considered. Vomiting may be observed during the adrenaline infusion.

Frequent checks of the serum potassium concentration should be made, because adrenaline, aminophylline, and β_2-agonists can cause hypokalaemia and predispose to cardiac arrhythmias.

Acute severe asthma seems to run a time course of approximately 24–48 hours. Do not abruptly cease administration of adrenaline, as sudden exacerbations of asthma can occur even after 24 hours. Gradually wean the patient from adrenaline, and be prepared to increase the infusion rate if deterioration occurs during the weaning process.

ANTIBIOTICS Antibiotics are rarely indicated for acute severe asthma. Use of these agents should be restricted to patients with bacteriologically proven infection or infiltrates seen on chest x-ray.

PHYSIOTHERAPY Physiotherapy is useful for patients in the recovery phase, when patients begin clearing mucous plugs. Intubated patients need aggressive physiotherapy in order to avoid atelectasis and lung collapse.

ARTIFICIAL VENTILATION

Indications

Artificial ventilation is a procedure of last resort and should be used only if medications fail. Asthmatic patients present difficult ventilatory challenges: Gas has to be forced in under pressure to an already over-distended chest and then has to escape passively through occluded airways. Serious complications of ventilation are common in these circumstances. The decision to ventilate is a clinical one, based on the patient's degree of exhaustion and the relative improvement achieved with more conservative measures.

Approach

ATTITUDE Reassure the patient, and explain what will happen.

OXYGENATION Pre-oxygenate with 100% oxygen.

INTRAVASCULAR VOLUME Pre-load the patient rapidly with 500 ml of colloid. During spontaneous breathing, these patients have very negative intrathoracic pressure, and venous return is enhanced. When positive-pressure ventilation is commenced, intrathoracic pressures increase, and venous return is severely impaired. Moreover, such patients often are dehydrated as a result of decreased oral intake, excessive sweating, and tachypnoea. Be prepared to infuse more fluid according to the cardiovascular response to positive-pressure ventilation.

INDUCTION AGENT Use an agent that will cause minimal cardiovascular depression (eg benzodiazepine plus narcotic), as well as a rapidly acting muscle relaxant to ensure adequate conditions for rapid-sequence intubation. Use cricoid pressure during intubation in order to prevent aspiration.

SEDATION Maintain sedation (eg midazolam and morphine) as a continuous intravenous infusion (see p. 114). Although morphine may release histamine, it is probably safe to use for sedation.

MUSCLE RELAXATION A muscle relaxant may be necessary (eg vecuronium, 8 mg initial dose, then an infusion of 5–10 mg/h) to prevent fighting against the ventilator and increasing the already high inspiratory pressures.

OXYGENATION Maintain with appropriate F_{IO_2} according to frequent determinations of blood gases and pulse oximetry.

VENTILATOR SETTINGS DO NOT OVER-VENTILATE OR AIM FOR 'NORMAL' $Paco_2$. Electively hypoventilate and tolerate high $Paco_2$ [keep $Paco_2$ < 90 mm Hg (12 kPa) and pH > 7.2 (63 mmol/L H^+)] in order to avoid high ventilatory pressures, barotrauma, and cardiovascular depression.

Each patient will need individual settings to maintain adequate oxygenation without over-distension of alveoli. As an initial setting, use

- a 1:1 inspiratory:expiratory ratio
- a low tidal volume (usually less than 400 ml)

Increase the ventilation by increasing the respiratory rate, but with an expiratory pause sufficient to allow for adequate lung emptying and to prevent 'stacking' of gas within the lung after each inspiration.

A slow inspiratory flow rate is optimal for low inspiratory pressures, but may not be sufficient for delivery of an adequate tidal volume. Reduce the inspiratory flow rate to as low a level as is compatible with adequate ventilation.

Keep peak inspiratory pressure less than 50 cm H_2O if at all possible.

CHEST X-RAY Inspect the patient and examine the chest x-ray for evidence of subcutaneous emphysema or mediastinal emphysema (Figure 19.11). This indicates extensive alveolar rupture and a high likelihood of pneumothorax formation; inform the staff, and have an intercostal catheter available, but do not insert it prophylactically.

OTHER POSSIBLE MEASURES

- Ketamine (20–40 $\mu g \cdot kg^{-1} \cdot min^{-1}$) may be useful for asthma that is unresponsive to other measures.
- Magnesium sulphate (1.2 g in 50 ml of isotonic saline, IV, over 20 minutes) has been reported to improve peak flow rates.
- Isoprenaline (0.05–0.6 $\mu g \cdot kg^{-1} \cdot min^{-1}$) has been used successfully in children.
- Halothane has been used as a last resort in ventilated patients with severe asthma. Care must be exercised to avoid cardiovascular de-

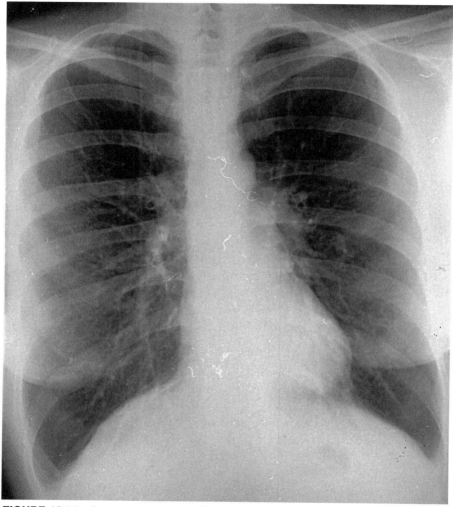

FIGURE 19.11 Acute severe asthma. Note over-distended lung fields.

pression and increased intracranial pressure. Ether, isoflurane, and enflurane have also been used.

• Manual chest compression during expiration may be needed in a minority of artificially ventilated patients in order to assist expiratory gas flow.

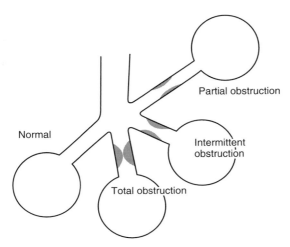

FIGURE 19.12 Model of alveoli in asthma.

• CPAP and PEEP have been used successfully in some centres, but the experience has been limited, and there is always the danger of over-inflating the lung further, causing serious cardiorespiratory sequelae. The PEEP levels will have to be high enough to keep airways open, but low enough to prevent alveolar over-distension. This may be difficult to achieve in a heterogeneous population of alveoli (Figure 19.12).

• Cardiopulmonary bypass may be successful in rare cases that are unresponsive to other measures.

CHRONIC AIRFLOW LIMITATION

Airflow can be limited because of narrowing of the airways or diminished elastic recoil in the lung. The clinical manifestations of these have been believed to be chronic bronchitis and emphysema, respectively. That may well be an inaccurate over-simplification. It is probably better to think of both diseases as forming part of the spectrum known as CAL, characterized by cough, dyspnoea, sputum production, airflow limitation, and impaired gas exchange. The lesions associated with CAL include

Acinus:
  emphysema

Bronchi:
  smooth-muscle hyperplasia
  mucous-gland enlargement
Bronchioles:
  narrowing and obliteration
  mucous plugging
  inflammation
  fibrosis

One or another of these lesions may dominate, but the usual picture is that the lesions occur in diverse combinations to varying degrees of severity. The reasons for such large variations among patients are unclear.

Many patients admitted to intensive care, for whatever reason, will have some degree of CAL, as smoking remains prevalent in many communities. For these patients, gas exchange will be compromised, and artificial ventilation will be associated with more complications. Some of these patients will be admitted primarily for an acute exacerbation of CAL. THE MOST IMPORTANT DECISION IN THE MANAGE-MENT OF THESE PATIENTS IS WHETHER OR NOT TO ADMIT THEM TO THE ICU. Increasingly the opinion is that the expensive resources in the ICU have little to offer patients with the severe limitations of respiratory reserve that result from advanced CAL.

The admission policy will depend on the severity of the chronic component and the extent of the acute component. A careful history usually will elicit a patient's previous exercise tolerance and quality of life. There may be little or no acute component, and in fact, the so-called deterioration may represent end-stage disease, at which point a diagnosis of 'dying' should be considered.

MANAGEMENT (Table 19.7)

Oxygen

There are certain individuals with severe CAL who are sensitive to even small increases in inspired oxygen concentration. For some reason, every medical student seems to remember that oxygen is dangerous in these circumstances, and therefore it is often delivered in only meagre and insubstantial amounts to all hypoxic patients. Oxygen-sensitive patients are rare, and yet our obsession with the

TABLE 19.7 MANAGEMENT OF CHRONIC AIRWAY LIMITATION IN INTENSIVE CARE

Consider carefully what intensive care can offer in terms of the reversible components of the presentation, especially when contemplating ventilation.

Give oxygen.

Correct any reversible component (eg drain a pneumothorax, treat infection).

Reduce the work of breathing (eg reduce sputum formation and bronchoconstriction).

Begin a trial of drug treatment (eg inhaled β_2-agonists and corticosteroids).

Reduce pain after surgery, and encourage early mobilization.

Use chest physiotherapy.

Begin a trial of CPAP.

Use mechanical ventilation.

potential danger from oxygen is responsible for widespread 'elective' hypoxia in hospitalized patients throughout the world.

In these days of readily available determinations of blood gases, these rare individuals can be recognized, and their inspired oxygen can be titrated carefully, whilst the remainder can survive in much safer circumstances with appropriate oxygenation. Oxygen is essential for optimal alveolar function and also helps to reduce pulmonary vasoconstriction and hypertension.

Correct any reversible components

Because the respiratory reserves of patients with CAL are minimal, reversing even small components of the disease can be beneficial. For example, even small pneumothoraces should be drained. The work of breathing can be decreased by reducing secretions and bronchoconstriction or by treating infections.

Drugs

The role of drugs in treating CAL is uncertain and depends on the degree of destruction of lung architecture. There has been little evaluation of the roles of drugs in treating acute exacerbations of CAL. Often the only way to determine their effectiveness is to try one or more drugs and evaluate the clinical effectiveness in each individual patient. Corticosteroids are sometimes helpful. Bronchodilators can be useful. Aerosol or intravenous β_2-adrenergic agents are more effective than intravenous aminophylline in the acute situation.

INHALED β_2-AGONISTS　The β_2-agonists have not been well evaluated regarding dosage and effectiveness in treating CAL, but they would seem to be worth a trial.

ANTICHOLINERGIC DRUGS　Nebulized ipratropium has bronchodilatory effects and may reduce the volume of sputum.

THEOPHYLLINE　The role of theophylline in treating CAL is not clear. Nevertheless, many patients are on long-term theophylline treatment.

CORTICOSTEROIDS　Corticosteroids may be worth a trial in patients with acute exacerbations of CAL.

Surgery

Thoracic or abdominal surgery, or even the insult of minor surgery, can reduce what little respiratory reserve is left in these patients, causing rapid deterioration in respiration function. This can be minimized by the following measures:

PAIN RELIEF　Provide adequate pain relief, especially local or regional analgesia peri-operatively, in order to encourage breathing and coughing and avoid sputum retention.

PERI-OPERATIVE PHYSIOTHERAPY

NASOTRACHEAL SUCTION　Use nasotracheal suction or minitracheostomy to facilitate sputum clearance.

INCENTIVE SPIROMETRY　Incentive spirometry and early mobilization can also help.

LOW-DOSAGE HEPARIN　Prophylactic use of low-dosage heparin can minimize the risk for thromboembolic phenomena.

Cardiac failure

Cardiac failure, with pulmonary and peripheral oedema, often can supervene in patients with CAL. It may be part of a primary process or secondary to right ventricular failure. The diagnosis is not easy, and interpretation of pulmonary oedema on a chest x-ray can be difficult because of distorted vascular markings and lung architecture.

Cardiac failure in these circumstances can be managed by cautious diuresis, use of β_2-agonist (eg salbutamol), and occasionally left- and right-side afterload reduction with nitroglycerin.

Continuous positive airway pressure

Dynamic hyperinflation of the lung is common in patients with CAL. The expiratory time is reduced to the point where complete exhalation cannot occur before the next inspiratory cycle is initiated. This leads to gas trapping at the end of expiration, also known as breath-stacking, occult PEEP, 'auto' PEEP, or 'intrinsic' PEEP ($PEEP_i$). The level of $PEEP_i$ may not be the same for each breath, nor can it be accurately predicted for each patient. It depends on factors such as lung compliance and resistance for any given airway diameter, inspiratory flow, and respiratory rate.

Intrinsic PEEP increases the work of breathing by acting as an inspiratory-threshold load. CPAP can counterbalance the effects of $PEEP_i$ and will reduce the work of breathing, as well as the sensation of dyspnoea. A well-designed CPAP circuit is essential (see p. 472). The level of CPAP should be titrated against the subjective improvement in the patient's responses (usually 5–10 cm H_2O). The level of applied PEEP should be less than the patient's $PEEP_i$.

Mask ventilation (see p. 476)

Pressure-support ventilation or IPPV via a nasal mask may preclude the need for intubation.

Mechanical ventilation

Artificial ventilation should be avoided, if possible, because of several considerations:

- Coughing reflex and clearing of secretions are reduced.
- Lung architecture is already disrupted and would be prone to further damage by positive airway pressure.
- Patients with CAL are notoriously difficult to wean from artificial ventilation.
- Unless there is a significant acute respiratory component, the prospect for long-term survival of these patients is poor.

APPROACH TO VENTILATION   Do not aim for 'normal' concentrations of blood gases. These patients often are severely hypoxic and hypercarbic at their best. Keep the Pa_{CO_2} at the patient's normal level. Encourage spontaneous breathing, and titrate the number of mechanical breaths against the patient's requirements. This is called intermittent mandatory ventilation (IMV) (see p. 472) and forms the basis for a continuous weaning process. For this technique to be successful, one must have a machine that allows efficient spontaneous breathing with minimum work (see p. 481). 'Pressure assist' or pressure support during inspiration may also help with weaning (see p. 473). Avoid excessive use of sedation or muscle relaxants, as that would prolong the already difficult weaning process. Tracheostomy may be needed if weaning from ventilation is delayed (see p. 27). An early introduction of enteral nutrition is important.

PULMONARY EMBOLISM

INCIDENCE IN THE ICU

It appears that whereas deep venous thrombosis (DVT) is relatively common in seriously ill patients, pulmonary embolism (PE) is rare. Nevertheless, patients outside of intensive care can develop life-threatening PE and may need support in the ICU.

PATHOPHYSIOLOGY

Pulmonary emboli usually are multiple. Acute obstruction of the pulmonary arterial tree will result in $\dot{V}/\dot{Q}$ abnormalities, hypoxia, and circulatory failure. Severe disturbances occur in about 10% of patients with PE (Table 19.8).

TABLE 19.8 DEGREES OF SEVERITY FOR PULMONARY EMBOLISM

Severity grade	Haemodynamic disturbance	Oxygenation	Clinical symptoms
I	Absent	Normal	Short-lasting
II	Mild	Normal	Moderate but persisting
III	Moderate	Abnormal	Severe
IV	Severe	Very abnormal	Shock

Diagnosis

Finding the source of the PE can be a frustrating and often futile exercise. Femoral and iliac veins can be sources of multiple emboli, and further investigation may be necessary in those circumstances.

PE is easily misdiagnosed. No single symptom or combination of symptoms is diagnostic. The classic clinical signs (dyspnoea, haemoptysis, and pleuritic chest pain) are uncommon. Determinations of arterial blood gases and serum enzymes show no consistent pattern on which a firm diagnosis could be made. However, a decrease in the platelet count is highly suggestive of PE.

There will be positive findings from chest x-ray in about 50% of patients (eg pulmonary haemorrhage or infarction, raised hemidiaphragm, atelectasis, oligaemia, pleural effusion). However, those features can accompany many illnesses in intensive care.

Transoesophageal echocardiography can demonstrate obvious right ventricular strain in cases of significant emboli.

More than 50% of patients with PE will have normal ECG patterns. Abnormal findings, such as right-side heart strain, frequently are transient, delayed, or non-specific.

When the findings from a perfusion lung scan are normal, the possibility of significant PE can almost be entirely excluded. However, in the presence of pre-existing lung abnormalities, lung scans can be very misleading.

The gold standard for diagnosis is pulmonary angiography, but that is a relatively invasive procedure. The difficulty lies in deciding which patients should be selected for angiography, as most of the other diagnostic methods have shortcomings.

MANAGEMENT

Most patients who survive for the first 30 minutes following PE will live, unless a further embolism occurs. One scheme for management is outlined in Figure 19.13.

Prophylaxis

Low-dosage heparin has not been demonstrated to decrease the incidence of PE in seriously ill patients, despite the many factors potentially predisposing them to venous thromboembolism. This may be related to the relatively high incidence of concurrent coagulopathy and thrombocytopenia. Graded compression stockings and sequential compression devices may reduce the incidence of DVT.

Supportive management

OXYGEN   Supplemental oxygen is almost always required.

CONTINUOUS POSITIVE AIRWAY PRESSURE   CPAP can improve gas exchange in patients with PE.

FLUID   Expansion of the intravascular volume to correct hypotension is necessary (see p. 61). If that fails, inotropes should be used.

INOTROPES   As in other forms of circulatory failure, finding the most suitable inotrope is a matter of trial and error (see p. 520).

• Dobutamine (see p. 522) can be used initially for mild haemodynamic disturbances, as it increases cardiac output and reduces pulmonary vascular resistance.

• Adrenaline or noradrenaline: Inotropes with vasoconstrictor activity are often used for more severe haemodynamic disturbances in order to maintain arterial blood pressure and vital-organ perfusion.

FIGURE 19.13 Management principles for patients with pulmonary embolism. (From Firoozan & Gray, 1993, with permission.)

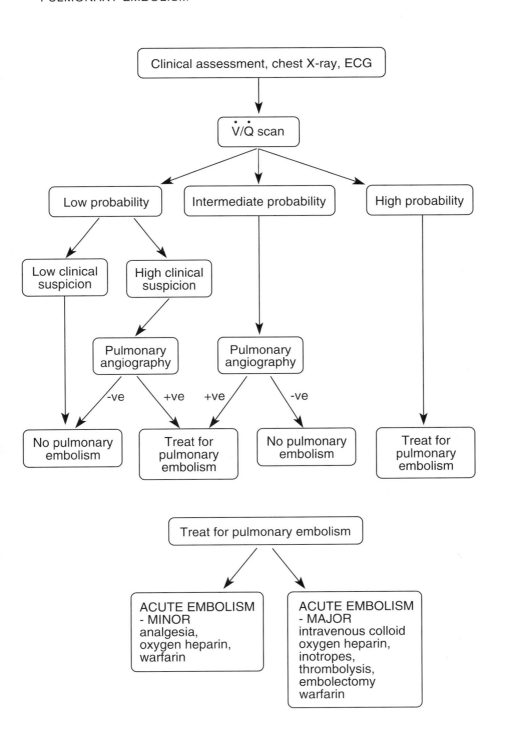

Definitive management

HEPARIN   Heparin will not dissolve an existing clot; it can only prevent extension. It can be given as an intermittent bolus every 4–6
hours or, preferably, via a continuous intravenous infusion. The dosage
can be selected empirically (eg 1,000 units per hour) or can be determined on the basis of tests such as the activated partial thromboplastin time (which should be about twice the control level), the clotting time, or the thrombin time, or a combination of all three. In a
case of proven PE, heparin is usually given for 7–10 days, followed
by a change to an oral anticoagulant for 3–6 months, with an overlap period of approximately 5 days when both drugs are given.

THROMBOLYTICS   The indications for thrombolytic treatment are not
yet settled. They probably should encompass patients with sustained
hypotension, shock, or acute right ventricular failure (RVF) and those
with obstruction to more than 50% of the pulmonary circulation. Heparin probably should be administered before and after the thrombolytic agent.
  Streptokinase   A bolus dose of 1 million units over 30 minutes
probably will be sufficient. However, some authorities recommend
100,000–200,000 units hourly for 24 hours.
  Allergic reactions occur in about 5% of patients. Most are mild and
can be minimized by giving hydrocortisone (100 mg IV) before the infusion. The possibility of anaphylactic reactions should be anticipated,
and they must be treated rapidly (see p. 131).
  Urokinase   A dose of 15,000 units per kilogramme probably will
be sufficient. Urokinase is as effective as streptokinase and appears
to be non-antigenic in humans. However, it is expensive and is not
available in all countries.
  Recombinant tissue plasminogen activator (rt-PA)   A dose
of 50 mg IV, repeated if necessary, has been used successfully in initial trials for PE.
  Contraindications and complications   Thrombolytic agents
should not be given to patients who have had surgery within the preceding 3–4 days (longer in cases of more complicated surgery, eg vascular surgery), nor to those who have other potential sites of bleeding, such as recent episodes of gastro-intestinal or cerebrovascular

haemorrhage. They should not be used during pregnancy, nor during the puerperium. Caution should be exercised in the presence of an existing coagulation deficit or thrombocytopenia. If bleeding occurs, the infusion should be stopped (the half-life of these agents is no more than 20 minutes), and fresh frozen plasma should be given.

INTERRUPTION OF THE INFERIOR VENA CAVA The use of various techniques such as clips, filters, and umbrellas can be considered after failure of anticoagulant treatment in the less severely ill, as well as for recurring cases of PE or when anticoagulation is considered hazardous.

EMERGENCY PULMONARY EMBOLECTOMY If thrombolytic treatment is contraindicated or is unsuccessful, there may be a place for embolectomy. Embolectomy should be considered in all cases of severe PE (eg patients with more than 50% occlusion of the pulmonary arteries and patients with continuing circulatory shock, hypotension, or RVF that has not responded 1 hour after the onset of PE or after thrombolytic treatment).

OBSTRUCTIVE SLEEP APNOEA

Obstructive sleep apnoea is defined as an absence of airflow lasting for at least 10 seconds and occurring more than 30 times during a 7-hour sleep. Sleep apnoea syndrome is divided into three groups:

obstructive: where airflow ceases despite continuation of abdominal and thoracic inspiratory movements.
central: where cessation of airflow is accompanied by cessation of respiratory efforts.
mixed: obstructive and central.

Obstructive sleep apnoea is by far the most common form, affecting 1–4% of the adult population.

CLINICAL FEATURES

- snoring (cardinal symptom)
- excessive daytime sleepiness (cardinal symptom)
- psychosocial problems and deterioration of intellectual function

- early morning headache
- arterial hypertension
- severe nocturnal hypoxia
- right-side heart failure and pulmonary hypertension
- polycythaemia
- obesity, hypothyroidism, acromegaly
- short, thick neck, retrognathia, nasal obstruction, and oropharyngeal mass
- often associated with excessive alcohol intake

DIAGNOSIS

Obtain a clinical history from patient and spouse. Night sleep studies are needed to confirm the diagnosis and to determine the method and urgency of treatment. Certain features are to be documented during sleep studies:

- continuous pulse oximetry and pulse-rate recovery
- continuous ECG
- continuous electromyogram of the diaphragm
- continuous oronasal airflow measurement (thermistor or pressure transducer)
- continuous sleep-state recording (EEG or electro-oculogram)
- continuous measurement of chest-wall and abdominal motions (inductive plethysmography)
- continuous recording of room noise
- cardiorespiratory investigation to determine extent of impairment

TREATMENT

General

- The patient must lose weight.
- The patient must abstain from alcohol and cigarettes.
- One must either rule out the presence of hypothyroidism and acromegaly or else treat those conditions.

Drugs

Naloxone, acetazolamide, medroxyprogesterone, theophylline, strychnine, and nicotine have all been tried, with little benefit, in patients with sleep apnoea.

Surgery

ANATOMIC OBSTRUCTION Surgical correction of any anatomic obstruction (eg nasal polyps, septal deviation, enlarged tonsils and adenoids) may cure some patients.

UVULOPALATOPHARYNGOPLASTY This procedure is designed to increase the cross-sectional area of the airway. The results are unpredictable.

TRACHEOSTOMY Tracheostomy should be considered in serious cases where other measures have failed.

Nasal CPAP

The principle of nasal CPAP is to provide a pressure at the collapsible segment of the upper airway that will be sufficient to counteract negative inspiratory pressures. The simplest system involves a blower, delivering air via a nasal mask. The system must have minimal inspiratory resistance during respiration. This form of treatment is becoming increasingly used for obstructive sleep apnoea.

TROUBLESHOOTING

HAEMOPTYSIS IN INTENSIVE CARE

Determine that there has been no iatrogenic trauma to upper airways as a result of the use of suction catheters, ETT, etc.

Blunt trauma and penetrating trauma can cause bleeding.

A pulmonary artery catheter can rupture a pulmonary vessel.

Look for pulmonary embolism.

Look for bleeding from carcinoma.

An infection such as tuberculosis can result in bleeding as it erodes into the pulmonary vessels.

Pulmonary oedema or long-standing mitral valve disease can result in haemoptysis.

Check coagulation/platelets.

FURTHER READING

General

Balk, R., & Bone, R. C. (1983). Classification of acute respiratory failure. *Medical Clinics of North America* 67:551–6.

Putman, C. E., & Goodman, L. (1983). Imaging in the critically ill or injured. In *Critical Care: State of the Art*, vol. 4, ed. W. C. Shoemaker & W. L. Thompson, pp. A1–63. Fullerton, CA: Society of Critical Care Medicine.

Repine, J. E. (1992). Scientific perspectives on adult respiratory distress syndrome. *Lancet* 339:466–9.

Hypoventilation

Kelly, B. J., & Luce, J. M. (1991). The diagnosis and management of neuromuscular disease causing respiratory failure. *Chest* 99:1485–94.

Upper-Airway Obstruction

Bogdonoff, D. L., & Stone, D. J. (1992). Emergency management of the airway outside the operating room. *Canadian Journal of Anaesthesia* 39:1069–89.

Cobley, M., & Vaughan, R. S. (1992). Recognition and management of difficult airway problems. *British Journal of Anaesthesia* 68:90–7.

Post-Operative Chest Complications

George, A., Chisakuta, A. M., Gamble, J. A. S., & Browne, G. A. (1992). Thoracic epidural infusion for postoperative pain relief following abdominal aortic surgery: bupivacaine, fentanyl or a mixture of both? *Anaesthesia* 47:388–94.

Lewis, G. A., Hopkinson, R. B., & Matthews, H. R. (1986). Minitracheostomy – a report of its use in intensive therapy. *Anaesthesia* 41:931–5.

Marshall, B. E., & Wyche, M. Q. (1972). Hypoxemia during and after anesthesia. *Anesthesiology* 37:178–201.

Atelectasis

Putman, C. E., & Goodman, L. (1983). Imaging in the critically ill or injured. In *Critical Care: State of the Art*, vol. 4, ed. W. C. Shoemaker & W. L. Thompson, pp. A1–63. Fullerton, CA: Society of Critical Care Medicine.

Cardiogenic Pulmonary Oedema

Bersten, A. D., Holt, A. W., Vedig, A. E., Skowronski, G. A., & Baggoley, C. J. (1991). Treatment of severe cardiogenic pulmonary edema with continuous airway pressure delivered by face mask. *New England Journal of Medicine* 325:1825–30.

Hillman, K. (1992). Acute cardiogenic pulmonary edema. In *Year Book of Intensive Care and Emergency Medicine*, ed. J. L. Vincent, pp. 185–93. Berlin: Springer-Verlag.

Adult Respiratory Distress Syndrome

Ashbaugh, D. G., Bigelow, D. B., Petty, T. P., & Levine, B. E. (1967). Acute respiratory distress in adults. *Lancet* 2:319–23.

Dellinger, R. P. (ed.) (1993). Adult respiratory distress syndrome: current considerations in future directions. *New Horizons* 1:463–650 (symposium issue).

Demling, R. H. (1993). Adult respiratory distress syndrome: current concepts. *New Horizons* 1:388–401.

Hickling, K. G. (1990). Ventilatory management of ARDS. Can it affect outcome? *Intensive Care Medicine* 16:219–26.

Knox, J. B. (1993). Oxygen consumption – oxygen delivery dependency in adult respiratory distress syndrome. *New Horizons* 1:381–7.

Kollet, M. H., Schuster, D. P. (1995). Medical progress: the adult respiratory distress syndrome. *New England Journal of Medicine* 332:27–37.

Staub, N. C. (1978). Pulmonary edema: physiologic approach to management. *Chest* 74:559–67.

Pneumonia

British Thoracic Society Research Committee (1987). Community acquired pneumonia in adults in British hospitals in 1982–83: a survey of aetiology, mortality, prognostic factors and outcome. *Quarterly Journal of Medicine* 62:195–220.

Cartier, F. (1987). Strategy in immunocompromised patients with pulmonary infiltrates. *Intensive Care Medicine* 13:87–8.

Chase, R. A., & Trenholme, G. M. (1986). Overwhelming pneumonia. *Medical Clinics of North America* 70:945–60.

Chastre, J., Fagon, J.-Y., & Lamer, C. H. (1992). Procedures for the diagnosis of pneumonia in ICU patients. *Intensive Care Medicine* 18:S10–17.

Meduri, G. U. (1990). Ventilator-associated pneumonia in patients with respiratory failure. A diagnostic approach. *Chest* 97:1208–19.

Meduri, G. U., Wunderink, R. G., Leeper, K. V. (1992). Management of bacterial pneumonia in ventilated patients. *Chest* 101:500–8.

Putman, C. E., & Goodman, L. (1983). Imaging in the critically ill or injured. In *Critical Care: State of the Art*, vol. 4, ed. W. C. Shoemaker & W. L. Thompson, pp. A1–63. Fullerton, CA: Society of Critical Care Medicine.

Unertl, K. E., Lenhart, F.-P., Forst, H., & Peter, K. (1992). Systemic antibiotic treatment of nosocomial pneumonia. *Intensive Care Medicine* 18:S28–34.

Aspiration

Britto, J., & Demling, R. H. (1993). Aspiration lung injury. *New Horizons* 1:435–9.

Putman, C. E., & Goodman, L. (1983). Imaging in the critically ill or injured. In *Critical Care: State of the Art*, vol. 4, ed. W. C. Shoemaker & W. L. Thompson, pp. A1–63. Fullerton, CA: Society of Critical Care Medicine.

Unilateral Lung Abnormalities

Hillman, K. M., & Barber, J. D. (1980). Asynchronous independent lung ventilation. *Critical Care Medicine* 8:390–5.

Powner, D. J., Eross, B., & Grenvik, A. (1977). Differential lung ventilation with PEEP in the treatment of unilateral pneumonia. *Critical Care Medicine* 5:170–2.

Acute Severe Asthma

Darioli, R., & Perret, C. (1984). Mechanical controlled hypoventilation in status asthmaticus. *American Review of Respiratory Disease* 129:385–7.

Editor (1986). Acute asthma. *Lancet* 1:131–3.

Hillman, K. M., & Bishop, G. (1993). Acute severe asthma. In *Pulmonary and Critical Care Medicine*, vol. 2, ed. R. C. Bone, pp. 1–20. St. Louis: Mosby.

Chronic Airway Limitation

Branthwaite, M. A. (1985). Acute on chronic respiratory failure. *Clinical Anaesthesiology* 3:831–47.

Ferguson, G. T., & Cherniack, R. M. (1993). Management of chronic obstructive pulmonary disease. *New England Journal of Medicine* 328:1017–22.

Thurleck, W. M. (1990). Pathophysiology of chronic pulmonary disease. *Clinics in Chest Medicine* 11:389–403.

Pulmonary Embolism

Duroux, P., Simonneau, G., Petitpretz, P., & Herue, P. L. (1984). Therapeutic approach to acute pulmonary embolism. *Intensive Care Medicine* 10:99–102.

Editor (1988). Management of venous thromboembolism. *Lancet* 1:275–7.

Firoozan, S., & Gray, H. H. (1992). Management of pulmonary embolism. *Thorax* 47:825–32.

Sors, H., Safran, D., Stern, M., Reynaud, P., Bon, J., & Even, P. (1984). An analysis of the diagnostic methods for acute pulmonary embolism. *Intensive Care Medicine* 10:81–4.

Obstructive Sleep Apnoea

Hanning, C. D. (1989). Obstructive sleep apnoea. *British Journal of Anaesthesia* 63:477–88.

Sullivan, C. E., & Issa, F. G. (1985). Obstructive sleep apnoea. *Clinics in Chest Medicine* 6:633–50.

20

VENTILATORY TECHNIQUES

- There will be an optimum ventilatory mode for each patient at each stage of that patient's disease.
- Because of the many serious disadvantages of positive-pressure ventilation, spontaneous respiration should be encouraged as soon as possible following acute respiratory failure.
- Weaning is a dynamic and continuous process that begins the moment a patient is artificially ventilated.
- 'Permissive hypercarbia' or 'elective hypoventilation' is an increasingly accepted practice – the need for oxygenation takes precedence over the need for optimal ventilation and carbon dioxide levels.

INTERMITTENT POSITIVE-PRESSURE VENTILATION

The lungs are designed to be inflated by the creation of a negative intrapleural pressure. Early artificial ventilators, such as the iron lung, followed that sound physiological method and created a vacuum around the chest to cause airflow.

The use of positive-pressure ventilation became widespread in the early 1950s, and its use has, in many ways, defined the practice of intensive care medicine. Intermittent positive-pressure ventilation (IPPV) is the commonest form of positive-pressure support used in intensive care: A certain tidal volume is delivered at a set rate to maintain a minute volume consistent with CO_2 elimination, while oxygenation is determined mainly by the fraction of inspired oxygen (F_{IO_2}).

Main indications for IPPV

1. failure of ventilation (eg caused by neuromuscular diseases such as tetanus or Guillain-Barré syndrome, or resulting from neuromuscular blocking drugs)

464

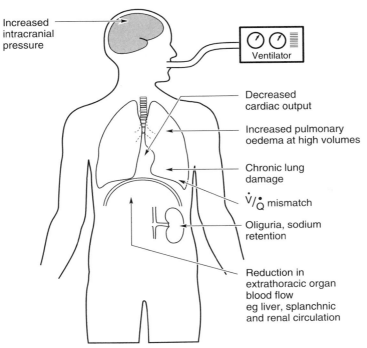

Increased intracranial pressure

Ventilator

Decreased cardiac output

Increased pulmonary oedema at high volumes

Chronic lung damage

$\dot{V}/\dot{Q}$ mismatch

Oliguria, sodium retention

Reduction in extrathoracic organ blood flow eg liver, splanchnic and renal circulation

FIGURE 20.1 Complications of positive intrathoracic pressure.

2. to facilitate carbon dioxide excretion (eg to reduce cerebral blood flow in patients with cerebral oedema secondary to head injury)

3. to reduce the work of breathing in patients with cardiorespiratory failure (eg the later stages of acute respiratory failure)

COMPLICATIONS OF POSITIVE INTRATHORACIC PRESSURE

The adverse effects of positive intrathoracic pressure are principally due to cardiovascular impairment and the direct effect of pressure on lung tissue (Figure 20.1).

Pulmonary effects of positive-pressure ventilation

When positive-pressure ventilation was first employed on a wide scale in the early 1950s, machines would simulate normal tidal volumes and rates. If the lungs were otherwise normal and the inflationary pressures were relatively low, lung damage due to positive pressure would be minimal. However, as the practice of ventilating patients with underlying lung disease became widespread, pulmonary barotrauma (lung damage secondary to excessive volume and pressure), causing alveolar over-distension, became an increasing problem.

The incidence of barotrauma increased even further with the advent of volume-cycled ventilators and the use of high levels of positive end-expiratory pressure (PEEP). Modern ventilators guarantee the delivery of a pre-set tidal volume, independent of the compliance or resistance of the lungs. This results in non-ventilation of some alveoli and over-distension of other, often normal, alveoli. It is not only high pressure that can damage lung tissue; high tidal volumes and alveolar over-distension can also result in rupture. In fact, excessive volumes may be more important than excessive pressures in causing alveolar over-distension and rupture. Alveolar over-distension also causes increased permeability pulmonary oedema. Ironically, that is often the problem for which the patient is being ventilated.

Gas from ruptured alveoli forms pulmonary interstitial emphysema, which travels in the adventitia of the pulmonary vessels (Figure 20.2). The gas bubbles coalesce along large vessels and migrate centrally to form mediastinal emphysema (ME). With further development of pulmonary interstitial emphysema and ME, the gas can burst through the mediastinal pleura to form pneumothoraces or can track along the fascia in the neck to form subcutaneous emphysema (SE) (Figure 20.3). Pneumothoraces and SE can occur together or independently in this setting. With increasing pressure, gas can track along the aorta and oesophagus to form pneumoretroperitoneum, pneumoperitoneum, and even air embolism (Figure 20.4).

It is important to recognize the presence of extra-alveolar gas, either clinically or on x-ray. ME can, for example, collect under tension in the mediastinum and cause cardiac tamponade. Both SE and ME are indicators of imminent risk for pneumothorax formation, unless ventilatory pressures and volumes can be reduced. Gas from a ruptured viscus must be differentiated from pneumoperitoneum and pneumoretroperitoneum.

The incidence of pulmonary barotrauma can be reduced by limiting peak inspiratory pressures to less than 35 cm H_2O, by reducing tidal volumes to less than 5–10 ml/kg, and by being more concerned with adequate oxygenation, rather than a 'normal' arterial pressure

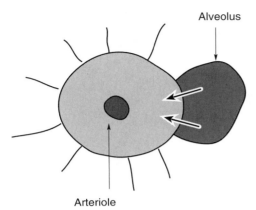

FIGURE 20.2 Origin of extra-alveolar air. Air under pressure moves from over-distended alveoli into the adventitia of pulmonary arterioles and venules. It moves along the adventitia toward the mediastinum as pulmonary interstitial emphysema.

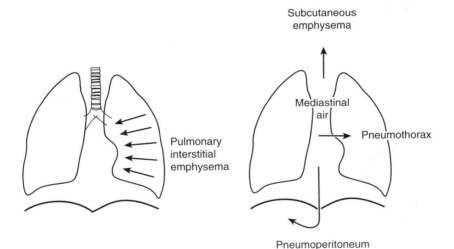

FIGURE 20.3 Forms of pulmonary barotrauma. Extra-alveolar air moves as pulmonary interstitial emphysema to form mediastinal emphysema. From there, under continued pressure, it can form SE, pneumothoraces, pneumoretroperitoneum, and pneumoperitoneum. (From Hillman, 1985, with permission of W. B. Saunders.)

of carbon dioxide (Pa_{CO_2}). The lungs are delicate structures that can easily be damaged by pressure and over-distension. Pulmonary barotrauma can also result in chronic lung damage or bronchopulmonary dysplasia as a result of rupture of the terminal airways and alveoli.

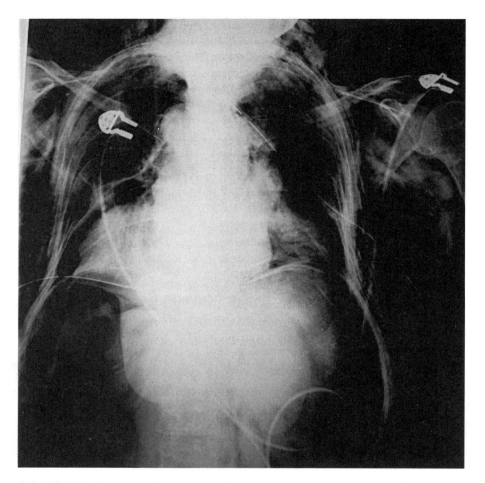

FIGURE 20.4 Pulmonary barotrauma, with massive extra-alveolar gas formation, including ME, SE, bilateral pneumothoraces (treated with intercostal catheters), and pneumoperitoneum.

Ventilatory techniques that can limit the adverse effects of excessive pressure are increasingly being used, and they are discussed in the next section of this chapter.

Relative hypoxia can also paradoxically occur when artificial ventilation is commenced. This is because of an exacerbation of mismatching between ventilation ($\dot{V}$) and perfusion ($\dot{Q}$). Pulmonary blood flow can be decreased as a result of positive pressure, and the distribution of ventilation is not the same as that which occurs during spontaneous respiration.

Cardiovascular effects of positive-pressure ventilation

Applying positive pressure to the lungs decreases venous return, which in turn decreases cardiac output and blood pressure, unless the body naturally compensates or there is a clinical intervention such as fluid infusion or inotrope administration. In addition to decreased arterial blood flow secondary to decreased cardiac output, there is increased venous return from extrathoracic organs. This is due to the fact that intrathoracic pressure (ITP) is impeding venous return. Decreased cerebral venous return can increase intracranial pressure, especially when the pressure is already abnormally high. As part of the body's normal responses to increased intrathoracic pressure and decreased venous return, there is also a tendency for sodium and water retention.

POSITIVE END-EXPIRATORY PRESSURE

PEEP is used to improve oxygenation (see p. 366). Adding PEEP to IPPV will improve oxygenation, probably by keeping alveoli open at the end of expiration and by recruiting non-ventilated alveoli.

The amount of PEEP needed to achieve optimal oxygenation usually varies between 5 and 20 cm H_2O, but pressures of up to 30 cm H_2O have been used. Because of the dangers associated with PEEP, there is an increasing tendency to use no more than 10 cm H_2O.

Optimal PEEP

The optimal level of PEEP is the airway pressure at which oxygen transport (the product of cardiac output and arterial oxygen content) will be maximal (see p. 366). Because PEEP decreases cardiac output and venous return to the heart, the compromise between improved oxygenation and reduced cardiac output is a matter of trial and error. Moreover, PEEP increases the peak inspiratory pressure (PIP), which is associated with increased pulmonary barotrauma and other complications (see p. 466). These adverse effects must be considered when determining the 'best' PEEP. Because in determining the opti-

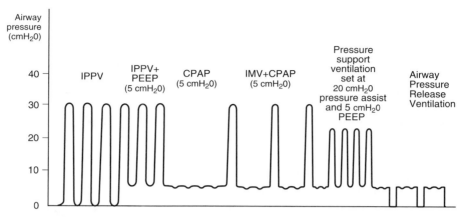

FIGURE 20.5   Different ventilatory modes.

mal PEEP, one must take all of these factors into account, it is, at best, an empirical estimate. One should aim for maximal alveolar recruitment, while avoiding over-distension and barotrauma. This is difficult because of the widespread heterogeneity throughout the lungs. The best PEEP probably is the lowest at which adequate oxygen delivery can be achieved.

CHOOSING THE RIGHT VENTILATORY MODE

In attempts to improve gas exchange, while avoiding the disadvantages of high intrathoracic pressure and alveolar over-distension, forms of ventilatory support other than IPPV and PEEP are increasingly being used (Figure 20.5). Many of these newer modes are incorporated into the ventilators being used in intensive care. They can provide many more ways of delivering a tidal volume under pressure, but they still have shortcomings regarding their ability to allow the patient to breathe spontaneously. Efficient spontaneous respiration is an essential requirement for successful use of continuous positive airway pressure (CPAP), intermittent mandatory ventilation (IMV), and pressure-support ventilation. It is in these spontaneous breathing modes where sophisticated and expensive ventilators still have problems. The problems are related to the ability of the machine to sense a spontaneous breath and rapidly respond with adequate flow rates. The pressure-support mode helps overcome this deficiency by enhancing each spontaneous breath with a predetermined pressure boost. As soon as artificial ventilation is commenced, one should begin planning a weaning strategy that will encourage spontaneous respiration.

The aim of ventilatory assistance has increasingly come to involve guaranteeing adequate oxygenation at safe pressures, with tolerable hypercarbia. Hypercarbia, by itself, may not be as harmful as was once thought. Hypercarbia causes peripheral vasodilatation, increases endogenous catecholamine release, and eventually can decrease the arterial pH. Relative contraindications to hypercarbia include intracranial abnormalities and cardiac arrhythmias. The rate of change of Pa_{CO_2} is as important as its absolute value. Sudden increases or decreases should be avoided. Where there is no definite contraindication to hypercarbia, oxygenation should be achieved at the lowest PIP. Another way of looking at this aim is that it is to limit the expansion of the lung during any single tidal volume. To achieve that, the difference between the end-expiratory pressure and PIP should be minimized. Ideally, that can be achieved with CPAP.

It is very difficult to clinically assess and compare different ventilatory modes. No large trial has shown one technique to be more effective than another. As is true for many aspects of intensive care medicine, **THERE PROBABLY IS A BEST VENTILATORY TECHNIQUE FOR A PARTICULAR PATIENT AT A PARTICULAR TIME, AND IT IS MORE LIKELY TO BE FOUND BY TRIAL AND ERROR THAN TO BE REVEALED BY DOGMA.** Moreover, the decision to choose one technique over another should depend on the skill of the driver rather than on the flashiness of the machine (Table 20.1).

CONTINUOUS POSITIVE AIRWAY PRESSURE

CPAP is more than spontaneous breathing with PEEP. Inspiration is also facilitated by a constant-pressure source (Figure 20.5). Perfect CPAP is achieved when airway pressure is constant throughout the respiratory cycle. This results in minimal work of breathing, increased lung compliance, and improved oxygenation, without the disadvantages of excessive inspiratory pressure associated with IPPV.

CPAP addresses the main problem of acute respiratory failure: OXYGENATION, as opposed to VENTILATION (see p. 360). Most patients with acute respiratory failure typically are hyperventilating and

TABLE 20.1 GUIDELINES TO ARTIFICIAL VENTILATION IN
INTENSIVE CARE

Use conventional IPPV when a patient has neuromuscular disease, when a
patient has been given excessive sedation or neuromuscular blocking
agents, or when the lung compliance or resistance problem is so severe
that the patient cannot ventilate adequately.

When a patient requires assisted ventilation, commence, when possible with
IMV and pressure assist. Then commence the weaning process to CPAP
as aggressively as you would wean a patient off inotropes. First wean the
ratio to about 4 breaths per minute; then reduce the pressure support.

Encourage spontaneous breathing modes such as CPAP, pressure assist, or
IMV, and accept a higher-than-normal $Paco_2$–permissive hypercarbia.

Maintain PEEP, usually between 5 and 15 cm H_2O.

Check the patient, ventilator, and circuit in an attempt to reduce the work of
breathing and facilitate spontaneous respiration.

hypocarbic. The failure of ventilation becomes increasingly evident as
the work of breathing increases, eventually leading to exhaustion. Often that can be avoided by employing CPAP early in the course of the
disease in order to increase lung compliance and decrease the work
of breathing.

It must be stressed that for CPAP to function efficiently as a form
of respiratory support, the circuit must provide almost constant positive pressure during both inspiration and expiration, with minimal
negative pressure swings during inspiration. The drop in pressure on
inspiration is proportional to the work of breathing. Currently, many
simple continuous-flow circuits with an appropriate reservoir bag or
a Venturi device offer more efficient CPAP than that available from
more expensive and sophisticated ventilators. This is because of the
limitations of the demand valves used in most ventilators. The work
of breathing with a demand valve often is considerably greater than
that needed with a continuous-flow system.

INTERMITTENT MANDATORY VENTILATION

IMV provides a spectrum of ventilatory support between total artificial ventilation, on the one hand, and CPAP or total spontaneous ventilation, on the other (Figure 20.5).

IMV combines conventional IPPV, which delivers a tidal volume at a predetermined frequency, with gas under pressure for spontaneous breathing. The number of mandatory ventilated breaths that the patient receives is titrated against the need for those breaths, as determined by arterial blood gases and clinical assessment. In between the predetermined mandatory breaths, the patient spontaneously breathes via CPAP. IMV is an ideal weaning mode, as the number of mandatory breaths can be reduced according to the patient's need.

SYNCHRONIZED IMV

During synchronized IMV (SIMV), the patient's positive-pressure breaths are synchronized with the inspiratory effort (Figure 20.5). If no inspiratory effort is sensed, a mandatory breath is delivered at a predetermined interval. Despite its theoretical appeal, there is no proven advantage of SIMV over IMV.

MANDATORY MINUTE VOLUME

Mandatory minute volume (MMV) ensures a predetermined minute volume, whether it is composed of spontaneous or mechanical breaths. The major disadvantage of MMV is that the set minute volume can be reached by various inadequate respiratory patterns (eg a minute volume of 6 litres could be made up of four large breaths of 1.5 litres each or 40 breaths of 150 ml each). Some of the more sophisticated ventilators overcome this problem by being programmed to disregard breaths below a certain tidal volume. However, IMV may be more useful than MMV, as it guarantees a minimal mechanically delivered tidal volume as well as a minute volume.

PRESSURE-SUPPORT VENTILATION (INSPIRATORY ASSIST)

This mode is available on many modern ventilators. Each spontaneous breath is sensed and assisted by a pre-set amount of positive pressure (Figure 20.5). It can be used in two ways. Firstly, low levels (2–10 cm H_2O) of 'pressure assist' are needed to overcome the high inherent work of breathing in many modern ventilators during spontaneous respiration. Secondly, high levels (5–50 cm H_2O) of assist can be used as a ventilatory mode in its own right. In other words, when the pressure assist is set higher than the PEEP level, a form of positive-pressure ventilation occurs. It is, in fact, patient-triggered, pressure-limited IPPV. When the assist level is the same as the PEEP level, it becomes CPAP. Obviously the patient must have an adequate spontaneous respiratory rate for this mode to be successful.

The tidal volume delivered will depend on the pre-set level of pressure as well as the underlying lung compliance and resistance. This can result in variable tidal volumes and variable rates of carbon dioxide excretion. However, there is now a trend toward tolerating moderate degrees of hypercarbia as a trade-off when guaranteeing adequate oxygenation at low inspiratory pressures.

Gradually decreasing the level of pre-set inspiratory pressure in the assist mode will add another dimension to weaning (see p. 478).

INVERSE-RATIO VENTILATION

The normal spontaneous inspiration:expiration (I:E) ratio is approximately 1:2. By increasing the I:E ratio to 3:1 or even 4:1, improvement in oxygenation at a lower mean airway pressure can be achieved, probably by gas trapping and a PEEP effect in the alveoli. The technique of reverse-I:E-ratio pressure-limited ventilation with small values of PEEP has been used successfully in patients with acute severe respiratory failure. It should be avoided in patients with acute asthma and used with caution in patients with chronic airway disease or any respiratory disease in which expiration may be delayed. Inverse-ratio ventilation is available on many modern ventilators, as well as any ventilator with separate inspiratory timing and expiratory timing. As is the case for all ventilatory modes, its exact clinical role is not known, but when IMV and pressure support have failed, it may give better ventilation for lower mean airway pressure than can conventional IPPV and PEEP. A patient will require heavy sedation with or without muscle relaxants for this technique to be successful.

AIRWAY-PRESSURE-RELEASE VENTILATION

This technique involves CPAP with intermittent releases of pressure (Figure 20.5). The intermittent release of pressure from the CPAP level is equivalent to expiration with passive exhalation of gas. The lungs are then reinflated to the CPAP level according to pre-set timing in combination with a special valve. The degree of ventilatory assistance provided by airway-pressure-release ventilation will be determined by the frequency and duration of pressure release, the CPAP level, the pressure-release level, the patient's lung-thorax compliance, and the flow resistance in the patient's airways and in the pressure-release valve. Preliminary results with this technique suggest improved gas exchange with lower mean intrathoracic pressures. However, it is still in its developmental stage and is not yet available on many ventilators.

HIGH-FREQUENCY POSITIVE-PRESSURE VENTILATION

High-frequency positive-pressure ventilation (HFPPV) is a controversial technique that uses small tidal volumes delivered at rapid rates. There are three main types:

- HFPPV, at a frequency of 60–120/min
- high-frequency jet ventilation (HFJV), at 60–300/min (the commonest mode used in clinical practice)
- high-frequency oscillation (HFO), at 300–1,800/min

Despite enormous interest in this area, its clinical application in adults currently is limited largely to use with bronchopleural fistulae, as well as rare cases in which other modes have failed. Currently, the equipment is complicated, the parameters are not easily monitored, and the gases are difficult to humidify.

SIGH

Many ventilators still have a 'sigh' function, supposedly simulating a physiological sigh or yawn. The purpose is to prevent atelectasis, which may occur during positive-pressure ventilation. The sigh mode is rarely used, nor probably needed, as PEEP and CPAP are effective for recruiting alveoli and preventing atelectasis.

INSPIRATORY WAVEFORMS

Although many ventilators provide inspiratory-waveform options such as square waves and accelerating or decelerating waves, none has been shown to have a distinct advantage over others in clinical practice. Moreover, the waveforms are generated within the ventilator and become modified in the ventilator tubing, the artificial airway, and the patient's own airway.

NEGATIVE-PRESSURE VENTILATION

Interest is being rekindled in this area as the adverse effects of positive-pressure ventilation are increasingly being realized. However the machinery is expensive and cumbersome and, as yet, is not well suited to many critically ill patients.

MASK VENTILATION

Non-invasive positive-pressure ventilation via mouth or nose has been used successfully in patients with neuromuscular weakness (eg Duchenne's muscular dystrophy), restrictive chest-wall defects, and chronic lung disease. It is usually used to provide support during sleep. Mask ventilation has also been used, with some success, for patients with acute lung injuries. One of two modes is commonly used: either pressure-support ventilation or patient-triggered volume-limited IPPV.

EXTRACORPOREAL TECHNIQUES

When conventional ventilation fails to oxygenate adequately or to remove carbon dioxide, extracorporeal techniques are sometimes used. Because they are expensive and time-consuming, with a high incidence of complications, we need good evidence that extracorporeal techniques make a difference in outcomes. Initial trials using extracorporeal oxygenation failed to show any difference in outcomes. Since then, the following two promising techniques have been reported.

Low-frequency positive-pressure ventilation with extracorporeal removal of CO_2

This technique is designed to protect the lung from the adverse effects of pressure by insufflating oxygen at low pressures, ventilating at very low rates, and removing CO_2 by an extracorporeal circuit. The results in patients with severe respiratory failure have been impressive, but the technique requires a high level of expertise, expensive equipment, and considerable manpower.

Intravascular oxygenation (IVOX)

This technique involves delivering oxygen via a device inserted into a large vein. Gas exchange occurs over the surface area of the device. The degree of gas exchange is limited by the size of the device and its surface area, and IVOX can only supplement the existing, albeit inadequate, gas exchange. It is expensive, and its use, so far, has been limited to less than 3 weeks. Systemic anticoagulation is required.

INDEPENDENT LUNG VENTILATION (see p. 437)
ADJUSTING THE VENTILATOR

Familiarize yourself with the particular ventilator used in your own ICU. Read the instruction manual; use it and discuss it. THEN READ THE INSTRUCTIONS MANUAL AGAIN.

BASIC PRINCIPLES

GUARANTEE VENTILATION   Watch the patient's chest movements initially, not the machine.

FIO2 AND PEEP LEVEL   Set levels to achieve optimal oxygenation (see p. 362). Where possible, keep the PEEP below 10 cm H_2O and the F_{IO_2} below 0.5.

INSPIRATORY PRESSURE   Wherever possible, reduce the PIP to less than 35 cm H_2O.

MONITOR   Both the low- and high-pressure alarms should be monitored in order to minimize barotrauma and warn of disconnection.

PORTABLE VENTILATORS

Transport of seriously ill ventilated patients is increasingly necessary, both between hospitals and within a hospital. The oxygen-powered, fluid-logic-controlled portable ventilators are ideally suited for this purpose. However, they are not suitable for spontaneous respiration, and a separate circuit and one-way valve should be incorporated for that purpose.

WEANING

Weaning is the process of gradually reducing a patient's dependence on ventilatory support. Because of the detrimental effects of artificial ventilation and positive intrathoracic pressure, patients should not be ventilated for any longer than is necessary.

Traditionally, weaning did not commence until the original disease process had been reversed and the F_{IO_2} and PEEP levels were low. Moreover, there had been an obsession with predicting which patients would be capable of being weaned. That is no longer necessary.

With increasing dependence on alternative modes of ventilation, weaning has now become a continual and dynamic process. In contrast with the former pattern of sedating, paralysing, and taking over the patient's ventilatory function totally, various ventilatory modes have been developed that encourage spontaneous breathing and are appropriate for a particular patient at a particular time in a given illness. A general approach (Table 20.2) is to correct as many of the reversible abnormalities as possible (eg electrolytes and fluid status), choose a ventilatory circuit and mode that will require minimal work for spontaneous breathing, and then give it a go! In other words, continually adjust the ventilatory mode and settings to the patient's needs. The number of breaths and the level of pressure assistance should be continually reduced, weaning the patient in the same way we continually wean from inotropes (ie based on regular patient assessments). There may still be a place for more aggressive weaning during the day, and resting the patient at night, with, for example, more mandatory breaths or higher levels of pressure support.

PATIENT ASSESSMENT DURING WEANING

VITAL SIGNS Signs such as respiratory rate, tidal volume, oxygen saturation levels, pulse rate, colour, and blood pressure must all be monitored carefully during weaning.

TABLE 20.2 OPTIMIZING THE WEANING PROCESS

Provide reassurance and explanation.

Treat any underlying disease, and correct any reversible problems (eg drain effusions).

Use maximum diameter for artificial airways.

Increase trigger sensitivity.

Adjust inspiratory support.

Use high flow rates or large, compliant reservoir bags.

Suction and attempt to reduce airway secretions.

Place patient in upright posture when possible.

Limit the length and weight of ventilator tubing.

Limit CO_2 production (eg fever).

Correct electrolyte and acid–base disorders.

Relieve pain.

Reverse bronchospasm.

Try to facilitate adequate sleep.

Ensure nutritional support.

PATIENT APPEARANCE Monitoring the clinical appearance of the patient is a useful way of assessing the success of weaning. Signs of increased work of breathing include tachypnoea, sweating, increased use of accessory muscles, obvious distress, and unco-ordinated respirations. Trained nursing and medical staff in intensive care can recognize these signs at an early stage and adjust the weaning process accordingly.

ARTERIAL CARBON DIOXIDE Monitoring the partial pressure of arterial carbon dioxide is another way of assessing weaning. There are many reasons why the $Paco_2$ can be higher than normal in the seriously ill, and as long as the arterial pH is above a certain limit (eg hydrogen-ion concentration < 63 nmol/L or pH > 7.2), a high $Paco_2$ is not necessarily unacceptable. During weaning, the $Paco_2$ will transiently rise, until the patient readjusts to levels of $Paco_2$ and pH that will determine the respiratory rate. Levels of $Paco_2$ commonly will be around 60–90 mm Hg (8–12 kPa) during weaning.

WEANING SEQUENCE

One should aim for the following as soon as possible:

1. Wean the patient from controlled ventilation to spontaneous breathing – CPAP.

2. Wean F_{IO_2} levels to less than 0.5.

3. Wean PEEP levels (not below 5 cm H_2O).

TECHNIQUES FOR WEANING

Intermittent mandatory ventilation (see p. 472)

IMV provides a natural basis for weaning. Patients should be encouraged to breathe spontaneously on CPAP during acute respiratory failure. When that is not possible, the number of mandatory breaths from the ventilator should be adjusted according to need. Similarly, and whenever possible, the number of mandatory breaths should be decreased in the same way that inotropes are increased or decreased to support cardiovascular function.

Pressure-support ventilation (see p. 473)

By gradually decreasing the pre-set amount of patient-triggered positive-pressure support, another dimension to weaning is possible. Many modern ventilators have this mode, as well as IMV, and the two usually are used together to facilitate weaning.

T-piece system

Weaning with a T-piece system involves alternating between breathing spontaneously through a T-piece circuit and using mandatory ventilation. The time period for each will vary according to the patient's condition. This all-or-none technique has been largely superseded by IMV and pressure-support ventilation. Unlike IMV, a T-piece circuit does not have the flexibility for a specific amount of controlled ventilatory support to be tailored for each patient.

THE WORK OF BREATHING

The work of breathing must be minimized if there is to be success in weaning. It may even be possible to avoid the use of ventilation if the work of breathing can be reduced. Many of the newer modes of ventilatory support can specifically decrease the work of breathing (eg CPAP and pressure-support ventilation), so that mandatory IPPV can be avoided. The work of breathing is related to the pressure generated by the respiratory muscles when displacing a volume of gas.

MEASURING THE WORK OF BREATHING

It is very difficult to get accurate measurements of the work of breathing in intensive care. The current techniques are complicated and require sophisticated technology. In clinical practice, patient observation is often used. If the work of breathing is excessive, the patient will look distressed, sweaty, and tachypnoeic with excessive use of the accessory muscles of respiration. If the patient is being ventilated or is on CPAP, the initial drop in inspiratory pressure necessary to achieve a spontaneous breath will correlate well with the work of breathing. A high negative pressure means increased work of breathing.

CLINICAL ASPECTS OF THE WORK OF BREATHING

To minimize the work of breathing, meticulous attention must be paid to the various patient- and equipment-related determinants. It is not simply a matter of increasing the pressure support or maintaining IPPV in order to 'rest the patient'. Often ventilation can be avoided, or weaning facilitated, by meticulously examining every component that may be contributing to increase the work of breathing.

Patient determinants

1. Airway (resistive forces)

  Secretions: Even minimal secretions can reduce the airway diameter and increase the work of breathing. Regularly perform airway suction and physiotherapy.

Bronchospasm: A decreased airway diameter is a crucial factor in causing increased resistance and increased work of breathing. Bronchospasm must be reversed with bronchodilators.

2. Chest wall and lung compliance (elastic forces) Treat any underlying disease [eg adult respiratory distress syndrome (ARDS), pneumonia, atelectasis] that decreases lung compliance. Sit the patient upright in order to increase compliance. Aggressively drain air pockets or pleural effusions.

3. Minute volume and CO_2 production The major determinant of the work of breathing is the minute volume. This can be reduced by decreasing physiological and anatomic dead space. Excessive CO_2 production can cause increased minute volume and should be limited by reducing fever and perhaps reducing the carbohydrate intake. Shivering, agitation, seizures, myoclonus, and any other cause of excessive muscle activity can also increase CO_2 production.

4. Expiratory work Increasingly it is being realized that expiration requires work in certain pathological conditions (eg asthma) and in all patients who are intubated and connected to breathing systems.

Resistance can be reduced by minimizing airway secretions and bronchospasm, as well as by reducing the length and increasing the diameter of artificial airways and circuits. Some PEEP valves (eg mushroom and scissor valves) have high expiratory resistance. PEEP levels should be increased when intrinsic PEEP is suspected (see p. 451).

Equipment determinants

1. Artificial airway The single most important equipment-related determinant of the work of breathing is the diameter of the artificial airway. A tube with the largest possible diameter should be employed. For this reason, orotracheal tubes and tracheostomy tubes have distinct advantages over nasotracheal tubes in spontaneously breathing patients. The larger the diameter of the tube, the less the resistance. Tracheostomy tubes of 8 mm for females and 9 mm for males will significantly reduce the work of breathing, as compared with tubes that are even one size smaller. The length of the tube and an absence of built-up secretions are also important. Similarly, kinks should be avoided, and angles minimized, and large connectors should be used.

2. Circuit and humidifier An increased length of tubing will cause increased resistance. Humidifiers with inspiratory underwater baffles should be avoided, and condenser humidifiers should be changed regularly.

3. CPAP devices A continuous-flow device usually will decrease the work of breathing, as compared with the demand-valve systems incorporated into modern ventilators. Large compliant reservoir bags are more effective than small non-compliant ones, and whereas high flow rates in the ventilator can decrease the work of breathing, turbulence can result if the flow is too high, thus increasing the work of breathing.

4. Ventilators Techniques such as pressure support (see p. 473) were developed to decrease the inherently high work of breathing with demand-valve systems. The demand valve should be adjusted to maximum sensitivity, and the peak inspiratory flow rate needs to be high (at least 4 times the minute volume, ie 50 L/min). A small amount of PEEP (3–5 cm H_2O) and pressure support should be used for all spontaneously breathing patients supported by a ventilator.

HUMIDIFICATION

Whenever the nose and mouth are bypassed, inspired gases should be humidified and heated artificially. The following are minimum requirements for humidification:

WATER CONTENT The 'absolute' or maximum humidity at a temperature of 37°C is 44 mg/L; this is achieved with normal nose breathing. For artificial ventilation, it is suggested that gases have a water content of at least 30–40 mg/L and be heated to 32–37°C in order to protect ciliary function.

RESISTANCE For spontaneous respiration, resistance should be minimal [<3 cm $H_2O \cdot L^{-1} \cdot s^{-1}$ (<0.29 kPa $\cdot L^{-1} \cdot s^{-1}$)].

SAFETY ALARMS Alarms are needed as protection against overheating and over-hydration in hot-water-bath humidifiers.

CONDENSER HUMIDIFIERS

A condenser humidifier consists of a tube containing material that conserves heat and water from the patient's expiratory efforts.

Advantages
- simple
- safe
- disposable

Disadvantages
- inefficient humidification with high flow rates and high F_{IO_2}
- increased dead space
- risk of infection
- increased risk of endotracheal-tube occlusion
- resistance can increase with use

Their main disadvantage – inefficient humidification – makes condenser humidifiers suitable only for short-term artificial ventilation, such as intra-operatively. The place of condenser humidifiers in the ICU has not been precisely determined. Because of the increased dead space and resistance, as well as the increased tendency for occlusion, they should be avoided during any long-term ventilatory mode that employs spontaneous breathing.

HOT-WATER-BATH HUMIDIFIERS

These devices provide the most common form of humidification in the ICU. Inspired gas passes over the water surface before delivery to the patient. Modifications can include increasing the surface area by using coils of absorbing paper and using heated delivery lines to prevent condensation.

The temperatures of the water bath and heating wires should be adjusted to achieve a delivery temperature of close to 37°C.

Disadvantages

Infection The water reservoir and tubing should be changed every 24–48 hours. Only sterile water should be used.

Over-heating Adequate alarm and safety devices should be employed to prevent over-heating and hyperpyrexia.

Inadequate humidification Flow rates for fully humidified gas as high as 60 L/min can be achieved with some of the more modern humidifiers. If higher flows are required, a dual system of gas delivery using two humidifiers may be necessary.

TROUBLESHOOTING

FIGHTING THE VENTILATOR

IS THE PROBLEM WITH THE PATIENT OR WITH THE VENTILATOR?

OBSERVE FOR THE AIR ENTRY.

TAKE THE PATIENT OFF THE VENTILATOR, AND 'BAG' THE PATIENT.

Patient

Listen for air entry.

Exclude the possibility of hypoxia and hypercarbia.

Check the chest x-ray.

Consider providing reassurance, relieving pain, or increasing the sedation.

Often a ventilated patient will be 'distressed' because of the increased work of breathing associated with the underlying lung disease: decreased lung compliance (eg ARDS, pneumonia) or increased resistance (eg asthma).

Ventilator

Is the airway patent? If in doubt, change the endotracheal tube or tracheostomy tube.

Check the ventilator function while 'bagging' the patient.

Check the circuit, including the humidifier (especially if using a heat-and-moisture humidifier, which can develop increased resistance over time).

Eliminate sources of increased work when the patient is spontaneously breathing (see p. 481):

Check the airway diameter and the length of the artificial airway. Ideally, adult males should have, as a minimum, a 9-mm-diameter tube, and adult women an 8-mm tube.

> CPAP systems: Spontaneous-breathing systems should have minimal respiratory-pressure swings (see p. 472).
> Check that the ventilator settings match the patient's needs (see p. 470). For instance, one may need to
> increase tidal volume
> increase pressure support
> decrease trigger threshold
> increase flow rate
> increase the number of breaths on IMV

FURTHER READING

General

Bushman, J. A. (1992). Ventilators and humidifiers. In *Scientific Foundations of Anaesthesia: The Basis of Intensive Care*, ed. C. Scurr, S. Feldman, & N. Soni, pp. 698–708. Oxford: Heinemann.

Perel, A., & Stock, M. C. (eds.) (1992). *Handbook of Mechanical Ventilatory Support*. Baltimore: Williams & Wilkins.

Rie, M. A., & Wilson, R. S. (1983). Acute respiratory failure. In *Care of the Critically Ill Patient*, ed. J. Tinker & M. Rapin, pp. 311–40. Berlin: Springer-Verlag.

Shapiro, B. A. (1984). Airway pressure therapy for acute restrictive pulmonary pathology. In *Textbook of Critical Care*, ed. W. C. Shoemaker, W. L. Thompson, & P. R. Holbrook, pp. 224–38. Philadelphia: Saunders.

Shapiro, B. A., & Cane, R. D. (eds.) (1987). Positive airway pressure therapy: IPPV and PEEP. *Anaesthesiology Clinics of North America* 5:695–913 (symposium issue).

Artificial Airways

Benjamin, B. (1993). Prolonged intubation of the larynx: endoscopic diagnosis, classification and treatment. *Annals of Otology, Rhinology and Laryngology (Suppl.)* 102:1–15.

Berlauk, J. F. (1986). Prolonged endotracheal intubation vs tracheostomy. *Critical Care Medicine* 14:742–5.

Mehta, S., & Michiewicz, M. (1985). Pressure in large-volume, low-pressure cuffs: its significance, measurement and regulation. *Intensive Care Medicine* 11:267–72.

Positive End-Expiratory Pressure

Kacmarek, R. M., & Goulet, R. L. (1987). PEEP devices. *Anaesthesiology Clinics of North America* 5:757–76.
Mancebo, J. (1992). PEEP, ARDS and alveolar recruitment. *Intensive Care Medicine* 18:383–5.

Complications of Positive Intrathoracic Pressure

Dreyfuss, D., & Saumon, G. (1992). Barotrauma is volutrauma, but which volume is responsible? *Intensive Care Medicine* 18:139–41.
Hillman, K. (1985). Pulmonary barotrauma. *Clinical Anaesthesiology* 3:877–97.
Vender, J. S. (1987). Complications and physiologic alterations of positive airway pressure therapy. *Anaesthesiology Clinics of North America* 5:807–19.

Alternative Modes of Ventilation

Froese, A. B. (1984). High frequency ventilation: a critical assessment. In *Critical Care: State of the Art*, vol. 5, ed. W. C. Shoemaker, pp. A1–55. Fullerton, CA: Society of Critical Care Medicine.
Gurevitch, M. J., van Dyke, J., Young, E. S., & Jackson, K. (1986). Improved oxygenation and lower peak airway pressure in severe respiratory distress syndrome. Treatment with inverse ratio ventilation. *Chest* 89:211–13.
Hickling, K. G., Henderson, S. J., & Jackson, R. (1990). Low mortality associated with low volume pressure limited ventilation with permissive hypercapnia in severe adult respiratory distress syndrome. *Intensive Care Medicine* 16:372–7.
Lawrence, P. J. (1985). Alternatives to intermittent positive pressure ventilation (IPPV). *Clinical Anaesthesiology* 3:849–75.
MacIntyre, N. R. (1986). Respiratory function during pressure support ventilation. *Chest* 89:677–85.
Mushin, W. W., Rendell-Baker, L., Thompson, P. W., & Mapleson, W. (eds.) (1980). *Automatic Ventilation of the Lungs*. Oxford: Blackwell.
Sassoon, C. S. H. (1991). Positive pressure ventilation. Alternate modes. *Chest* 100:1421–9.
Slutsky, A. S. (1991). High frequency ventilation. *Intensive Care Medicine* 17:375–6.
Stock, M. C., Downs, J. B., & Frolicher, D. A. (1987). Airway pressure release ventilation. *Critical Care Medicine* 15:462–5.
Willatts, S. M. (1985). Alternative modes of ventilation. Part I. Disadvantages of controlled ventilation: intermittent mandatory ventilation. *Intensive Care Medicine* 11:51–5.

Willatts, S. M. Alternative modes of ventilation. Part II. High and low frequency positive pressure ventilation, PEEP, CPAP, inverse ratio ventilation. *Intensive Care Medicine* 11:115–22.

Work of Breathing

Marini, J. J. (1986). The physiologic determinants of ventilator dependence. *Respiratory Care* 31:271–82.
Marini, J. J., Rodriguez, R. M., & Lamb, V. T. (1986). Bedside estimation of the inspiratory work of breathing during mechanical ventilation. *Chest* 89:902–9.
Stock, M. C. (1992). The oxygen cost of breathing. *Chest* 10:1486–7.

Portable Ventilators

Phillips, G. D., Coates, D. L. B., Runciman, W. B., & Vedig, A. E. (1983). Versatile portable respirator. *Anaesthesia and Intensive Care* 10:281–2.

Humidification

Ogina, H., Kopotic, R., & Mannino, F. L. (1985). Moisture-conserving efficiency of condenser humidifiers. *Anaesthesia* 40:990–5.
Poulton, T. J., & Downs, J. B. (1981). Humidification of rapidly flowing gas. *Critical Care Medicine* 9:59–63.

21

CARDIORESPIRATORY MONITORING

- There is no single value for any physiological variable that can be said to be the normal value. Measurements should be interpreted more in terms of being adequate or inadequate.
- Continuous monitoring of oxygenation is indispensable in intensive care.
- It is important to understand the limitations of sophisticated invasive monitoring and the value of clinical observations and simple monitoring.

The heart and lungs together are responsible for pumping oxygenated blood to the tissues. The process of monitoring the effectiveness of oxygenation cannot be broken apart and divided between the cardiovascular and respiratory systems.

Although intensive care medicine traditionally has been associated with sophisticated, expensive, and invasive techniques, that orientation is now being critically examined. There is a trend toward simpler, continuous monitoring techniques that are non-invasive.

It is important to display physiological variables clearly and to interpret their significance accurately. A single flowchart will facilitate documentation and interpretation. However, such information can reflect only an instant in time. Continuous displays of measurements such as ECG, pulse oximetry, and intravascular pressures are often employed to track the more useful information revealed by trend data.

Current techniques for cardiorespiratory monitoring often are limited to global and relatively crude measurements. The obsession in the 1970s with generating numbers derived from the pulmonary artery catheter has been largely superseded by the desire to achieve continuous, non-invasive monitoring. However, even the new devices designed for that purpose usually have been limited to measurements of global functions, such as arterial oxygen saturation, blood pressure, and expired volume of carbon dioxide. More complex and more invasive measurements, such as determining the relationship between oxygen delivery (Do_2) and oxygen consumption ($\dot{V}o_2$), are difficult to perform, prone to inaccuracies, and hard to interpret, and at best they tell us about the whole body, rather than the status of individual tissues (see p. 376). It is to be hoped that the next major breakthrough in monitoring will bring us practical, inexpensive, non-invasive means to achieve continuous monitoring of cardiorespiratory function at the tissue or cellular level (Table 21.1).

NON-INVASIVE MONITORING

HEART RATE AND RHYTHM

Although it can be affected by many factors in the seriously ill, the heart rate remains a valuable source of information and a parameter that is easy to measure. Most seriously ill patients are connected to an ECG monitor with a continuously displayed ECG trace, with alarms to detect the extremes of heart rate. In addition to heart rate, ECG monitoring can detect arrhythmias and pacemaker functioning, and ST-segment analysis can reveal myocardial ischaemia.

BLOOD PRESSURE

Vital organs depend on autoregulation for their blood flow. The kidney, heart, and brain need effective driving pressures across their vascular beds for adequate perfusion. Non-invasive and invasive techniques for measuring blood pressure correlate well. There are increasing numbers of automatic devices that can display non-invasively measured blood pressure.

PERIPHERAL/CORE TEMPERATURE DIFFERENCE

The relative 'coolness' of distal limbs can serve as a rapid and useful guide to peripheral perfusion. Measuring the central temperature and comparing it to the measured peripheral temperature (eg temperature of the big toe) probably is not necessary. Estimating the degree of coolness of the periphery (eg toes, feet, lower half of the leg) can give an empirical impression of circulatory status. The difference between peripheral and central temperatures cannot be used to dis-

TABLE 21.1   NON-INVASIVE AND INVASIVE CARDIORESPIRATORY MONITORING

Non-invasive cardiorespiratory monitoring
Pulse rate and rhythm
Blood pressure
Peripheral perfusion
Temperature (core/peripheral difference)
Urine output
Echocardiography
Non-invasive cardiac output
Radionuclide imaging
Respiratory rate and character
Tidal volume
Pulse oximetry
Capnography
Chest radiograph
Fluid balance
Invasive cardiorespiratory monitoring
Central venous pressure
Arterial pressure monitoring
Pulmonary artery catheterization
Pulmonary artery pressure
PAWP
Cardiac output
Oxygen consumption
Oxygen delivery
Mixed venous oximetry
Lung water

criminate among cardiac failure, hypovolaemia, and other forms of cardiovascular failure and cannot be quantified.

URINE OUTPUT

Hourly measurements of urine output can give an excellent reflection of general tissue perfusion. This method loses some of its value in the presence of drugs, such as diuretics, or when renal function is compromised.

RESPIRATORY RATE AND TYPE OF BREATHING

Simple measurements or observations of respiratory rate and type of breathing can provide information about the disease process, as well as the effects of drugs and lung mechanics.

TIDAL VOLUME

Tidal volume is relatively easy to measure in a spontaneously breathing, intubated patient. Most ventilators have mechanisms for measuring and displaying tidal volume and minute volume. However, even more important than tidal volume or minute volume is the end product of effective ventilation: adequate gas exchange (see p. 353).

CHEST RADIOGRAPH (see Chapter 18)

A chest x-ray should be obtained at least once each day for all seriously ill patients. Additional x-rays will be needed following major changes in clinical status or following intubation and central-line placement. The radiography should be performed, whenever possible, with the patient sitting upright, so that abnormal fluid and air collections can be seen. The chest x-ray can allow for effective monitoring of fluid status, as lung water content will correlate reasonably well with chest x-ray density.

FLUID BALANCE (see p. 59)

Fluid balance has some bearing on intravascular-fluid status, but there are many better and more direct measurements. Although fluid balance can give an excellent indication of the fluid losses from certain sites (eg nasogastric contents, wounds), the net figure measured every 24 hours can be misleading, as there are many 'unseen' inputs and outtakes that are not measured (eg water of oxidation, insensible losses). Furthermore, a single net figure cannot indicate which of the body's fluid spaces is depleted, nor what fluid should be used for replenishment (see Chapter 4).

TISSUE PERFUSION

Doppler laser devices for measuring blood flow in the skin may become more widely employed. Currently, we estimate general tissue perfusion on the basis of parameters such as urine output and peripheral skin temperature.

TISSUE pH

The presence of compensated shock is difficult to detect with global measurements of variables such as blood pressure, pulse rate, cardiac output, $\dot{V}o_2$, and Do_2. Moreover, compensated shock can result in ischaemia of organs such as the gastro-intestinal tract (GIT). The GIT is selectively impaired in patients who are in shock. It is one of the first organs to be affected and one of the last to be restored by resuscitation. Measurement of GIT perfusion is therefore important and can be estimated on the basis of the intramural pH (pH_i). This is indirectly measured by tonometry: A catheter with a Silastic balloon at its tip is introduced into the stomach or into the sigmoid colon. The balloon is filled with saline and allowed to equilibrate with the luminal Pco_2, which is assumed to be the same as the Pco_2 of the superficial mucosa. Determination of the arterial bicarbonate concentration will allow calculation of the pH_i, using the Henderson-Hasselbalch equation. This measurement reflects splanchnic tissue oxygenation and is an indirect and early means to estimate global tissue oxygenation.

Transcutaneous Po_2 monitoring can also provide an early and accurate non-invasive indicator of the adequacy of oxygen delivery to the skin (see p. 508).

CAPNOGRAPHY

A capnometer measures the concentration of carbon dioxide (CO_2), usually by infrared analysis. A device that continuously records and displays CO_2 concentrations as a waveform is a capnograph – the tracing or recording paper being called a capnogram (Figure 21.1). Capnography is the study of the shape of the curve that shows the changing concentrations of CO_2 in expired gas. The alveolar CO_2 will

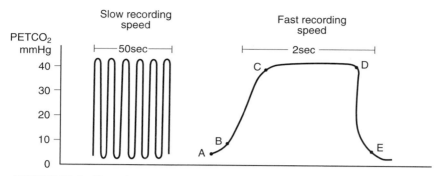

FIGURE 21.1 Normal capnogram.

depend on the amount produced by the body and on the adequacy of transport to and across the lungs.

POTENTIAL USES OF CAPNOGRAPHY IN INTENSIVE CARE

• Capnography can be used to select optimal ventilator settings and reduce the need for invasive blood-gas analysis.

• At intubation, a normal end-tidal CO_2 can help confirm tracheal placement of the ETT.

• End-tidal CO_2 monitoring can warn of sudden changes in the breathing system because of leaks, disconnections, or obstruction.

• Capnography can give an indication of the efficiency of the weaning process.

• Capnography can provide information about hypoventilation and hyperventilation, apnoea, and periodic breathing.

• CO_2 elimination and physiological dead space can be measured by measuring the CO_2 fraction in mixed expired gases. This can give an indication of metabolic activity.

• A reduction in cardiac output will be accompanied by a reduction in expired CO_2. This can result from any form of shock. Air embolism or blockage of the pulmonary capillaries due to any cause can also decrease the expired CO_2. Mixed venous CO_2 is more dependent on changes in alveolar ventilation than on cardiac output. A difference between the concentrations of arterial CO_2 and mixed venous CO_2 is most likely to be produced by low cardiac output. Tissue hypoxia can be assumed when this difference exceeds 10 ml/dl.

There are limitations to capnography with regard to the predictability of the correlation between end-tidal CO_2 and $Paco_2$. In patients with respiratory failure or rapidly changing cardiovascular conditions, that correlation is even less reliable. Although capnography theoretically should have many uses in the ICU, it has not yet universally replaced intermittent arterial Pco_2 monitoring in the way that pulse oximetry has come to be used as a continuous form of oxygenation monitoring (see p. 507).

PULSE OXIMETRY

Pulse oximetry is discussed in detail elsewhere (see p. 507).

ECHOCARDIOGRAPHY

Echocardiography is increasingly being used to assess cardiac function (Table 21.2). It can be used to diagnose abnormalities of structure (eg valves, pericardial effusions) as well as to assess functioning by directly revealing wall movement and defining the chamber dimensions throughout the cardiac cycle, thereby allowing estimation of the ejection fraction. The technique also can be used to diagnose pulmonary embolism (see p. 452), valvular infections, and aortic dissection. Its use in the ICU has been limited because of the distortion of ultrasound waves passing through air and bone. In up to 30% of seriously ill patients, hyperinflated lungs due to underlying abnormalities or secondary to ventilation can cause inadequate images. The use of transoesophageal echocardiography (TOE) will give a much cleaner image of the heart and may increasingly be used for assessment of the critically ill.

NON-INVASIVE DETERMINATION OF CARDIAC OUTPUT

There are many techniques for non-invasive determination of cardiac output. One technique employs Doppler ultrasound velocimetry in conjunction with ultrasound echo imaging of the ascending aorta in order to determine stroke volume. The product of stroke volume and heart rate is then used to determine cardiac output. All of these measurements are non-invasive. However, this technique involves many assumptions and has inherent inaccuracies, and as yet there is no universal agreement on its correlation with more established techniques.

TABLE 21.2 APPLICATIONS OF TRANSOESOPHAGEAL ECHOCARDIOGRAPHY

Continuous intraoperative monitoring (eg myocardial ischaemia, adequacy of surgical repair)

Thoracic aortic abnormality (eg dissection, aneurysm)

Valvular function (particularly the mitral valve)

Excluding infective endocarditis and its complications

Intracardiac masses (eg thrombi, tumours)

Coronary artery disease

Congenital heart disease

RADIONUCLIDE IMAGING

The use of radionuclide imaging is rapidly expanding in intensive care, and these procedures can be performed at the bedside with portable cameras. The principle is to use an unstable structure (a radionuclide) that emits energy as it assumes a more stable structure. That energy is recorded on film, after which the signal is amplified and converted into electrical energy and finally analysed by computer. It can be used in the following applications:

TESTS FOR MYOCARDIAL-PERFUSION TISSUE INJURY These tests can use a variety of isotopes [eg thallium 201, ^{99m}Tc-pyrophosphate (^{99m}Tc-PYP)] to make 'hot-spot' scans. These are mainly used to define the area of damage in suspected cases of myocardial infarction.

ECG-GATED CARDIAC SCINTIGRAPHY After the patient's blood cells have been labelled and reinjected, a camera linked to an ECG monitor collects data from many cardiac cycles. Left and right ventricular volumes can be estimated, ejection fractions calculated, and heart-wall motion assessed.

INVASIVE MONITORING

MONITORING OF ARTERIAL BLOOD PRESSURE

Direct measurement of arterial pressure is common in the ICU, both for continuous monitoring and for blood sampling. It is therefore lit-

TABLE 21.3 SOME LIMITATIONS OF CARDIORESPIRATORY MEASUREMENTS AND MONITORING

Haemoglobin saturation

Only measured saturations should be used when calculating the shunt equation and D_{O_2} and $\dot{V}_{O_2}$, as there can be large differences between measured and calculated oxygen saturations.

Arterial pressure

Direct monitoring is more accurate than indirect pressure measurement.

The femoral artery is the best site for accurate pressure measurements.

Short, non-compliant catheters and extension tubing should be used.

Avoid bubbles and clots in the system.

Atrial pressures

With the patient supine, the mid-axillary line is the standard place for atrial pressure measurement.

The pulmonary artery waveform display is necessary to detect inadvertent wedging and over-wedging and to visualise respiratory variations.

End-expiratory readings should be used.

PAWP measurements should be from a proximal branch of the pulmonary artery in a West zone III part of the lung.

Remember the limitations of PAWP as representative of left ventricular end-diastolic volume or lung capillary pressure.

Cardiac output

The temperature difference between injectate and blood temperature should be maximal.

Standardize injections to end-expiration.

---

tle trouble to connect a transducer and monitor the arterial blood pressure continuously. Directly measured arterial pressure may vary from that measured indirectly. Both techniques have inherent inaccuracies, and, as with most measurements, the trend should be looked at, rather than an absolute reading (Table 21.3).

ARTERIAL CATHETERS The modified Allen test is rarely used now to assess collateral flow before insertion of a catheter. Usually a catheter will be inserted into the radial artery, but the dorsalis pedis, brachial, axillary, and femoral arteries can also be used. There does not appear to be a higher incidence of infection with femoral artery cannulation.

If there are no signs of infection, the catheter does not need to be changed routinely.

The main complication of arterial catheterization is thrombosis. It is common, but it rarely causes serious morbidity. The catheter should be removed immediately if there are any signs of ischaemia. Complications such as emboli, haemorrhage, infection, and inadvertent injection of drugs are much rarer. Very small amounts of air can travel retrogradely into cerebral vessels, and so great care must be exercised, especially during flushing.

CENTRAL VENOUS PRESSURE

In most cases, a seriously ill patient will have a line inserted into a central vein to facilitate drug and fluid infusion. As with arterial monitoring, the central venous line can also be used for pressure monitoring.

The central venous pressure (CVP) is normally 0–8 mm Hg (0–1.1 kPa), but there are many possible causes of right-side heart dysfunction and high pulmonary artery pressure in the critically ill. This can mean that the 'normal' CVP is high. A HIGH CVP MAY BE A REFLECTION OF PULMONARY ABNORMALITY, HIGH PULMONARY ARTERY PRESSURE, OR HIGH VENTILATORY PRESSURE, RATHER THAN A REFLECTION OF CARDIAC DYSFUNCTION OR INTRAVASCULAR VOLUME DISTURBANCE. Moreover, the CVP can be high, normal, or low in the presence of hypovolaemia. Trends, rather than single readings, must be looked at. Right atrial pressure often is not a reflection of left atrial pressure in the seriously ill.

A catheter can be inserted from the cubital fossa or directly from the thorax via the subclavian or internal jugular vein. The femoral vein can also be used. Complications of central venous cannulation can include pneumothorax, arterial puncture, haemothorax, nerve damage, air embolism, catheter embolism, cardiac perforation and tamponade, venous thrombosis, and embolism, as well as infection. These complications are common, but serious complications occur in fewer that 2% of these patients, and death is extremely uncommon.

A chest x-ray should always be obtained after insertion of a central catheter, to check for positioning and complications (eg pneumothorax, mediastinal bleeding). If infection is suspected, the catheter should be removed, the skin site should be swabbed, and material adhering to the tip or intradermal section should be cultured.

PULMONARY ARTERY CATHETER

No other instrument is so strongly associated with the practice of intensive care medicine as the flow-directed pulmonary artery (PA) catheter. To 'Swan' a patient, or to put in a 'Ganz', has become one of the hallmarks of our specialty. It became an impressive and unusual skill amongst those practising in the ICU. The mystique became exaggerated because of the enormous numbers of figures and amounts of data that could be generated from a few measurements. Such abundant figures often served to complicate a simple picture. The catheter itself probably was over-used. As in the case of many innovations in medicine, we are now critically redefining the role of the PA catheter. It is expensive and needs complicated machinery to support it; it also requires valuable labour time to insert it and maintain it. That, of course, could be justified if it could be shown to significantly affect patient outcomes. Unfortunately, that has never been demonstrated. Furthermore, measurements of parameters such as pulmonary artery wedge pressure (PAWP) may be of limited value in the critically ill, and many of the derived variables, such as pulmonary vascular resistance, may be meaningless.

INDICATIONS The indications for insertion of a PA catheter have not been defined. The rates at which PA catheters are used vary for different ICUs and between different countries. Some physicians insert them whenever a central line is needed; others never use them. We await studies demonstrating the usefulness of PA catheters and detailing the precise indications for their use.

There are two situations in which a PA catheter may prove useful:

1. where there is difficulty with fluid replacement, especially in patients in whom cardiac function is also compromised (see p. 511); this is particularly important in patients with pulmonary oedema and renal failure

2. where oxygen supply and demand need to be more precisely defined (see p. 376)

COMPLICATIONS The complications of using a PA catheter can include all the complications associated with insertion of central venous catheters (see p. 498), as well as arrhythmias (usually terminated by

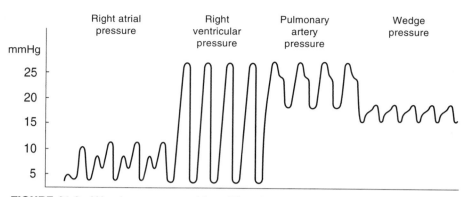

FIGURE 21.2 Waveforms generated by a PA catheter as it is floated into the pulmonary artery.

withdrawal), bundle branch block, pulmonary infarction, pulmonary artery rupture and knotting, and damage to the endocardial structures of the heart.

The risks begin to outweigh the potential benefits after 48 hours, and the catheter should be removed as soon as possible after that time.

PULMONARY ARTERY WEDGE PRESSURE

A PA catheter is inserted in the same way as a central venous catheter. A distal balloon is inflated to facilitate its passage through the right side of the heart into the pulmonary artery (Figure 21.2). When the balloon is wedged in a small branch of the pulmonary artery, the distal lumen should be measuring a pressure that is a reflection of the left atrial pressure, assuming that there is a continuous column of fluid from the tip of the catheter to the left atrium. This assumption may be affected by factors such as alveolar pressure and the zone of the lung where the tip resides. The catheter tip should be placed in zone III of the lung, confirmed by a chest x-ray showing the tip below the left atrium. Alternatively, one can be reasonably sure of correct positioning if the PAWP reading is not markedly affected by a sudden increase or decrease in positive end-expiratory pressure (PEEP). Even when the catheter is correctly positioned, it can be difficult to assess left ventricular preload by PAWP. This is particularly

TABLE 21.4 CONDITIONS THAT CAN RESULT IN DISCREPANCIES BETWEEN PAWP AND LEFT VENTRICULAR END-DIASTOLIC PRESSURE

Mitral valvular disease
Aortic incompetence
IPPV + PEEP
Increased intrathoracic pressure from any cause
Left-to-right intracardiac shunt
Increased pulmonary artery resistance
Tachycardia
Chronic airflow limitation
Catheter not placed in West zone III
Non-compliant left ventricle
Reduced pulmonary vasculature (eg pulmonary embolism or pneumonectomy)

TABLE 21.5 ASSUMPTIONS IN THE MEASUREMENT OF PAWP

Left ventricular end-diastolic volume
↓ Normal LV compliance
Left ventricular end-diastolic pressure
↓ Normal mitral valve
Left atrial pressure
↓ Normal airway pressure
Pulmonary artery wedge pressure
↓ Normal pulmonary vascular resistance
Pulmonary artery diastolic pressure
↓ Right side of heart equals left side
Central venous pressure

the case in the critically ill, where the relationship between end-diastolic pressure and volume (compliance) is non-linear (Tables 21.4 and 21.5).

As a guideline, however, a PAWP of more than 18 mm Hg will be associated with increased lung water in patients with cardiogenic pulmonary oedema. In non-cardiogenic pulmonary oedema (ARDS), the accumulation of lung water will increase as the PAWP increases. However, reduction of preload can lead to decreased cardiac output and generalized ischaemia, especially renal insufficiency in the critically ill. Often, therefore, an increase in lung water will be accepted as the price for adequate tissue perfusion.

CARDIAC OUTPUT

Cardiac output is usually measured by the thermodilution method, using a PA catheter with a thermistor near the tip. A known volume of cold fluid is injected near the right atrium, and the blood flow is calculated from the temperature drop sensed by the thermistor in the pulmonary artery after mixing has occurred. The cardiac output or index can be used as a prognostic indicator and guide to treatment. The adequacy of cardiac output must be judged in light of whether or not oxygen delivery (DO_2) is adequate. Sepsis and trauma are commonly associated with a high cardiac output. It is better to avoid thinking in terms of a 'normal' cardiac output – it is either adequate or inadequate for DO_2 (Table 21.6) (see p. 362).

MIXED VENOUS OXYGEN SATURATION

The mixed venous oxygen saturation ($S\bar{v}O_2$) can be measured intermittently as a sample taken from the PA catheter or continuously by a modified PA catheter with a sensing device at its tip. $S\bar{v}O_2$ reflects the status of oxygen supply and consumption (Table 21.7). The oxygen supply is dependent on cardiac output, haemoglobin concentration, and arterial oxygen saturation. The demand side of the equation depends on cellular extraction of oxygen. Normal $S\bar{v}O_2$ is approximately 60–80%. A decreasing $S\bar{v}O_2$ indicates that the demand is becoming greater than the supply.

When the compensatory mechanisms for matching oxygen demand and supply are exhausted, at approximately 40% of normal levels, lactic acidosis is likely to occur. A sudden significant decrease in $S\bar{v}O_2$ (10–20%) indicates that an urgent clinical review is necessary. An increase in $S\bar{v}O_2$ indicates that the arterial oxygen supply has increased or that the demand has decreased (eg hypothermia, paralysis, sedation); septic shock can also be associated with an increase in $S\bar{v}O_2$, because of decreased tissue oxygen extraction. This may paradoxically occur in the presence of hypotension. Despite its theoretical advan-

TABLE 21.6 SOME MEASURED AND CALCULATED HAEMODYNAMIC VARIABLES WITH NORMAL RANGES

Parameter	Measurement	Normal
Systemic blood pressure (mean)	Direct	120/80 (mean 95) mm Hg [15.9/10.6 (12.5) kPa]
Pulmonary artery pressure (mean) (PAP)	Direct	20/10 (mean 13) mm Hg [2.6/1.3 kPa]
Heart rate (HR)	Direct	80 ± 10 beats/min
PAWP	Direct	10 ± 2 mm Hg (1.3 ± 0.3 kPa)
CVP	Direct	0–8 mm Hg (0–1.1 kPa)
Cardiac index (CI)	Direct	3.0 ± 0.5 L $\cdot$ min^{-1} $\cdot$ m^{-2}
Stroke volume index	CI/HR $\times$ 1,000	40 ± 7 ml $\cdot$ beat^{-1} $\cdot$ m^{-2}
Systemic vascular resistance index (SVRI)	$\dfrac{MAP^a - CVP}{CI} \times 80$ dyn-s $\cdot$ cm^{-5}	1,760–2,600 dyn-s $\cdot$ cm^{-5} $\cdot$ m^{-2}
Pulmonary vascular resistance index (PVRI)	$\dfrac{PAP - PAWP}{CI} \times 80$ dyn-s $\cdot$ cm^{-5}	45–225 dyn-s $\cdot$ cm^{-5} $\cdot$ m^{-2}
O$_2$ consumption ($\dot{V}O_2$)	Direct, or CI $\times$ (CaO$_2$ − C$\bar{v}$O$_2$) $\times$ 10	100–170 ml $\cdot$ min^{-1} $\cdot$ m^{-2}
O$_2$ delivery	CI $\times$ (CaO$_2$) $\times$ 10	520–720 ml $\cdot$ min^{-1} $\cdot$ m^{-2}
O$_2$ extraction	(CaO$_2$ − C$\bar{v}$O$_2$)/CaO$_2$	22–30%

^{a}Mean arterial pressure.

TABLE 21.7 MIXED VENOUS OXYGEN SATURATION

$S\bar{v}o_2$ describes the adequacy of oxygen delivery relative to oxygen consumption
Major determinants:
O_2 consumption
cardiac output
Normal values:
$S\bar{v}o_2$, 60–80%
$P\bar{v}o_2$, 33–55 mm Hg (4.4–7.3 kPa)

tages, the clinical indications for $S\bar{v}o_2$ monitoring are far from clearly defined.

DUAL OXIMETRY

Dual oximetry consists in simultaneous measurements of arterial oxygenation using pulse oximetry and mixed venous oximetry with a modified PA catheter. Dual oximetry provides real-time values for arterial and mixed venous oxygen saturations. When the oxygen supply is estimated by pulse oximetry, variations in $S\bar{v}o_2$ can be more easily interpreted as either decreases in oxygen supply or increases in oxygen demand.

OXYGEN CONSUMPTION AND DELIVERY

Sequential measurements of cardiac output, oxygen consumption ($\dot{V}o_2$), and Do_2 will reveal the point at which further increases in cardiac output will not increase $\dot{V}o_2$ or Do_2. Simultaneous measurements of oxygen extraction will identify patients who have a failure in oxygen utilisation, such as occurs in severe sepsis. This concept is discussed in more detail in Chapter 13.

LACTATE, PYRUVATE, AND THE LACTATE/PYRUVATE RATIO

When Do_2 fails to match $\dot{V}o_2$, anaerobic metabolism occurs, and lactate is generated. However, the relationship between serum lactate and tissue oxygenation in the seriously ill is complex.

MONITORING GAS EXCHANGE

CARBON DIOXIDE

Carbon dioxide levels are determined by CO_2 production and elimination and offer a reflection of the adequacy of ventilation. The partial pressure of CO_2 in arterial blood (Pa_{CO_2}) can be measured by intermittent sampling of arterial blood gases. End-tidal expired CO_2, which is a reflection of alveolar CO_2, can be continuously measured and displayed using capnography (see p. 493). Tissue CO_2 levels can be continuously monitored with transcutaneous electrodes. Monitoring of ventilatory function is considered elsewhere (see p. 357).

OXYGENATION

One of the primary aims of intensive care medicine is to provide adequate oxygenation to cells. To monitor the efficiency and adequacy of oxygenation, we first need to measure the inspired oxygen concentration, expressed as a fraction (F_{IO_2}) or percentage (Table 21.8). This is then compared to the oxygenation of arterial blood expressed as a partial pressure (Pa_{O_2}) or concentration (Ca_{O_2}). Normal Pa_{O_2}/F_{IO_2} values are 500–600 mm Hg (66.7–80 kPa). In patients with severe respiratory failure, values can fall as low as 40–50 mm Hg (5.3–6.7 kPa). The amount of oxygen used by tissues can then be estimated by comparing the arterial oxygen concentration and the mixed venous oxygen partial pressure or concentration ($P\bar{v}_{O_2}$ or $C\bar{v}_{O_2}$). The lungs are responsible for efficient oxygenation, and their efficiency can be expressed as the alveolar–arterial difference in partial pressures of oxygen ($PA_{O_2} - Pa_{O_2}$) or the percentage of venous admixture or shunt ($\dot{Q}_S/\dot{Q}_T$). The normal $P(A-a)_{O_2}$ is less than 50 mm Hg (6.6 kPa), breathing 100% oxygen. In the most severe forms of respiratory failure, values can be as high as 550 mm Hg (73.1 kPa). The percentage of venous admixture or shunting is normally less than 10%. Inadequate oxygenation causes cells to undergo anaerobic metabolism and produce lactate. Lactate can therefore be a measure of inadequate oxygenation (see p. 504).

Oxygenation can be monitored by intermittent sampling of arterial blood gases, measuring Pa_{O_2} and comparing it to F_{IO_2}. The frequency of blood-gas sampling may need to be increased in hypoxic

TABLE 21.8 OXYGEN MEASUREMENTS

F_{IO_2}	Fraction of inspired oxygen
P_{IO_2}	Partial pressure of inspired oxygen: $(760 - 47) \times F_{IO_2}$ mm Hg $[(101.3 - 6.2) \times F_{IO_2}$ kPa$]$
P_{AO_2}	Partial pressure of oxygen in the alveoli: $P_{AO_2} = P_{IO_2} = -P_{aCO_2}/RQ$
P_{aO_2}	Partial pressure of oxygen, arterial
S_{aO_2}	Oxygen saturation of haemoglobin (Hb)
C_{aO_2}	Oxygen content = (Hb concentration) $\times$ (% saturation) $\times$ 1.34
$(A-a)D_{O_2}$	Alveolar-arterial oxygen gradient: $P_{AO_2} - P_{aO_2}$; normal value, 15–35 mm Hg (0.13–4.7 kPa)
P_{aO_2}/F_{IO_2}	Similar information as $(A-a)D_{O_2}$, but results are in the direction opposite to $(A-a)D_{O_2}$
$S\bar{v}_{O_2}$	Mixed venous oxygen saturation
$P\bar{v}_{O_2}$	Partial pressure of oxygen, mixed venous blood
$\dot{Q}_S/\dot{Q}_T$	Venous admixture or shunt: $$\frac{\dot{Q}_s}{\dot{Q}_T} = \frac{Cc'_{O_2} - Ca_{O_2}}{Cc'_{O_2} - C\bar{v}_{O_2}}$$ $$\frac{\text{shunt flow}}{\text{total flow}} = \frac{\text{end pulmonary capillary } O_2 \text{ content} - \text{arterial } O_2 \text{ content}}{\text{end pulmonary capillary } O_2 \text{ content} - \text{mixed venous } O_2 \text{ content}}$$ For practical purposes, $Cc'_{O_2} = C_{AO_2}$
Lactate	Adequacy of oxygen consumption relative to O_2 demand
pH_i	Intramucosal pH (measures tissue oxygenation)
RQ	Respiratory quotient

patients. Continuous monitoring of tissue oxygenation would be more appropriate in those circumstances. Continuous tissue oximetry (pulse oximetry) to measure oxygen saturation is a simple, relatively inexpensive, and accurate way to monitor peripheral saturation. Although pulse oximeters are subject to some shortcomings, they provide a convenient and reliable way to monitor oxygenation, and they are now almost mandatory for all hypoxic patients .

$P\overline{v}O_2$ can be monitored continuously with specially adapted PA catheters (see p. 502). Transcutaneous monitoring of oxygen tension ($PtcO_2$) is a relatively inexpensive and non-invasive form of monitoring. However, it is a reflection of oxygenation only when skin perfusion is adequate and constant, and it has now been largely superseded by pulse oximetry (see below).

Oxygen monitoring

MONITORING INSPIRED OXYGEN CONCENTRATION The concentration of inspired oxygen can be estimated from the gas flow rates or measured directly in the delivery tubing. Too much or too little oxygen will cause tissue damage.

MONITORING OXYGEN TENSION Oxygen tension is measured by polarographic electrodes either in vitro using intermittent arterial blood-gas samples or in vivo by continuous intravascular or transcutaneous techniques.

MONITORING OXYGEN SATURATION (PULSE OXIMETRY) The relationship between the saturation of oxygen on haemoglobin (SaO_2) and the oxygen tension (PaO_2) is expressed by the oxyhaemoglobin dissociation curve. Saturation can be measured invasively using an arterial blood-gas sample or non-invasively using pulse oximetry. Both methods use the principles of spectrophotometry. The non-invasive technique is becoming the standard technique for continuous monitoring of oxygenation in the ICU. Pulse oximeters have lightweight, accurate, and reliable skin sensors. However, they may not adequately detect arterial waveforms when tissue perfusion is inadequate. Moreover, pulse oximeters cannot determine other forms of haemoglobin, such as carboxyhaemoglobin or methaemoglobin, which, if present, will result in over-estimation. Pulse oximeters can also be affected by skin pigmentation, jaundice, dyes and pigments, external light sources, and anaemia (Table 21.9). Another major disadvantage is that the accuracy of pulse oximeters is ±3–5%, which can result in large errors on the flat part of the oxyhaemoglobin dissociation curve. Thus,

TABLE 21.9 FACTORS THAT CAN INTERFERE WITH
OXIMETER ACCURACY

False-high O$_2$ saturation levels
Elevated methaemoglobin
Elevated carboxyhaemoglobin
Hypothermia
Ambient light
False-low O$_2$ saturation levels
Skin pigment
Elevated serum lipids
Nail polish
Ambient light
Poor signal detection
Motion
Poor peripheral perfusion
Hypothermia
Malposition

going from a Pao_2 of 60 mm Hg (8 kPa) (90% saturation) to a Pao_2 of 100 mm Hg (13.3 kPa) (98% saturation) represents only an 8% difference in saturation. Therefore, within the normal range of oxygenation, pulse oximeters can be relatively inaccurate. Moreover, saturation levels below 80% also have limitations, and care should be taken with their interpretation. This may be related to the difficulty in calibrating and developing algorithms below this saturation level. Until better calibration algorithms are available, oximeters should be considered unreliable at levels below 70%.

MONITORING TRANSCUTANEOUS PO$_2$ This technique uses heated polarographic electrodes fixed to the skin surface. Oxygen diffuses from the skin and equilibrates with a contact liquid between the skin and electrode membrane.

There is poor correlation between $Ptco_2$ and Pao_2 when skin perfusion falls; $Ptco_2$ tracks respiratory function when the circulation is adequate, and circulatory function when oxygenation is adequate. In other words, it is not a reflection of circulatory function nor of respiratory function, but rather a measurement to be interpreted in its own right. The conjunctival oxygen tension ($Pcjo_2$) is the oxygen tension in the conjunctival bed and has the same disadvantages. Both $Pcjo_2$ and $Ptco_2$ provide early and accurate indications of decreased peripheral perfusion.

CONTINUOUS MONITORING OF OXYGENATION IN INTENSIVE CARE IS BECOMING AS COMMON AND AS INDISPENSABLE AS CONTINUOUS ECG MONITORING.

FURTHER READING

Bernstein, D. P. (1987). Non-invasive cardiac output, Doppler flowmetry, and gold-plated assumptions. *Critical Care Medicine* 15:886–8.

Calvin, J. E., Driedger, A. A., & Sibbald, W. J. (1981). Does the pulmonary capillary wedge pressure predict left ventricular preload in critically ill patients? *Critical Care Medicine* 9:437–43.

Curley, F. J., & Smyrnios, N. A. (1990). Routine monitoring of critically ill patients. *Journal of Intensive Care Medicine* 5:153–74.

Donovan, K. D. (1985). Invasive monitoring and support of the circulation. *Clinics in Anaesthesiology* 3:909–53.

Fiddian-Green, R. G. (1991). Should measurements of pH and Po_2 be included in the routine monitoring of intensive care unit patients. *Critical Care Medicine* 19:141–3.

Goldenham, P. D., & Kazemi, H. (1984). Cardiopulmonary monitoring of critically ill patients. Parts 1 and 2. *New England Journal of Medicine* 311:717–20, 776–80.

Gravenstein, J. S., & Paulus, D. A. (eds.) (1987). *Clinical Monitoring Practice*, 2nd ed. Philadelphia: Lippincott.

Lysak, S. Z., & Prough, D. S. (1987). Monitoring of patients receiving airway pressure therapy. *Anaesthesiology Clinics of North America* 5:821–41.

Neil, S. G., Lam, A. M., Turnbull, K. W., & Tremper, K. K. (1987). Monitoring of oxygen. *Canadian Journal of Anaesthesia* 34:56–63.

Peter, J. L. (1982). Current problems in central venous catheter systems. *Intensive Care Medicine* 8:205–8.

Robin, E. D. (1985). The cult of the Swan-Ganz catheter. *Annals of Internal Medicine* 103:445–9.

Sharpe, M., Driedger, A. A., & Sibbald, W. J. (1985). Non-invasive clinical investigation of the cardiovascular system in the critically ill. *Critical Care Clinics* 1:507–32.

Snyder, J. V., & Pinsky, M. R. (eds.) (1987). *Oxygen Transport in the Critically Ill*, 2nd ed. Chicago: Year Book.

Sprung, C. L., Drescher, M., & Schein, R. M. H. (1985). Clinical investigation of the cardiovascular system in the critically ill: invasive techniques. *Critical Care Clinics* 1:533–46.

Tee, E. A., & Shah, P. M. (1992). Transoesphageal echocardiography. *Journal of Intensive Care Medicine* 7:113–26.

22

ACUTE CARDIOVASCULAR FAILURE

> • Continuous correction of the intravascular volume is one of the most important manoeuvres in intensive care.
> • Inotropes and vasopressors should be titrated against desired effects – there is a right combination at a right dose for each patient at different times during the illness.
> • Early signs of poor peripheral perfusion must be rapidly and aggressively corrected.

This chapter describes the general principles of treating acute cardiovascular failure. Specific problems (eg cardiogenic shock) are discussed elsewhere.

PATHOPHYSIOLOGY

Acute cardiovascular failure occurs when there is insufficient blood flow to meet tissue demands. Either the heart is inefficient or the vascular tree fails to deliver the blood effectively to the tissues. This can be due to a primary heart problem (eg valvular rupture) or can be secondary to a systemic process (eg septic shock) (Table 22.1).

CARDIAC OUTPUT

cardiac output = heart rate × stroke volume

Stroke volume

Stroke volume is dependent on preload, afterload, and contractility.

PRELOAD Preload is a measure of the end-diastolic length of muscle fibres prior to contraction. It is usually estimated on the basis

TABLE 22.1   CAUSES OF ACUTE CARDIOVASCULAR FAILURE

Common causes

Endocardial: acute valvular insufficiency

Myocardial: ischaemia, infarct, arrhythmias, heart block, cardiomyopathy

Pericardial: tamponade, aortic dissection

Outside the heart: pulmonary embolus, pulmonary hypertension secondary to acute respiratory disease

Secondary causes

Other disease processes, sepsis, overdose, phaeochromocytoma

of ventricular filling pressures. Optimizing the preload is the first therapeutic manoeuvre in acute cardiovascular (CVS) failure. Initially the heart is very responsive to preload, but during late CVS failure an increase in preload will not increase cardiac output (Figure 22.1).

AFTERLOAD   Afterload is the force that impedes or opposes ventricular contraction. For a normal heart, impedance to ejection is due mainly to systemic vascular resistance (SVR). In many forms of acute CVS failure, SVR will be high because both stimulation of the sympathetic nervous system and the presence of angiotensin II will be causing vasoconstriction. A high SVR may maintain blood pressure, but is not advantageous for blood flow.

CONTRACTILITY   Contractility is a measure of the change in the force of contraction over a given time period; contractility is independent of preload and afterload. It is difficult to estimate in the clinical situation – the ejection fraction may be a useful approximation.

Heart rate

When the stroke volume cannot be increased, because of a diseased myocardium, the heart rate must increase to maintain cardiac output. However, an increased heart rate will lead to decreased diastolic filling of the coronary arteries and therefore to a decrease in the oxygen supply to an already stressed myocardium.

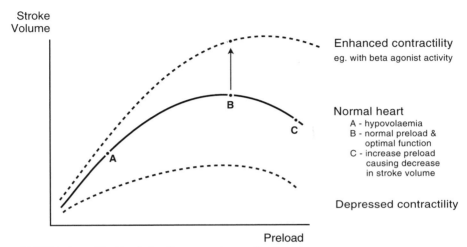

FIGURE 22.1 The Frank-Starling curve for cardiac function.

Because an increase in heart rate often is a compensatory mechanism, pharmacological intervention to lower the heart rate may also lower cardiac output.

Myocardial oxygen balance

An imbalance between myocardial oxygen supply (MDo_2) and myocardial oxygen demand ($M\dot{V}o_2$) can impair ventricular performance:

$$MDo_2 = (\text{coronary blood flow}) \times (\text{Hb concentration}) \times (\% \text{ saturation}) \times 1.34$$

Determinants of coronary blood flow
- aortic diastolic pressure
- heart rate
- myocardial extravascular compression

Major determinants of $M\dot{V}o_2$
- heart rate
- preload
- afterload
- contractility

Note that the heart rate is involved in determining both supply and demand.

The lower limit of coronary autoregulation is 40–70 mm Hg; subendocardial ischaemia will occur below that value.

The balance $M\dot{V}O_2/MDO_2$ can be important. For instance, dobutamine will increase cardiac output (increase MDO_2) but will also increase heart rate and contractility, which will increase $M\dot{V}O_2$.

Vasodilators will off-load the heart and increase cardiac output, but will also decrease diastolic pressure and thus decrease MDO_2.

BLOOD PRESSURE

The blood pressure is critical for maintenance of an effective driving pressure across the vascular beds. It is a function of cardiac output and SVR:

blood pressure = cardiac output × SVR

Cardiac output and blood pressure should not be thought of in terms of normal or abnormal. A better concept is their adequacy or inadequacy to maintain end-organ function.

The amount of pressure or flow (cardiac output) required must be determined on an individual-patient basis. For example, if a patient was previously hypertensive, then the autoregulation curve for the kidneys will be shifted to the right, and a higher mean arterial pressure will be needed to maintain function.

TYPES OF HEART FAILURE

Forward versus backward

These are old terms, but they are sometimes useful. Forward failure and backward failure can occur simultaneously in a given patient (eg cardiogenic shock).

FORWARD FAILURE The major problem is decreased cardiac output, with oliguria, confusion, and hypotension.

BACKWARD FAILURE The main problems are increased pressure and volume 'behind' the failing cardiac chamber, leading to pulmonary oedema, increased jugular venous pressure (JVP), hepatomegaly, and peripheral oedema.

Systolic versus diastolic

SYSTOLIC FAILURE   This is failure to pump. Forward failure and backward failure are examples of this.

DIASTOLIC FAILURE   Approximately one-third of patients with acute heart failure will show normal systolic function on echocardiography. Diastolic failure is failure of the ventricle to relax and allow filling: Left ventricular end-diastolic pressure (LVEDP) will be high, but left ventricular end-diastolic volume (LVEDV) will be reduced, the ejection fraction will be increased, and cardiac output may be normal.

Diastolic dysfunction can be difficult to define via a pulmonary artery catheter, which can be used to measure pressures, not volumes; echocardiography is useful. Because treatment for systolic and diastolic dysfunction can be quite different, estimations of their separate functions are important.

Right versus left

RIGHT-SIDE HEART FAILURE   Right-side heart failure (see p. 542) features high right-side pressures, slightly lower or equal left-side pressures, and normal findings on chest x-ray.

LEFT-SIDE HEART FAILURE   Left-side heart failure (see p. 597) involves both forward failure and backward failure, as described earlier.

AUTONOMIC NERVOUS SYSTEM

The sympathetic nervous system (SNS) is important because of its physiological control over the cardiovascular system and because many of the pharmacological agents used in treating diseases are designed to manipulate various parameters via the SNS (Figures 22.2 and 22.3).

In a patient with acute heart failure, the SNS is activated by hypotension and angiotensin II to produce tachycardia, vasoconstriction, and increased contractility.

Myocardial receptors

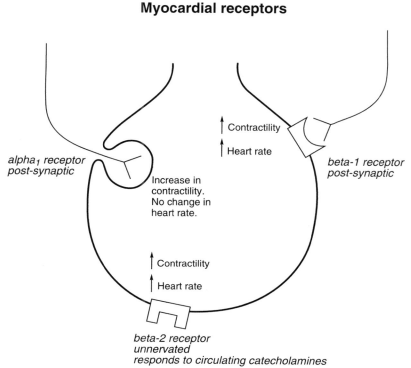

FIGURE 22.2   Myocardial receptors.

The classic model of the SNS may not apply in the presence of disease states, and the actions of the SNS may be different during an acute state than during a chronic state. Therefore, selection of vasoactive drugs remains empirical, by trial and error, with various combinations often being needed.

TREATMENT OF ACUTE CARDIOVASCULAR FAILURE

CLINICAL PRESENTATION

The signs and symptoms at presentation will depend on the underlying cause (eg a patient with mitral valve rupture will present with

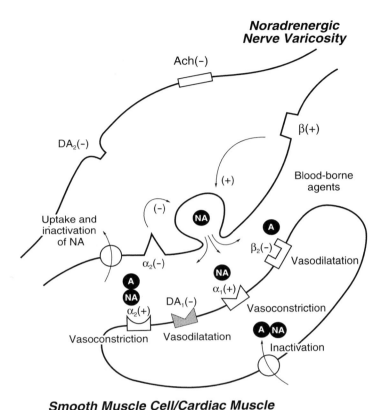

FIGURE 22.3 Interactions between the adrenergic nervous system and circulating cate-cholamines on smooth muscle and cardiac muscle.

rapid-onset pulmonary oedema). Ischaemia or infarction can have a slow onset, with initial dyspnoea and pain (Table 22.1). LVEDV and LVEDP will rise, heart rate will increase, and stroke volume will decrease. Cardiac output will be largely unchanged.

As the left ventricle fails, dyspnoea, tachypnoea, tachycardia, hypotension, confusion, and oliguria will appear, along with poorly perfused peripheries. These correspond to a further increase in left ventricular volume, a decrease in stroke volume, and a decrease in cardiac output (Table 22.2).

TABLE 22.2 DIFFERENCES BETWEEN ACUTE AND CHRONIC
HEART FAILURE

1. Retention of sodium and water is a feature of chronic heart failure, not acute heart failure.
2. Patients with acute heart failure are normovolaemic or relatively hypovolaemic, as a result of increases in hydrostatic pressure causing acute intravascular fluid loss, whereas patients with chronic heart failure are hypervolaemic, as a result of salt and water retention.
3. Cardiomegaly occurs in patients with chronic heart failure, but not necessarily in those with acute heart failure.
4. Acute pump failure can expose the pulmonary circulation to sudden increases in pressure, resulting in severe pulmonary oedema.

These differences are important because treatment strategies such as use of digoxin and diuretics may have little place in the treatment of acute heart failure, as opposed to chronic congestive heart failure.

MANAGEMENT

Reversible causes

Reverse any immediately reversible causes of cardiovascular failure, such as arrhythmias, pericardial tamponade, hypovolaemia, or valvular disease (Table 22.3).

Preloading

The most common cause of transient hypotension and inadequate tissue perfusion in the seriously ill is hypovolaemia (eg rewarming after surgery, vasodilatation secondary to sepsis, fluid loss as a result of polyuria, or other occult fluid losses). The effect of hypovolaemia on blood pressure will be exacerbated by high intrathoracic pressures, secondary to ventilatory support, that will decrease venous return and cardiac output.

FLUID CHALLENGE Give fluid or blood (depending on the haemoglobin concentration) as a bolus of 200–500 ml immediately. Assess responses. A further bolus or constant infusion (50–300 ml/h) may be required.

TABLE 22.3 PRINCIPLES OF TREATMENT FOR ACUTE CARDIOVASCULAR FAILURE

> 1. Reverse any immediately reversible causes (eg tamponade, arrhythmias, bleeding, valvular disease).
> 2. Fluid challenge: If hypovolaemia is suspected, give 200–500 ml of intravenous fluid or blood (depending on the haemoglobin concentration).
>
>   Depending on the responses of intravascular measurements (eg pulse rate, blood pressure, urine output, CVP, PAWP, peripheral perfusion), commence infusion at 50–200 ml/h, and adjust frequently.
> 3. Inotropes and vasopressors: After the intravascular volume has been replenished, catecholamine support may be needed.
>
>   There will be a best drug combination at the best dosage for each patient at any given stage of the illness.
>
>   A therapeutic challenge must be given, and its efficacy must be assessed by cardiovascular measurements (eg cardiac output, blood pressure, preload measurements, serum lactate, mixed venous oxygen saturation, urine output) taken before and after the drug challenge.
>
>   **THE CORRECT DOSAGE OF INOTROPE OR VASOPRESSOR MUST BE ASSESSED CLINICALLY AT THE BEDSIDE, OFTEN ON A MINUTE-TO-MINUTE BASIS.**
> 4. Vasodilation
>
>   Afterload reduction is sometimes useful for heart failure or hypertension.
> 5. Other measures (eg pacemakers, IABP).

Fluid replenishment should be charted on an hourly basis, with intermittent boluses as necessary, modified frequently according to the intravascular measurements of blood volume: pulse rate, urine output, blood pressure, cardiac output, central venous pressure (CVP), pulmonary artery wedge pressure (PAWP), and peripheral perfusion. Fluid such as colloid or blood is preferable to crystalloids when titrating against intravascular measurements, as less volume is needed, and they cause less peripheral and pulmonary oedema (see Chapter 4). Seriously ill patients often require large amounts of intravascular fluid.

The patient's preload is best judged on the basis of the response to a fluid load, rather than on the basis of a single reading, such as right (CVP) or left (PAWP) atrial pressure.

Following a fluid challenge, there may be clues that the patient's preload could be further optimized:

- a minimal change or no change in PAWP
- an increase in cardiac output
- improvements in terms of blood pressure and urine output
- a decrease in heart rate

Conversely, there may be clues that no more preload will be beneficial:

- high PAWP (>20 mm Hg)
- decreased Sao_2 (may mean alveolar flooding)
- no change in cardiac output

If the preload is optimized, but the haemodynamics still have not improved, then inotropes and vasopressors will be required to increase cardiac output and blood pressure.

Inotropes and vasopressors

Inotropes increase contractility, whereas vasopressors increase SVR by increasing peripheral vasoconstriction. Most exogenous catecholamines will increase both inotropic activity in the heart and vasoconstriction in the peripheral vasculature (Table 22.4).

FACTORS AFFECTING THE CHOICE OF AN INOTROPE OR VASOPRESSOR

- The chosen end point against which the drug will be titrated (eg heart rate, cardiac output, blood pressure, peripheral perfusion).
- An underlying disease state.
- The variability of responses according to age.
- Fashion: Pharmaceutical companies can exert enormous pressure on physicians. Many clinicians have been conditioned to use the latest and most expensive drugs (eg dopexamine and dobutamine, instead of older and cheaper drugs such as adrenaline and noradrenaline).
- The exact actions of most drugs on the heart and vessels in humans are uncertain, even when in a state of good health. Most experimental work has been performed on animals. However, the differences in

TABLE 22.4 SELECTIVITY OF CATECHOLAMINES FOR ADRENERGIC RECEPTORS

Catecholamine	α_1	α_2	β_1	β_2	DA[a]
Adrenaline	+ +	+ +	+ + +	+ + +	0
Noradrenaline	+ + +	+ + +	+ + +	+	0
Isoprenaline	0	0	+ + +	+ + +	0
Dopamine	0 to + + +	+	+ + to + + +	+ + +	+ + +
Dobutamine	0 to +	0	+ + +	+	0
Dopexamine	0	0	0 to +	+ + +	+

[a]DA, dopaminergic receptor.
Source: From Zaritsky and Chernow (1983), with permission.

the autonomic nervous systems of the various species make any comparison difficult.

• Catecholamines have varying dose-dependent effects that are even more unpredictable in disease states.

• Adrenergic desensitization or down-regulation of adrenoceptors can occur in disease states.

Therefore, any drug should be empirically tested at a certain dosage in a particular patient at a particular time during the disease. Specific end points should be used as guidelines to efficacy, with either the dosage being adjusted accordingly or the drug changed. There have been few controlled clinical trials comparing catecholamines for efficacy in seriously ill patients.

THE CHOICE BETWEEN CATECHOLAMINES IS MORE DEPENDENT ON THE CLINICAL CIRCUMSTANCES OF THE PATIENT THAN ON THE PHARMACEUTICAL CHARACTERISTICS OF THE DRUGS.

ONE OF THE PRIMARY GOALS IN TREATING THE SERIOUSLY ILL IS TO CORRECT HYPOTENSION. The dangers of hypotension probably have been under-estimated. This is related to recent attention being focused on flow assessment in terms of cardiac output rather than in terms of pressure, as well as an obsession with decreasing the afterload in an attempt to increase cardiac output. This focus overlooks the fact that vital-organ perfusion is critically dependent on an adequate pressure.

INOTROPES ARE LIKE FLUIDS – A CHALLENGE SHOULD BE GIVEN, AND THE RESPONSE MEASURED AND EVALUATED. There appears to be a point of maximum effect from inotrope infusions, above which increasing the dosage will have little impact. There is little evidence of any linear response to dosage changes in the seriously ill.

PRACTICAL GUIDELINES TO INOTROPE/VASOPRESSOR CHOICE

If a patient's blood pressure is relatively normal and there is a primary problem with oxygen delivery (DO_2) after a fluid challenge has failed, then a drug that will primarily increase the cardiac output, such as dobutamine, with or without low-dosage dopamine, may be appropriate. If the arterial blood pressure is low, despite an adequate preload, drugs such as adrenaline or noradrenaline, in combination with low-dosage dopamine, may offer useful combinations of first choice. Despite the theoretical danger of excessive vasoconstriction as a result of using vasopressors, the increased blood pressure often increases, rather than decreases, peripheral perfusion to the skin, kidneys, and other organs.

Inotropes/vasopressors (Table 22.5)

Dobutamine   Dobutamine will increase cardiac output when filling pressures are normal or high, with little change in blood pressure. Although predominantly a selective β_1-agonist, dobutamine also has β_2 activity that causes peripheral vasodilation and possibly hypotension. Dobutamine is associated with tachycardia, which in patients with ischaemic heart disease can cause myocardial ischaemia. Dobutamine can be useful to match DO_2 with consumption ($\dot{V}O_2$) (see p. 376).

Dopamine   Dopamine has a wide spectrum of actions, ranging from dopaminergic at low dosages to β and α effects as the dosage increases. It is often used for its action on renal and mesenteric blood flow at low dosages. However, it is now thought that any improvement in renal function probably is due to the drug's inotropic and diuretic actions, not specific dopaminergic actions. At higher dosages, its actions can simulate those of other drugs, such as dobutamine or adrenaline, depending on the proportions of its α and β actions (Table 22.4).

Adrenaline   Adrenaline is cheap and has a wide spectrum of β_1, β_2, and α actions. It increases cardiac output and blood pressure.

Noradrenaline   Noradrenaline has a spectrum similar to that of adrenaline, but it is more efficient for increasing the blood pressure through its predominant α effects. It has less β action than adrenaline. It is useful in patients with septic shock.

Isoprenaline   Isoprenaline has pure β effect only. Classically it has been used to increase the heart rate during bradycardias. However, it also decreases coronary perfusion by β_2 vasodilation. Adrenaline probably is a better drug.

Dopexamine   Dopexamine is a synthetic analogue of dopamine, with the theoretical advantage of having dopaminergic activity without α effects. Care must be taken not to compromise the myocardial oxygen balance, because by decreasing myocardial perfusion pressure, dopexamine will increase the oxygen demand and lower its supply.

Phosphodiesterase inhibitors   These act at a cellular level to inhibit phosphodiesterase, resulting in an increased concentration of cyclic adenosine monophosphate. Theoretically these drugs are inotropes and vasodilators, but their predominant action is vasodilation. The exact roles for this group of drugs in acute heart failure are yet to be defined. There are two types of compounds in this group of drugs: the imidazole derivatives and the bipyridine derivatives. The bipyridine derivatives include amrinone and milrinone. Amrinone causes potent vasodilation of the systemic and pulmonary arterial and venous beds. It also has mild inotropic effects. Amrinone may be effective in treating right-side heart failure, as it off-loads the right ventricle and increases right ventricular contractility. Currently it is usually used in combination with other inotropes and vasopressors. Hypotension and reflex tachycardia can occur if amrinone is used by itself. It has a long elimination half-life that is further prolonged in patients with renal failure. Milrinone is about 15 times as potent as amrinone and has a similar pharmacological profile.

The imidazole derivatives are the other group of phosphodiesterase inhibitors. They include enoximone and piroximone. They have actions similar to those of amrinone and milrinone and also are best used in combination with a drug such as adrenaline, in order to enhance stroke volume. The duration of action of the imidazole deriva-

TABLE 22.5 INFUSION RATES FOR DRUGS ACTING ON THE
CARDIOVASCULAR SYSTEM

Drug	Concentration	Rates and comments
Dopamine	200–800 mg in 500 ml	1–5 μg · kg^{-1} · min^{-1} ('renal dose') 6–15 μg · kg^{-1} · min^{-1} (mainly β effects)
	200 mg in 50 ml (in syringe pump)	>15 μg · kg^{-1} · min^{-1} (increasingly α effects) <50 μg · kg^{-1} · min^{-1} is often needed for severe sepsis; as the effects are predominantly α in this dosage range, it may be better to use adrenaline or noradrenaline
Dobutamine	250–500 mg in 500 ml 250 mg in 50 ml (in syringe pump)	2.5–10 μg · kg^{-1} · min^{-1}
Noradrenaline	4–20 mg in 500 ml	Noradrenaline should be titrated against the patient's response
	2 mg in 50 ml (in syringe pump)	This is extremely variable and can be as high as 15 mg/h in severe sepsis; commence at 0.5 μg · kg^{-1} · min^{-1} (approximately 2 mg/h)
Adrenaline	5–20 mg in 500 ml	Adrenaline should be titrated against the patient's response
	4 mg in 50 ml (in syringe pump)	This is extremely variable; as much as 20 mg/h may be necessary for severe sepsis; commence at 0.5 μg · kg^{-1} · min^{-1} (approximately 2 mg/h)
Isoprenaline	2–4 mg in 500 ml	0.02–0.10 μg · kg^{-1} · min^{-1}
	2 mg in 50 ml (in syringe pump)	Titrate against heart rate for complete heart block; adrenaline is probably a better drug
Phentolamine	50 mg in 500 ml	Commence at 0.1 mg/min, increasing every 5 min, to a maximum of 2 mg/min; as the major effect is on peripheral resistance, its main use is for hypertension

(continued)

Sodium nitroprusside	50 mg in 500 ml	Commence at 0.5 $\mu g \cdot kg^{-1} \cdot min^{-1}$, increasing every 5 minutes by 0.2 $\mu g \cdot kg^{-1} \cdot min^{-1}$, up to a maximum of 8 $\mu g \cdot kg^{-1} \cdot min^{-1}$; avoid excess drug during prolonged administration
	More concentrated solutions can be used in higher dosages	Thiocyanate levels must be kept lower than 10 mg/dl
Nitroglycerin	50–100 mg in 500 ml	Commence at 400 μg/h, and increase by 400 μg every 5 minutes; its major effect is on venous capacitance; headache can be a problem with higher dosages
Milrinone	10 mg in 50 ml	Loading dose 50 μg/kg; maintenance dosage 0.3–0.75 $\mu g \cdot kg^{-1} \cdot min^{-1}$
Amrinone		Loading dose 0.75–3.0 mg/kg over 10–30 minutes; maintenance dosage 10 $\mu g \cdot kg^{-1} \cdot min^{-1}$
Enoximone		Loading dose 0.5 mg/kg; maintenance dosage 2.5–10 $\mu g \cdot kg^{-1} \cdot min^{-1}$
Dopexamine	50 mg in 50 ml	0.5–10 $\mu g \cdot kg^{-1} \cdot min^{-1}$; vasodilation and inotropy; reflex tachycardia may be a problem

tives is much longer than that for the bipyridine derivatives. It has been suggested that enoximone may be more effective than dobutamine for overcoming the condition of a β-blocked heart, but the therapeutic roles for these drugs still are far from clear.

INOTROPES AND VASOPRESSORS CAN BE USED AS TEMPORARY MEANS OF SUPPORT WHILE DEFINITIVE TREATMENT IS DELIVERED OR WHILE THE PATIENTS HEAL THEMSELVES.

Vasodilatation

A decrease in resistance to left ventricular ejection will increase the stroke volume. This is particularly important in patients with pure heart failure, characterized by low cardiac output and high SVR. Vasodilators can act predominantly on the arterial circulation, decreasing the afterload, or on the venous circulation, decreasing the preload. A lower preload is particularly important in a patient with cardiogenic pulmonary oedema (see p. 397).

The major factor limiting the use of vasodilators is hypotension, which results in decreased rather than increased perfusion.

VASODILATING DRUGS

Sodium nitroprusside   Sodium nitroprusside causes arterial and venous dilation.

Phentolamine   Phentolamine is an α-receptor antagonist that acts mainly on the arterial circulation.

Nitroglycerin   Nitroglycerin acts mainly on the venous circulation, with arterial effects at higher dosages.

Phosphodiesterase inhibitors

Vasodilators should be carefully titrated against whatever effect is required (eg cardiac output). The dosage should be increased incrementally, while not allowing the blood pressure to fall rapidly below the patient's normal pressure range.

DIURETICS

Diuretics are useful for chronic heart failure and acute left ventricular failure. They should not be used in patients with right-side heart failure and diastolic dysfunction, as a high preload is necessary to maintain cardiac output.

OTHER FORMS OF SUPPORT

Cardiac pacing

Cardiac pacing is used infrequently in ICUs, as compared with coronary care units.

INDICATIONS

Bradyarrhythmias
- profound bradycardia (with symptoms)

- sinus arrest (with symptoms)
- complete atrioventricular block (with slow escape rhythm)

Tachyarrhythmias

- termination of supraventricular or ventricular tachycardias resistant to drug treatment, by overdrive pacing, as an alternative to cardioversion

Although most temporary pacemakers are inserted transvenously, the oesophageal and percutaneous routes are increasingly being used.

Percutaneous pacing pads are placed on the anteroposterior chest, much as for defibrillation, and the output is increased until cardiac pacing is achieved. Because a high output is necessary to pace the heart through the thick chest wall, synchronous stimulation of skeletal muscle usually occurs. High levels of discomfort and pain often accompany percutaneous pacing. It should be a temporary measure while waiting for transvenous pacing.

Intra-aortic balloon pump

The intra-aortic balloon pump (IABP) improves the myocardial oxygen supply by diastolic augmentation of aortic pressure and reduces the afterload by a sudden deflation of the balloon during systole. The balloon is timed to inflate just after the dicrotic notch of the arterial pressure trace and is deflated by triggering from the R wave of the ECG or from the arterial pressure waveform. The IABP can be inserted either percutaneously or as a formal surgical procedure.

The question of who benefits from use of the IABP has few clear-cut answers. The technique provides short-term benefits for post–myocardial infarction patients with acute ventricular septal defects or mitral valve insufficiency, as well as for post–cardiac surgery patients. Thus far, patients with cardiogenic and septic shock have shown no long-term benefits from use of the IABP. The best use of the IABP is as a bridge to transplantation or coronary artery grafting.

Ventricular-assist devices

These are either roller pumps or centrifugal pumps that assist ventricular output. Their main uses are before or after cardiac transplantation and to wean patients off cardiopulmonary bypass. Their complications are many (eg bleeding, coagulopathy, infection).

TROUBLESHOOTING

INOTROPE SELECTION

The best inotrope combination and dosage will vary (sometimes rapidly) according to the patient's condition. Avoid belonging to the school of single-inotrope use. Use different combinations and dosages according to the desired effects.

What is the problem?
PRESSURE (eg hypotension)
FLOW (decreased cardiac output)
Do_2/Vo_2 mismatch

Is there anything correctable?
Cardiac tamponade
Arrhythmia

Have you optimized the preload?

Features of main inotropes
Dobutamine
• Increases cardiac output and Do_2
• Blood pressure: no change, or decreased
• Used mainly to increase oxygen delivery in patients with normal blood pressure
• Useful for matching Do_2 and $\dot{V}o_2$
Dopamine
• Specifically increases renal and mesenteric blood flow when used at low dosages
• Mimics dobutamine when used at medium dosages, and adrenaline at higher dosages
• Often used in combination with other inotropes for its specific renal and mesenteric actions
Adrenaline
• Increases blood pressure

- Guarantees perfusion pressure for vital organs, sometimes at the expense of tissue perfusion
- Despite the theory, ventricular arrhythmias and oliguria are uncommon complications
- A good all-purpose inotrope, especially when there is decreased blood pressure (eg sepsis)

Noradrenaline

- Similar to adrenaline, but with greater peripheral vasoconstrictor effects
- Useful for refractory hypotension, especially in patients with sepsis

Isoprenaline

- Similar to dobutamine, but causes marked tachycardia
- Very little used in the ICU

Dopexamine

- Dopamine without the vasoconstriction
- Inotrope and vasodilator

Amrinone/milrinone

- Mild inotrope, mainly a vasodilator
- Used to off-load the heart when blood pressure is adequate

FURTHER READING

Bryan-Brown, C. (1988). Blood flow to organs: parameters for function and survival in critical illness. *Critical Care Medicine* 16:170–6.

Chernow, B., & Roth, B. L. (1986). Pharmacologic manipulation of the peripheral vasculature in shock: clinical and experimental approaches. *Circulatory Shock* 18:141–55.

Desjars, P., Pinaud, M., Potel, G., Tasseau, F., & Touze, M. D. (1987). A reappraisal of norepinephrine therapy in human septic shock. *Critical Care Medicine* 15:34–137.

Kantrowitz, A., Cardona, R. R., & Freed, P. S. (1992). Percutaneous intra-aortic balloon counterpulsation. *Critical Care Clinics* 4:819–37.

Mohan, P., Hii, J. T. Y., & Wuttke, R. D. (1991). Acute heart failure determinants of outcome. *International Journal of Cardiology* 32:365–75.

Robotham, J. L., Takata, M., Berman, M., & Harasawa, Y. (1991). Ejection fraction revisited. *Anesthesiology* 74:172–83.

Sibbald, W. J. (ed.) (1985). Symposium on cardiovascular crises in the critically ill. *Critical Care Clinics* 1:433–731 (symposium issue).

Zaloga, G. P., Prielipp, R. C., Butterworth, J. F., et al. (1993). Pharmacologic cardiovascular support. *Critical Care Clinics* 9:335–62.

Zaritsky, A., & Chernow, B. (1983). Catecholamines, sympathomimetics. In *The Pharmacologic Approach to the Critically Ill Patient*, ed. B. Chernow & C. R. Lak. Baltimore: Williams & Wilkins.

23

SPECIFIC CARDIOVASCULAR PROBLEMS

ARRHYTHMIAS

Cardiac arrhythmias are common problems in the ICU. The causes, predisposing factors, clinical significance, and management strategies for arrhythmias in the ICU are often different from those for patients with primary cardiac disease in the more classic setting of coronary care units (CCUs). This section will concentrate on arrhythmia management only as it relates to the ICU (Table 23.1).

Arrhythmias in the ICU can be classified into two categories:

• Some arrhythmias result from irritant affects on an essentially normal heart. They are usually supraventricular. Management is dependent on identification and alteration of the predisposing factors, such as hypoxia, hypokalaemia, sepsis, central-line irritation, and inadvertent boluses of concentrated drugs through central lines.

• Arrhythmias in the second grouping occur as a result of myocardial ischaemia caused by an imbalance between oxygen supply and oxygen demand. These arrhythmias are the same as those seen commonly in patients with primary heart disease. These arrhythmias can be either supraventricular or ventricular in origin.

INITIAL MANAGEMENT OF ARRHYTHMIAS

Resuscitation

If the cardiovascular system is severely compromised, immediate cardiopulmonary resuscitation (CPR) and cardioversion should be instituted.

TABLE 23.1   AETIOLOGY OF ARRHYTHMIAS IN THE ICU

Common factors in the seriously ill
Hypokalaemia
Hypomagnesaemia
Acidosis
Hypoxia
Sepsis, pancreatitis, multitrauma, multiorgan failure
Pro-arrhythmic effects of antiarrhythmic drugs (eg digoxin)
Inotropic drugs (inadvertent purges of adrenaline)
Irritation from central line or pulmonary artery catheter
Microshock
Underlying patient factors
Coronary artery disease
Congenital heart disease
Valvular heart disease
Hyperthyroidism
Hypothyroidism
Phaeochromocytoma

Cardioversion

Cardioversion is the treatment of choice in the presence of haemodynamic compromise due to a tachyarrhythmia, whether it is supraventricular or ventricular (Table 23.2):

Ventricular fibrillation (VF)	200–360 J
Ventricular tachycardia (VT)	200–360 J
Supraventricular tachycardia (SVT)	20–200 J
Atrial flutter	50–200 J
Atrial fibrillation (AF)	50–360 J

Cardioversion can itself cause VF, sinus arrest, or increased atrioventricular (AV) node block. Patients who are receiving drugs that block conduction across the AV node (eg digoxin, calcium-channel blockers, β-blockers) can develop sinus arrest after cardioversion. Synchronous DC cardioversion for supraventricular arrhythmias decreases the risk of inducing ventricular tachyarrhythmias.

TABLE 23.2 ELECTIVE CARDIOVERSION

1. Give nothing orally for at least 4 hours.
2. Have intravenous cannulae in situ.
3. Use sedative/anaesthetic drugs with minimal cardiovascular depressant activities.
4. Select synchronous mode for cardioversion, apart from VF or very rapid SVT and VT.
5. Select lower-range energy levels initially, and increase if unsuccessful.

CONTRAINDICATION: Dislodgement of an intracardiac mural thrombus can occur, particularly if the rhythm disturbance has been long-standing. If the need for cardioversion is not urgent, echocardiography should be performed to exclude a thrombus, and anticoagulation should be commenced if necessary.

Cardiac pacing

Cardiac pacing is especially useful for bradyarrhythmias in the presence of cardiovascular instability. For example:

- complete AV block, with slow escape rhythm
- profound sinus bradycardia
- sinus arrest

Cardiopulmonary resuscitation may be necessary to support the circulation before the pacing device is inserted. Drug treatment may also be useful for bradyarrhythmias (see p. 537). Temporary transcutaneous pacing is increasingly being used as an emergency technique in intensive care.

Correction of underlying cause

ELECTROLYTES Potassium is particularly important. Hypokalaemia is common in the seriously ill, and it should be corrected with aggressive measures. **HYPOKALAEMIA IS A POTENT CAUSE OF VENTRICULAR AND SUPRAVENTRICULAR ARRHYTHMIAS.** Keep the serum potassium concentration on the higher side of normal (ie >4.0 mmol/L). Other electrolytes, including MAGNESIUM, should also be measured frequently and corrected.

OXYGEN DELIVERY TO THE MYOCARDIUM Maintain adequate oxygen delivery (DO_2) to the heart by attention to the following parameters:

• coronary perfusion pressure (diastolic pressure minus right atrial pressure)
• haemoglobin concentration
• oxygen saturation
• coronary blood flow

CENTRAL LINES Closely monitor the insertion of pulmonary artery catheters. Any central line within the heart can cause mechanical irritability and arrhythmias.

BOLUSES OF ARRHYTHMOGENIC DRUGS Arrhythmias can be caused by boluses of the many potent and concentrated drugs delivered to seriously ill patients. Check the delivery device and the protocols for flushing central lines. The dead space in delivery tubing can contain concentrations of drug.

MICROSHOCKS The measures taken to ensure electrical safety in modern ICUs make the likelihood of microshocks rare.

SPECIFIC TREATMENT FOR ARRHYTHMIAS (Tables 23.3 and 23.4)

Sinus tachycardia

Sinus tachycardia is very common in intensive care and almost always is a physiological response to underlying disease (eg fever, pain, sepsis). Treatment should be directed at the underlying cause, not the arrhythmia (see p. 564).

Atrial fibrillation

AF tends to be a very common accompaniment of any severe illness, especially sepsis (see p. 188), but also pneumonia, pancreatitis, multitrauma, and multiorgan failure. **HYPOVOLAEMIA AND SEPSIS CAN PRECIPITATE AF IN THE SERIOUSLY ILL.** Potentially correctable factors include atrial distension, hypoxia, electrolyte abnormalities, thyrotoxicosis, and drug side effects.

Cardioversion often is not successful in this setting. The ventricular rate should be controlled with digoxin or amiodarone, and the underlying cause treated. These patients invariably have compromised cardiovascular function as a result of the underlying disease, and the arrhythmia should be treated as soon as possible.

DIGITALIZATION Patients with acute rapid AF should be digitalized in order to reduce the ventricular response rate. Digoxin is usually ineffective for inducing reversion of AF to sinus rhythm. Check the potassium level; it should be greater than 4.0 mmol/L.

• Loading dose: Give digoxin at 0.5–1.0 mg IV, over 20 minutes, or 0.25 mg IV, every 2 hours. Total dose should be no more than 1.5 mg in 24 hours

• Maintenance dosage: 0.25 mg IV, daily, modified according to regularly measured levels, especially in the presence of compromised renal and hepatic functions

VERAPAMIL Verapamil can be used together with digitalization to control rapid AF. Both drugs block AV conduction.

• **Bolus:** Give boluses of 1 mg IV each minute, up to a total of 20 mg or until there is a satisfactory response or an untoward response in heart rate or blood pressure.

• **Infusion:** If repeated boluses of verapamil are needed, an infusion through a central venous line can be used at a rate of 5–20 mg/h to maintain the heart rate between 80 and 110 beats per minute.

In some patients, this will induce reversion to sinus rhythm, and it will control the ventricular response in others.

If the heart rate remains stable for more than 3 hours with verapamil treatment at less than 5 mg/h, an attempt to discontinue the infusion can be made.

Verapamil should be used cautiously in patients with compromised left ventricular function. Always commence with small doses, and monitor the cardiovascular system carefully.

TABLE 23.3 TREATMENT OF ARRHYTHMIAS

Arrhythmia	Diagnostic hints	Treatment	Additional comments
Ventricular premature beats	Irregular, broad-complex ventricular beats.	Nil if haemodynamically stable. Monitor.	Often occurs with right-side heart catheterization and reperfusion after thrombolysis.
Ventricular tachycardia	Broad-complex tachycardia. Evidence of AV dissociation clinically and on ECG.	Cardioversion. Lignocaine. Procainamide.	Often due to myocardial ischaemia. Reverse abnormalities such as hypokalaemia.
Ventricular fibrillation	Irregular broad-complex tachycardia. No discrete QRS morphology. Cardiorespiratory arrest.	DC cardioversion. Adrenaline.	Terminal event unless treated. Usually due to myocardial ischaemia.
Torsade des pointes	Polymorphic QRS complexes that change in amplitude and cycle length. QT interval > 0.60 second.	Remove underlying causes. DC cardioversion. β-blockers for congenital prolonged QT syndrome.	Due to prolonged QT syndrome (congenital, hypokalaemia, hypomagnesaemia, antiarrhythmics, phenothiazines, antidepressants).
Multifocal atrial tachycardia	Discrete P waves of variable morphology and variable P-R interval.	Treat underlying cause. Often resistant to cardioversion.	Associated with pulmonary disease, particularly chronic lung disease.
Paroxysmal supraventricular tachycardia	Narrow-complex tachycardia. P waves often inverted or retrograde. Carotid sinus massage may cause reversion.	As for atrial flutter.	Common accompaniment of sepsis. History of Wolff-Parkinson-White syndrome contraindicates drugs that block AV conduction. Often resistant to cardioversion and digoxin in the ICU.

AV junctional tachycardia	Narrow-complex tachycardia. No P waves or retrograde P waves. Rate slowed with carotid sinus massage.	Exclude digoxin toxicity. Atrial pacing. Lignocaine. β-blocker.	If due to digoxin, cardioversion should not be attempted. Often occurs after AMI and cardiac surgery.
Atrial flutter	Flutter waves, II, III, aVF. Regular R:R interval, often at 150 bpm, indicating 2:1 AV block.	Cardioversion. Rapid atrial pacing. Verapamil if rate > 140 bpm. Digitalization if rate < 140 bpm. Amiodarone. Adenosine.	Rate > 140 bpm needs urgent reversion, with either intravenous treatment or cardioversion.
Atrial fibrillation	Irregular R-R interval, with no discrete P waves.	As for atrial flutter.	Common accompaniment of sepsis.
Sinus bradycardia	Sinus rate < 60 bpm.	Correct hypoxia. Atropine, 0.3–0.6 mg. Adrenaline, 1-mg increments IV. Pacemaker.	Almost invariably associated with hypoxia in ICU. Check for drugs that impair AV conduction. Manifestation of sick-sinus syndrome. May be normal in athletes.
Sinus arrest	Prolonged pause between P waves. Usually reverts spontaneously.	Treatment not usually necessary. Stop digoxin. Pacemaker.	Usually due to excessive vasovagal stimulation. Check digoxin level.

TABLE 23.4 DRUGS USED TO TREAT ARRHYTHMIAS

Drug	Indications	IV dose	Complications	Interactions
Lignocaine	VT VF	1.5 mg/kg over 1–2 minutes. Dose may be repeated at 20-minute intervals up to a total dose of 300 mg.	Convulsions. Allergy. Cardiovascular system collapse, with bradycardia. Toxicity, with hepatic dysfunction.	Anticonvulsants may increase hepatic metabolism. Additive cardiodepressant effect with phenytoin.
Procainamide	PAT[a] AF VT	7–10 mg/kg, at a rate no greater than 50 mg/min to a total dose of 1,000 mg.	Hypotension. Widening of QRS complex. Prolonged PR interval. Hypersensitivity.	Contraindicated in patients with AV block and torsade des pointes.
Adenosine	Cardioversion of narrow-complex tachycardia Diagnosis of wide-complex tachycardia.	0.05 mg/kg by rapid IV injection via large peripheral vein. Further doses up to a total of 20 mg.	Avoid in those with asthma. Avoid in those with Wolff-Parkinson-White syndrome. Transient flushing, chest discomfort, and dyspnoea.	Dipyridamole blocks cellular uptake and thereby increases adenosine levels.

Drug	Indication	Dose	Side effects	Precautions
Verapamil	Cardioversion of narrow-complex tachycardia Slowing of ventricular rate in AF.	1 mg/min, up to 20 mg.	Hypotension. Acceleration of ventricular response rate in pre-excitation syndrome.	AV-node block with β-blockers. Asystole with cardioversion. Decreased sensitivity with hypokalaemia.
Digoxin	As for verapamil.	0.5–1.0 mg IV over 30 minutes; 0.25 mg IV every 2 hours, to a total dose of no more than 1.5 mg in 24 hours.	Virtually any arrhythmia. Acceleration of ventricular response rate in pre-excitation syndrome.	Calcium-channel blockers and amiodarone will increase digoxin levels. Caution in those with renal dysfunction.
Amiodarone	Narrow- or broad-complex tachycardia.	5 mg/kg over 1 hour in 250 ml of 5% dextrose. Followed by repeat infusions of 12 mg $\cdot$ kg^{-1} $\cdot$ d^{-1} for up to 7 days, or until oral treatment can be started.	Hypotension. Long-term use leads to corneal deposits, photosensitivity, thyroid disorders, interstitial pneumonitis, hepatotoxicity, nausea, and vomiting.	Long half-life. Potentiates bradycardia with calcium-channel blockers and β blockers.
Sotalol	Narrow- or broad-complex tachycardias. Atrial fibrillation and flutter.	0.5–1.5 mg/kg over 10 minutes. May be repeated after 6 hours.	Pure β-blocker. Hypertension, bradycardia, cardiac failure.	Prolongs QT interval; therefore should not be given with drugs that prolong QT interval (quinidine, disopyramide).

[a]Paroxysmal atrial tachycardia.

AMIODARONE

- Emergency dose: 150–300 mg IV, rapidly.
- Otherwise, infuse 5 mg/kg IV over 1 hour in a dilute solution of 250 ml of 5% dextrose. Repeat 4–6-hourly if required.
- The total dose should not exceed 1,200 mg over 24 hours.
- The maintenance dosage should be 12 mg $\cdot$ kg^{-1} $\cdot$ d^{-1}.

Amiodarone can cause AV block, sick sinus syndrome, and hypotension in the short term. Other side effects include corneal deposits, skin photosensitivity, hyperthyroidism or hypothyroidism, and pulmonary interstitial fibrosis.

SOTALOL   Sotalol is a non-selective β-blocker and a class III antiarrhythmic agent. Its dose should be 0.5–1.5 mg/kg over 10 minutes, repeated after 6 hours.

Supraventricular tachycardia

Like AF, SVT is a common accompaniment of severe illness in intensive care, and it does not necessarily indicate underlying primary heart disease. Predisposing factors include sepsis, multiorgan failure, and hypovolaemia. SVT can be exacerbated by electrolyte disorders such as hypokalaemia and hypomagnesaemia.

Cardioversion often is not successful in this setting. If the cardiovascular system is compromised, then cardioversion should be attempted initially (20–200 J). Otherwise, attempt to reverse any predisposing factors and control the rate with drugs.

VERAPAMIL   The use of verapamil is discussed elsewhere (see p. 535).

DIGOXIN   Digoxin treatment is discussed elsewhere (see p. 535).

ADENOSINE   A rapid intravenous bolus of 0.05 mg/kg, increasing to a maximum dose of 20 mg, is successful in correcting SVT in over 90% of cases. Its half-life is very short (<2 seconds), and its side effects few: transient dyspnoea, flushing, and chest pain. Contraindications include AF with ventricular pre-excitation, patients with asthma, and those taking dipyridamole.

TABLE 23.5 BROAD-COMPLEX TACHYARRHYTHMIAS

90% of broad-complex tachycardias are VT.	
SVT	**VT**
No AV dissociation.	AV dissociation.
Regular P waves may be seen.	P waves may be seen marching through ventricular complexes.
Previous ECG with bundle branch block.	Previously normal ECG.
No fusion or capture beats.	Fusion and capture beats may be evident.
QRS width < 0.14 second.	QRS width > 0.14 second.
No concordance in V_1–V_6.	Concordance in V_1–V_6.
Same axis compared to previous ECG without arrhythmia.	Different axis compared to previous ECG without arrhythmia.

PROCAINAMIDE Give 7–10 mg/kg IV over 10 minutes, followed by an infusion of 1–4 mg/min.

CARDIAC PACING Over-ride atrial pacing may be necessary for patients in whom drugs and cardioversion have been ineffective.

Ventricular tachycardia and fibrillation

These are uncommon arrhythmias in seriously ill patients in the ICU, as opposed to patients with primary ischaemic heart disease. Rapid defibrillation will improve outcomes. For VT and VF treatment protocols, see Chapter 10.

Broad-complex tachyarrhythmias of uncertain origin

In some patients there may be little clinical or ECG evidence to differentiate VT from SVT with aberrant conduction. More than 90% of cases will be VT. When in doubt, treat the arrhythmias as VT, and refer the patients electively for electrophysiological studies at a later date (Table 23.5).

IMMEDIATE TREATMENT

1. Attempt rapid defibrillation, commencing at 200 J and increasing to 360 J, if the patient is haemodynamically compromised.

2. Lignocaine (1.5 mg IV stat, followed by IV infusion at 1–4 mg/min) may be effective if the rhythm is VT. Lignocaine will not aggravate SVT.

3. Procainamide 7–10 mg/kg IV over 10 minutes, followed by infusion at 1–4 mg/min) may be effective whether the wide-complex tachycardia is ventricular or supraventricular. It will not affect VT.

4. Adenosine, as rapid boluses at 0.05 mg/kg IV, is a relatively safe antiarrhythmic that can be used in these circumstances and may be successful in correcting SVT.

5. Although intravenous verapamil is highly effective in terminating SVT, its use should be avoided in patients who have a broad-complex tachyarrhythmia of unclear cause.

Some complications of antiarrhythmic drugs

Combinations of antiarrhythmics can be dangerous, as drug interactions can occur. It is better to give one drug to its limit of safety, and attempt cardioversion should that fail.

With the exceptions of amiodarone and digoxin, all antiarrhythmics are negatively inotropic and, when given intravenously, can cause hypotension.

All antiarrhythmics have pro-arrhythmic properties. Drugs such as quinidine, flecainide, encainide, digoxin, amiodarone, calcium-channel antagonists, and β-blockers can either exacerbate existing arrhythmias or cause new ones. The risk of pro-arrhythmic effects is increased with the use of multiple drugs.

RIGHT VENTRICULAR FAILURE

Our understanding of right ventricular function is not as extensive as our understanding of left ventricular function. However, the function of the right ventricle is an important consideration in the seriously ill. For example, both underlying lung disease and artificial ventilation can cause right ventricular strain.

TABLE 23.6 SITUATIONS IN WHICH RIGHT VENTRICULAR DYSFUNCTION MAY OCCUR IN INTENSIVE CARE

Acute on chronic lung disease.
Pulmonary embolism.
Acute respiratory failure causing pulmonary hypertension (eg ARDS, pneumonia, aspiration).
Right ventricular infarction, especially in association with inferior infarction.
Positive end-expiratory pressure and ventilation.
Cardiac contusion.

Right ventricular failure can be difficult to diagnose. Its features include an elevated jugular venous pressure with a positive Kussmaul sign, hepatic congestion, right ventricular heave, and a loud P_2 on auscultation. Haemodynamic monitoring will reveal the combination of low pulmonary artery wedge pressure (PAWP) and high central venous pressure (CVP). The chest x-ray will show clear lung fields. A dilated, poorly functioning right ventricle will be seen on transoesophageal echocardiography.

Acute increases in pulmonary artery pressure as a result of various lung disorders can lead to increases in right ventricular afterload, right ventricular volume, right ventricular wall stress, and oxygen consumption (Table 23.6). High pulmonary artery pressures can cause ballooning of the **RIGHT VENTRICLE,** which in turn can cause a paradoxical right-to-left septal shift – the so-called internal-tamponade effect or ventricular interdependence, which can in turn compromise left ventricular contraction.

CLINICAL APPROACH TO RIGHT VENTRICULAR DYSFUNCTION

CORRECT THE CORRECTABLE Treat any underlying condition, such as adult respiratory distress syndrome (ARDS), pulmonary embolism, or infection, in an attempt to reduce pulmonary artery pressure and right ventricular work.

INCREASE RIGHT VENTRICULAR PRELOAD The first response to most acute episodes of hypotension in the ICU should be to increase the preload with colloid or blood (see p. 61). Increasing the preload of the right ventricle will similarly improve right ventricular function in many cases. This is an important manoeuvre, especially in the presence of right ventricular infarction. Drugs that can reduce right ventricular preload (diuretics, vasodilators) should be avoided.

DECREASE RIGHT VENTRICULAR AFTERLOAD   Although the option of decreasing the right ventricular afterload sounds attractive, it has certain disadvantages. Firstly, achieving pulmonary vasodilation with agents such as sodium nitroprusside, hydralazine, or prostacyclin will not cure the underlying parenchymal abnormality and may over-ride the hypoxic vasoconstrictive response, worsening the hypoxia. Secondly, it may decrease systemic blood pressure and therefore coronary perfusion pressure. Because of increased wall tension, the right ventricle is particularly sensitive to decreased coronary perfusion pressure.

INOTROPES AND VASOPRESSORS   Both adrenaline and noradrenaline have been shown to improve coronary blood flow and right ventricular contractility. This can be particularly important for the acute right ventricular load associated with pulmonary embolism.

HYPERTENSIVE CRISES

AETIOLOGY

Hypertensive crises are most commonly seen in ICUs in the following settings:

• Post operation (eg post cardiac bypass, vascular surgery, or with any prolonged surgery, and in association with inadequate analgesia).
• Iatrogenic (due to inadvertent administration of a vasopressor or flushing of a central line with a fluid containing a vasopressor agent).
• Autonomic disorders such as poliomyelitis, tetanus, and Guillain-Barré syndrome (see p. 627).
• Hypertension is often seen in association with acute cardiorespiratory events such as pulmonary oedema, acute severe asthma, angina pectoris, and myocardial infarction.
• Paradoxical hypertension or a labile blood pressure often occurs in

association with hypovolaemia, particularly in previously hypertensive patients or in patients suffering from autonomic disorders. It seems that the brittle cardiovascular system associated with such conditions over-reacts to intravascular volume depletion.

• Hypertension secondary to increased intracranial pressure accompanying any intracerebral catastrophe (see p. 569).

• In association with diseases such as renal dysfunction, phaeochromocytoma, thyrotoxicosis, and pre-eclampsia.

• In association with poisoning or abuse of illicit drugs (eg amphetamines, monoamine oxidase inhibitors, cocaine) (see Chapter 16).

• Primary hypertension (not commonly seen now because of improved long-term antihypertensive control). It is occasionally seen as a rebound phenomenon after clonidine or β-blocker withdrawal or in non-compliant patients.

MANAGEMENT

Clinical evaluation

Determine the duration of hypertension, the history of onset of the current crisis, and the patient's current drug regimen.

Determine target-organ involvement via history and physical examination, paying particular attention to the optic fundi, central nervous system, renal function, and cardiorespiratory system (Table 23.7).

Initial investigations should include 12-lead ECG, chest x-ray, biochemistry, urinalysis, full blood count, and CT scan if the patient is confused or if there are focal neurological signs.

General measures

Confirm blood-pressure reading – check cuffs, transducers, and other measuring equipment.

Decide whether the hypertension is a true emergency (eg in association with pre-eclampsia) or whether it can be controlled electively (eg long-standing hypertension with minimal acute effects on target organs). It is the presence or absence of acute or progressive target-organ dysfunction that will determine whether or not immediate

TABLE 23.7 TYPES OF HYPERTENSIVE EMERGENCIES AND
TREATMENT RECOMMENDATIONS

Type of hypertensive emergency	Recommended treatment	Drugs to avoid
Hypertensive encephalopathy	SNP,[a] labetalol, diazoxide	β-blockers, methyldopa, clonidine, SNP, and other cerebral vaso-dilators if intracranial pressure is raised
Cerebral infarction	No treatment, SNP, labetalol	β-blockers, methyl-dopa, clonidine
Intracerebral haemorrhage, subarachnoid haemorrhage	No treatment, SNP, labetalol	β-blockers, methyldopa, clonidine
Myocardial ischaemia, myocardial infarction	Nitroglycerin, labetalol, calcium antagonists, SNP	Hydralazine, diazoxide, minoxidil
Acute pulmonary oedema	SNP and loop diuretic, nitrogly-cerin and loop diuretic	Hydralazine, diazoxide, β-blockers, labetalol
Aortic dissection	SNP and β-blocker; β-blocker and trimetha-phan; labetalol	Hydralazine, diazoxide and minoxidil
Eclampsia	Hydralazine, diazoxide, labetalol, calcium antagonists, SNP	Trimethaphan, diuretics, β-blockers
Acute renal insufficiency	SNP, labetalol, calcium antagonists	β-blockers, trimethaphan
Microangiopathic haemolytic anaemia	SNP, labetalol, calcium antagonists	β-blockers

[a]SNP, sodium nitroprusside.
Source: Adapted from Calhoun and Oparil (1990), with permission.

treatment of the hypertension is required, not the absolute value of the blood pressure.

Reverse the reversible (eg alleviate post-operative pain, reduce anxiety, check gas exchange, and exclude the possibility of a full bladder or inadvertent vasopressor infusion). It is important always to check for hypovolaemia as a paradoxical cause of hypertension.

Primary malignant hypertension is a diagnosis of exclusion. Its onset is over days or weeks, on a background of long-standing hypertension.

Approach to severe hypertension

LONG-STANDING SEVERE HYPERTENSION MUST BE TREATED SLOWLY AND SMOOTHLY. The faster the rate of rise in systemic pressure, the faster the reduction can be safely achieved. The organs most at risk from hypertension are the heart, kidney, and brain. They are autoregulated at a high baseline pressure in patients with long-standing hypertension (Figure 23.1). Organ autoregulation will adjust to a lower arterial pressure at a slow rate. The pressure must be monitored carefully during this adjustment stage. THE ARTERIAL PRESSURE SHOULD BE REDUCED SLOWLY OVER 3–4 DAYS, IN ORDER TO PREVENT RELATIVE HYPOTENSION AND ISCHAEMIA IN ORGANS NORMALLY ACCUSTOMED TO HIGH PRESSURE. As a guide, the lower limit of cerebral autoregulation is 25% below the resting mean arterial pressure (MAP). Hence, the aim of immediate treatment is to reduce the MAP by 20–25%, over minutes to hours, depending on the nature of the emergency. Aim for a pressure reduction to approximately 160/110 mm Hg within the first 48 hours, or aim to reduce the mean pressure by no more than 30% in the first 24 hours, especially if hypertension has been long-standing.

Continuous monitoring of arterial pressure and cardiac, renal, and cerebral functions is mandatory.

Correct the hypovolaemia that often accompanies severe hypertension because of sodium and water losses. The circulation will become angiotensin-dependent in these circumstances. IT IS IMPORTANT NOT TO USE DIURETICS NOR INHIBITORS OF ANGIOTENSIN-CONVERTING ENZYME (ACE) INITIALLY, AS DANGEROUS LEVELS OF HYPOTENSION CAN RESULT.

Autoregulation in normal and hypertensive patients

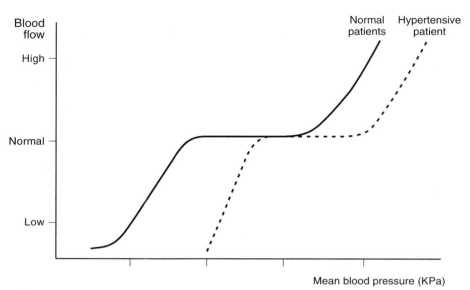

FIGURE 23.1 Autoregulation in normal and hypertensive patients.

Drug usage in severe hypertension

Administer small doses of antihypertensive drugs while closely monitoring arterial pressure, pulse rate, and cardiac, renal, and cerebral functions. It is not possible to predict the critical diastolic pressure at which coronary perfusion will be compromised in any given individual. Thus, the arterial pressure should be lowered in a gentle fashion in order to avoid myocardial ischaemia.

Short-acting drugs should be used initially, in order to prevent prolonged hypotension.

There is no single drug of choice for severe hypertension. At present, the most commonly employed agents are as follows:

SODIUM NITROPRUSSIDE (SNP) Give a continuous intravenous infusion (50 mg/50 ml), commencing at 5 μg/min and going up to a maximum of 500 μg/min (0.5–10 μg · kg^{-1} · min^{-1}), **SLOWLY AND SMOOTHLY,** in order to avoid precipitous decreases in arterial pressure. Measure the plasma thiocyanate, and look for unexplained metabolic acidosis in cases of prolonged high-dosage infusion. Use SNP cautiously in patients with hypertensive encephalopathy, as it can cause a rise in intracranial pressure.

NITROGLYCERIN Nitroglycerin, at 5–100 μg/min as an intravenous infusion, may be useful in hypertensive patients with acute left ventricular failure, acute coronary insufficiency, and post-operative hypertension. Remember that nitroglycerin has its main vasodilatory action on the venous circulation, not the arterial circulation, and therefore will not have a major effect on severe hypertension.

NIFEDIPINE Give 5 mg initially, sublingually, and then 5–10-mg boluses at intervals that can range up to 30 minutes. It can also be given orally at 5–30 mg at intervals of up to 30 minutes. However, sudden decreases in blood pressure can occur with higher doses, especially if orally administered.

HYDRALAZINE Give 10–20 mg IV at 15-minute intervals. Repeat as necessary, or commence a continuous intravenous infusion at 5–30 mg/h titrated against response.

INHIBITORS OF ANGIOTENSIN-CONVERTING ENZYME ACE inhibitors can cause profound vasodilation and sudden hypotension when used in patients with long-standing hypertension. They should be used for long-term control of hypertension, not as a first-line treatment.

• Captopril: It has been suggested that 6.25 mg can be given as an initial oral dose. However, when there is doubt, give one-quarter that dose, and observe the response. Gradually increase the dosage, according to the patient's responses, at intervals of 8 hours or 12 hours.

• Enalapril: Similarly, an initial dose of 2.5 mg orally has been suggested. This can also cause severe hypotension. If in doubt, give one-quarter of that dose as a maximum, and observe the response; then continue with the 0.6-mg doses one or two times daily, and increase the dosage as necessary.

LABETALOL Give an intravenous bolus of 20–80 mg every 5–10 minutes, up to a total of 300 mg; or give an intravenous infusion commencing at 10 mg/h and titrating against the patient's responses. Exercise caution in patients with heart failure or phaeochromocytoma.

PHENTOLAMINE Give an intravenous bolus of 5–10 mg every 5–15 minutes or an intravenous infusion (5–500 μg/min). Along with SNP, it is the drug of first choice for treating a severe adrenergic storm, and it may have advantages over SNP for patients with encephalopathy, as it does not increase cerebral blood flow. Phentolamine use is often associated with compensatory tachycardia.

β-BLOCKERS β-blockers are used mainly as adjuncts to treatment initially. Avoid them or use them carefully in patients with phaeochromocytoma and heart failure.

DIAZOXIDE Diazoxide can be unpredictable when used as a bolus dose and can cause increases in heart rate. The suggested dose is 50–100 mg as a bolus intravenous injection within 30 seconds, every 5–15 minutes, up to a total of 600 mg, until the desired effect is achieved.

Drugs such as methyldopa, prazosin, trimethaphan, and clonidine can also be used.

Hypertensive encephalopathy

Hypertensive encephalopathy is a rare but serious sequela to severe hypertension. The intracranial pressure is elevated in these circumstances. Many antihypertensive drugs (such as nitroprusside and hydralazine) will cause a further increase in intracerebral pressure (ICP) by causing cerebral vasodilation.

A slow infusion of an α-blocker such as phentolamine or labetalol may be best employed initially.

Further treatment of hypertension

Avoid fluid retention as the arterial pressure decreases with the gradual introduction of diuretics.

Aim for monotherapy, although two or three drugs in combination occasionally are necessary.

Reconsider the possibility of a secondary cause of hypertension (eg

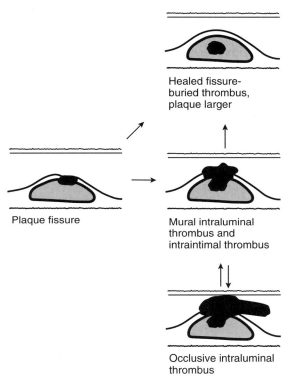

Healed fissure-
buried thrombus,
plaque larger

Plaque fissure

Mural intraluminal
thrombus and
intraintimal thrombus

Occlusive intraluminal
thrombus

FIGURE 23.2 Pathophysiology of ischaemic heart disease. Plaque fissuring is probably responsible for many of the manifestations of ischaemic heart disease. The plaque fissure can heal (top) or can go on to form thrombosis that partially occludes the coronary artery (middle), causing symptoms of unstable angina. Complete obstruction (bottom) can also occur, resulting in total occlusion and myocardial infarction if there is no collateral flow. (From Fuster et al., 1990, with permission of the American Heart Association.)

phaeochromocytoma, renal artery stenosis) if the arterial pressure remains resistant to treatment.

ACUTE MYOCARDIAL INFARCTION

Ischaemic heart disease is very common in the Western world, especially among older populations (Figure 23.2). Many seriously ill patients being treated in ICUs probably have concurrent coronary artery disease. Cardiac ischaemia or acute myocardial infarction (AMI) po-

TABLE 23.8　DIAGNOSIS OF ACUTE MYOCARDIAL INFARCTION

---

1. ECG

ST-segment elevation > 1 mm in relevant leads.

T waves flatten and invert within hours to days of AMI.

Q waves usually develop over the first 1–2 days.

ECG changes may be minimal or non-existent in the presence of pre-existing abnormality such as left bundle branch block.

2. Cardiac enzymes

CK-MB isoenzyme activity:

>4% of CK-MB level

>14 units/L (glass-bead assay)

>40 μg/L (radioimmunoassay)

Elevation 6 hours after AMI.

Peak activity 10–30 hours.

3. Radioisotope imaging

Technetium pyrophosphate imaging or 'hot-spot' scan can help to identify acute damage secondary to AMI.

4. Cardiac ultrasound

Can usually identify segmental dyskinesia consistent with AMI.

---

tentially can complicate the clinical courses of many patients being managed in the ICU. This text will not deal exhaustively with the management of myocardial ischaemia or AMI. There are many good text-books covering this area. However, because coronary artery disease is so common in our community, some aspects of its presentation and management in the seriously ill will be discussed here (Table 23.8).

Clinical features of AMI in intensive care

• If conscious, the patient may complain of typical chest pain. However, peri-operative infarcts often are silent.

• Typical changes on 12-lead ECG.

• A new bundle branch block.

• Increases in cardiac enzymes.

• ST-segment elevation on continuous ECG monitoring.

• Sudden onset of ventricular arrhythmia (eg VT or VF).

• Sudden changes in arterial blood pressure (hypotension or hypertension).

• Any change in heart rate (sinus tachycardia caused by increased pain and anxiety, or sinus bradycardia due to intracardiac conduction delays).

• Increasing requirements for analgesia or sedation.

• Onset of cardiogenic shock (hypotension and decreased peripheral perfusion) (see p. 555).

• Sudden onset of pulmonary oedema.

Diagnosis of AMI

• Maintain a high index of clinical suspicion.

• 12-lead ECG changes: Remember that the classic changes of AMI may not occur for up to 24 hours and may be non-specific.

• Cardiac enzymes: There may be other explanations for many of these enzyme elevations in the seriously ill; what is required for diagnostic purposes is a rise in the specific cardiac enzyme CPK-MB.

• Echocardiography may demonstrate abnormal wall motion typical of AMI.

Treatment of AMI

Thrombolytics, anticoagulants, and antiplatelet drugs have all been shown to be useful in patients with AMI (Table 23.9). However, the seriously ill often have contraindications to their use (Table 23.10). Treatment should take the following factors into account:

• Size of AMI: The extent of the ECG changes, the sizes of the cardiac enzyme changes, and echocardiography can give an indication of infarct size.

• Coagulation profile: Measure the baseline prothrombin time, activated partial thromboplastin time, and platelet count.

• Presence of major bleeding predisposition (eg recent surgery).

• Presence of major intravascular lines (remember that it is better to insert these prior to administration of thrombolytic agents).

TABLE 23.9   APPROACH TO THROMBOLYTIC TREATMENT OF ACUTE
MYOCARDIAL INFARCTION

---

1. Aspirin, 150–300 mg.

2. Streptokinase, 1.5 million units over 1 hour

THEN

Aspirin, 75 mg

+

Heparin, 12,500 units SC twice daily after 24 hours.

CONSIDER

Heparin IV or repeat thrombolysis for recurrent cardiac pain or reoc-
clusion.

3. If there is streptokinase allergy, or was exposure to streptokinase between
5 days and 1 year previously:

Recombinant tissue plasminogen activator (rt-PA), 100 mg, as follows:

10 mg IV, stat

THEN

50-mg IV infusion over 1 hour

THEN

40-mg IV infusion over 2 hours

THEN

Aspirin, 75 mg

Full heparinization IV after rt-PA infusion, 24,000–30,000 units/24 hours,
check activated partial thromboplastin time.

Management otherwise is supportive (Table 23.11). Relieve any pain.
Aim to maintain normal oxygenation, systemic arterial pressures, cardiac output, and haemoglobin levels in order to provide adequate oxygen levels to the myocardium. Myocardial oxygen demand can be reduced by measures such as avoiding tachycardia and reducing cardiac
afterload. Insertion of a pulmonary artery catheter, particularly in patients with already compromised oxygen demand/supply ratios, may
help with titration of drug regimens.

The roles for early β-blockers and calcium-channel blockers have
not been determined in the critically ill.

TABLE 23.10 THROMBOLYTIC TREATMENT

Indications

Patient presenting within 24 hours of major symptoms suggestive of AMI

ECG: ST elevation of at least 1 mm in standard leads or at least 2 mm in two adjacent precordial leads

Absolute contraindications

Active haemorrhage

Recent central nervous system (CNS) infarction, haemorrhage, surgery, trauma, or malignancy (<3 months)

Relative contraindications

Recent non-CNS surgery (<10 days)

Recent trauma (<10 days)

Recent gastro-intestinal haemorrhage

Recent external cardiac massage

Coagulation disorders

Pregnancy or <10 days post partum

Severe hypertension (diastolic blood pressure > 130 mm Hg)

Conditions with potential for CNS embolism (eg bacterial endocarditis)

CARDIOGENIC SHOCK

Cardiogenic shock reflects failure of the heart as a pump. Its clinical signs are as follows:

1. Hypotension: systolic pressure less than 90 mm Hg, or 30 mm Hg below the 'normal' systolic pressure.

2. Manifestations of low cardiac output, such as

- oliguria
- confusion, coma, agitation
- peripheral vasoconstriction
- high systemic vascular resistance (SVR), high PAWP

The commonest cause is acute myocardial infarction. Other causes are listed in Table 23.12.

TABLE 23.11   MANAGEMENT OF ACUTE MYOCARDIAL INFARCTION

Oxygen at 4–6 L/min may marginally improve myocardial oxygenation.

Continuous ECG monitoring for 24–48 hours, if uncomplicated.

Pain relief: liberal use of narcotics in the acute stage; morphine, 2.5–5.0 mg IV, titrated against pain relief.

Nitrates: Reduce preload and myocardial oxygen demand and improve collateral flow. They may exacerbate hypotension.

Thrombolytic agents, aspirin, and anticoagulants if no contraindication.

Aspirin, 150–300 g/d.

Streptokinase or rt-PA.

Heparin.

Immediate investigation of post-AMI unstable angina not responding to nitrates, β-blockers, or calcium-channel blockers, with a view to definitive measures such as angioplasty or coronary artery bypass grafting.

Other drugs: β-blockers instituted early may limit infarct size and reduce long-term mortality.

Observe and treat complications (eg unstable angina, heart failure, pulmonary oedema, pericarditis, arrhythmias, and mechanical complications such as ruptured papillary muscle, ruptured intraventricular septum, or left ventricular aneurysm).

TABLE 23.12   CAUSES OF CARDIOGENIC SHOCK

Acute myocardial infarction

Cardiomyopathy

Valve rupture

Aortic dissection

Cardiac tamponade

Acute pericarditis

PATHOPHYSIOLOGY

The pathophysiology of cardiogenic shock is both fascinating and frustrating. The mortality remains greater than 80%, despite many new interventions (eg acute angioplasty and drugs).

A large, acute anterior myocardial infarction is the most common cause of cardiogenic shock: The cardiac output decreases, leading to hypotension and decreased end-organ perfusion. Left ventricular end-diastolic pressure rises, and pulmonary venous pressure increases, which then leads to pulmonary oedema. This results in hypoxia, decreased lung compliance, and increased work of breathing. The myocardial oxygen supply is compromised secondary to low Sao_2 and low diastolic blood pressure.

These patients usually have a high PAWP and are severely hypoxic secondary to pulmonary oedema, so that left ventricular preload cannot be increased. However, decreasing the left ventricular preload can cause worsening of the hypotension, as a failing heart usually is very dependent on preload.

The cardiac afterload usually is very high, and it would be advantageous to off-load the heart. However, that normally results in hypotension and decreased coronary perfusion. Combinations of inotropes and vasodilators may work.

With limited options in regard to altering preload or afterload, increasing the contractility is the only option. This may increase cardiac output, but at the expense of increasing the myocardial oxygen demand and possible extension of the infarct!

MANAGEMENT

Reverse the reversible

CORRECT HYPOVOLAEMIA Patients with acute heart failure are sometimes hypovolaemic. This is related to aggressive diuretic treatment and is secondary to loss of protein-rich pulmonary oedema fluid into the lungs. Furthermore, a high filling pressure is needed for a failing heart. Aim to keep PAWP > 18 mm Hg (2.4 kPa). Patients with inferior infarctions and right ventricular involvement are especially dependent on a high filling pressure for optimum cardiac output.

CORRECT ELECTROLYTE AND ACID–BASE DISTURBANCES

EXCLUDE OR CORRECT, WHERE POSSIBLE:
- mitral regurgitation secondary to ruptured papillary muscle
- ventricular septal rupture
- pericardial effusion
- any other surgically reversible lesion

- arrhythmias
- pulmonary embolism

General supportive measures

PAIN   Treat pain or anxiety with continuous intravenous infusion of opiates.

OXYGENATION   Increase the oxygen delivery by

- simple face mask
  OR
- CPAP, via a mask or endotracheal tube (ETT), especially in the presence of pulmonary oedema, to keep $Pao_2 > 80$ mm Hg (10.00 kPa) (see p. 397)

LOW-DOSAGE DOPAMINE   Give dopamine at 1–3 μg $\cdot$ kg^{-1} $\cdot$ min^{-1} to encourage renal and mesenteric blood flow.

MONITORING   Monitor arterial blood pressure, pulse rate, and specific indices of organ function, such as hourly urine output, peripheral skin perfusion, and level of consciousness. Pulmonary artery catheterization, with measurement of PAWP and cardiac output, can help to optimize ventricular filling pressures.

ANTICOAGULATION   Consider the use of full-dosage heparin, especially if there is a large anterior infarction; otherwise, use 'low' subcutaneous doses of heparin.

PRINCIPLES OF DRUG MANAGEMENT   The aim is to increase end-organ perfusion without adversely affecting the remaining cardiac function. This can be difficult. For each beneficial effect of an intervention or drug, usually there will be an adverse effect. The mortality from cardiogenic shock is 70–100% and has not changed markedly in the past 10 years, despite many new interventions and drugs. This is related to the vicious spiral of pathophysiology and limited treatment options.

VASODILATOR TREATMENT   It is difficult to use vasodilator treatment when the arterial pressure is already low, as a further decrease will reduce coronary perfusion and exacerbate myocardial dysfunction. Sodium nitroprusside and nitroglycerin can be cautiously commenced as a continuous infusion. However, further hypotension must be avoided.

VASOPRESSOR AND INOTROPIC TREATMENT Increasing the contractility of the remaining heart muscle with inotropes, such as with noradrenaline, adrenaline, and dopamine, will also increase peripheral vascular resistance and afterload. This may increase arterial pressure and coronary blood flow, but it will simultaneously increase cardiac oxygen consumption. An inotrope with mainly β activity, such as dobutamine, may be more appropriate. However, it can increase oxygen consumption by increasing the heart rate, and it may decrease coronary perfusion and arterial blood pressure as a result of peripheral vasodilation.

Vasodilators, inotropes, and vasopressors must be carefully balanced when treating cardiogenic shock. Careful monitoring and titration of the drugs, with an understanding of their actions, is essential. There may be a drug combination that will be ideal for a given patient. A combination of α effects to increase coronary perfusion pressure and β effects to increase cardiac output is often necessary. In the presence of pump failure secondary to severe obstructive coronary artery disease, coronary autoregulation is limited, and coronary blood flow becomes dependent on perfusion pressure. It is crucial, therefore, not to decrease blood pressure in these circumstances.

Other techniques

POSITIVE INTRATHORACIC PRESSURE The use of positive intrathoracic pressure in the form of continuous positive airway pressure (CPAP) or intermittent positive-pressure ventilation (IPPV) may be effective, especially in the presence of hypoxia and pulmonary oedema. CPAP must be delivered through an efficient circuit via a mask, nasal prongs, or ETT (p. 472).

CPAP has unique abilities to improve gas exchange and decrease respiratory work, in addition to decreasing preload and afterload. In other words, cardiac function potentially can be improved without increasing myocardial oxygen demand.

INTRA-AORTIC BALLOON PUMP The intra-aortic balloon pump (IABP) can be inserted directly or percutaneously into the femoral artery using the Seldinger technique. Use of the IABP results in increased coronary perfusion, as well as decreased afterload, and can temporarily improve cardiac function.

As is the case with drugs, neither IABP nor CPAP has been demonstrated to influence long-term outcomes for patients in cardiogenic shock.

ARTERIAL RECANALIZATION If shock occurs within 6 hours of the onset of pain, recanalization should be attempted, with thrombolysis, percutaneous transluminal angioplasty, or coronary artery surgery. Use of the IABP may be necessary for temporary support until definitive treatment can be instituted.

AORTIC DISSECTION

PATHOPHYSIOLOGY

Aortic dissection occurs as a result of a tear in the intima of the aorta, usually against a background of hypertension and atheroma. Pressure within the aorta forces the blood to dissect within the intimal plane. The blood forms a false lumen. It can then rupture back through the intima, further along the aorta, or even rupture through the media and adventitia.

During the formation of a false lumen, many complications can occur. For example, the aortic valve can be disrupted, causing aortic incompetence. When coronary arteries are involved, myocardial ischaemia and infarction can occur.

CLINICAL PRESENTATION

Pain is usually a marked feature of sudden dissection. Pain usually begins retrosternally and radiates to the back, as well as to wherever the dissection extends (eg legs, abdomen, limbs, face). Branches of the aorta, such as the carotid, subclavian, renal, and mesenteric arteries, may be involved, causing a wide range of signs and symptoms, such as stroke, loss of peripheral pulses, and bowel ischaemia. Abdominal pain, bloody diarrhoea, and oliguria will indicate involvement of the splanchnic and renal circulations. The aortic valve can also be involved, causing aortic incompetence.

Important considerations in the differential diagnosis are acute myocardial infarction, cholecystitis, and pancreatitis.

INVESTIGATIONS

• Monitor with 12-lead ECG recordings.

• Perform routine haematology and biochemistry tests.

• A chest x-ray may show evidence of a widened mediastinum.

• Whereas angiography is widely held to be the gold-standard investigative tool, contrast-enhanced computed tomography (CT), magnetic-resonance imaging (MRI), and combined transthoracic-transoesophageal echocardiography have all been shown to have similar sensitivities and specificities in the right hands.

Certain diagnostic information is required:

(a) Confirm the presence of dissection.

(b) Determine whether the dissection involves the ascending aorta (type A) or the descending aorta (type B).

(c) Determine the extent of the dissection, the sites of entry and re-entry, the extent of involvement of other arteries, and the presence or absence of thrombus in the false lumen. Information on aortic insufficiency and pericardial effusion should also be obtained.

All four diagnostic techniques have strengths and weaknesses in these areas.

MANAGEMENT

• The diagnosis must be rapidly confirmed, and then the type and extent of dissection must be defined.

• Early cardiothoracic surgical consultation is essential, especially if there are mechanical complications such as aortic valve involvement.

• Use antihypertensive medication, if indicated (see p. 544). Sodium nitroprusside (see p. 548) and β-blockers often are needed to control the hypertension.

TABLE 23.13   CAUSES OF PERICARDIAL EFFUSION

Haemorrhage
Cardiac surgery
Trauma (blunt and penetrating)
Anticoagulation
Aortic dissection
Malignancy
Infection
Tuberculosis
Viral infections
AIDS
Pericarditis
Post irradiation
Uraemic

OUTCOME

The prognosis is poor, with mortality of 25% within the first hour, 50% cumulative mortality at 1 week, and 90% mortality at 1 year in untreated or unrecognized cases.

CARDIAC TAMPONADE

Cardiac tamponade occurs when there is accumulation of fluid or air in the pericardium, causing impaired filling of the ventricles and therefore decreased cardiac output.

PATHOPHYSIOLOGY

It is important to distinguish between pericardial effusion and cardiac tamponade. Pericardial effusion is a collection of fluid in the pericardial space that does not necessarily impede cardiac function. The effusion may be blood, transudate, or exudate, usually having been accumulated chronically (Table 23.13).

On the other hand, cardiac tamponade occurs when the pericardial fluid or gas impairs cardiac filling and output: Both right and left ventricular filling pressures are increased, but filling volumes are decreased. Initially this is compensated for by an increase in heart rate. As the tamponade worsens, cardiac output decreases.

As little as 250 ml of fluid can cause acute cardiac tamponade, whereas under chronic conditions, greater amounts of pericardial fluid can accumulate, as the cardiovascular system can slowly adjust.

CLINICAL FEATURES

1. Tachycardia and hypotension:
- low-volume pulse
- pulsus paradoxus > 10 mm Hg

2. Poor peripheral perfusion

3. Dyspnoea

4. Signs of impaired ventricular filling:

(a) Right ventricle:
- increased jugular venous pressure or CVP
- hepatomegaly (in chronic cases)
- ascites, pleural effusions (in chronic cases)
- peripheral oedema (in chronic cases)

(b) Left ventricle:
- low cardiac output
- high PAWP (classically, PAWP equals CVP, which equals pericardial pressure)

5. Muffled heart sounds

6. ECG:
- tachycardia
- small complexes
- signs of atrial enlargement

7. Chest x-ray:
- cardiomegaly (if chronic)
- oligaemic lung fields (if acute)

INVESTIGATIONS

Echocardiography is diagnostic and not only will detect pericardial effusion but also will document ventricular function.

MANAGEMENT

Cardiac tamponade is a medical emergency, and drainage of the pericardial effusion is a priority. In the first instance, pericardiocentesis should be performed under ultrasound guidance, either by using a Seldinger technique to pass a catheter into the pericardial space or by aspirating the effusion with a needle.

Some patients may require thoracotomy and surgical drainage of the effusion.

A fluid bolus will initially increase cardiac output. Inotropes usually are ineffective.

TROUBLESHOOTING

SINUS TACHYCARDIA

Sinus tachycardia rarely needs specific treatment. BEWARE OF SPECIFICALLY REDUCING THE RATE, AS THE CARDIAC OUTPUT AND ARTERIAL BLOOD PRESSURE MAY DEPEND ON A HIGH HEART RATE.

Exclude the possibilities of hypoxia and hypercarbia.

Consider the problem of increased work of breathing (eg partially occluded endotracheal tube, bronchospasm, pulmonary oedema, or circuit, humidifier, or ventilator malfunction).

Consider the possibility of infection (eg catheter infection, pneumonia, sinusitis, intra-abdominal sepsis, urinary-tract infection).

Ensure that there is no pain, distress, or distended bladder.

Consider the possibility of occult bleeding.

Often sinus tachycardia is a non-specific accompaniment of multiorgan failure.

Often sinus tachycardia is a non-specific accompaniment of severe trauma.

Check the use of drugs (eg β_2-agonists, inotropes).

Exclude the possibility of myocardial ischaemia or infarction.

Consider the presence of alcohol or other drug withdrawal.

FURTHER READING

Arrhythmias

Aronson, J. K. (1985). Cardiac arrhythmias: theory and practice (editorial). *British Medical Journal* 290:487–8.

Edwards, J. D., & Kishen, R. (1986). Significance and management of intractable supraventricular arrhythmias in critically ill patients. *Critical Care Medicine* 14:280–2.

Rogrove, H. J., & Hughes, C. M. (1992). Defibrillation and cardioversion. *Critical Care Clinics* 8:839–64.

Schoenfeld, P. (1993). Management of severe tachyarrhythmias. In *Yearbook of Intensive Care and Emergency Medicine*, ed. J. L. Vincent, pp. 431–43. Berlin: Springer-Verlag.

Sharma, A. D., & Kleen, G. J. (1985). Pathophysiology and management of atrial and ventricular arrhythmias in the critically ill. *Critical Care Clinics* 1:677–97.

Wood, M., & Ellenbogen, K. A. (1989). Bradyarrhythmias: emergency pacing and implantable defibrillation devices. *Critical Care Clinics* 5:551–68.

Right Ventricular Pathophysiology

Hurford, W. E., & Zapol, W. M. (1988). The right ventricle and critical illness: a review of anatomy, physiology and clinical evaluation of its function. *Intensive Care Medicine* 14:448–57.

Suter, P. M. (1985). Right ventricular pathophysiology in the critically ill. *Clinical Anaesthesiology* 3:899–907.

Vincent, J. L. (ed.) (1988). Right ventricular ejection fraction. *Intensive Care Medicine* 14:447–501 (symposium issue).

Wiedemann, H. P., & Matthay, R. A. (1985). Acute right heart failure. *Critical Care Clinics* 1:631–59.

Hypertensive Crises

Calhoun, D. A., & Oparil, S. (1990). Treatment of hypertensive crisis. *New England Journal of Medicine* 323:1177–83.

McRae, R. P., & Liebson, P. R. (1986). Hypertensive crisis. *Medical Clinics of North America* 70:749–67.

Rubenstein, E. B., & Escalante, C. (1989). Hypertensive crisis. *Critical Care Clinics* 5:477–96.

Acute Myocardial Infarction

Fuster, V., Stein, B., Ambrose, J. A., Badmion, L., Badmion, J. J., & Chesebro, J. H. (1990). Atherosclerotic plaque rupture and thrombosis. *Circulation (Suppl. II)* 82:1147–59.

Acute Myocardial Infarction

International Society and Federation of Cardiology and World Health Organisation Task Force on Myocardial Reperfusion. (1994). Reperfusion in acute myocardial infarction. *Circulation* 90:2091–102.

Cardiogenic Shock

Alpert, J. S., & Becker, R. C. (1993). Mechanisms and management of cardiogenic shock. *Critical Care Clinics* 9:205–18.

Goldberg, R. H., Gore, J. M., Alpert, J. S., et al. (1991). Cardiogenic shock after acute myocardial infarction. *New England Journal of Medicine* 325:1117–22.

Rasanen, J., Vaisanen, I., Heikkila, J., & Nikki, P. (1985). Acute myocardial infarction complicated by left ventricular dysfunction and respiratory failure. The effects of continuous positive airways pressure. *Chest* 87:158–62.

Roberts, R. (1988). Inotropic therapy for cardiac failure associated with acute myocardial infarction. *Chest (Suppl.)* 93:22–4.

Aortic Dissection

Anonymous (1988). Acute aortic dissection. *Lancet* 2:827–8.

Cigarroa, J. E., Isselbacher, E. M., DeSanctis, R. W., & Eagle, K. A. (1993). Diagnostic imaging in the evaluation of suspected aortic dissection. *New England Journal of Medicine* 328:35–43.

Khandheria, B. K. (1992). Aortic dissection. The diagnostic dilemma resolved. *Chest* 101:303–4.

24

ACUTE INTRACRANIAL DISASTERS

- Attention to the basic principles, such as airway, breathing, and circulation, is crucial in the management of all patients with intracranial abnormalities.
- Management of patients with increased intracranial pressure (ICP) must be based on a thorough understanding of intracranial pathophysiology.
- Manoeuvres designed to reduce ICP, such as hyperventilation and the use of barbiturates and mannitol, should be reserved for short-term reduction of a high ICP, rather than being part of long-term management.

The complexities of intracranial function largely remain mysteries. Compared with our knowledge of organs and structures such as the heart, lungs, limbs, and gut, our knowledge of the brain is relatively crude.

No matter what the cause of the intracranial catastrophe, there are certain principles of management that are held in common:

1. Ensure an adequate supply of well-oxygenated blood under a reasonable head of pressure (eg attention to the basic details of airway, ventilation, oxygenation, and cardiovascular support).

2. Make more space inside the head, if possible [eg remove tumour, drain blood or cerebrospinal fluid (CSF), reduce oedema].

3. Study the basic principles of intracranial pathophysiology, and learn how to work with them – for example, the way cerebral blood flow (CBF) varies with metabolic activity and Pa_{CO_2}, and the concepts of intracranial compliance and autoregulation.

PATHOPHYSIOLOGY

Although the brain contributes only 2% of the total weight of a human body, it receives 15% of the cardiac output and accounts for

15–20% of the total oxygen consumption. Cerebral ischaemia occurs when there is an inadequate oxygen supply resulting from a critical reduction in CBF, haemoglobin concentration, or oxygen saturation in the blood. The brain is heterogeneously vulnerable to ischaemia. The most vulnerable zones are the cerebellum, parts of the hippocampus, the basal ganglia, and the boundary zones between major intracranial vessels.

Another unique feature of the brain that tends to make it vulnerable to certain insults is that the intracranial contents are confined within a rigid bony box. That affords considerable protection for the brain, but at the cost of subjecting it to high pressures within its confining box when there is intracranial swelling.

INTRACRANIAL VOLUME

The contents of the cranium are as follows:

- cells   85%
- CSF   10%
- blood volume   5% (150 ml)

Cells

Cells account for most of the intracranial content. Apart from removing brain tissue or shrinking it with diuretics, the cell mass cannot be decreased.

Cerebrospinal fluid

In the presence of increased ICP, CSF production is decreased, and CSF absorption is increased, and the remainder that cannot be accommodated is squeezed into the spinal canal. Thus, draining the CSF in an attempt to make more space, in addition to being technically difficult, usually is futile – hydrocephalus being an exception to this principle. Failure to image the ventricles on a CT scan is a common feature in patients with increased ICP. If excessive CSF is present, it can be drained by ventriculostomy. The initial compensation mechanism for increased ICP is displacement of CSF into the spinal cord. Because epidural analgesia involves the use of large volumes of fluid,

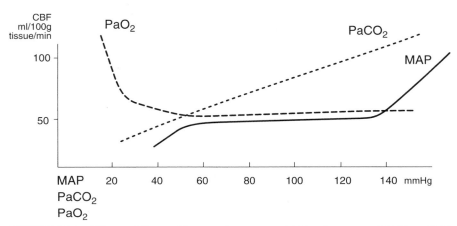

FIGURE 24.1   Effects of $Paco_2$, Pao_2, and mean arterial blood pressure (MAP) on CBF.

which can interfere with spinal CSF flow, it should be avoided in patients suspected of having increased ICP.

Blood volume

The volume of intracranial blood is approximately 150 ml, and although it is the smallest component of the intracranial contents, it is the most amenable to therapeutic manipulation. The aim is to decrease the CBF in an attempt to make more space within the cranium. Altering $Paco_2$ is the main way of manipulating the CBF (Figure 24.1). However, the CBF must not be reduced below the critical level necessary for adequate cellular perfusion. An increase in $Paco_2$ will cause an increase in the CBF, which in turn will increase the ICP and can result in ischaemia. Conversely, a decrease in $Paco_2$ will reduce the CBF, and if that reduction is severe enough, it can also cause ischaemia. This represents a fine therapeutic line. Intracranial blood flow is well controlled over a wide range of systemic pressures by a phenomenon known as autoregulation (see p. 575).

INTRACRANIAL PRESSURE

As the intracranial volume increases, compensation takes place, and the ICP remains stable up to a point at which decompensation begins

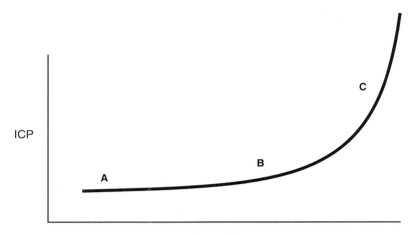

FIGURE 24.2   Relationship between ICP and intracranial volume.
A   As the intracranial volume increases on this part of the curve, compensation occurs, and the ICP rises little.
B   Compensation is increasingly ineffective.
C   At this point on the curve, a small increase in intracranial volume will cause a great rise in ICP. For a patient functioning on this part of the curve, meticulous care is mandatory in order to avoid catastrophic ischaemia. Similarly, small decreases in volume will result in large decreases in pressure.

to occur, and then the ICP rises dramatically (Figure 24.2). On that part of the intracranial compliance curve where the pressure suddenly increases, a small increase in volume will cause a dramatic increase in the ICP and will further reduce cerebral perfusion. Similarly, meticulous care of a patient who is functioning on this part of the curve can be rewarding. Any small decrease in intracranial volume that can be achieved (eg by sitting the patient up, keeping the head straight, using adequate sedation) can have a dramatic effect in bringing the ICP down. **METICULOUS NURSING CARE IS CRUCIAL TO OUTCOMES FOR PATIENTS WITH INCREASED ICP.**

The cerebral perfusion pressure (CPP) is equivalent to the mean arterial blood pressure (MAP) minus the ICP. The aim of treatment is to maintain CPP at more than 60 mm Hg (8.0 kPa) with an adequate MAP and a low ICP. If measures aimed at reducing the ICP fail to maintain an adequate CPP, then the MAP should be increased.

To achieve this, volume loading and vasopressors should be considered.

CPP = MAP − ICP

ICP values:

0–15 mm Hg (0–2.0 kPa)	normal
15–20 mm Hg (2.0–2.7 kPa)	equivocal
20–40 mm Hg (2.7–5.3 kPa)	moderately increased
40 mm Hg (>5.7 kPa)	severely increased

Increases in the ICP often are related to events in the immediate environment. Even in normals, the ICP can transiently rise to high levels. During manoeuvres such as physiotherapy and endotracheal suction, the ICP can rise to very high levels.

FAILURE OF THE ICP TO RAPIDLY RETURN TO NORMAL LEVELS AFTER A TRANSIENT RISE INDICATES DECREASED INTRACRANIAL COMPLIANCE.

Like many aspects in the management of seriously ill patients, ICP monitoring has not been demonstrated to affect outcome. However, it does keep the staff aware of the factors that can affect the ICP for better or worse, in addition to being a guide to CPP (Table 24.1). Moreover, because these patients often are rendered unconscious, clinical signs of an increased ICP are almost non-existent, and without direct measurements of ICP there would otherwise be no indication of its level. So long as attention is not focused on any absolute values for ICP, and it is seen in its clinical context, then ICP is as useful as many other forms of invasive monitoring. A good trace usually indicates adequate ICP performance. However, if there is doubt about the trace, changes in ICP should be sought via a Valsalva manoeuvre, coughing, or occlusion of the internal jugular veins.

ICP MONITORING

Indications for ICP monitoring

Monitoring should be considered for patients who are comatose and have CT signs of significantly increased ICP, such as midline shift or third-ventricle or cisternal compression, and who have potentially re-

TABLE 24.1   ADVANTAGES OF MONITORING ICP

Can be useful as a continuous means of monitoring heavily sedated patients, when there is no other means of assessing the level of consciousness.

Any procedures that can cause severely elevated ICP can be identified, and thereafter modified or avoided. This is very useful for assisting the staff in managing these patients.

The CPP can be determined as a guide to cerebral perfusion, and it should be maintained at more than 60 mm Hg (8.0 kPa).

The ICP will track the progression of the cerebral oedema and give an indication as to when to cease sedation, wean from ventilation, and assess neurological status.

The ICP is a guide to prognosis. Patients without intracranial haematomas who have ICP values consistently above 40 mm Hg (5.3 kPa) have a grim prognosis.

If the ICP rises to more than 25 mm Hg (3.3 kPa) for more than 5 minutes and the arterial blood pressure is constant, short-term manoeuvres probably should be employed to reduce ICP, after obvious reversible factors have been attended to (eg hypoxia, hypercarbia, intracranial bleeding) and the pressure measurement checked.

versible diseases [eg head injury, subarachnoid haemorrhage (SAH), intracerebral haematoma, meningitis, encephalitis, fulminant hepatic failure, Reye's syndrome or cerebral oedema from other causes].

Types of monitoring

INTRAVENTRICULAR   Intraventricular monitoring is the gold standard for ICP monitoring. However, it can be difficult to locate the ventricles in the presence of increased ICP, and the risk of infection is higher than in the other forms of ICP monitoring. The infection rate increases after 5 days in situ, and infection is almost invariable after 10 days. A decrease in the patient's level of consciousness or clinical state may accompany infection.

SUBDURAL AND EXTRADURAL   Extradural monitoring in adults is often damped, as compared with subdural monitoring. There are many commercial products available that can measure both extradural and subdural pressures. Alternatively, a narrow catheter, such as an infant feeding catheter, can be inserted into the epidural or subdural space. The column of fluid in the catheter can be transduced and displayed in the most convenient form. Monitoring of both subdural and extradural pressures is damped, compared with intraventricular monitoring, and in rare cases it can be associated with bleeding.

CEREBRAL MONITORING

Apart from measurement of ICP and the use of electroencephalography (EEG), the parameters of cerebral function that one might wish to monitor are relatively inaccessible. It is usually assumed that if well-oxygenated blood with a normal haemoglobin is supplied to the brain at a reasonable MAP, then cerebral autoregulation will meet the brain's oxygen needs. This assumes that there is no vessel obstruction and no increased ICP. Normal findings on global measurements of cardiorespiratory function usually will guarantee adequate cerebral function. However, more accurate means for monitoring cerebral function are becoming increasingly available, and they may provide more than our current assumptions and our relatively crude monitoring of the oxygenation of brain tissue.

BRAIN ELECTRICAL ACTIVITY   Measurement of voltage using a cerebral-function monitor (CFM) with biparietal electrodes will give an indication of the general level of the brain's electrical activity. This can be useful in testing for brain death and detecting convulsive activity, and it can serve as a general guide to treatment with sedative drugs.

EVOKED POTENTIALS   An evoked potential provides a measure of the ability of the nervous system to receive and respond to an external stimulus. Evoked potentials can sensitively reveal the quantitative responses to auditory, visual, or somatosensory stimulation. They are more accurate for predicting outcome for patients in coma than is a CT scan, ICP monitoring, or clinical examination. Evoked potentials are particularly useful in assessing cerebral function in the presence of drugs, for, unlike the ECG, evoked-potential responses are not altered by the presence of drugs. Assessment of cerebral ischaemia and confirmation of brain death are also feasible with evoked potentials.

CEREBRAL BLOOD FLOW Measurement of cerebral blood flow usually is based on a technique to determine the clearance of xenon 133 from the brain, as detected by scintillation counters positioned over the scalp after intracarotid injection. Because of technical difficulties, it has mainly been used as a research tool.

FLOW VELOCITY Transcranial Doppler (TCD) ultrasound is a commercially available non-invasive technique often used to measure flow velocity in the middle cerebral artery. It is a useful technique for detecting severe stenosis, assessing collateral circulation, and evaluating vasospasm after SAH.

JUGULAR VENOUS SATURATION The oxygen content of blood obtained from the jugular venous bulb ($Cjvo_2$) is the cerebral equivalent of the oxygen content of mixed venous blood. The cerebral metabolic rate for oxygen ($CMRO_2$), CBF, arterial oxygen content (Cao_2), and $Cjvo_2$ are related according to the following equations:

$$CMRO_2 = (CBF)\,(Cao_2 - Cjvo_2)$$
$$Cjvo_2 = Cao_2 - \frac{CMRO_2}{CBF}$$

Retrograde cannulation of the jugular bulb is technically simple, and measurement of $Cjvo_2$ or continuous monitoring of jugular venous saturation ($Sjvo_2$) is possible. Both measurements offer only global average estimates of the degree of cerebral ischaemia and, as such, have limitations.

NEAR-INFRARED SPECTROSCOPY This provides another indirect measure of brain metabolism. Near-infrared light will penetrate the skull, and during its transmission through the brain tissue it will undergo changes in wavelength that will be proportional to the relative concentrations of oxygenated haemoglobin in the tissue beneath the field. This may become a practical, non-invasive technique for continuous cerebral monitoring.

CEREBRAL OEDEMA

Cerebral oedema is an abnormal extravascular accumulation of fluid in the brain, in either the intracellular or the interstitial compartment. It should not be confused with other causes of increased intracranial volume, such as vascular congestion, tumour, or hydrocephalus. Cerebral oedema is a non-specific accompaniment of many disorders, such as head injury, tumour, and infection. The division of cerebral oedema into vasogenic (vascular damage, or damage to the blood–brain barrier) and neurogenic (direct cellular damage) forms is of little clinical importance, as common insults such as global ischaemia and head injury are accompanied by both forms of oedema, and the clinical differentiation is, in any case, impossible.

Cerebral oedema can be detected on CT scan or by monitoring the results of oedema, such as clinical signs or direct measurement of ICP. The signs of increased ICP seen on CT scan can include reduced CSF, loss of gyri and sulci, loss of grey/white differentiation, and flattening of the basal cisterns.

PRINCIPLES OF MANAGING INCREASED ICP (Table 24.2)

The initial assessment and investigation of a patient with increased ICP are discussed in the section on coma (see p. 569). As with all aspects of treating intracranial disasters, attention to basic principles is crucial (eg monitoring the airway, ventilation, oxygenation, intravascular volume, and blood pressure).

AUTOREGULATION

Autoregulation normally operates as an excellent mechanism for maintaining CBF over a wide range of MAP (approximately 60–160 mm Hg). REMEMBER THAT IN HYPERTENSIVE PATIENTS, THE AUTOREGULATION CURVE WILL BE SHIFTED TO THE RIGHT (ie they will maintain a constant flow at a higher-than-normal MAP, but CBF will decrease at a pressure that would be considered normal in a nonhypertensive patient).

Autoregulation, unfortunately, may be compromised by the underlying intracranial abnormality. CBF may then passively follow changes in arterial pressure and ICP. Therefore, never assume that autoregulation offers full protection against fluctuating blood pressure. METICULOUSLY AVOID HYPOTENSION AND HYPERTENSION. Hypertensive surges associated with pain, endotracheal intubation and suctioning, procedures that involve turning the patient, and so

TABLE 24.2 PRINCIPLES OF MANAGEMENT OF
INTRACRANIAL DISASTERS

1. Ensure an adequate airway. Intubate if necessary.
2. Ensure adequate ventilation. Use artificial ventilation if necessary.
3. Ensure adequate cardiovascular function, oxygenation, and haemoglobin concentration. Correct acidosis.
4. Reverse any reversible abnormality (eg drain intracranial blood, treat seizures, hydrocephalus, or infection).
5. Keep the arterial blood pressure within 'normal' limits. Hypotension will cause a decreased CPP, and hypertension can cause 'breakthrough oedema', increased ICP, and consequently decreased CPP.
6. Avoid hypertensive surges, and guarantee sedation with continuous intra-venous narcotics and intermittent boluses of narcotics immediately be-fore procedures such as physiotherapy, turning, or suction. Lignocaine (1.5 mg/kg IV) may help to reduce an elevated ICP during intubation. Continuous infusion of lignocaine (7 mg/min IV) may also help to re-duce ICP and maintain CPP over the longer term.
7. Facilitate jugular venous drainage:
   Sit the patient up at 30° to 45°, and maintain arterial blood pressure. Avoid the head-down position.
   Keep the head straight.
   Avoid securing the artificial airway with tape that can cause constriction around the neck.
8. In order to avoid the problems of coughing, straining, or 'fighting' the ven-tilator, use continuous intravenous narcotic infusion and muscle relax-ants if necessary.
9. Avoid the use of high ventilatory pressures, which would decrease cere-bral venous drainage.
10. Avoid excessive crystalloid treatment. Maintain intravascular volume.
11. Consider ICP monitoring if high pressures are suspected (on the basis of observing the waveform and whether or not the ICP increases with brief bilateral jugular compression).
12. Avoid drugs that would cause a rise in ICP (eg volatile anaesthetic agents, nitrates, ketamine).
13. Use hyperventilation as a short-term manoeuvre; otherwise keep Pa_{CO_2} at 30–40 mm Hg (4–5.3 kPa).
14. Consider diuretics (eg mannitol, 0.3 g/kg, 8-hourly), with or without a loop diuretic, as a temporary measure to reduce ICP.

(continued)

15. If measures aimed at reducing ICP fail, consider a further increase in intravascular volume and the use of vasopressors in an attempt to increase the MAP and therefore the CPP.
16. Consider the development of reversible intracranial pathological conditions (eg a new haemorrhage, or hydrocephalus).
17. Consider 'coma therapy' if diuretics fail to halt severe increases in ICP:

Barbiturates: Give intermittent boluses or a continuous infusion of thiopentone or phenobarbitone. The effects of both take 6–7 days to wear off; so modify the neurological assessment.

Lignocaine, at 1.5 mg/kg IV as a stat dose, and continuous infusion at 7 mg/min, may decrease the ICP.

Phenytoin, in addition to controlling seizures, may decrease the ICP. Give 15 mg/kg over 1 hour as a loading dose, and 5 mg/kg daily as a single intravenous dose over 1 hour.

forth, can cause a sudden increase in cerebral blood volume and may increase oedema formation across a damaged blood–brain barrier. An extra bolus of sedation (eg 5–10 mg morphine, 25–100 mg thiopentone) may be required before any of these procedures is performed, in order to attenuate the hypertensive response.

Lignocaine (1.5 mg/kg) has been recommended, before intubation and tracheal suction, in order to prevent hypertensive surges. Blood pressure should otherwise be maintained at 'normal' or premorbid levels.

FACILITATE VENOUS DRAINAGE

Occlusion of the cerebral venous drainage can cause acute and dangerous increases in cerebral blood volume and ICP (eg coughing, straining, and fighting the ventilator can all cause dangerous increases in ICP by impeding venous return).

Depending on how much pressure is transmitted intracranially, intermittent positive pressure ventilation (IPPV) and positive end-expiratory pressure (PEEP) can also cause increases in ICP.

Taping the endotracheal tube, tracheostomy tube, or nasotracheal tube too tight can cause partial occlusion of the jugular veins in the neck and can increase ICP.

Venous occlusion will be accentuated by allowing the head to turn, even slightly. Keep the head absolutely straight if the patient's ICP is high.

Beware of hard collars, as used for patients suspected of having cervical spine injuries, as they can also increase ICP.

As long as the MAP is maintained at a normal value, position the patient sitting up at 30° to 45°, in order to facilitate venous drainage. Avoid the head-down position whenever possible, even for medical procedures. It is important to maintain the MAP in the desired range when placing a patient head-up in an effort to achieve an adequate CPP.

CARBON DIOXIDE

The Pa_{CO_2} largely determines the CBF, and therefore the cerebral blood volume, because of its rapid effect on the extracellular-fluid hydrogen-ion concentration (ECF [H^+]). The cerebral blood volume will change by approximately 4 ml for every change in Pa_{CO_2} of 5 mm Hg (0.6 kPa). Below a Pa_{CO_2} of 25 mm Hg (3.3 kPa), there is a danger of causing cerebral hypoperfusion. Therefore, the suggested ideal Pa_{CO_2} in these circumstances is 25–35 mm Hg (3.3–4.7 kPa). However, normally there is almost full adaptation to the new Pa_{CO_2} and a return to the same CBF within 4 hours. If the Pa_{CO_2} returns to 'normal' levels, a dangerous increase in CBF can result, as the co-called normal Pa_{CO_2} will then be equivalent to hypercarbia. The 'ideal' Pa_{CO_2} in patients with elevated ICP values is not known, and perhaps hyperventilation should be reserved for use as a temporary measure when the ICP rises suddenly. Otherwise the Pa_{CO_2} should be kept at 35–40 mm Hg (4.7–5.3 kPa). Similarly, acidosis should be avoided, as it can also increase CBF, independent of Pa_{CO_2}.

OXYGENATION

Hypoxia [Pa_{O_2} < 50 mm Hg (6.7 kPa)] can cause an increase in CBF. Maintaining an airway and guaranteeing ventilation and oxygenation are therefore essential for management of an elevated ICP.

DIURETICS

Of all the diuretics, mannitol has become the one most frequently used in clinical practice. Like hyperventilation, it can only buy time, and certainly it is no substitute for the definitive measures needed to reduce intracranial volume, such as drainage of a subdural or extradural haematoma. It should be given as a bolus at 0.3 g/kg over 15 minutes, and then no more frequently than 8-hourly. Higher doses will cause rapid increases in the circulating blood volume and CBF, yielding a paradoxical increase in ICP. Mannitol should not be used at all if the serum osmolality is greater than 330 mOsm/L. A loop diuretic, such as frusemide, will reduce ICP, probably by its diuretic effect, in addition to reducing CSF formation. It can enhance the action of mannitol. Frusemide should be used in small doses (0.2–0.3 mg/kg), repeated as necessary in order to avoid sudden diuresis leading to hypovolaemia, hypotension, and decreased CPP.

FLUID RESTRICTION

Excessive intravenous administration of crystalloid can exacerbate cerebral oedema. Achieve 'euvolaemic dehydration' by maintaining the intravascular volume and CPP with blood or colloid, and otherwise limit fluids to less than 1,500 ml, or approximately two-thirds of the patient's normal maintenance fluid intake, over 24 hours. Maintain the serum sodium concentration at the upper limit of normal, as hyponatraemia can potentiate cerebral oedema.

AVOID DRUGS THAT CAUSE INCREASES IN ICP

• Most of the volatile anaesthetic agents (eg halothane, ethrane, but not isoflurane)
• Nitrous oxide
• Ketamine
• Sodium nitroprusside
• Nitroglycerin

MAINTAIN COLLOID ONCOTIC PRESSURE WITHIN NORMAL LIMITS

A low colloid oncotic pressure (COP) theoretically can encourage movement of fluid from the intravascular space and worsen cerebral oedema. Maintaining a normal serum albumin usually will maintain a normal COP.

DECREASED METABOLIC ACTIVITY OF THE BRAIN: 'COMA THERAPY' OR 'BRAIN PROTECTION'

Although a decrease in metabolic activity is an attractive goal, it is clinically difficult to achieve. 'Coma therapy', using large intravenous doses of anaesthetic agents, such as the barbiturates and etomidate, has, in the past, been used in order to reduce ICP. Although the ICP can be reduced in the short term, these drugs often cause cardiovascular depression and immunosuppression and do not appear to have made any impact on outcome. In clinical practice, the metabolic activity of the brain is most effectively influenced by aggressive control of seizures (see p. 616). There may still be a place for drugs that can specifically decrease the ICP, when all other efforts have failed, or in specific conditions such as Reye's syndrome. High fever should be actively treated, as it can increase the cerebral metabolic rate. A relative degree of central hypothermia (35–36°C) may, in turn, decrease the cerebral metabolic rate and oxygen demand. However, excessive hypothermia must be avoided, as it predisposes to unpredictable haemodynamic effects, impairments of drug metabolism, and increased rates of infection (see p. 156). It has also been suggested that glucose-containing solutions should be avoided during the early stages of treating head injuries, in an attempt to decrease brain metabolic activity by decreasing the supply of metabolic substrate. Some of the drugs used to decrease cerebral metabolism and ICP are as follows:

PHENYTOIN   In addition to helping to control seizures, phenytoin may have some value for 'cerebral protection'. The loading dose should be 15 mg/kg IV, over 1 hour, then 5 mg/kg IV daily as a single dose over 1 hour. Because of the cardiovascular depressant effects of phenytoin, its rate of infusion should be decreased in the presence of hypotension.

LIGNOCAINE   Lignocaine (1.5 mg/kg IV initially, followed by IV infusion at 5 mg/min) can significantly decrease ICP and improve CPP in the short term, especially before interventions such as intubation and physiotherapy.

BARBITURATES Intermittent or continuous intravenous infusions of barbiturates (eg thiopentone or phenobarbitone) are sometimes employed to control severe increases in ICP. Their effects of immunosuppression and cardiovascular depression, along with the absence of good data supporting their effectiveness, have limited the use of barbiturates for treating increased ICP. After cessation of treatment, the effects of large doses of barbiturates can take up to 1 week to wear off, and so neurological assessment can be difficult.

INTRAVENOUS ANAESTHETIC AGENTS Etomidate can reduce ICP; however, etomidate predisposes to infection if used over the long term, and so it is no longer used for that purpose. Propofol will decrease CBF and ICP in certain patients. However, its effects on the immune system have not been investigated, and studies of its efficacy have not been performed on a large scale in seriously ill patients.

OTHER DRUGS

Corticosteroids have been used extensively for management of intracranial abnormalities. Their current uses are limited to patients with certain brain tumours, brain abscesses, and meningoencephalitis (see p. 612). They have little, if any, place in the acute treatment of head injuries. The indications for prophylactic use of anticonvulsants in patients with head injuries are controversial.

SURGICAL PROCEDURES

Procedures to remove brain tissue or part of the bony cranium are sometimes used to decrease severe elevations in ICP.

MISCELLANEOUS

- Institute prophylaxis for stress ulcers (see p. 31).
- Seek an early return to enteral feeding (see p. 32).
- Give antibiotics for documented infection or as prophylaxis in patients with skull fractures (see p. 606). Prophylactic antibiotics are sometimes used during ICP monitoring.
- Neurogenic pulmonary oedema is a rare condition in patients with

elevated ICP, possibly associated with a sympathetic storm. It should be treated as for acute respiratory failure (see Chapter 17).

• In patients with diabetes insipidus (see p. 71), match urine output with hypo-osmolar fluids, and consider giving desmopressin acetate (DDAVP), 1–5 units IM, 4–6-hourly, according to control of the polyuria.

FURTHER READING

Busija, D. W., & Heistad, D. D. (1984). Factors involved in the physiological regulation of the cerebral circulation. *Reviews of Physiology, Biochemistry, and Pharmacology* 101:161–211.

Hall, R., & Murdoch, J. (1990). Brain protection: physiological and pharmacological considerations. Part II: The pharmacology of brain protection. *Canadian Journal of Anaesthesia* 37:762–77.

Jones, R. F. C., Dorsch, N. W. C., Silverberg, L. I. D., & Torda, T. A. (1981). Pathophysiology and management of raised intracranial pressure. *Anaesthesia and Intensive Care* 9:336–51.

Mathern, G. W., Martin, N. A., & Becker, D. P. (1987). Cerebral ischaemia: clinical pathophysiology. In *Critical Care: State of the Art*, ed. F. B. Cerra & W. C. Shoemaker, pp. 13–42. Fullerton, CA: Society of Critical Care Medicine.

Murdoch, J., & Hall, R. (1990). Brain protection: physiological and pharmacological considerations. Part I: The physiology of brain injury. *Canadian Journal of Anaesthesia* 37:663–71.

Prough, D. S., & Michenfelder, J. D. (1987). Cerebral blood flow and metabolism: implications for clinical monitoring. In *Critical Care: State of the Art*, ed. F. B. Cerra & W. C. Shoemaker, pp. 43–70. Fullerton, CA: Society of Critical Care Medicine.

Siesjo, B. K. (1984). Cerebral circulation and metabolism. *Journal of Neurosurgery* 60:883–908.

Trubuhovich, R. V. (ed.) (1979). Management of acute intracranial disasters. *International Anesthesiology Clinics* 17:1–448 (symposium issue).

25

SPECIFIC INTRACRANIAL PROBLEMS

COMA

Coma, or a decreased level of consciousness, is a common condition in intensive care. Consciousness depends on both the reticular activating system (RAS), which is responsible for general alertness, and the cerebral cortex, which is responsible for the quality of behaviour. The cause of coma must be localized to one of two sites: the brainstem or the cerebral hemispheres, or their connections. Coma usually is defined as a score of 9 or less on the Glasgow coma scale (GCS).

CAUSES OF COMA

The causes of coma are many (Table 25.1). There is a mnemonic aid to assist in the diagnosis:

A   alcohol
E   epilepsy
I   infection
O   overdose
U   uraemia and other metabolic causes

T   trauma, tumour, temperature
I   insulin
P   psychiatric
S   strokes and other vascular causes

COMA IN INTENSIVE CARE

Although there are many possible causes of coma, the commonest in the setting of the ICU usually fall into these categories:

(a) coma related to a primary brain lesion (eg head injury, global hypoxia)

TABLE 25.1 AETIOLOGY OF COMA

CORTICAL
Structural
Diffuse axonal injury
Tumour
Vascular
Cerebrovascular accidents (haemorrhage or infection)
Subarachnoid haemorrhage
Arteriovenous malformation
Global ischaemic injury
Trauma
Subdural haemorrhage
Extradural haemorrhage
Multiple petechial haemorrhage
Contracoup injury
Infection
Cerebral abscess
Meningoencephalitis
Metabolic
Hypoxia
Hypercarbia
Hypoglycaemia
Hepatic failure
Renal failure
Rapid changes in serum osmolality
Electrolyte disorders
Endocrine abnormalities
Other
Hypothermia
Hypotension and shock
Poisons
Drugs
Seizure
Psychiatric disorders
RETICULAR ACTIVATING SYSTEM
Brain herniation
Tumour
Haemorrhage
Cerebrovascular injury

(b) coma resulting from a systemic illness [eg hepatic encephalopathy, multiorgan failure (MOF), shock, sepsis]

(c) coma resulting from drugs (eg drugs used for analgesia or sedation, or drug poisoning)

The combination of (b) and (c) is common and is often called 'ICU coma'. It affects the elderly more severely than the young, but it is completely reversible.

Specific syndromes important in the ICU

VEGETATIVE STATE A vegetative state is a syndrome of diffuse cortical damage in which there is preservation of brain-stem activity, such as eye opening and muscle movements, but with no voluntary control of the movements. It is usually a long-term, often permanent, state associated with primary injuries such as head injury and global ischaemia.

LOCKED-IN SYNDROME The locked-in syndrome is a state of quadriplegia and paralysis of the lower cranial nerves, with a normal level of consciousness. These patients can communicate only by blinking and eye movement. It is important to distinguish it from true coma. The syndrome is rare, and survival is uncommon.

PSYCHOGENIC COMA Psychogenic coma is recognized on the basis of the patient's apparent unresponsiveness, despite normal findings on electroencephalographic (EEG) and brain-stem tests.

ASSESSMENT OF COMA

THE INITIAL ASSESSMENT AND TREATMENT OF COMA MUST BE CARRIED OUT SIMULTANEOUSLY. ASSESS AND CONTROL THE AIRWAY, BREATHING, AND CIRCULATION, AND EXCLUDE HYPOGLYCAEMIA.

History

The history is all-important in the assessment of coma. A diagnosis often can be made rapidly by talking to witnesses. Of particular im-

TABLE 25.2   GLASGOW COMA SCALE

Eye opening:	
spontaneous	4
to speech	3
to pain	2
nil	1
Best motor response:	
obeys commands	6
localizes pain	5
withdraws from pain	4
abnormal flexion	3
extensor response	2
nil	1
Verbal response:	
oriented	5
confused conversation	4
inappropriate words	3
incomprehensible sounds	2
nil	1

portance are the circumstances surrounding the onset of coma (eg headache, trauma, seizures), together with a history of previous illnesses (eg diabetes, drug abuse, epilepsy).

Neurological assessment

A full neurological examination should be carried out, but the initial focus should be on diagnosing conditions that need rapid treatment, such as:

- localizing signs in trauma patients
- signs of increased intracranial pressure (ICP)
- meningism
- seizures

LEVEL OF CONSCIOUSNESS   Firstly, assess the patient's level of consciousness. The GCS is widely accepted as the standard method (Table 25.2). Coma is usually defined as a GCS score of less than 9. It is usually documented in shorthand, according to eye movement (E), motor response (M), and verbal response (V), such as E3M4V3, giving a total GCS score for this patient of 10. Of the three components of the GCS, the motor response gives the most useful prognostic information. Applying a painful stimulus in the supraorbital region can cause nerve damage, and on the sternum it can cause unsightly bruising. Nailbed pressure is more satisfactory.

The advantage of the GCS is that it provides a standardized, easily reproducible assessment of the level of consciousness, as opposed to the use of ill-defined words such as 'semiconscious' or 'rousable'. Its disadvantages include its inability to note localizing signs and its lack of documentation of pupil size and reaction. These must be specified separately.

MOTOR FUNCTION Motor examination will give us two important pieces of information: focal signs and positioning. When assessing motor function, it is important to compare the left and right sides. Asymmetry in muscle tone, power, or reflexes is highly suggestive of a focal lesion. Plantar reflexes are not specific, and most comatose patients will have bilateral Babinski signs regardless of the causes of their conditions.

BRAIN-STEM REFLEXES

Pupils Pupils should be assessed for size, reactivity, and equality. Unreactive (but not necessarily dilated) pupils suggest a severe brain-stem abnormality, and a large unilateral pupil indicates tentorial herniation causing a third-nerve palsy. Remember that a small percentage of the population will normally have unequal pupils and that severe facial injuries can be associated with pupil damage. Small pupils usually result from a pontine lesion or ingestion of opiates.

Pain Application of a painful stimulus below the neck should cause a cranial nerve response, such as grimacing. In the presence of brain death, bizarre spinal reflexes can sometimes occur in response to painful stimuli.

Corneal reflex Absence of a corneal reflex indicates deep coma.

Gag reflex Stimulate the back of the throat, or pass a suction catheter down the endotracheal tube (ETT) if the patient is intubated, in order to test for a gag or cough reflex. Beware of eliciting a gag reflex in an unconscious patient with an unprotected airway.

Vestibulo-ocular (caloric) reflexes Firstly, examine the external auditory canals for patency and an intact tympanic membrane. If ice-cold water (20 ml) is then slowly syringed into each canal, nystagmus should be provoked within 20–30 seconds. The so-called doll's-eye movement will test the same pathways in a less satisfactory fashion, but may be dangerous if there is a question of cervical spine injury.

Abnormal respiratory patterns Like plantar reflexes, Cheyne-Stokes respiration is a non-specific sign. Complete apnoea is part of the spectrum of total brain-stem failure (see p. 618).

GENERAL EXAMINATION A complete, thorough general examination should be performed on all coma patients, looking for

- needle marks
- signs of trauma
- signs of chronic disease (alcoholism, renal failure)
- signs of muscle damage (eg compartment syndrome)

INVESTIGATIONS

Rapidly exclude

- hypoglycaemia
- hypoxia
- hypercarbia
- electrolyte abnormalities
- drug overdose

Further evaluation may require CT scan, lumbar puncture, angiography, EEG, or magnetic-resonance imaging.

MANAGEMENT OF COMA (Table 25.3)

Take measures to keep the patient alive until a diagnosis can be made. The general principles of management for the critically ill apply (see p. 10). Management procedures for specific causes of coma are dis-

TABLE 25.3 ACUTE MANAGEMENT OF COMA

Use supportive measures while making the diagnosis.
Maintain a clear airway – intubate if there is any doubt.
Ventilate if there is doubt about respiration.
Maintain 'normal' blood pressure.
Restore intravascular volume.
Correct hypoxia and anaemia.
Give 50 g of glucose intravenously if hypoglycaemia cannot be excluded.
Give thiamine, 50 mg IV.

cussed elsewhere: head injuries (see p. 599), meningitis (see p. 610), poisoning (see Chapter 16).

Airway

Maintaining a clear airway and preventing aspiration are the first priorities in the management of coma. Lateral posturing and supplemental oxygen often will be sufficient if the gag reflex is adequate. If not, intubation is mandatory.

Ventilation

Ventilation assistance should be instituted if there is doubt about adequate respiration, or it can be used as a short-term measure to decrease ICP by decreasing the partial pressure of arterial carbon dioxide ($Paco_2$) and cerebral blood flow (CBF).

Blood flow and oxygenation

Adequate cerebral perfusion with well-oxygenated blood is essential. Maintain a normal arterial blood pressure, if possible, replenish the intravascular volume, and correct hypoxia and anaemia.

Drugs

If there is any concern that the coma is related to hypoglycaemia, 50 g of glucose should be administered intravenously. Thiamine and

TABLE 25.4 FLOW THRESHOLD FOR CEREBRAL ISCHAEMIA

Normal	50 ml/min[a]
EEG abnormalities	20–25 ml/min
Evoked-response failure	15–20 ml/min
Cell death starts to occur	10–15 ml/min

[a]Flow per 100 g of tissue.

naloxone are often given as first-line drugs, in order to counteract any involvement of alcohol or narcotics.

PROGNOSIS

The best indicators of survival are certain factors related to the cause of the coma, the patient's age, the best motor response, the duration of coma, the absence of intracranial haemorrhage, and the state of the somatosensory evoked potentials. As a general rule, and apart from head injuries, among patients who are more than 20 years of age and who have been in coma for more than 2 weeks, the mortality approaches 100%.

GLOBAL ISCHAEMIA

'Global ischaemia' is a term that implies generalized cerebral damage due to insufficient blood flow, usually as a result of cardiorespiratory arrest (Table 25.4). The term 'global ischaemia' also implies damage secondary to severe hypoxia, hypotension, or anaemia, or following insults such as carbon monoxide poisoning.

Some aspects of the pathophysiology of cerebral ischaemia are becoming clearer. For example, whereas complete functional recovery cannot be expected after more than 7 minutes of normothermic global anoxia, some neurons can survive 1 hour of circulatory arrest. The duration, as well as the degree of ischaemia, will also affect cellular survival.

The complex series of events that ultimately result in cell death may one day be amenable to specific treatment. However, despite a wealth of experimental data, we seem to have only limited, often anec-

TABLE 25.5 SUMMARY OF MANAGEMENT FOR GLOBAL ISCHAEMIA[a]

Protect the airway.
Prevent hypoxia.
Prevent hypercarbia.
Facilitate cerebral venous drainage.
Maintain a 'normal' blood pressure for that patient.
Position the patient sitting up at an angle of 30° to 45°, keeping the head straight, and avoid constricting tape around the neck.
Avoid hypertensive surges.
Avoid drugs that can cause an increase in ICP.
Maintain 'euvolaemic dehydration' (ie avoid excessive use of clear fluid, but maintain intravascular volume).
Treat epilepsy aggressively.

[a]For further details, see Chapter 24.

dotal, information on the efficacy of active treatments for global ischaemia. In the meantime, caution must be exercised when extrapolating from animal data to clinical treatment.

Brain swelling and elevated ICP are not as severe in patients with global ischaemia as they can be, for example, in patients with severe head injuries. Therefore, ICP monitoring and osmotherapy are rarely indicated.

The only undisputed therapeutic principle is to improve the cerebral oxygen demand:supply ratio. Rapid restoration and maintenance of cerebral perfusion and arterial oxygenation are crucial. The general principles of management are as for any intracranial disaster (see p. 576) (Table 25.5).

Drugs such as antioxidants, free-radical scavengers, steroids, barbiturates, lazaroids, calcium-channel blockers, and prostaglandin inhibitors have, so far, not been demonstrated to influence recovery from global ischaemia.

PROGNOSIS (Table 25.6)

The most important clinical advances in the management of global ischaemia have been in the prognostic guidelines. These have obvi-

TABLE 25.6 GLOBAL ISCHAEMIA: VERY POOR PROGNOSTIC SIGNS

Initially
No pupillary light reflex
At 24 hours
Motor response – no better than flexor
No spontaneous eye movement (neither orienting nor roving conjugate)
Absence of corneal response
At 3 days
Motor response – no better than flexor
No cranial nerve reflexes
At 1 week
Not obeying commands
No eye movements (neither orienting nor roving conjugate)

ous importance for the decision whether active treatment should be continued or withdrawn. Patients in coma after cardiac arrest and global ischaemia are commonly seen in the ICU. The major question is whether or not, after all the efforts of resuscitation, the patient will remain in a persistent vegetative state (PVS). Their indiscriminate maintenance of patients in a PVS remains one of the more legitimate criticisms leveled against ICUs. Only approximately 10% of such patients will ever regain any sort of independent function following a coma resulting from global ischaemia. Many patients will remain in a PVS, with spontaneous eye opening and normal brain-stem reflexes, but without cognition – 'the lights are on, but nobody is at home'.

Careful and frequent neurological examinations should be performed as a guide to prognosis. One needs to regularly assess pupillary light reflex, motor response, spontaneous eye movement, and corneal reflex with regard to prognosis, especially in the first 72 hours after the onset of coma. The rate of clinical improvement should be taken into consideration. Guidelines regarding prognosis usually can be formulated after 72 hours.

To prevent unnecessary suffering by patients and relatives, it is important not to prolong advanced supportive measures indefinitely when there is little hope.

EEG: Although burst suppression, α waves, and predominantly delta patterns are indicators of a poor prognosis, there are no specific features of global ischaemia that are reflected on EEG.

Regarding sensory evoked potentials (SEPs), absence of a cortical response at 8 hours is a bad prognostic sign.

A patient's age and sex, the presence or absence of spontaneous eye opening, and the presence or absence of post-anoxic seizures do not correlate well with neurological outcome.

CEREBRAL INFARCTION

Acute cerebrovascular events can lead to infarction or haemorrhage. Cerebral infarction usually results from thrombosis or embolism. Patients with cerebral thrombosis and cerebral embolism are not routinely admitted to the ICU, because active monitoring and support can rarely change the course of the disease. Brain infarction is not amenable to many interventions in the ICU, apart from special circumstances such as a post-operative complication of carotid artery endarterectomy.

Strokes are very common in our community. An ageing population with high incidences of hypertension and arteriosclerosis is being treated in our ICUs. These patients can coincidentally develop cerebral infarction, precipitated by events such as hypotension, hypoxia, or atrial fibrillation, whilst being treated in the ICU for other conditions. Early mobilization and rehabilitation in a specialized unit will offer the best outcome for patients with cerebral infarction.

Investigation

The most important investigation in a patient with cerebral infarction is a CT scan, in order to exclude other pathological conditions such as intracranial haemorrhage, especially if the question of using anticoagulation is being considered. However, it may be several days before there will be evidence of infarction visible on CT scans, and there are certain areas of the brain, such as the brain-stem, that are always difficult to visualize with CT. Therefore, magnetic-resonance imaging (MRI) may be a better screening procedure.

TREATMENT

Support

General supportive measures such as physiotherapy, maintenance of a good airway, prevention of pressure areas, and nutritional support are the mainstays of treatment. Low-dosage heparin or 'antithrombotic' stockings may reduce the associated high incidence of deep venous thrombosis. The role of antiplatelet treatment has not, as yet, been established.

Surgery

Surgical procedures such as carotid endarterectomy are useful as preventive measures, but have no place in the management of acute stroke. There is considerable doubt about the effectiveness of extracranial-intracranial anastomoses for prevention of strokes.

Hypertension

Beware of acutely reducing a patient's blood pressure after a stroke, unless it is much higher than 'normal', and even then, act cautiously. Hypertension is common after stroke and may be a reflex phenomenon that can help to maintain blood flow.

Other Drugs

Drugs such as corticosteroids, 21-amino steroids, osmolar agents, or naloxone should be avoided until evidence for their efficacy is demonstrated. Thrombolytics for acute management of stroke are currently undergoing trials. The therapeutic window is very narrow. Tissue salvage is optimal within 45 minutes. After 4 hours, the incidence of associated parenchymal haemorrhage is high.

SPONTANEOUS INTRACRANIAL HAEMORRHAGE

Cerebral infarction secondary to thrombosis or embolism accounts for approximately 85% of strokes, and spontaneous intracranial haemorrhage accounts for a further 10–12%.

INTRACEREBRAL HAEMORRHAGE

Intracerebral haemorrhage is usually the result of systemic hypertension, but it can also result from other intracranial abnormalities, such as arteriovenous malformations, tumours, or infection. The di-

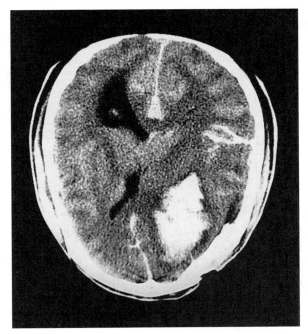

FIGURE 25.1 CT scan showing intracranial haemorrhage, with surrounding oedema and midline shift.

agnosis is best made by CT scan, which may also help in the decision whether or not evacuation of the haematoma is indicated (Figure 25.1). Most cases are treated conservatively, but surgical evacuation may be indicated if the haematoma is within the cerebellum or elsewhere and is causing a mass effect, with increased ICP or hydrocephalus. The prognosis largely depends on local extent of destruction due to haemorrhage, rather than on the level of ICP.

SUBARACHNOID HAEMORRHAGE

'Subarachnoid haemorrhage' (SAH) refers to bleeding within the subarachnoid space, rather than the brain parenchyma, and usually that is the result of rupture of a cerebral aneurysm. The peak incidence of SAH occurs in the fourth to sixth decades of life. The classic manifestations are abrupt onset of headache, a variable period of uncon-

TABLE 25.7   GRADING OF SUBARACHNOID HAEMORRHAGE

Grade I	Asymptomatic or minimal headache and slight nuchal rigidity
Grade II	Moderate to severe headache, nuchal rigidity, no neurological deficit other than cranial nerve palsy
Grade III	Drowsiness, confusion, mild focal deficit
Grade IV	Stupor, moderate to severe hemiparesis, possible early decerebrate rigidity and vegetative disturbances
Grade V	Deep coma, decerebrate rigidity, moribund appearance

sciousness, vomiting, neck stiffness, and focal signs (Table 25.7). A preceding or 'sentinel' headache occurs in about 25% of patients.

Confirmation is usually by CT scan. Lumbar puncture often will cause acute deterioration, especially if there is significant intracerebral bleeding. Lumbar puncture should therefore be performed after a CT scan. If CT scanning is unavailable, lumbar puncture should be used only if there are no signs of elevated ICP. Exanthochromia of the cerebrospinal fluid (CSF) results from breakdown of haemoglobin and can be seen if blood has been present in the CSF for at least 6 hours.

Outcome

Of those patients admitted to hospital, approximately half will die within the first 2 weeks if surgery is not performed. Approximately one-third will survive without major disability. The major complications are rebleeding and vasospasm (Table 25.8).

Whenever possible, these patients should be rapidly transferred to a specialized neurosurgical unit. The aim of treatment is to prevent further haemorrhage and to manage the sequelae of the haemorrhage, such as vasospasm and cerebral oedema.

Investigation

SERIAL CT SCANS   A CT scan is essential in order to determine the site and extent of bleeding, as well as any associated oedema, infarction, or hydrocephalus. CT scans will reveal 90–95% of these haem-

TABLE 25.8 MORTALITY ASSOCIATED WITH SUBARACHNOID HAEMORRHAGE

Initial haemorrhage	50%
Vasospasm	20%
Rebleeding	13%
Surgery	4%
Other	11%

orrhages if the studies are performed within 5 days of the bleeding. The pattern of the subarachnoid blood on a CT scan may suggest the likely location of the ruptured aneurysm.

ANGIOGRAPHY Angiography is needed to demonstrate the anatomy of the aneurysm and its association with parent vessels, as well as to define the presence of vasospasm and to exclude multiple aneurysms.

CEREBRAL IMAGING Imaging with radionuclides may help to identify patients with poor cerebral perfusion and vasospasm.

Management

GENERAL PRINCIPLES The general principles of care for an unconscious patient (see p. 589) and the principles of care associated with an elevated ICP (see p. 575) apply to these patients. However, beware of bringing hypertension under control too rapidly. Hypertension may herald the onset of further haemorrhage, but a high pressure may also be needed to maintain an adequate CBF, especially in the presence of vasospasm. Reduce the blood pressure (eg >200 mm Hg systolic) cautiously if it is high. β-blockers are the drugs of choice.

VASOSPASM OR DELAYED CEREBRAL ISCHAEMIA Vasospasm is responsible for much of the morbidity and mortality associated with SAH. It generally develops between the 5th and 14th days after the SAH, with a peak incidence around days 7–10. There is a 30–40% incidence of clinically detected vasospasm, and a 60–80% incidence seen on angiography. The incidence of vasospasm is correlated with the extent of haemorrhage. The pathophysiology is not well understood. The diagnosis is made on clinical grounds and can be confirmed by angiography, Doppler ultrasound, or CBF studies. Symptoms include an insidious decrease in the level of consciousness and fluctuating focal neurological signs. Angiography can worsen the vasospasm. There have been many vasolytic agents used in attempts to relieve the vasospasm, but their effectiveness has not been unequivocally demonstrated. The calcium-channel blockers, especially nimodipine, appear promising for prevention and treatment of vasospasm. After the aneurysm is clipped, induction of hypertension and hypervolaemia can be used to increase cerebral perfusion pressure (CPP). Cerebral autoregulation will be impaired in the ischaemic area, and blood flow possibly will change with blood pressure. Aim for a pressure 20–40 mm Hg (2.6–53. kPa) higher than the premorbid systolic blood pressure.

REBLEEDING   Rebleeding occurs in 15–20% of patients. Its peak incidence occurs within the first 24 hours, with a second peak at 1 week. This is related to clot breakdown. Antifibrinolytics such as ϵ-aminocaproic acid (EACA) have been suggested as possibilities to reduce the incidence of further haemorrhage. However, EACA can also cause intracerebral and systemic venous thrombosis, as well as vasospasm, and we await the results of further trials of its efficacy. The mortality associated with rebleeding is approximately 20%.

SURGERY   As with most other aspects of SAH, there is controversy over when to surgically clip the aneurysm. As a general principle, patients with grade IV or V aneurysms are treated conservatively, and patients with grades I–III aneurysms should have early angiography, followed by surgery. The surgical mortality among good-risk patients should be less than 5% in either case.

OTHER COMPLICATIONS   Cardiac arrhythmias, myocardial ischaemia, and pulmonary oedema can sometimes occur in patients with SAH. This is probably related to massive catecholamine release. Hydrocephalus occurs in about one-third of these patients and may need surgery and drainage. Convulsions occur in about 5% of SAH patients.

SUMMARY   Treatment of patients with SAH is difficult because of our lack of knowledge about the pathophysiology and the rates of success with specific management techniques. For example, guidelines regarding the control of blood pressure include warnings about hypertension causing further bleeding, as well as suggestions about the possible benefits of induced hypertension in the presence of vasospasm. More data are needed on the use of drugs in patients with vasospasm and rebleeding, as well as the timing of surgery.

SEVERE HEAD INJURY

Primary head injury

Primary head trauma occurs at the moment of impact and includes scalp lacerations, skull fractures, and brain injury.

Secondary head injury

Secondary damage can occur as a result of oedema from injured cerebral tissue, bleeding from torn intracranial blood vessels, or exacerbation of primary damage. Some of the causes of secondary brain injury are

- hypoxia
- hypercarbia
- hypoglycaemia
- seizures

TREATMENT OF SEVERE HEAD INJURY IS AIMED AT LIMITING THE SECONDARY DAMAGE, WHICH OCCURS MAINLY IN THE FIRST 8 HOURS.

Intracranial haemorrhage (Figures 25.2 and 25.3)

Extradural haematoma Extradural haematoma occurs between the dura and inner table of the skull, usually as a result of laceration of the middle meningeal artery.

Subdural haematoma Subdural haematoma occurs between the inner table's dural surface and the thin meninges covering the brain. The bleeding usually is venous in origin and is associated with contusion of the underlying brain.

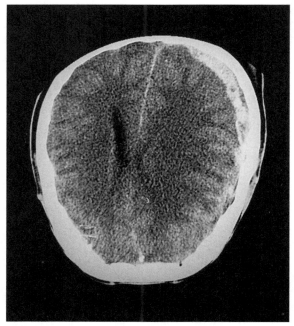

FIGURE 25.2   CT scan showing subdural haematoma and midline shift as a result of trauma.

Intracerebral haematoma   Intracerebral haematomas are variable in size, number, and location, depending on the force of impact.

INITIAL MANAGEMENT

For more details on the principles to be outlined next, see Chapter 14.

Airway

Often in these patients the level of consciousness will be impaired, leading to airway obstruction. This can be exacerbated by facial fractures and bleeding. Initially, attempt chin-lift and jaw-thrust manoeurvres, or insert an oropharyngeal airway tube. If there is doubt about the airway, INTUBATE.

Intracranial Haemorrhage

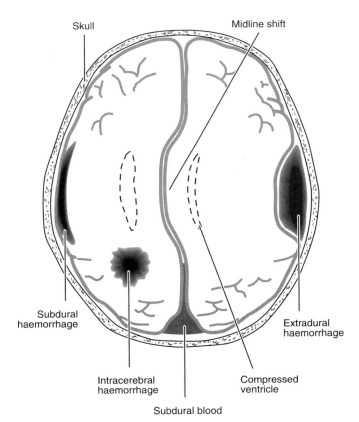

FIGURE 25.3 Intracranial haemorrhage.

TECHNIQUE FOR INTUBATION

• Keep the head in a neutral position during airway manoeuvres, until any cervical spine fractures have been ruled out. This can be achieved by in-line immobilization or by use of a hard collar.

• Avoid nasal intubation if it is suspected that there may be base-of-skull fractures.

• Avoid aspiration: Always be prepared to encounter a full stomach, and use rapid-sequence intubation, with pre-oxygenation and cricoid pressure.
• Sedate the patient adequately, in order to prevent hypertensive surges during instrumentation. Hypertensive surges can aggravate intracranial bleeding and cerebral oedema. During intubation, keep the patient well sedated in order to prevent coughing and straining, for the same reason. In the short term, an intubating dose of a drug such as thiopentone is useful for preventing hypertensive surges. However, in the presence of hypovolaemia and cardiovascular instability, the dose will have to be modified in order not to decrease the blood pressure and CPP.
• Insert an orogastric tube at the same time. This can be changed to a nasogastric tube once base-of-skull fracture is ruled out.

Ventilation

All patients with serious head injuries require artificial ventilation. This should be rapidly instituted, especially when the head injuries are associated with chest injuries or with hypercarbia and hypoxia. Aim for a Pao_2 greater than 90 mm Hg (12 kPa) and a $Paco_2$ of 30–35 mm Hg (4–4.6 kPa).

Hyperventilation is a short-term measure that will decrease ICP by decreasing CBF. However, CBF will rapidly adapt to a lower $Paco_2$ and return to a former baseline. This can give a false sense of security. If the $Paco_2$ then rises to a so-called normal level, this represents hypercarbia, with increases in CBF and ICP. After artificial hyperventilation, care should be exercised when returning to 'normal' levels of $Paco_2$, so that the CBF can adjust to a new level of $Paco_2$.

Cerebral blood flow

Hypovolaemia and hypotension should be reversed as soon as possible, in order to establish adequate CPP and CBF. Acute injury diminishes the brain's ability to withstand changes in Pao_2 and CPP. Hyperventilation that leads to $Paco_2$ values less than 25 mm Hg (3.3 kPa) should be avoided, as it may cause cerebral ischaemia.

Hypotension in the presence of cerebral trauma is NOT due to the brain injury. The most likely cause is hypovolaemia (exacerbated by mannitol and other diuretics). Other possible causes of hypotension include concurrent use of drugs and cardiac dysfunction related to contusion or coincidental infarction.

Haemoglobin

Significant bleeding should be rapidly treated with blood infusion. Beware of under-estimating blood loss from scalp wounds, which can account for early and rapid loss of blood at the site of injury.

Sedation

Sedation during ventilation is often necessary to achieve pain relief and to prevent hypertensive surges, coughing, and straining, all of which will increase ICP. A continuous infusion of narcotics and benzodiazepines, with muscle relaxants as necessary, is safe, effective, and inexpensive.

Routine use of intravenous anesthetic agents such as barbiturates, once claimed to offer 'brain protection', is becoming less fashionable because of the dangers of cardiovascular depression and immune suppression.

The argument that sedation will obscure neurological signs is offset by the disadvantages of having a restless patient on a ventilator, with surges of increased ICP.

Priorities in management

Head injuries often occur in the setting of multitrauma, and management priorities need to be established. For example, if a patient is hypotensive, despite ongoing blood and colloid infusion, laparotomy/thoracotomy may be needed before a CT scan of the head. If the patient is stable, cranial CT can be done before definitive treatment is undertaken.

DIAGNOSIS, ASSESSMENT, AND FURTHER TREATMENT (Table 25.9)

A FULL AND THOROUGH GENERAL EXAMINATION OF PATIENTS WITH MULTITRAUMA MUST BE PERFORMED AS SOON AS POSSIBLE IN ORDER TO RULE OUT OTHER INJURIES (SEE CHAPTER 14).

TABLE 25.9 MANAGEMENT OF SEVERE HEAD INJURIES

Secure the airway. If in doubt, intubate, with in-line immobilization of head and neck (see p. 243).

Stabilize the cervical spine with a hard collar until the possibility of fracture or dislocation is ruled out.

Sedate and paralyse all patients for intubation. Prevent coughing and gagging, which can cause acute increases in ICP.

Artificially ventilate to ensure normal oxygenation and relative hypocarbia: 35 mm Hg (4.6 kPa).

Maintain normal MAP and keep CPP > 60 mm Hg (8.0 kPa) (see p. 570). CPP = MAP − ICP. Hypotension is almost always a result of blood loss, not an intracranial abnormality.

CT scan

• Clinical signs are notoriously inaccurate for determining intracranial abnormalities.

• Either rule out or treat intracranial haematomas.

Facilitate cerebral venous drainage

• Sit patient up at an angle of 30° or more.

• Avoid compressing the internal jugular veins with ill-fitting hard collars and devices for artificial-airway fixation.

• Avoid high levels of PEEP and high ventilatory pressures, unless absolutely necessary.

• Avoid high intra-abdominal pressures, which can increase right ventricular filling pressure and ICP.

Avoid hypertensive surges before procedures such as endotracheal suction and physiotherapy (eg bolus of sedation ± lignocaine, 1.5 mg/kg) (see p. 577).

Avoid excessive fluid intake – maintain normal intravascular volume with colloid/blood, and use two-thirds of maintenance fluid requirements.

If there are sustained increases in ICP [eg > 20 mm Hg (>3 kPa)], despite the foregoing measures, consider

• hyperventilation

• mannitol, 0.3 g/kg, with or without frusemide, 40 mg IV

• another CT scan

• phenytoin, 15 mg/kg IV, loading dose, plus 5 mg kg^{-1} d^{-1} IV

• barbiturates (eg thiopentone, 50-mg IV increments)

Neurological examination

Document the patient's level of consciousness according to the GCS (see p. 586). Examine the external scalp for obvious fractures. Fractures of the orbital and maxillofacial structures usually can be detected by palpation. A bloody discharge from the nose or ear will indicate leakage of CSF. Bruising over the mastoid bone (Battle's sign) and periorbital haematoma (raccoon's eyes) will suggest a base-of-skull fracture.

The sizes and reactions of pupils should be tested, and one should look for evidence of decortication or decerebration and evidence of lateralizing signs in the limbs. Ongoing neurologic assessment should be updated frequently. This should consist of a clinical examination, recording the GCS score, pupil size and reaction, tone, reflexes, and cranial nerve function. This can be difficult in severely traumatized patients, especially those who have been given high doses of drugs for sedation and muscle relaxation. Pupil dilation is a reliable but late neurological sign. ICP monitoring may be useful in these patients (see p. 571). A well-designed and time-coded flowchart is helpful for neurological assessment.

CT scanning

Any serious head injury should be investigated with a CT scan as soon as the patient is resuscitated and relatively stable. The only exception is when rapid neurological deterioration occurs and CT is not immediately available, in which case immediate surgery may be indicated.

As a general guide, all patients with GCS scores of 9 or less should be scanned. Patients with GCS scores of 13 or more can simply be observed for signs of neurological deterioration. The decision whether or not to scan a patient with a GCS score between 10 and 12 is controversial. Any patient with localizing signs should have a CT scan, regardless of GCS score. Up to 20% of patients with GCS scores of 13 or more will show some abnormality on a CT scan, of which only a small number will require neurosurgical intervention.

All patients going for CT scanning should be accompanied by personnel skilled in advanced resuscitation.

Nutrition

Early enteral feeding is desirable. However, in many cases there will be an ileus and excessive gastric aspirate in a patient with severe head injuries, even in the absence of abdominal trauma. Duodenal or jejunal feeding often will be more successful.

Surgery

Obviously, significant intracranial haemorrhage should be evacuated surgically as soon as possible. The delay between injury and operation is the single most important determinant of prognosis. Meticulous management of the patient along the lines already outlined must be maintained during transport to and from the CT facility, as well as during the operative procedure (see p. 575).

Skull fractures

Skull x-rays still are usually obtained for head injuries, but the presence or absence of fractures will have little bearing on outcome, except as an indicator of a higher-than-otherwise incidence of intracranial bleeding. Depressed fractures usually require elevation, and if compound, they will also need antibiotic cover.

Basal fractures often are complicated by tearing of the dura mater, with CSF leakage and possible cranial nerve damage. Prophylactic antibiotics may be indicated (benzylpenicillin, 600 mg IV, 6-hourly, or co-trimoxazole, 600 mg IV, 12-hourly, until the leak stops). The most common organism is *Streptococcus pneumoniae*. Surgery may be indicated for persistent CSF leaks.

CEREBRAL OEDEMA

Most patients with head injuries develop some degree of cerebral oedema. This can vary from minor concussion to rapidly advancing, life-threatening generalized oedema. The general principles of treatment for cerebral oedema are outlined in Chapter 24. They are summarized here:

VENTILATION   The time during which a patient needs to be ventilated is variable. On the basis of ICP and CT-scan evidence, the acute stage for intracranial oedema causing compression appears to be between 2 and 15 days. The advantages and disadvantages of ventilation for each patient must be assessed on a daily basis. Remember that reducing the Pa_{CO_2} is only a short-term measure for reducing CBF and ICP – they both usually return to baseline value within 4 hours.

It is advisable to keep the Pa_{CO_2} around 35 mm Hg (4.7 kPa) so that hyperventilation can be kept as a reserve measure in case of further increases in ICP. As we learn more about head injuries, we may be able to define certain subgroups of patients in whom hyperaemia is an important feature, in which case hyperventilation may be more effective by reducing CBF and ICP.

SEDATION   Sedate with continuous intravenous narcotics and neuromuscular blocking agents if necessary. Straining and coughing should be avoided, as they can cause acute elevations in ICP. Boluses of sedatives should be tried before procedures such as turning or physiotherapy (see p. 576).

FACILITATE VENOUS DRAINAGE   Sit the patient up at an angle of 30° to 45°. Make sure that the blood pressure is maintained, in order to guarantee adequate cerebral perfusion.

HEAD POSITION   Avoid any head turning or tying the ETT tightly with a constricting bandage.

EPIDURAL ANALGESIA   Avoid epidural analgesia, as it can interfere with CSF drainage from the ventricles and consequently exacerbate any increase in ICP.

AVOID HYPOTENSION OR HYPERTENSION

MANNITOL   Give mannitol, 0.3 g/kg, no more than three or four times per day, to control persistently high ICP. A loop diuretic may also be useful.

INTRAVENOUS FLUIDS   Maintain the intravascular volume with colloid or blood while giving a minimum amount of 5% dextrose

(1,000–1,500 ml/d) – the principle of so-called euvolaemic dehydration.

SEIZURES   Treat seizures aggressively (see p. 613).

SHORT-TERM MANOEUVRES TO DECREASE ICP
• hyperventilation
• mannitol, 0.3 g/kg

If those measures fail try:

• lignocaine, 1.5 mg/kg IV
• barbiturates: 25–100-mg IV boluses of thiopentone, with or without continuous infusion of 2 g in 500 ml of isotonic saline, titrated against the effect achieved
• phenytoin, 15 mg/kg, over 1 hour, then 5 mg/kg IV as a single daily dose (monitor the levels)

OTHER DRUGS   So far, other drugs, such as corticosteroids, have had little impact on outcome following head injuries. A new group of amino steroid drugs called lazaroids are currently being tested, with some early success reported in patients with head injuries.

SYNDROME OF INAPPROPRIATE ADH SECRETION   SIADH is discussed elsewhere (see p. 70).

OUTCOME

Most head injuries are minor, with the patients being admitted only for short-term observation. However, many patients with even minor head injuries suffer long-term effects, such as headaches, emotional disturbances, and personality changes. Other symptoms such as cognitive dysfunction, fatigability, depressive symptoms, anxiety, flattening of affect, and slowness of thinking are very common. The more serious the initial head injury is, the more profound these symptoms are.

The facilities and services for rehabilitation of patients with head injuries usually are not as good as those for their acute management.

Unfortunately, there are few early and accurate predictors of outcome following head injuries. About one-third of patients with severe head injuries die, one-third experience good recovery, and one-third are variously disabled. Many of the so-called good recoveries have the long-term disabilities just mentioned. This is an enormous burden on society as well as on the relatives and friends of patients. Increasing age of the patient and the severity of the GCS score correlate with a poor prognosis. When a patient is in coma for more than 6 hours, the chance of death or PVS increases by about 3.6% for each year by which that patient's age exceeds 35 years, so that by the age of 75, a patient in coma for more than 6 hours has almost a 100% chance of dying or being left in a PVS.

VIRAL ENCEPHALITIS

Apart from herpes simplex encephalitis (HSE), most of the common viral infections of the central nervous system (CNS) tend to be relatively benign. The diagnosis usually is made on the basis of history and examination and often is one of exclusion. The specific viruses often are difficult to isolate.

CLINICAL FEATURES

- headache
- vomiting
- fever
- seizures
- signs of increased ICP
- neck stiffness
- drowsiness
- focal neurological signs

CSF

- findings often normal
- increased protein content
- glucose may be normal to low
- elevated white-cell count (especially lymphocytes)

EEG   EEG findings are non-specific.

CT SCAN   CT can show only non-specific changes.

HERPES AND SIMPLEX ENCEPHALITIS

HSE is the most common form of sporadic encephalitis, and it entails very high mortality and morbidity.

Diagnosis

HSE can show a higher incidence of focal EEG abnormalities than other forms of viral encephalitis, as well as more temporal-lobe involvement seen on CT scanning and MRI. However, those examinations may yield only normal findings during the early stages of the disease. Moreover, abnormalities are not specific for HSE. Specific herpes simplex viral antibody titres are accurate, but delayed. Antigen detection using a polymerase chain-reaction (PCR) technique is proving sensitive for early detection of HSE infection. Because the antiviral agents originally used in patients with HSE had many side effects, a specific diagnosis by brain biopsy was thought to be essential. That is no longer believed to be necessary.

Treatment

The mortality from HSE approaches 70%. This depressing outcome may be favourably influenced by early administration of acyclovir (10 mg/kg, 8-hourly, for 10 days), a specific antiviral agent. The absence of serious side effects from this agent and the high morbidity and mortality associated with HSE suggest that acyclovir should be used in any patient suspected of having viral encephalitis who has focal clinical features, while waiting for confirmation with viral antibody tests. The management of patients with elevated ICP in association with encephalitis follows the general principles for elevated ICP due to any cause, as discussed in Chapter 24.

BACTERIAL MENINGOENCEPHALITIS

CLINICAL FEATURES

- fever
- headache
- signs of increased ICP
- neck stiffness
- decreasing level of consciousness
- photophobia
- seizures

It is important to make a rapid diagnosis of bacterial meningitis, as it involves high morbidity and mortality. These patients can deteriorate and even die within hours of presentation.

MANAGEMENT

The sooner antibiotics are started, the better the patient outcome. There is good evidence to suggest that antibiotics should be commenced as soon as the disease is suspected, even in the pre-hospital setting.

LUMBAR PUNCTURE   If a patient has been admitted before the commencement of antibiotics and is neurologically stable, lumbar puncture ideally should be performed before antibiotic treatment is commenced. Because of the danger of an elevated ICP and coning, CT should be performed before lumbar puncture is attempted. However, normal findings on CT scan do not guarantee normal ICP. If, because of local circumstances, these investigations would cause unreasonable delay, blind antibiotic treatment must be commenced.

Classically, the CSF will be purulent or cloudy and will have

- increased protein content
- increased polymorphonucleocytes
- decreased glucose content

ORGANISMS   The causative organisms in children more than 3 months old and in adults usually are *Haemophilus influenzae* type B, *Neisseria meningitis,* or *Streptococcus pneumoniae*. It is usually a disease of childhood, but it can sometimes occur in adults.

If antibiotics were given before the organism was identified, pneumococcal or *Haemophilus* antigens may be detected in the urine. Alternatively, a PCR test can be performed on the CSF at a later time.

Bacterial identification often can be made on the basis of Gram staining. While waiting for identification and sensitivities, the following antibiotic treatment should be commenced:

- pencillin: 1.2–2.4 g IV, 4-hourly, for adults
         60 mg/kg IV, 4-hourly, for children

OR

• ampicillin: 1.2–2.4 g IV, 4-hourly, for adults
            60 mg/kg IV, 4-hourly, for children
+

• cefotaxime: 50 mg/kg IV, 4-hourly (adults and children)

The antibiotics may need modification when sensitivities become known.

Prophylaxis, in the form of rifampicin, 20 mg/kg (maximum 600 mg), should be given daily for 4 days to all people who have had close contact with patients who have meningococcal meningitis.

Strains of *H. influenzae* that are resistant to ampicillin and chloramphenicol have been identified, as have strains of *S. pneumoniae* that are resistant to penicillin. High doses of third-generation cephalosporins, such as cefotaxime or ceftriaxone, are indicated in these cases.

The question of the optimal duration of antibiotic treatment has not been resolved. Most authorities recommend a 7–10-day course.

CORTICOSTEROIDS   Although the findings from clinical trials are equivocal, there is some evidence that corticosteroids may be useful in treating meningitis, decreasing the hearing loss and other neurological sequelae. Seriously ill adults and children may benefit from dexamethasone (0.15 mg/kg), given 15–20 minutes before antibiotic treatment is commenced.

COMPLICATIONS   The complications of meningitis include seizures, PVS, extensive brain infarction, oedema, brain abscesses, and venous sinus thrombosis. A CT scan will reveal many of these complications. The mortality among adults who have *S. pneumoniae* meningitis remains around 20–30%, with neurological morbidity affecting over half of all survivors.

Other CNS infections

MENINGITIS AFTER NEUROSURGERY   This is usually caused by Gram-negative aerobic bacilli. It can be treated with ampicillin plus cefotaxime.

NEONATAL MENINGITIS   Neonatal meningitis is discussed elsewhere (see p. 765).

RARER FORMS OF MENINGITIS   In searching for the causes of the rarer forms, *Mycobacterium tuberculosis, Pseudomonas* spp., fungi, and other rarer organisms should be considered, especially in an immunocompromised host.

BACTERIAL BRAIN ABSCESS   Bacterial abscesses usually are associated with sinusitis, otitis, cranial trauma, or metastatic infection. Appropriate use of antibiotics, the general principles of management for elevated ICP (see p. 569), and surgical drainage or excision are the mainstays of treatment.

STATUS EPILEPTICUS

Epilepsy is a chronic disorder, or group of disorders, characterized by seizures that usually recur unpredictably in the absence of consistent provoking factors (Table 25.10). The seizures are characterized by excessive and hypersynchronous discharges of cortical neurons. Status epilepticus is a medical emergency. The brain is at risk from cerebral oedema, hypoxia, and direct neuronal damage, and the lungs are at risk from aspiration. Status epilepticus is defined as the occurrence of seizures that persist for a prolonged period (more than 30 minutes) or occur so frequently that recovery between attacks is not possible.

COMPLICATIONS OF STATUS EPILEPTICUS

Intracerebral

During any type of seizure there is increased electrical activity, as well as increased neurotransmitter release, increased oxygen consumption in the brain, and increases in CBF and cerebral oedema. The molecular events include increases in intracellular calcium, arachidonic acid, metabolites, prostaglandins, and leukotrienes. The more prolonged the seizure, the worse these effects are. Permanent brain damage can occur after 60 minutes of continuous convulsions.

TABLE 25.10   CAUSES OF TONIC-CLONIC STATUS EPILEPTICUS

First presentation
Drug overdose (eg phenothiazines, theophylline, tricyclic antidepressants)
Drug withdrawal (eg after prolonged midazolam use in the ICU)
Metabolic disorder (eg electrolyte disturbances, hypoglycaemia, renal and hepatic dysfunction)
Global ischaemia
Head injury
Cerebrovascular disease
Infection (eg brain abscess, meningoencephalitis)
Intracerebral tumour
Inflammatory arteritis
Eclampsia
Embolism (fat or air)
Background of epilepsy
Inadequate treatment (eg non-compliance or drug reduction)
Alcohol or drug withdrawal
Pseudo–status epilepticus

Airway

During a seizure, the airway is compromised by extreme muscle activity and increasing intragastric pressure, as well as by the loss of consciousness and decreased airway reflexes. Moreover, the drugs used to treat status epilepticus will compromise the airway further. If there is any hint of aspiration, or doubt about airway competence, intubation should be performed early.

Muscle activity

Excessive muscle activity can significantly increase oxygen consumption and can cause hyperthermia, excessive fluid loss, rhabdomyolysis, and hyperkalaemia, as well as renal failure.

Ventilation

Discoordinate muscle activity often impairs ventilation, causing hypoxia and hypercarbia. Induction of paralysis and artificial ventilation may be necessary. Whereas paralysis will prevent muscle activity, it will not affect the intracerebral epileptic activity. Therefore, what is needed is either continuous EEG monitoring or only partial paralysis, so that ongoing abnormal muscle activity can be detected.

Other complications

Hyperglycaemia or hypoglycaemia can occur. Autonomic dysfunction, sweating, hypertension, and hypotension can all occur in patients with status epilepticus.

MANAGEMENT OF EPILEPSY (Table 25.11)

Status epilepticus is a medical emergency. The physiological disturbances during epilepsy are life-threatening. Urgent treatment is required.

Resuscitation

Airway, breathing, circulation. As with any other medical emergency, the first priority is to secure the airway. If necessary, intubation should be performed. Hypoxia and hypercarbia should be corrected with adequate ventilation and oxygenation (see p. 578). Vascular access must be secured, and hypotension, acid–base abnormalities, and electrolyte disorders corrected where necessary.

All patients who are having seizures must be continuously observed in an appropriate area. Every possible precaution must be taken against aspiration, and if necessary, the patient's airway must be protected by intubation.

Diagnosis, monitoring, and further management

Restoration of cerebral oxygenation with adequate resuscitation is as important as the use of anticonvulsant drugs and must be performed simultaneously with drug administration.

The cause of the epilepsy should be investigated and corrected as soon as possible. A history often will suggest the diagnosis.

Glucose (50 ml of 50% glucose) should be given intravenously if the possibility of hypoglycaemic coma cannot be excluded.

Laboratory determinations of blood glucose, urea, electrolytes, blood

TABLE 25.11   MANAGEMENT OF EPILEPSY

---

1. EPILEPSY MUST BE AGGRESSIVELY AND RAPIDLY TREATED. EPILEPSY IS
   A MEDICAL EMERGENCY.

2. MAINTAIN AIRWAY, BREATHING, CIRCULATION.

3. Drugs

• diazepam, IV increments of 5 mg/min, up to a total of 50 mg

OR

• clonazepam, 2 mg/min

+

phenytoin, 20 mg/kg IV, over 1–4 hours (<50 mg/min), depending on the cardiovascular status, as a loading dose

THEN

• phenobarbitone, 100 mg/min IV, up to 20 mg/kg

OR

• thiopentone, 25–400 mg IV, over 5 minutes, then 2 g in 500 ml, titrated as
an infusion, up to 5 g/d

OR

• sodium valproate, 200–800 mg rectally every 6 hours

4. Rule out or treat reversible causes of epilepsy (eg hypoglycaemia, electrolyte disturbances) while resuscitation is continuing.

5. Use neuromuscular blocking agents only in the presence of excessive
   muscle spasm, which can cause complications such as hyperthermia and
   rhabdomyolysis.

---

count, osmolality, toxicology screening, anticonvulsant drug levels,
and arterial blood gases are necessary in the first instance. Give thiamine (1 mg/kg IV) if there is a suggestion of alcohol abuse. Monitor
respiration, arterial blood pressure, ECG, and continuous EEG (where
possible).

Definitive tests can be performed when the patient is stable: lumbar puncture, CT scan, EEG.

Anticonvulsant treatment

INITIAL TREATMENT

• diazepam, 5 mg/min IV, or clonazepam, 2 mg/min IV, until seizures
cease

• SIMULTANEOUSLY give phenytoin, 20 mg/kg IV, over 1–4 hours (<50 mg/min) as a loading dose, and then give 5 mg/kg IV daily, as a single dose over 1 hour, with monitoring of levels. Beware of cardiotoxicity, hypotension, and bradycardia. Give slowly, with continuous ECG monitoring. If the patient has been on phenytoin, its concentration should be measured first.

FURTHER TREATMENT There are many other drugs that have been recommended for intractable epilepsy, including amylobarbitone, paraldehyde, and even halothane. The latter should be avoided, because it will cause increases in CBF and ICP. As epilepsy has such disastrous consequences, there is a sound argument for trying a drug such as a barbiturate (thiopentone or phenobarbitone intravenously) if diazepam and phenytoin fail. Intubation, ventilation, and intravenous fluid replacement are indicated at this stage.

1. Barbiturates:

• phenobarbitone, 100 mg/min IV, until seizures cease, as a loading dose of up to 20 mg/kg.

• thiopentone (2.5% solution), 25–400 mg IV, over 5 minutes, or until seizures cease; then 2 g in 500 ml of isotonic saline titrated against effect, as a dose of up to 5 g/d. Beware of hypotension and accumulation; barbiturates such as thiopentone can take many days to be metabolized. The level of consciousness will be depressed until the drug is metabolized and excreted, making neurological assessment difficult.

2. Alternatively, or in addition to diazepam, phenytoin, and thiopentone:

• sodium valproate, 200–800 mg, can be given rectally every 6 hours.

• propofol infusion, 5–100 mg $\cdot$ kg^{-1} $\cdot$ h^{-1}, until seizures are controlled.

Other measures

TEMPERATURE Hyperthermia should be aggressively treated with fanning, tepid sponging, axillary ice packs, and antipyretics via the nasogastric tube or rectally. For more aggressive measures, see Chapter 11.

EXCESSIVE MUSCLE MOVEMENT Muscle movement should be reduced with muscle relaxants if necessary. As little drug as possible should be used, unless continuous EEG recording is available in order to clinically monitor the effects of anticonvulsant treatment. Otherwise the potentially fatal situation could arise wherein one successfully treats the muscular manifestations, but the cerebral epileptiform activity continues unabated.

SUPPORTIVE MEASURES The airway, breathing, and circulation must be constantly monitored. Give prophylaxis against stress ulceration (see p. 31). Beware of the possibility of a supervening nosocomial infection, such as pneumonia or sepsis, especially if using large doses of intravenous barbiturates.

RE-EVALUATE Re-evaluate the cause of the epilepsy if it continues. Further investigation may be required (eg lumbar puncture or CT scan).

BRAIN DEATH

'Brain death' is said to occur when there is irreversible loss of consciousness and loss of brain-stem reflexes, including cessation of respiratory-centre function. This is associated with irreversible cessation of intracranial blood flow.

Clinical confirmation of brain death is all that is legally required in many countries. Angiography may be required if one or more of the clinical tests cannot be performed.

There are certain essential steps that must be taken before brain death can be declared. It is important to be meticulous about these steps, as once brain death is declared, organ donation may be contemplated, and further treatment would be futile.

DIAGNOSIS OF BRAIN DEATH

Preconditions

1. The patient is deeply comatose.

2. The patient is being artificially ventilated, because spontaneous respiration has ceased.

3. There is no doubt that the patient's condition is due to irremediable structural brain damage. A diagnosis is essential. Head injury and intracranial haemorrhage account for approximately 80% of cases. Other cases include global ischaemia, infection, and brain tumour.

Exclusion of reversible causes

DRUG INTOXICATION Long-acting drugs, such as barbiturates, especially if used in large doses, make neurological assessment difficult. The hypometabolism that often accompanies brain death can decrease the rate of metabolism of drugs. Adequate time for drug metabolism must therefore be allowed. Drug levels should be measured, where possible, and concentrations of sedative drugs must be at less than the therapeutic range before testing is contemplated. There must be no residual effect of neuromuscular blocking drugs.

HYPOTHERMIA Patients with brain-stem dysfunction often become hypothermic. Testing can be done only when the core temperature is 35.0°C or greater.

METABOLIC AND ENDOCRINE DISTURBANCES Normal metabolic and endocrine status must be established. Electrolytes, acid–base status, and blood glucose must be within normal ranges.

Confirmatory tests

The following observations will determine the state of brain-stem reflexes and respiratory-centre function. These observations and tests should be performed only after the foregoing conditions have been met.

• Pupils not responding to light, direct or consensual.
• No corneal reflex.
• Vestibulo-ocular reflexes absent when 20 ml of ice-cold saline is injected into the patient's external ear, after ensuring a clear canal and an intact eardrum.
• No response to painful stimuli within the cranial nerve distribution when stimulated below the neck.

• No gag reflex.

• No respiratory movements after disconnection from the ventilator in the presence of a Pa_{CO_2} of more than 50 mm Hg (6.7 kPa). In order to avoid hypoxia during testing, the patient should be insufflated with low flow rates of 100% oxygen (3–5 L/min), preferably with 5 cm H_2O positive end-expiratory pressure. Because of hypometabolism, the Pa_{CO_2} may not rise to adequate levels before 5–10 minutes.

Definitive diagnosis

The criteria for a definitive diagnosis of brain death vary for different countries. Angiography, EEG, and tests of evoked potentials are not necessary adjuncts for a diagnosis of brain death in most countries. The number of examinations required, the timing between examinations, and the number of separate assessors and their qualifications also vary between countries.

RELATIVES

The confidence and trust of the patient's relatives should be sought during this trying period. It must be emphasized that a diagnosis of brain death is equivalent to a diagnosis of death, and the decision to withdraw support is purely a medical one, not one the relatives need bear in any way.

TRANSPLANTATION

Consent for transplantation must be gained from the relatives. They should be approached only after the diagnosis of brain death, and then they must be given a certain amount of time and, if necessary, further information with which to make the decision.

Keeping the cadaveric organs well perfused, once the diagnosis of brain-stem death has been made and organ transplantation is being considered, can be a real challenge. Large fluid losses secondary to polyuria, as well as hypotension, bradycardia, and hypoxia, can all compromise the functioning of potential donor organs. Adequate perfusion often necessitates large amounts of colloid and inotropes in order to maintain an adequate pressure. Encouraging mesenteric and renal blood flow with low-dosage dopamine may help to maintain liver and kidney functions.

FURTHER READING

Coma

Plum, F., & Posner, J. B. (eds.) (1980). *The Diagnosis of Stupor and Coma,* 3rd ed. Philadelphia: Davis.

Teasdale, G., & Jennett, B. (1974). Assessment of coma and impaired consciousness – a practical scale. *Lancet* 2:81–4.

Brain Death

Conference of Medical Royal Colleges and Their Faculties in the United Kingdom (1975). Diagnosis of brain death. *British Medical Journal* 2:1187–8.

Pallis, C. (1982). ABC of brainstem death. Diagnosis of brainstem death I. Diagnosis of brainstem death II. *British Medical Journal* 285:1558–60, 1641–4.

Pallis, C. (1983). Reappraising death. *British Medical Journal* 286:284–7.

Global Ischaemia

Safar, P. (1985). Cerebral resuscitation after cardiac arrest: a review. *Circulation (Suppl. 4)* 75:138–53.

Smith, G., & McDowall, D. G. (eds.) (1985). Symposium on brain ischaemia–its prevention and treatment. *British Journal of Anaesthesia* 57:1–120.

Acute Cerebrovascular Events

Auer, L. M. (1991). Outcome following early surgical repair of ruptured cerebral aneurysms – a critical review of 238 patients. *Surgical Neurology* 35:152–8.

Hopkins, L. N., & Long, D. M. (eds.) (1980). *Clinical Management of Intracranial Aneurysms.* New York: Raven Press.

Kistler, J. P., Ropper, A. H., & Heros, R. C. (1984). Therapy of ischaemic cerebral vascular disease due to artherothrombosis. *New England Journal of Medicine* 311:27–34, 100–6.

Severe Head Injury

Jennett, H. B., & Teasdale, G. (eds.) (1981). *Management of Head Injuries.* Philadelphia: Davis.

Marion, D. W. (1991). Complications of head injuries and their treatment. *Neurological Clinics of North America* 2:411–24.

Moss, E., Gibson, J. S., McDowall, D. G., & Gibson, R. M. (1983). Intensive management of severe head injuries. *Anaesthesia* 38:214–15.

Pascucci, R. C. (1988). Head trauma in the child. *Intensive Care Medicine* 14:185–95.

White, R. J., & Likavec, M. J. (1992). The diagnosis and initial management of head injury. *New England Journal of Medicine* 327:1507–11.

Meningoencephalitis

Quagliarello, V., & Scheld, W. M. (1992). Bacterial meningitis: pathogenesis, pathophysiology and progress. *New England Journal of Medicine* 327:864–72.

Tunkel, A. R., & Scheld, W. M. (1991). Acute therapy of bacterial meningitis. *Journal of Intensive Care Medicine* 6:229–37.

Werner, L. P., & Fleming, J. D. (1984). Viral infections of the nervous system. *Journal of Neurosurgery* 61:207–24.

Epilepsy

Delgado-Escuela, A. V., Wastetlain, C., Treiman, D. M., & Porter, R. J. (1982). Management of status epilepticus. *New England Journal of Medicine* 306:1337–40.

Scheuer, M. L., & Pedley, T. A. (1990). The evaluation and treatment of seizures. *New England Journal of Medicine* 323:1468–74.

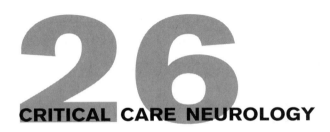

CRITICAL CARE NEUROLOGY

MYASTHENIA GRAVIS

Myasthenia gravis is a neuromuscular disorder characterized by weakness and fatigability of voluntary muscles. The weakness is exacerbated by effort and improved by rest, and it affects, in order of decreasing frequency, the ocular, bulbar, neck, limb, girdle, distal limb, and trunk muscles.

It is a classic autoimmune disease marked by the presence of heterogeneous acetylcholine receptor antibody (IgG) in approximately 90% of symptomatic patients. The antibodies react with the receptor, block its action, and accelerate receptor degradation. As a result, fewer receptors can be activated, causing muscle weakness.

DIAGNOSIS

Clinical suspicion and the finding of skeletal-muscle fatigability with repetitive exercise will support the diagnosis. The diagnosis can be confirmed by complete reversibility of muscle fatigue after intravenous administration of the rapidly acting anticholinesterase drug edrophonium (5–10 mg IV, over 1 minute, should produce an effect within 10 minutes).

Electrophysiological testing will demonstrate progressive declines in muscle action potentials with repetitive stimulation of a motor nerve.

TREATMENT

Definitive treatment aims to reduce antibody production and/or increase the effect of unaffected acetylcholine receptors.

ANTICHOLINESTERASES A longer-acting anticholinesterase, pyridostigmine, is titrated against patient response, using a starting dosage of 60 mg orally four times daily. Excessive use of anti-cholinesterases can cause a cholinergic crisis, with progressive muscle weakness as well as muscarinic effects, such as abdominal colic, diarrhoea, small pupils, lacrimation, and excessive salivation.

THYMECTOMY   Among all patients with myasthenia gravis, 75% have thymic abnormalities. Most have thymic hyperplasia, but up to 15% have thymomas. It is thought that the thymus may be involved in initiating development of the autoantibodies that attack the postsynaptic acetylcholine receptor.

Thymectomy is especially useful in patients who are young at the onset of disease. Complete remission or improvement occurs in about 80% of patients without a tumour of the thymus, although it may take 3–5 years to gain the full benefit.

CORTICOSTEROIDS   Corticosteroids can be used in patients for whom thymectomy has not been successful, in patients who are seriously ill before thymectomy, and occasionally for those with ocular myasthenia. Steroids can take several weeks to achieve their optimum effects and may even cause an initial deterioration.

AZATHIOPRINE   Azathioprine should be reserved for patients with severe myasthenia who do not respond to other forms of treatment. It should be used in association with plasma exchange.

PLASMAPHERESIS   Plasmapheresis can produce dramatic short-term improvement. It should be reserved for use in severely ill patients while other forms of treatment are taking effect.

MYASTHENIA GRAVIS IN INTENSIVE CARE

Myasthenic patients often are admitted to the ICU for elective ventilation after thymectomy or incidental surgery (Table 26.1). Prolonged paralysis can occur in some patients, even after the use of reduced doses of anticholinesterase drugs and in the presence of neuromuscular drugs. Patients can also be admitted for myasthenic or cholinergic crisis.

In patients with deteriorating myasthenia gravis, it is important to differentiate between myasthenic crisis and cholinergic crisis. This can be determined by the response to intravenous edrophonium, 5–10

TABLE 26.1 EVALUATION OF THE NEED FOR RESPIRATORY
SUPPORT IN PATIENTS WITH NEUROMUSCULAR DISEASE

Parameter	Normal	Borderline	Failure
Forced vital capacity	>15 ml/kg	10–15 ml/kg	<10 ml/kg
Negative inspiratory force	>−40 mm Hg	−25–40 mm Hg	<−25 mm Hg
Airway integrity	Eats and drinks normally; no difficulty in articulating	Cannot handle fluids well, but manages with oral suctioning; noticeable impairment of speech	Obstruction of airway in certain positions; intermittent aspiration of secretions
Chest x-ray	Absence of atelectasis	Presence of subsegmental atelectasis	Major atelectasis or infiltrate

Source: From Malkoff (1993), with permission of Williams & Wilkins.

mg IV, given in 2-mg increments. Patients in myasthenic crisis will
show rapid improvement in terms of their symptoms, whereas those
in cholinergic crisis will deteriorate.

Whatever the reason myasthenic patients are in the ICU, they usually have decreased respiratory and bulbar muscle function, and many
of the aspects of management for myasthenic and cholinergic crises
are the same.

Management

AIRWAY Rectify a compromised airway with an endotracheal tube
(ETT).

VENTILATION Artificial ventilation will be necessary if respiratory
muscles are ineffective. Ventilation should be regularly assessed by
measurements of parameters such as peak flow, vital capacity, and
tidal volume.

RESPIRATORY COMPLICATION Atelectasis, pneumonia, aspiration,
and sputum retention ideally should be prevented or treated aggres-

sively by early physiotherapy, as well as early intubation and ventilation, where indicated (see Chapter 20).

SUPPORTIVE CARE A return to enteral feeding, prophylaxis against stress ulceration and deep venous thrombosis, and provision of emotional support (see Chapter 5) are essential for these patients.

ANTICHOLINESTERASES Each patient should be stabilized on the optimal dosage of anticholinesterase, either oral pyridostigmine or intravenous neostigmine, given continuously or intermittently, as titrated against muscle strength, especially the bulbar and respiratory groups. Intravenous edrophonium, 2–10 mg, in between doses can be used as a guideline to the optimal dosage. Give intravenous edrophonium in 2-mg increments, pausing in between, especially if there is a suspicion of cholinergic crisis.

After thymectomy, patients may have markedly reduced anticholinesterase requirements within the first 48 hours.

CHOLINERGIC CRISIS Atropine, intravenously or preferably orally, can be titrated against the muscarinic or parasympathomimetic manifestations of a cholinergic crisis.

CONCURRENT DRUG TREATMENT If possible, avoid drugs that might make the condition worse, such as non-depolarizing muscle relaxants, aminoglycosides, quinine, quinidine, procainamide, lignocaine, and propranolol.

WEANING Carefully assess the strength of bulbar and respiratory muscles during weaning from ventilatory and airway support (see p. 478) in order to decide when artificial ventilation can be ceased and the patient extubated. Objective measurements of parameters such as expiratory flow rates and vital capacity can be used to monitor progress. Tracheostomy may be required if intubation is prolonged (see p. 27).

Weaning from the ventilator, for some patients, may be impossible without corticosteroids. Azathioprine or plasmapheresis may be indicated when the response to anticholinesterase drugs is unsatisfactory.

GUILLAIN-BARRÉ SYNDROME

PATHOPHYSIOLOGY

Guillain-Barré syndrome is an antibody-mediated attack on peripheral nerves. A peripheral neuropathy results, with lymphocytes and macrophages surrounding endoneural vessels, with adjacent demyelination. The inflammation probably is based on an aberrant response to an immunological stimulus mediated by primary lymphocytic T-cell activity.

CLINICAL FEATURES

Guillain-Barré syndrome is an inflammatory demyelinating polyneuropathy that often presents with dramatic onset of muscle weakness and autonomic signs. Despite the acute nature of this disorder, patients occasionally require ventilatory support for months or even years. Some cases never completely resolve.

Typically, the syndrome is heralded by paraesthesia of the fingertips and toes, followed within days by a progressive, symmetrically ascending, flaccid motor paralysis. This may remain localized to the lower limbs, or it can extend to the trunk and respiratory muscles, as well as to the cranial nerves. Tendon reflexes are absent in the affected areas. Pain is common, especially in the large muscles of the upper legs and back. However, usually there is only minimal sensory loss.

The clinical course can be described in four phases:

PRODROMAL PHASE The prodromal phase develops over days or weeks, with over 60% of patients having had a preceding viral illness. Other cases are associated with vaccination or gastro-intestinal-tract infection.

EXTENSION OF NEUROLOGICAL DEFICITS This phase is relatively constant and lasts about 2 weeks.

PLATEAU PHASE The plateau phase can be unpredictable, but usually lasts from a few days to a few weeks, or even longer in about 10%

of cases. The maximum effects occur within 2 weeks of onset in about 50% of cases, and within 4 weeks in 90% of cases.

RECOVERY PHASE Most patients recover within 6 months. However, only about 15% of patients have no residual deficits. About 65% have persistent minor problems, such as weakness or distal numbness. Permanent disabling weaknesses or other severe neurological deficits occur in about 5–10%. About 5% of patients develop chronic relapsing polyneuropathy, with further bouts of demyelination.

CLINICAL VARIANTS Variants of Guillain-Barré syndrome include

- Fisher's syndrome (ophthalmoplegia, ataxia, areflexia, with little weakness)
- weakness without paraesthesia or sensory loss
- pure ataxia
- facial paresis with paraesthesia
- pharyngeal-cervical-brachial weakness

DIAGNOSIS

The diagnosis of Guillain-Barré syndrome is usually made on clinical grounds. Cerebrospinal fluid (CSF) typically shows normal pressure, few or no cells, and an elevated protein concentration. Protein levels may be normal initially, and the cell count is occasionally increased. The major reason for lumbar puncture is to exclude other conditions, not to make a positive diagnosis of Guillain-Barré syndrome. Abnormalities of nerve conduction occur early and demonstrate the characteristic findings of demyelination, including conduction block (causing motor weakness) and spontaneous discharges in demyelinated sensory nerves (causing paraesthesia and pain). However, normal findings on nerve conduction studies do not exclude the diagnosis.

MANAGEMENT IN INTENSIVE CARE

Meticulous supportive care is the mainstay of treatment for Guillain-Barré syndrome in the ICU. This includes prevention of aspiration and respiratory infections, avoiding the complications of intubation and tracheostomy, and commencing prophylaxis for deep venous thrombosis. Because the underlying disease is largely reversible, and the complications largely avoidable, successful outcomes can be achieved by excellent supportive care.

The immediate dangers are increasing bulbar weakness and impaired ventilation. Respiratory function must be tracked by serial measurements of parameters such as vital capacity and negative inspiratory effort, rather than by using arterial blood-gas analysis. Test and chart three separate groups of muscles (bulbar, limb, and respiratory) on a regular basis.

Airway

If in doubt about the airway, intubate the patient before complications occur. Support the patient's respiration with artificial ventilation before widespread collapse and infection occur. Approximately 20–30% of patients will require intubation and mechanical ventilation.

DO NOT USE SUXAMETHONIUM TO FACILITATE INTUBATION. IT IS UNNECESSARY AND CAN CAUSE MASSIVE RELEASE OF POTASSIUM FROM DENERVATED MUSCLE, LEADING TO CARDIAC ARREST.

Ventilation

Ventilatory failure usually occurs when the vital capacity falls below 20 ml/kg. Patients who need artificial ventilation usually require it for 4–8 weeks, and sometimes for several months.

Tracheostomy should be considered early in order to facilitate nursing care and reduce the complications involved in using an ETT (see p. 27).

Because artificial ventilation is often prolonged, maintain meticulous airway toilet. Regular checking of the airway cuff pressures is required.

General support

Institute general measures such as enteral feeding, physiotherapy, prophylaxis against stress ulceration, and provision of emotional support.

These patients usually are fully conscious; explain every manoeuvre, and discuss the proposed management and progress with them. It is important to provide stimulation directly from the staff and from audiovisual aids, in addition to encouraging frequent and flexible visits from relatives and friends.

Because of the danger of pulmonary emboli, all ventilated patients should receive low-dosage heparin (5,000 units subcutaneously three times daily). Other prophylactic techniques, such as compression stockings, may also be useful.

Patients with Guillain-Barré syndrome usually have moderate to severe pain that is muscular in origin. Patients should be carefully questioned about this possibility and given appropriate and generous oral or parenteral pain relief.

Cardiovascular complications

Autonomic instability is common in these patients, resulting in tachyarrhythmias and severe blood-pressure fluctuations. They are often precipitated by stimulation of the patient. Intravenous sedation, volume loading with fluid, and α- or β-adrenoceptor blockade may be necessary to treat these complications. Similar treatment may be required prophylactically before procedures. The same strategies are used for the autonomic instability in patients with tetanus and are discussed in detail with that topic (see p. 634).

Hyponatraemia

Hyponatraemia, possibly due to inappropriate secretion of antidiuretic hormone (ADH) is sometimes seen. Avoidance of hypovolaemia and excessive water administration usually will correct the abnormality. Rarely, hypertonic saline is needed.

Other treatment

CORTICOSTEROIDS Corticosteroids should not be used in patients with Guillain-Barré syndrome.

FRESH FROZEN PLASMA Use of fresh frozen plasma probably is of no benefit.

PLASMAPHERESIS Early use of plasmapheresis will reduce the duration and severity of the acute phase of the disease and may accelerate recovery, as well as shorten the period of artificial ventilation. Albumin, rather than fresh frozen plasma, is the replacement fluid of choice. The optimal number of plasma exchanges and the scheduling of changes are not known. A commonly employed treatment is five courses over 10 days. Several issues remain unresolved: Which group of patients can benefit most from plasmapheresis? Does it reduce overall mortality? Moreover, plasmapheresis is not without complications, such as increased bleeding and activation of complement and fibrinolysis.

INTRAVENOUS IMMUNE GLOBULIN Use of immune globulin may speed recovery and decrease the need for ventilatory support. It may be as effective as plasmapheresis, with less severe complications. The amount suggested is 0.4 g/d, divided into five doses.

CRITICALLY ILL POLYNEUROPATHY

Critically ill polyneuropathy may be another manifestation of multiorgan failure (MOF) (see Chapter 9). It involves impairment of peripheral nerve function, including the cranial nerves. It can affect both motor and sensory functions.

Critically ill polyneuropathy is a difficult diagnosis to make, as the patients often are unconscious or sedated, and thus tests of their sensations and motor functions are almost impossible. The syndrome can be manifest as failure to be weaned from the ventilator, or it can become obvious as the patient recovers. Because it is so difficult to diagnose, its incidence has not been accurately documented, but it may affect up to 70% of patients with MOF.

This diagnosis is made after one excludes all other possible causes for the polyneuropathy. It is important to remember that there are many potential causes of polyneuropathy (Tables 26.2 and 26.3).

The finding of primary axonal degeneration of mainly motor fibres, but also sensory fibres, without inflammatory change, and with a relatively normal CSF, can distinguish this neuropathy from Guillain-Barré syndrome. The precise cause remains obscure. Recovery occurs spontaneously. In addition to a thorough clinical examination, studies of nerve conduction and electromyography (EMG) studies may be

TABLE 26.2   DISORDERS OF NEUROMUSCULAR FUNCTION

Level	Associated clinical features	Nerve conduction	EMG findings
Upper motor neuron	Weakness Hyperreflexia Increased muscle tone May have sensory and autonomic changes	Normal	Normal
Lower motor neuron	Weakness Atrophy Flaccidity Hyporeflexia Fasciculations Bulbar involvement No sensory changes	Normal	Denervation potentials of giant motor units
Peripheral neurons	Weakness Flaccidity Hyporeflexia Bulbar involvement Sensory and autonomic changes	Reduced	Denervation potentials in axonal neuropathies
Myoneural junction	Fluctuating weakness Fatigability Ocular and bulbar involvement Normal reflexes No sensory changes	Normal	Change in amplitude of the response to repetitive nerve stimulation
Muscle	Weakness, usually proximal Normal reflexes No sensory or autonomic changes Often have pain	Normal	Small motor units

necessary to document the syndrome. The creatinine phosphokinase (CPK) levels will be normal or only slightly elevated.

There have been increasing reports of motor neuropathy and/or myopathy in patients receiving neuromuscular blocking agents and

TABLE 26.3 NEUROMUSCULAR DISORDERS IN THE SERIOUSLY ILL

Condition	Clinical features	Electrophysiology	Morphology
Guillain-Barré syndrome	Mainly motor neuropathy	Consistent with primary demyelinating polyneuropathy	Primary demyelination of nerve and inflammation; invariable denervation of muscle
Nerve compression due to positioning, plasters, etc.	Motor and sensory features	Consistent with primary degeneration	Fibre atrophy on muscle biopsy
Cachectic myopathy	Diffuse muscle wasting	Normal	Type II fibre atrophy on muscle biopsy
Critically ill polyneuropathy	None, or else signs of mainly motor neuropathy	Consistent with primary axonal degeneration of mainly motor fibres	Primary axonal degeneration of nerve; denervation atrophy of muscle
Neuromuscular blocking agents	Persistent quadriplegia for up to 2–3 weeks	Neuromuscular transmission deficit and/or axonal motor neuropathy	Normal or denervation atrophy on muscle biopsy

Source: Adapted from Bolton (1992).

steroids, especially patients being ventilated for severe asthma. However, there is, as yet, no direct evidence linking those drugs to the observed weakness.

TETANUS

FEATURES

Tetanus is caused by *Clostridium tetani,* an anaerobic, Gram-positive spore-forming bacillus. Clostridial spores, which are endemic in soil and dirt, develop into the vegetative form of the organism when introduced into the anaerobic environment of devitalized tissue. *C. tetani* itself does not cause tissue damage or evoke an inflammatory response, but rather produces an exotoxin, tetanospasmin.

The exotoxin forms an irreversible bond with synaptosomes, both in the spinal cord and in the central nervous system. The toxin ascends intra-axonally in motor and autonomic nerve fibres. The exact site of action has not been elucidated, but some evidence suggests that it mainly depresses the inhibitory influence from Renshaw cells (inhibitory interneurons). This leads to paroxysmal muscle spasm, often triggered by minimal sensory input.

The centripetal spread of toxin is more rapid with increased doses of toxin. A rapid onset of symptoms suggests inoculation by a larger dose of exotoxin and increased severity of disease.

The first symptoms usually are stiffness in the back muscles, abdominal muscles, and masseters, followed by dysphagia and eventually generalized muscle spasms. Most muscles are eventually affected. The respiratory pattern and breathing can be compromised by general muscle spasms leading to hypoventilation and even respiratory arrest. Tetanus varies from a very mild disease, with minimal muscle spasm, to a fulminant variety characterized by severe recurrent spasms and autonomic over-activity.

The mortality from tetanus remains high (10–50%), despite management in the ICU. Nowadays, death often occurs as a result of autonomic over-activity, with arrhythmias, hypotensive and hypertensive crises, and myocardial ischaemia, rather than as a result of respiratory failure.

DIAGNOSIS

The diagnosis is made on the basis of the clinical history and observation of muscle spasms. The organism can be cultured from the suspected infection site.

TREATMENT

Eradication of the source

- Vigorous drainage and debridement of the suspected site of infection are important.
- Penicillin G, 3–6 million units per day, IV, for approximately 10 days.
- Use erythromycin if the patient is allergic to penicillin.
- Immobilization of the wound area.

Neutralization of toxin

There is some doubt about the efficacy of human tetanus immunoglobulin, because the exotoxin rapidly becomes fixed on the nervous tissue and therefore will not be modified if symptoms are already present.

However, immunoglobulin is still commonly given: 3,000–10,000 units of human tetanus immunoglobulin, diluted with saline, as a slow intravenous infusion over 15 minutes.

Human immunoglobulin can be given intrathecally (250 units) in an attempt to neutralize unbound exotoxin more effectively, although there is no conclusive evidence that it is useful. Preservatives such as phenol must not be used in this situation.

Supportive Care

AIRWAY The airway must be protected, and intubation performed early, if there is any doubt about airway patency. Intubation is often necessary to facilitate ventilation and to prevent aspiration. Tracheostomy usually is considered when the course of the disease runs longer than 2–3 weeks.

VENTILATION   Some ventilatory assistance (see Chapter 20) will almost certainly be required in most patients, because of inefficient respiration resulting from muscle spasms or from the drugs given to control the spasms. As muscle spasms are controlled with sedation and muscle relaxants, total respiratory support may become necessary, rather than the use of modes that employ spontaneous ventilation, such as intermittent mandatory ventilation (IMV) or continuous positive airway pressure (CPAP) (see Chapter 20).

CONTROL OF SPASMS

Benzodiazepines   A benzodiazepine such as diazepam (intermittent intravenous doses or infusion of 5–10 mg/h) is often used as a first-line drug because it has muscle-relaxing and sedative properties. Shorter-acting benzodiazepines probably are equally as effective.

Narcotics   Narcotics should be used liberally, especially in the presence of spasms, which can be quite painful (eg intermittent or continuous intravenous infusion of morphine, 2–20 mg/h) (see p. 116).

Non-depolarizing muscle relaxants   Use these only if other drugs fail to control the spasms. Continue diazepam and/or narcotics during administration of muscle relaxants. Give them either as intermittent intravenous boluses or as a continuous infusion (see p. 119). **DEPOLARIZING MUSCLE RELAXANTS ARE CONTRAINDICATED, AS THEY CAN CAUSE ACUTE HYPERKALAEMIA AND CARDIAC ARREST.**

FEEDING   Start enteral feeding early. Parenteral feeding is necessary only if enteral food is not tolerated (eg as a result of autonomic dysfunction and ileus).

FLUIDS   Fluid requirements should be met by adequate enteral nutrition. Otherwise, use a maintenance intravenous regimen. Hypovolaemia should be rapidly corrected. Hypertension, paradoxically, can be caused by hypovolaemia during autonomic dysfunction.

THROMBOSIS AND EMBOLISM   Begin prophylaxis against venous thrombi and pulmonary embolism, using subcutaneous heparin (5,000 units, two or three times daily). Antithrombotic stockings may also be useful.

OTHER GENERAL SUPPORTIVE MEASURES Supportive measures such as chest physiotherapy and prophylaxis against stress ulceration (see Chapter 2) are necessary.

PATIENT AND RELATIVES Patients with tetanus who are not being heavily sedated often are fully aware. They need constant reassurance from the attending staff and relatives.

Autonomic over-activity

Cardiovascular instability is characterized by over-activity of the sympathetic and parasympathetic nervous systems, including tachycardia, labile and elevated blood pressure, variable skin blood flow, fever, hypersalivation, arrhythmias, and even cardiac standstill. It usually presents some days after the onset of muscle spasms. The over-activity can persist for many hours, but more often it is intermittent and of short duration. Autonomic over-activity can be associated with mortality of more than 50%.

MANAGEMENT Intravenous sedative agents such as benzodiazepines and phenothiazines usually are required. General anaesthetic agents have also been used. The aim of treatment is complete inhibition of both somatic and autonomic over-activity without producing hypotension or hypothermia. Suggested regimen: diazepam, 20 mg, 4–6-hourly, and additional increments are required. In severe uncontrollable cases, intravenous diazepam may need to be supplemented with thiopentone, at a starting dosage of 25 mg IV, hourly, by continuous infusion. Sedation is usually required for at least 2–3 weeks. Muscle relaxants usually are necessary only for control of severe spasms, and they always must be used in conjunction with sedation.

Increase sedation (eg diazepam) before any procedure that can precipitate autonomic dysfunction. Other measures also need to be considered:

CORRECT HYPOVOLAEMIA Paradoxical hypovolaemia is commonly associated with hypertension and a labile blood pressure.

INTRAVENOUS β-BLOCKERS Intravenous β-blockers (either intermittent or continuous) must be used with caution, and only if sympathetic over-activity is still present after maximum sedation. Use a short-acting agent such as esmolol, and titrate it against an effect. Beware of unopposed α activity when using β-blockers.

INTRAVENOUS α-BLOCKERS Intravenous α-blockers (either intermittent or continuous) for hypertension must be used with caution, and only after correcting hypovolaemia and after failure of maximum sedation and β-blockers. Chlorpromazine is the most commonly used drug.

CONTINUOUS LUMBAR EPIDURAL BLOCKADE Lumbar epidural blockade with local anaesthetic or morphine has also been used to control labile blood pressure. Hypovolaemia should be aggressively reversed with fluid infusion before epidural drugs are commenced.

MAGNESIUM SULPHATE Magnesium sulphate by intravenous infusion can be used if other measures have failed: 70 mg/kg over 5 minutes, then infusion to keep the serum magnesium at 2.5–4 mmol/L, measuring serum levels every 4 hours. Ventilation is mandatory in these patients.

ATROPINE Atropine by intravenous infusion, titrated against response, can be used if parasympathetic symptoms are predominant.

FURTHER READING

General

Benson, C. A., & Harris, A. A. (1986). Acute neurological infections. *Medical Clinics of North America* 70:987–1011.

Bleck, P., & Klawan, S. (1985). Neurological emergencies. *Medical Clinics of North America* 70:1167–84.

Editor (1986). Plasma exchange for neurological disorders. *Lancet* 2:1313–14.

Kelly, B. J., & Luce, J. M. (1991). The diagnosis and management of neuromuscular diseases causing respiratory failure. *Chest* 99:1485–94.

Malkoff, M. D. (1993). Neuromuscular disease. In *Pathophysiologic Foundations of Critical Care*, ed. M. R. Pinsky & J.-F. A. Dhainaut, pp. 778–88. Baltimore: Williams & Wilkins.

Myasthenia Gravis

Scadding, G. K., & Harvard, C. W. H. (1982). Pathogenesis and treatment of myasthenia gravis. *British Medical Journal* 285:1000–12.

Guillain-Barré Syndrome

Bolton, C. F. (1992). Neuropathies in the critical care unit. *British Journal of Hospital Medicine* 47:358–60.

Ferner, R., & Barnett, M. (1987). Management of Guillain-Barré syndrome. *British Journal of Hospital Medicine* 38:525–30.

Hund, E. F., Borel, C. O., Cornblath, D. R., Hanley, D. F., & McKhann, G. M. (1993). Intensive management and treatment of severe Guillain-Barré syndrome. *Critical Care Medicine* 21:433–46.

Ropper, A. H. (1992). The Guillain-Barré syndrome. *New England Journal of Medicine* 326:1130–6.

Critically Ill Polyneuropathy

Bolton, C. F. (1993). Neuromuscular abnormalities in critically ill patients. *Intensive Care Medicine* 19:309–10.

Hinds, C. J., Yarwood, G. D., & Coakley, J. H. (1994). Acquired neuromuscular abnormalities in intensive care patients. In *Yearbook of Intensive Care and Emergency Medicine,* ed. J.-L. Vincent, pp. 655–67. Berlin: Springer-Verlag.

Zochodne, D. W., Bolton, C. F., Wells, G. A., et al. (1987). Critical illness polyneuropathy. *Brain* 110:819–42.

Tetanus

Rothstein, R. J., & Baker, F. J. (1978). Tetanus. Prevention and treatment. *Journal of the American Medical Association* 240:675–6.

Trudillo, M. J., Catillo, A., Espana, J. V., Guevarra, P., & Eganez, H. (1980). Tetanus in the adult. *Critical Care Medicine* 8:419–23.

27

ACUTE RENAL FAILURE

- Most acute renal failure in the ICU is potentially preventable.
- Rapid restoration of renal blood flow and arterial blood pressure is crucial.
- Old and 'sick' kidneys (eg patients with chronic renal impairment) are particularly vulnerable to acute insults.

ACUTE RENAL FAILURE IN INTENSIVE CARE

PATHOPHYSIOLOGY

Acute renal failure (ARF) occurs when there is a temporary and usually reversible failure of the kidney's ability to excrete the waste products of metabolism.

The kidney is usually an innocent bystander in the critically ill – the common causes of ARF in the ICU are renal ischaemia secondary to hypotension and hypovolaemia and nephrotoxic drugs, sometimes in combination.

ARF in the seriously ill is commonly referred to as 'acute tubular necrosis', and usually it is marked by oliguria and uraemia. The term 'cortical necrosis' is reserved for irreversible renal failure resulting from prolonged ischaemia.

Among the difficulties of dealing with ARF have been our lack of suitable animal models for experimental studies and our failure to define its precise pathophysiology. We know that ARF involves patchy tubular cell necrosis, cell swelling, and loss of the brush border. The cellular debris coalesces with protein to form intraluminal casts, which impede tubular flow. However, the glomerulus is also affected. This may be related to pre-glomerular vasoconstriction. The combination of back-pressure from tubular obstruction and pre-glomerular vasoconstriction decreases the net glomerular transcapillary pressure gradient to almost zero, resulting in little or no filtrate formation (Figure 27.1).

Pathophysiology of acute renal failure

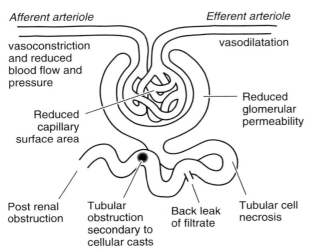

FIGURE 27.1 Pathophysiology of acute renal failure, which often is multifactorial. Some or all of these factors may play roles.

The renal medulla is relatively vulnerable to hypoxic injury, as compared with the cortex. Because the tubular work load is determined by the glomerular filtration rate, ARF may be a physiologically based, short-term response, designed to minimize medullary hypoxic damage. The reduced tubular and glomerular functions can be viewed as an effort to protect the ischaemic medullary ascending limb from further hypoxic injury. This results in reduced ability to concentrate urine.

Following ischaemic damage, usually there is an 'oliguric phase' lasting about 2 weeks, but this can continue for up to 60 days. The return of renal function is heralded by a 'diuretic phase', marked by increasing urine output. This may be due in part to removal of excess water and salt, but it can also be a reflection of impaired tubular function, which sometimes remains for weeks or months. A modified diuretic phase can occur after renal insufficiency and relative oliguria.

AETIOLOGY OF ACUTE RENAL FAILURE IN THE SETTING OF AN ICU

The causes of renal failure often are divided into 'pre-renal', 'renal', and 'post-renal' causes (Table 27.1). Hypotension in the presence of chronic renal insufficiency or chronic hypertension is a particularly dangerous combination. Post-renal causes of renal failure are uncommon in the ICU. However, a kinked or blocked catheter can be a spurious cause of anuria or oliguria. The commonest 'renal' causes of renal failure in intensive care are related to drugs and toxins. The aminoglycoside antibiotics are the drugs best known for causing direct nephrotoxicity in the ICU, but others have been implicated. Toxins such as those found in patients with septicaemia have also been implicated in ARF.

Acute renal failure in the ICU is often multifactorial. For example, the factors contributing to sepsis can include hypotension, a direct nephrotoxic effect of septicaemia, and possibly drugs, especially the aminoglycosides. Whatever their causes, cases of ARF usually have similar pathophysiologies and clinical courses in the ICU. Renal biopsy is indicated only if the cause of the ARF is uncertain.

Ultrasound or nuclear medicine studies may give some idea of renal size if chronic renal disease is suspected. Small kidney size indicates chronic renal insufficiency. Although glomerulonephritis is rare in the setting of intensive care, proteinuria, haematuria, and the presence of casts point to that possibility.

Rhabdomyolysis is becoming increasingly common in intensive care and usually is found in association with prolonged immobility following a drug overdose, intravenous narcotic abuse, trauma, alcoholism, or an infective process (see p. 298). Obvious limb damage, with muscle necrosis, is common. Rhabdomyolysis is marked by myoglobinuria, a rapid and profound rise in the serum concentration of creatine phosphokinase, and the presence of pigmented casts in the urinary sediment. There will be a grossly increased solute load, combined with decreased renal function. The prognosis for complete recovery in this type of ARF is excellent.

NON-OLIGURIC RENAL FAILURE Non-oliguric renal failure is characterized by normal or increased urine output in the presence of

TABLE 27.1 MAJOR CAUSES OF ACUTE RENAL FAILURE IN THE ICU

PRE-RENAL CAUSES

Decreased effective circulating volume

Hypovolaemia, eg
  Haemorrhage
  Gastro-intestinal loss
  Skin loss
  Polyuria

Volume redistribution
  Peripheral vasodilatation, eg
  Sepsis and anaphylaxis
'Third-space' loss, eg
  Peritonitis
  Pancreatitis
  Ascites

Decreased cardiac function, eg

Congestive heart failure
Cor pulmonale
Vascular heart disease
Pericarditis, tamponade

Renal vascular disease, eg

Dissecting aortic aneurysm
Thromboembolic disease

RENAL CAUSES

Nephrotoxins

Aminoglycosides
Cephalosporins, penicillins,
  tetracyclines, quinolone,
  sulphonamides
Frusemide/aminoglycoside
  combination
Amphotericin B, polymyxin, iodinated
  radiographic contrast solutions,
  antineoplastic drugs
Immunotherapy (eg interferon)
Hypercalcaemia, hyperuricaemia
Free haemoglobin and myoglobin
Heavy metals, glycols, organic
  solvents

Septicaemia

Combination of cardiovascular failure,
  intravascular volume redistribution,
  and nephrotoxicity

Other renal causes

Acute interstitial nephritis
Microvascular (eg malignant,
  hypertension, DIC)
Glomerulonephritis secondary
  to systemic disease (eg
  systemic lupus erythe-
  matosus, vasculitis,
  endocarditis)
Acute-on-chronic renal failure
Renal vein thrombosis
  (eg hypercoagulable states)
Papillary necrosis (eg diabetes,
  sickle-cell disease)
Hepatorenal failure
Thrombotic microangiopathy
  (eg scleroderma, malignant
  hypertension)

POST-RENAL CAUSES, eg

Blocked or kinked urinary catheter
High intra-abdominal pressure from any trauma cause
Bilateral ureteric pathology

uraemia. The pathophysiology is similar to that seen in classic ARF. However, while the production of urine, albeit not of good quality, makes fluid balance easier, the prognosis for patients with non-oliguric renal failure requiring repeated dialysis is the same as for those with oliguric renal failure. There have been suggestions that drugs such as mannitol and frusemide might be able to convert olig-uric to non-oliguric renal failure, but as yet it is uncertain which, if any, of these drugs have this action, what dosages should be employed, in which types of renal failure they could be successful, and at what stage in the disease process the drugs might be effective.

INVESTIGATIONS

ROUTINE INVESTIGATIONS   The diagnosis of ARF is usually clinical: uraemia in the presence of suggestive clinical circumstances (eg sep-sis or hypotension). Daily determinations of serum creatinine, urea, and electrolytes, including sodium, calcium, phosphate, and magne-sium, should be performed. Routine haemoglobin and blood counts should be done. Because active intervention may be required, more frequent estimations of serum potassium and arterial blood gases may be needed when ARF is suspected.

URINALYSIS   There can be higher concentrations of protein in the presence of glomerular disease than in renal failure of pre-renal or post-renal origin.

Glomerular lesions usually are associated with a urinary sediment that contains cells, casts, and cellular debris.

Drug-induced acute interstitial nephritis can occur in the intensive care setting. It is suggested by the presence of white cells, white-cell casts, and eosinophils in the urine and can be associated with fever, rash, and peripheral eosinophilia.

URINE SODIUM CONCENTRATION AND OSMOLALITY   Classically, renal hypoperfusion is associated with avid retention of sodium by the body, with minimal excretion in the urine (usually less than 20 mmol/L). In patients with intrinsic renal disease, the excretion of sodium in the urine typically is higher than 40 mmol/L.

Similarly, decreased renal perfusion is associated with high osmo-lality of the urine (>400 mOsm/L), whereas with intrinsic renal disease, the urine osmolality typically is 300–400 mOsm/L. In the presence of dopamine and diuretics, urinary electrolytes are difficult to interpret.

OTHER INVESTIGATIONS   In patients in whom the causes of ARF are unclear, renal ultrasound is the investigation of first choice, because it provides information about chronicity in terms of kidney size, in addition to excluding obstruction. It is a highly sensitive, but non-specific, detector of dilatation of the collecting system, and it is most useful as a screening method for discriminating between chronic obstruction and acute obstruction. Intravenous pyelography may be useful for defining renal anatomy and ruling out the possibility of obstruction. A CT scan may provide more detail regarding a site of obstruction. The use of contrast medium can exacerbate renal disease. If vascular occlusion is suspected, radionuclide imaging or angiography can be performed. Renal biopsy should be performed only if the cause remains unclear, if glomerular disease or interstitial nephritis is suspected, or if there is prolonged ARF (4–6 weeks).

MANAGEMENT

PREVENTION

The onset of ARF in intensive care usually occurs days after the precipitating event. It is crucial to apply the basic principles of rapid cardiorespiratory resuscitation **OUTSIDE** as well as inside the ICU, in order to prevent renal failure. For example, multitrauma victims must be rapidly transfused, and peri-operative patients must be kept well hydrated. The degrees of ischaemic insults that individual kidneys can tolerate will vary considerably. 'Old' kidneys and hypertensive kidneys cannot tolerate ischaemic insults as well as young healthy kidneys. **MANY CASES OF ARF COULD HAVE BEEN AVOIDED IF HYPOVOLAEMIA AND HYPOTENSION HAD BEEN CORRECTED WITHIN MINUTES, RATHER THAN HOURS.** The management of ARF represents an enormous drain on resources and considerably increases the ICU mortality figures.

The aim of preventive manoeuvres is to continually provide ideal homeostatic conditions in which healthy kidneys can operate (Table 27.2).

TABLE 27.2   PREVENTION OF ACUTE RENAL FAILURE

Maintain renal perfusion
Begin rapid and efficient resuscitation
Correct hypovolaemia
Avoid hypoxia
Correct low cardiac output
Maintain patient's normal blood pressure
Avoid abdominal tamponade
Diagnose and aggressively treat septicaemia
Avoid high intrathoracic pressure
Use low-dosage dopamine or dobutamine infusion
Avoid or closely monitor nephrotoxic drugs
Exclude obstruction of urinary tract
Other possible drugs
   Mannitol
   Frusemide

Renal perfusion

HYPOVOLAEMIA   In many instances, rapid correction of hypovolaemia is all that is required to prevent ARF. This is best achieved with a rapid infusion of fluids (see Chapter 4). Hourly urine output is a critical measurement for all seriously ill patients, and it must always be **MONITORED AND MAINTAINED.**

CARDIAC OUTPUT   Restoring cardiac output depends on manipulating the preload, afterload, and contractility of the heart (see Chapter 22).

Hypotension

Blood pressure must be restored rapidly. This is particularly important in previously hypertensive patients. 'Hypotension' is a relative term. Always note a patient's preadmission pressure or theoretically 'normal' blood pressure, and aim for that level. The blood flow to the kidneys is autoregulated according to the patient's normal blood-pressure range, and a 'normal' pressure may be too low in previously hypertensive patients. This is often the case with the elderly, when a combination of decreased renal function and a moderate degree of pre-existing hypertension makes them particularly prone to develop ARF during hypotensive insults.

INOTROPES   In some situations, such as septicaemia, it is difficult to increase the blood pressure, despite an adequate preload and good cardiac function. The use of a drug with vasoconstrictive properties, such as adrenaline or noradrenaline, may paradoxically increase rather than decrease renal blood flow and urine output. This is related to an increase in renal perfusion pressure. The combination of adrenaline or noradrenaline, in order to increase blood pressure, together with low-dosage or 'renal'-dosage dopamine (1–3 μg $\cdot$ kg^{-1} $\cdot$ min^{-1}), to increase renal blood flow, is commonly used for this purpose. However, there is some suggestion that the α-mediated vasoconstruction overrides any dopamine-mediated vasodilation.

LOW-DOSAGE DOPAMINE   The status of low-dosage (1–3 μg $\cdot$ kg^{-1} $\cdot$ min^{-1}) dopamine is changing. It was thought to stimulate specific dopaminergic receptors, causing renal vasodilation and promoting diuresis and sodium excretion. However, at such low dosages, dopamine enhances renal plasma flow by a global increase in cardiac output and mean arterial pressure, rather than a specific dopaminergic-mediated renal vasodilation. Dobutamine has been shown in some trials to be as effective as or more effective than dopamine for increasing the urine output and preventing a rise in creatinine. Dopamine has few side effects at low dosages and is still widely used in attempts to prevent renal failure and promote urine output.

ABDOMINAL TAMPONADE   Abdominal tamponade due to excessive bleeding, intra-abdominal fluid, severe ileus, or intestinal obstruction can cause renal impairment because of the combination of decreased arterial supply and decreased venous drainage, as well as ureteric obstruction.

As a guide to the severity of abdominal tamponade, and as a guide to surgical intervention, the intra-abdominal pressure should be measured in all seriously ill patients when the abdomen feels tense. The intravesical pressure is an accurate reflection of intra-abdominal pressure and is easily measured (see p. 699). Decreased renal blood flow and oliguria can occur with pressures as low as 20 cm H_2O. This will progressively worsen until total anuria eventually supervenes.

There is urgent need to relieve the tamponade by laparotomy. The abdomen may have to be left open, with packs, or closed, using a Marlex graft. The combination of oliguria and abdominal tamponade due to bleeding is a difficult diagnostic and therapeutic dilemma. It is often assumed that the oliguria is related to hypovolaemia, rather than to the tamponade itself. Moreover, relief of the tamponade may be impossible when the intra-abdominal bleeding cannot be controlled by the usual surgical techniques. Bilateral nephrostomy to facilitate urine drainage may also be performed in cases of severe abdominal tamponade causing deterioration in renal function.

POSITIVE INTRATHORACIC PRESSURE   Positive-pressure ventilation, especially with high levels of positive end-expiratory pressure (PEEP), can reduce renal blood flow by up to 20%. Ventilatory modes using lower mean intrathoracic pressures, such as continuous positive airway pressure (CPAP) or intermittent mandatory ventilation (IMV), may result in improved renal perfusion (see Chapter 20).

Aovid or closely monitor nephrotoxic drugs

Drugs can exacerbate or cause renal failure by direct nephrotoxicity or interstitial nephritis. Drugs that can exacerbate renal failure include those that can contribute to hypotension or hypovolaemia, such as diuretics and vasodilators.

DIRECT NEPHROTOXICITY   Aminoglycoside antibiotics are the drugs best known to cause nephrotoxicity in intensive care. Levels should be monitored closely when they are used (see p. 204). Other drugs that have been implicated in the intensive care setting include the tetracyclines, methotrexate, cisplatin, cephalosporins, ethylene glycol, amphotericin B, radiographic contrast agents, and non-steroidal anti-inflammatory agents. Although the angiotensin-converting enzyme (ACE) inhibitors are not directly nephrotoxic, they can predispose to ARF, especially in patients with long-standing hypertension. This is related to their pronounced vasodilatory effect on the efferent arteriole of the kidney, reducing the glomerular capillary pressure.

Drugs for preventing renal failure

One of the great dilemmas in treating ARF is whether or not to use mannitol and loop diuretics. Except in special circumstances, such as in the presence of damage due to myoglobinuria or haemoglobinuria (see p. 298), neither has been shown to prevent ARF, and both have certainly been abused. Oliguria is not due to a lack of either drug, and too often the automatic response to oliguria is to use frusemide. The theoretical basis for their use supposedly is related to their ability to increase renal blood flow and encourage tubular fluid flow. Mannitol may encourage necrotic debris to be washed away, but it has also been implicated in causing ARF, presumably by exacerbating hypovolaemia as a result of its diuretic effect. The 'diuretic challenge' or 'kick start' with loop diuretics usually is based on the premise that it may do some good and probably will not do any harm. However, both loop diuretics and mannitol have side effects that are exacerbated by their accumulation in patients with renal failure. Furthermore, diuresis will worsen renal insufficiency related to hypovolaemia. At best, diuretics may convert an oliguric renal failure to a non-oliguric one, once all other reversible causes have been excluded. Neither mannitol nor loop diuretic has consistently been shown to alter the course of ARF, nor improve survival.

So-called cytoprotective agents may become important in reducing the initial damage and encouraging more rapid recovery by reducing reperfusion injury. Calcium-channel blocking agents, prostacyclin, xanthine oxidase inhibitors, and pentoxifylline may become useful in the future.

Exclude obstruction

Acute onset of renal failure, with total anuria, and in the absence of shock, should direct the diagnostician's attention to the urinary tract, in order to exclude obstruction along its length. Always flush the catheter, in order to exclude obstruction. Remove the urinary catheter if there is doubt about obstruction, especially in the presence of blood clot or sediment. Ultrasound or pyelography with computed tomography (CT) should be employed to rule out obstruction within the urinary tract. If this is unsuccessful, a retrograde uretero-pyelogram may be necessary.

MANAGEMENT OF RENAL FAILURE

The functions of the kidneys are to maintain fluid and electrolyte homeostasis and to excrete the waste products of metabolism. The following are immediate considerations that precede the decision whether or not and when to use dialysis.

WATER RETENTION   Water retention results in peripheral and pulmonary oedema. Fluid restriction should be used only in the presence of established ARF. Restriction of fluid in the presence of hypovolaemia will increase the likelihood of the renal insufficiency becoming established.

HYPERKALAEMIA   The rate of rise of the potassium concentration will depend on the degree of oliguria, the amount of tissue trauma, and the presence and extent of haemolysis, protein catabolism, and sepsis.

ACIDOSIS   Acidosis usually is not a problem in the early stages of ARF. If it becomes significant [eg hydrogen-ion concentration ≥ 80 mmol/L (pH < 7.1)], then bicarbonate can be given (50 ml of 8.4% solution) as a temporary measure. Dialysis should be started early.

HYPONATRAEMIA   Hyponatraemia usually is not a major problem. It is related to water retention, rather than an absolute decrease in body sodium. Sodium-containing solutions are not indicated (see p. 73).

BLOOD UREA   The rate of increase in the urea concentration will depend on the degree of hypercatabolism – usually 5–10 mmol $\cdot$ $L^{-1} \cdot d^{-1}$.

SERUM CREATININE   The rate of increase will depend on the degree of muscle breakdown – usually 0.05–0.20 mmol $\cdot L^{-1} \cdot d^{-1}$.

CALCIUM AND PHOSPHORUS METABOLISM   Hyperphosphataemia and hypocalcaemia can occur in ARF.

INFECTION   Among patients with ARF there is a general increase in severe infections, including septicaemia (see p. 182).

STRESS ULCERATION There may be an increased incidence of stress ulceration among ARF patients (see p. 31).

NEUROLOGICAL COMPLICATIONS Alterations in mental status are early findings in patients with ARF, with progression from somnolence to disorientation and coma.

Dialysis

Clearly, the foregoing are all temporary measures, and if the renal failure progresses, dialysis is indicated. Uncontrolled hyperkalaemia, uraemia, acidosis, and fluid accumulation are indications for dialysis. Strict indications for the commencement of dialysis can be misleading. The rate of rise of urea and creatinine is more important. A blood urea concentration of 35 mmol/L and serum creatinine concentration of 0.60–0.80 mmol/L are guidelines for commencement of dialysis. Aim to keep the blood urea below 30 mmol/L. Dialysis should be instituted earlier, rather than later, and should be carried out more aggressively in hypercatabolic states, such as sepsis, trauma, or rhabdomyolysis.

Dialysis should be continued until there is recovery of renal function. In non-oliguric renal failure, recovery is heralded by increasing urine output, and in both oliguric and non-oliguric renal failure by a 'plateauing' of urea and creatinine concentrations. The urinary catheter should always be removed if there is significant oliguria, as it is simply an extra source of infection.

COMPLICATIONS OF ACUTE RENAL FAILURE

GASTRO-INTESTINAL-TRACT BLEEDING This can be a serious problem in patients with ARF, and measures should be taken to prevent it (see p. 31).

SEPTICAEMIA The major cause of mortality among patients with ARF is septicaemia. Meticulous attention should be paid to the prevention, detection, and treatment of septicaemia (see Chapter 13).

FEEDING Where possible, enteral feeding should be encouraged in patients with ARF. The use of peritoneal dialysis (PD) does not interfere with intestinal absorption. If enteral feeding is not possible, parenteral nutrition (see p. 89) should be considered, as long as there is adequate removal of fluid and urea.

DRUG TREATMENT IN ACUTE RENAL FAILURE Drugs normally handled by the kidney often need to be given in modified amounts during ARF. Consideration should also be given to the efficiency of drug removal by haemodialysis, PD, or haemofiltration.

RECOVERY AND PROGNOSIS

Acute tubular necrosis will last approximately 2–3 weeks – rarely more than 2 months.

If complete anuria lasts for more than 4–5 weeks, then the likelihood of irreversible cortical necrosis increases, and further investigation is necessary.

Patients can rapidly become dehydrated in the polyuric phase of renal recovery. Measure the urinary electrolytes, and replace them with an equivalent solution – usually 0.45% saline solution.

The mortality from ARF in intensive care is more than 50%. Despite many advances, the mentality regarding ARF with multiorgan failure has changed little over the past 20 years.

MODE OF DIALYSIS

The mode of renal replacement treatment will be determined by the clinical circumstances and by the hospital facilities available. Intermittent haemodialysis (HD) is still commonly used, but it requires specialized nursing staff and facilities. Peritoneal dialysis (PD) and haemofiltration can be employed in most ICUs, and they have certain advantages over HD for use in the seriously ill. Increasingly, continuous dialytic techniques, such as continuous haemofiltration and haemodiafiltration, are being used in ICUs.

HAEMODIALYSIS

Haemodialysis works on the principle of diffusion of molecules across a semipermeable membrane. The movement of molecules occurs largely as a result of a concentration gradient and the nature of the membrane. Haemodialysis is an efficient technique for removing waste products and correcting electrolyte imbalances.

Haemodialysis is less efficient than PD or haemofiltration for removing water, but ultrafiltration can be employed in conjunction with HD for rapid and efficient removal of water. Ultrafiltration involves fluid movement as a result of pressure. The high return pressure when using 'single-needle' dialysis encourages the use of ultrafiltration.

Hypotension is invariably associated with HD in the critically ill. Bicarbonate dialysate, rather than acetate, will decrease this complication. Hypotension decreases the efficiency of dialysis.

Highly trained nursing staff are required for HD. In these days of decreasing resources and increasing demand for HD, this poses a problem for hospital renal services. Furthermore, patients in the ICU often require long and difficult dialysis every second day, or even daily. If a patient is hypercatabolic, requiring more frequent HD, further strain is placed on the nursing staff of the renal unit.

It is beyond the scope of this book to describe the technique of HD in detail, as it is usually performed by specialized staff from outside the ICU.

PERITONEAL DIALYSIS

Peritoneal dialysis works in a manner similar to that of HD. The capillaries in the peritoneal membranes are used as a semipermeable membrane, and exchange occurs as a result of diffusion, according to the concentration gradient between the capillaries and the peritoneal fluid. Movement of water occurs according to the osmolality of the peritoneal fluid.

Peritoneal dialysis is not as efficient as HD for removing waste products, but is more efficient for removing fluid. This has certain advantages in the ICU, with its problems of pulmonary and peripheral oedema. Furthermore, with efficient fluid removal, adequate space can be made for parenteral nutrition, blood products, and colloid.

It may be an added advantage to use PD for renal failure in the presence of peritonitis or pancreatitis. However, patients in intensive care commonly have concurrent lung abnormalities. Increased abdominal pressure due to the dialysate can cause elevation of the diaphragm and basal atelectasis. This can worsen the existing hypoxia and compromise ventilation. Aggressive physiotherapy, sitting the patient upright, or using CPAP via a mask or cuffed endotracheal tube can be used to help prevent basal atelectasis.

TECHNIQUE

1. The peritoneal catheter should be a soft, Silastic, Tenkhoff-type catheter, inserted in the midline, 3 cm below the umbilicus, preferably by a surgeon experienced in the technique under sterile conditions in the operating theatre. Suturing the catheter onto the top of the bladder will improve the efficiency of the procedure. Commence PD intraoperatively to prevent blockage: Initially, use small-volume (500-ml) cycles (20 minutes) to run in, 20 minutes of dwell time, 20 minutes to run out) in order to minimize leakage and scrotal oedema.

2. Add heparin, 500 units per litre, for the first 48 hours, and whenever infection is present, in order to decrease the incidence of fibrin formation and catheter occlusion.

3. After 24 hours, conduct hourly exchanges of either 1 or 2 litres of peritoneal dialysate (20 minutes run in, 20 minutes dwell time, 20 minutes run out) for as long as renal failure persists. Continuous PD will ensure adequate removal of waste products as well as continuous fine tuning of fluid removal.

4. Having recently had a laparotomy is not necessarily a contraindication to PD. These wounds usually will not leak if they are made waterproof by suturing with continuous nylon and the volume used is less than 500 ml hourly for the first 48 hours. If drains are employed during the laparotomy, PD is not, of course, possible.

5. Varying concentrations of glucose in the dialysate (usually 1.5%, 2.5%, 4.5%) will determine the rate of removal of fluid. The 1.5% solution usually results in neutrality – no fluid loss. Resulting hyperglycaemia may require an insulin infusion. Potassium can be added in an appropriate concentration to the dialysate (usually 3.5 mmol/L) or given directly to the patient in intravenous form.

TROUBLESHOOTING   POOR DRAINAGE IS THE COMMONEST PROBLEM WITH PD. Inadequate drainage usually is related to malpositioning of the catheter or fibrin clotting in the catheter lumen. Addition of 500 units of heparin to each litre of dialysate can help prevent fibrin clots, and flushing of the catheter can dislodge fibrin clots. Unfortunately, an occasional 'rogue' catheter will fail to drain, whatever is done. This necessitates early surgical replacement.

INFECTION of the dialysate can present as peritonism, cloudy dialysate, fibrin aggregates, or clinical deterioration of the patient. It is relatively common during prolonged PD in intensive care. Gram staining and culturing should be performed daily on the dialysate. In the presence of infection, antibiotics should initially be added to the dialysate: penicillins or cephalosporins (200 mg/L) and/or aminoglycosides (5 mg/L). Heparin (500 units/L) should also be added to the dialysate, in the presence of infection, to prevent fibrin aggregation.

DISADVANTAGES OF PERITONEAL DIALYSIS

- Technical problems with fluid drainage.
- Leakage around catheter site.
- Peritonitis.
- Basal atelectasis and interference with ventilation.
- Hyperglycaemia.
- Peritoneal dialysis is not as efficient as HD for removing waste products of metabolism.
- Peritoneal fluid can leak out of peritoneal space to form oedema.

ADVANTAGES OF PERITONEAL DIALYSIS

- Can be performed by non-specialized staff in the ICU.
- Very efficient for removing fluid.
- Can control metabolic disturbances in most patients.
- No special dialysis equipment required.

HAEMOFILTRATION AND HAEMODIAFILTRATION
(Figure 27.2)

Haemofiltration is a relatively recent technique that passes extracorporeal blood across a filter. The filter has a polyacrylnitrile or polycarbonate membrane, with a pore size similar to that of a normal glomerulus. A filtrate of blood, similar to glomerular filtrate in composition, is formed from the hydrostatic pressure across the membrane. The movement of fluids and small molecules is due to convection, not diffusion as in HD. The hydrostatic pressure is generated either by the pressure difference between a large artery and vein or artificially by a roller pump. An extracorporeal circuit containing the filter is connected either between a larger artery and vein or between

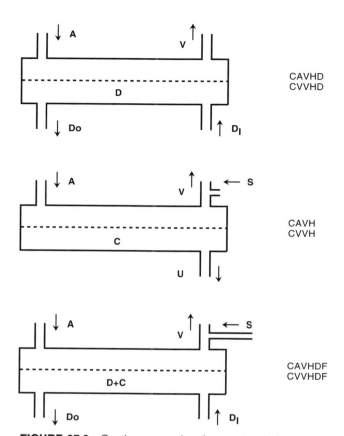

FIGURE 27.2 Continuous renal replacement techniques.

A	'arterial' blood
V	'venous' blood
U	ultrafiltrate
S	substitution fluid
D_I	dialysate inflow
Do	dialysate outflow
D	diffusion
C	convection
CAVH	continuous arteriovenous haemofiltration
CVVH	continuous venovenous haemofiltration
CAVHD	continuous arteriovenous haemodialysis
CVVHD	continuous venovenous haemodialysis
CVVHDF	continuous venovenous haemodiafiltration
CAVHDF	continuous arteriovenous haemodiafiltration

two large veins if a roller pump is used. Prevention of clotting in the system is achieved by heparinization (500–1,500 units/h) or by prostacyclin infusion.

Whereas the filter acts like an artificial glomerulus, there is no equivalent to a renal tubule in this system. In order to achieve elimination of urea, creatinine, and other products of metabolism, the filtrate [blood − (red blood cells + large molecules such as protein)] is replaced by a fluid whose composition is similar to that of the filtrate, but without waste products (eg Ringer's lactate). Therefore, to achieve relatively normal levels of urea and creatinine, a large fluid turnover is needed. Depending on the catabolic rate, a fluid turnover of 10–40 L/d may be needed. Haemodiafiltration largely overcomes this problem by employing a filter with a membrane that is capable of dialysis, using diffusion as in conventional haemodialysis, as well as convection as in haemofiltration. Haemofiltration and/or haemodiafiltration are increasingly being used as the dialytic techniques of choice in ICUs.

INDICATIONS FOR HAEMOFILTRATION AND HAEMODIAFILTRATION

- Dialysis.
- Fluid removal.
- Treating peripheral and pulmonary oedema.
- Drug and toxin removal.

ADVANTAGES OF HAEMOFILTRATION AND HAEMODIAFILTRATION AS FORMS OF DIALYSIS

- Very efficient and versatile for removing fluid and products of metabolism.
- Can be installed and operated by intensive care staff.
- Very stable cardiovascular system during haemoperfusion.

DISADVANTAGES OF HAEMOFILTRATION AND HAEMODIAFILTRATION

- Expensive filters and disposable circuits.
- Extracorporeal circuits require special skills for their operation and can involve complications such as air embolism and hypothermia.
- Thrombocytopenia is very common.

• Facilitating flow can be technically difficult (eg correct anticoagulation and catheter position).

CONTINUOUS ARTERIOVENOUS HAEMOPERFUSION

Kits are available for continuous arteriovenous haemoperfusion (CAVH) – they consist of large-bore arterial and venous catheters (usually inserted in the femoral vessels) with tubing connected to a filter. As CAVH can remove large volumes of fluid, it can be used for dialysis, for fluid removal, or in conjunction with conventional haemodialysis.

TECHNIQUE

1. Insert the large-bore cannulae into a large artery and vein (usually femoral).

2. Give a bolus of heparin (eg 5,000 units IV).

3. Connect the primed (including heparin) extracorporeal circuit and the filter.

4. Establish blood flow through the circuit.

5. Give continuous heparin infusion (500–1,500 units/h) or prostacyclin infusion to minimize clot formation in the filter. The infusion rate can be titrated against measurements of heparin activity, such as APPT.

6. The filtrate flow can be increased by

• lowering the filtrate collection container

• applying suction to the filtrate

• increasing arterial pressure or decreasing venous pressure

• inserting the line for the replacement fluid before the filter (ie on the 'arterial' side), rather than after the filter

• adjusting the heparin or prostacyclin infusion to prevent clotting and to facilitate blood flow through the filter

7. Accurately record the volumes of filtrate and fluid replacement. The next hourly fluid replacement is determined by the previous hourly amount of filtrate and the concurrent patient requirements (Figure 27.3):

fluid replacement/unit time = filtrate/unit time $- \chi$

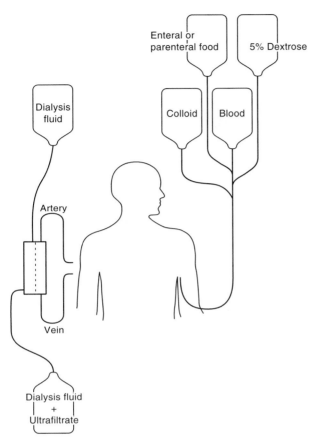

FIGURE 27.3 Fluid management during continuous dialytic treatment. The amount of ul-trafiltrate should be empirically adjusted on an hourly basis (eg 100–300 ml/h) against an es-timation of the body's fluid-retention status. The other fluids should be titrated separately ac-cording to separate end points (eg colloid against intravascular measurement, blood against haemoglobin, 5% dextrose against serum sodium, and food according to nutritional status). There is little point in adding all of these fluids together when considering fluid balance.

where χ is determined by the patient's needs. This is estimated on the basis of the state of hydration of the patient and the amount of fluid otherwise being infused. It normally varies between 50 and 200 ml/h to maintain a neutral fluid balance, but larger amounts can be removed when peripheral or pulmonary oedema is excessive.

8. Alternatively, commercial balance beams can be employed. These will automatically replace an adjustable and predetermined amount of fluid, depending on the filtrate flow.

9. The filtrate is equivalent to glomerular filtrate or the interstitial component of the extracellular fluid compartment. Apart from normal exchange-fluid replacement, the intravascular fluid volume may have to be replaced by colloid or blood in order to efficiently maintain the circulating volume and colloid osmotic pressure.

DISADVANTAGES

• It is difficult to insert a large-bore cannula into the femoral artery. This can cause bleeding, distal ischaemia (especially in patients with peripheral vascular disease), and arteriovenous fistulae at the sites of the cannulae.

• The filtrate flow is limited by the arteriovenous pressure gradient. Hypotension will limit filtrate flow. The efficiency of dialysis is dependent on filtrate flow and on the fluid turnover matching the clearance of waste products.

• In spite of heparinization, clots frequently accumulate in the filter, causing a decreasing filtrate flow. Clot formation in the filter is mainly dependent on platelet function. Some degree of thrombocytopenia is almost invariable with all varieties of haemofiltration and haemodiafiltration. It is relatively common to have platelet counts as low as $50,000 \times 10^9$ or even lower. This usually does not require active intervention.

• The lives of these filters are largely unpredictable, and they are expensive to replace. Ensure that the flow rate is adequate, and increase the heparin infusion rate.

Continuous venovenous haemofiltration

Continuous venovenous haemofiltration (CVVH) uses the same principle of filtration as CAVH. The major differences between CAVH and CVVH are as follows:

• CVVH uses a double-lumen venous catheter or two separate venous lines. Any large vein can be used for this purpose.

• The hydrostatic pressure and flow are created by a roller pump –

the same device used during haemodialysis. The pump is usually equipped with air-bubble and venous-pressure monitors and alarms.

TECHNIQUE

1. Insert a large-bore double-lumen venous catheter (eg 'vascath') into a large vein. Flow usually is more efficient through the femoral or internal jugular vein, rather than the subclavian vein.

2. Prime the extracorporeal circuit and filter as for CAVH.

3. Insert extracorporeal tubing into the roller pump, and adjust the flow rate between 50 and 200 ml/min.

4. It is advisable to keep the flow rate constant and adjust the filtrate formation by a simple gate clamp on the filtrate line, in order to avoid clot formation in the filter. Replacement of fluid into the prefilter line can also increase the filtrate flow and the filter life.

5. Aim for filtrate removal of approximately 1–2 L/h in catabolic patients, and otherwise adjust according to serum creatinine and urea levels. Creatinine clearance ideally should be 10–20 ml/min, blood urea less than 15 mmol/L, and serum creatinine less than 200 μmol/L.

6. Use continuous heparin infusion (500–1,500 units/h) or prostacyclin infusion to minimize clot formation in the filter, as for CAVH (see p. 658).

7. Remove filtrate and replace it according to fluid needs:

replacement fluid/unit time = filtrate loss/unit time − χ

where χ is determined by the patient's needs. This would normally vary between 50 and 200 ml/h to accommodate for other fluid being given concurrently and to compensate for the fluid retention associated with seriously ill patients. However, a net loss of up to 400 ml/h may be necessary to actively reduce pulmonary and peripheral oedema. The filtrate is equivalent to the interstitial component of the extracellular fluid space. The intravascular volume should be meticulously maintained by infusions of colloid or blood while net fluid removal from the interstitial space is being achieved with haemofiltration.

8. Fluid replacement can be performed as in CAVH (see p. 658). However, because of the increased filtrate removal possible with CVVH, balance beams that automatically deliver replacement fluid make nursing easier. With the balance beam, net fluid loss per cycle can be predetermined and adjusted.

9. Monitor and record the flow rate, the venous pressure in the system, and the filtrate and replacement amounts.

Advantages of CVVH compared with CAVH

- Only venous access is required for CVVH.
- Filtrate formation is independent of arteriovenous pressure.
- Higher and more predictable filtrate flows are possible. This is important in hypercatabolic or fluid-overloaded patients, because extracorporeal blood flow is readily adjustable, and filtrate flow and fluid turnover can be tailored to waste-product removal. Urea and creatinine levels are controllable in most hypercatabolic patients with CVVH.
- A longer filter life is possible with CVVH because of more consistent flow rates.

Continuous arteriovenous or venovenous haemodialysis (CAVHD, CVVHD) and haemodiafiltration (CAVHDF, CVVHDF)

Solute transfer and elimination occur by convection with CAVH and CVVH, whereas they occur by diffusion in CAVHD and CVVHD. The principles of convection and diffusion are combined in haemodiafiltration (CAVHDF or CVVHDF). This is achieved by infusing dialysate fluid through the ultrafiltrate compartment of a filter capable of dialysis, counter-currently to blood flow. Thus, a single filter acts as a haemodialyser and provides haemofiltration.

TECHNIQUE

1. Establish vascular access using either an arteriovenous entry, as in CAVH (see p. 658) or venous entry (see p. 660). Alternatively, a Scribner shunt can be inserted by means of a surgical cut down onto the radial artery in the forearm or the posterior tibial artery in the leg. These shunts can provide adequate blood flow (50–200 ml/min) even with relatively low mean blood pressure.

2. The extracorporeal circuit is set up as for CAVH (see p. 658) and CVVH (see p. 661). Prior to connection, the system is primed with approximately 2 litres of heparinized saline (5 units of heparin per millilitre), ensuring that there is no air in the system.

After the circuit is connected to the patient, warmed isotonic peritoneal dialysis fluid is infused into the dialysate compartment of the haemodialyser at a rate of 1–2 L/h. A potassium concentration of 4 mmol/L is usually required in the dialysate to minimize potassium loss. The combined dialysate and ultrafiltrate is measured hourly. Ultrafiltrate volume is calculated by subtraction of the volume of dialysate infused and an appropriate volume replaced according to the patient's needs.

Alternatively, instead of peritoneal dialysis fluid, a commercially available haemodiafiltration fluid may be used.

3. The extracorporeal circuit is kept anticoagulated in the same manner as for CAVH and CVVH (see p. 658).

4. The efficiency of the filter can be monitored by daily comparison of the urea concentration in the patient's serum and that in the dialysate/ultrafiltrate solution. As the filter becomes less efficient, there will be a reduction in the dialysate/ultrafiltrate urea concentration. When there is a significant difference between the two, particularly if the patient's serum urea is rising, the haemodialyser should be changed.

5. An insulin infusion may be necessary to prevent hyperglycaemia from the net uptake of glucose from the dialysis fluid. Phosphate, magnesium, and calcium should be measured at least once daily and replaced accordingly.

ADVANTAGES

• Efficient solute removal by diffusion across the membrane in the same way as haemodialysis.

• Efficient and flexible fluid removal through haemofiltration.

• All of the convenience and advantages associated with CAVH and CVVH (see p. 662).

TROUBLESHOOTING

OLIGURIA

Pre-renal   A pre-renal cause of oliguria is the commonest by far.
Hypovolaemia
- Intravenous fluid will correct most oliguria in the ICU.
- Give a fluid bolus, and increase the rate of fluid infusion.
- Think about possible causes for the hypovolaemia.
- THEN GIVE MORE FLUID.
Hypotension
- Correct hypovolaemia.
- Restore blood pressure to the patient's 'normal' level.
- Vasopressors and/or inotropes may be required.
- Commence 'renal'-dose dopamine.

Renal

Nephrotoxic drugs
- Check levels (eg aminoglycoside antibiotics)
- Avoid where possible (eg radio-contrast drug)
Sepsis
Myoglobin (see p. 298)

Post-renal

No catheter, kinked catheter, blocked catheter
Increased intra-abdominal pressure (see p. 699)
Bilateral ureteric obstruction (eg trauma, tumour)

FURTHER READING

Brezis, M., & Epstein, F. H. (1989). A closer look at radiocontrast-induced nephropathy. *New England Journal of Medicine* 320:179–81.

Corwin, H. L., & Bonventre, J. V. (1988). Acute renal failure in the intensive care unit. *Intensive Care Medicine* 14:10–16, 86–96.

Dickson, D., & Hillman, K. (1989). Continuous renal replacement therapy. *Anaesthesia and Intensive Care* 18:76–92.

Finn, W. F. (1990). Diagnosis and management of acute tubular necrosis. *Medical Clinics of North America* 74:873–91.

Levinsky, N. G. (1977). Pathophysiology of acute renal failure. *New England Journal of Medicine* 296:1453–8.

Myers, B. D., & Moran, S. M. (1986). Hemodynamically mediated acute renal failure. *New England Journal of Medicine* 314:97–105.

Schrier, R. W. (ed.) (1986). *Renal and Electrolyte Disorders*, 3rd ed. Boston: Little, Brown.

Vendegna, T. R., & Anderson, R. J. (1994). Are dopamine and/or dobutamine renoprotective in intensive care unit patients? *Critical Care Medicine* 22:1893–4.

Walker, R. (1994). Aminoglycoside nephrotoxicity: recent developments. *New Zealand Medical Journal* 107:54–5.

28

CRITICAL CARE GASTROENTEROLOGY

FULMINANT HEPATIC FAILURE

Fulminant hepatic failure is defined as encephalopathy due to massive hepatic necrosis within 8 weeks of the onset of the primary illness, with no evidence of previous liver disease. This excludes subacute hepatic necrosis, acute-on-chronic hepatic failure, and chronic hepatic encephalopathy. It is a relatively rare disease.

AETIOLOGY

• Viral causes: the viruses that cause hepatitis A, B, C, D, E, and non-A, non-B, as well as Epstein-Barr virus, herpes simplex virus, and cytomegalovirus (CMV). Viral causes account for over 70% of all cases of fulminant hepatic failure.

• Paracetamol poisoning.

• Idiosyncratic drug reactions: antituberculous drugs, methyldopa, monoamine oxidase inhibitors, halothane hepatitis.

• Direct drug toxicity: carbon tetrachloride, yellow phosphorus.

• Ischaemia, hypoxia (Budd-Chiari syndrome, lymphoma, heatstroke, shock).

• Acute fatty liver of pregnancy.

• Wilson's disease.

CLINICAL FEATURES

The diagnosis can be difficult, especially in the early stages. Patients usually do not have signs of chronic liver failure, such as spider naevi and palmar erythema.

ENCEPHALOPATHY is the hallmark of this disease, and disturbance in the level of consciousness may be the only presenting feature.

The clinical course may be played out over hours or days.

ENCEPHALOPATHY Many factors have been implicated, but as yet no definite cause of the encephalopathy has been found. Ammonia, free fatty acids, phenols, bilirubin, bile acids, mercaptans, false neuro-transmitters, benzodiazepine analogues, and γ-aminobutyric acid (GABA) are some of the implicated compounds.

Stages of encephalopathy
Grade I: mood changes and confusion
Grade II: drowsiness and increase in muscle tone
Grade III: stuporous but rousable
Grade IV: unrousable to maximum stimulation

There are no specific clinical or EEG features that can be used to dif-ferentiate this encephalopathy from those associated with other meta-bolic disturbances.

Encephalopathy is associated with cerebral oedema – THIS IS THE CAUSE OF DEATH. Over 80% of patients with grade IV encephalopa-thy have cerebral oedema. The sequela of the cerebral oedema – elevated intracranial pressure (ICP) – should be monitored, and at-tempts should be made to decrease it. One must rule out the pres-ence of hypoglycaemia, acid–base or electrolyte disturbances, and hy-poxia, as these contribute to the severity of the encephalopathy.

BLEEDING DIATHESIS Most of the clotting factors are manufactured in the liver, and therefore their levels usually will be decreased. The prothrombin time is always prolonged – it is a good marker of liver function and clinical course. Platelets are reduced in number and func-tion. Gastro-intestinal-tract (GIT) haemorrhage may occur.

HEPATORENAL SYNDROME The 'hepatorenal syndrome' is renal fail-ure that occurs in patients with liver disease in the absence of other causes. It usually occurs in patients with chronic hepatic insufficiency, usually in association with ascites, and often is associated with a sep-sis-like syndrome, with peripheral vasodilatation and increased car-diac output. Hepatorenal syndrome is exacerbated by hypovolaemia and hypotension, especially in association with fluid loss secondary to diuretic treatment and aggressive paracentesis. Most patients with hepatorenal syndrome die. That it is related to the liver failure is em-phasized by the fact that renal function recovers after liver transplantation. Apart from liver transplantation there is no definitive treatment.

ELECTROLYTES Hypokalaemia occurs early. Hyperkalaemia associated with renal failure may supervene. Hyponatraemia may occur in the latter stages.

ACID–BASE DISTURBANCES Respiratory alkalosis is common in the early stages. Lactic acidosis occurs in over half of all these patients, especially in the latter stages.

HYPOGLYCAEMIA Hypoglycaemia can occur and probably is due to failure of gluconeogenesis.

CARDIOVASCULAR FAILURE Hypotension, with a high cardiac output and vasodilatation, is common. The pathophysiology is similar to that for septicaemia.

RESPIRATORY FAILURE The airway may be compromised because of coma. Adult respiratory distress syndrome (ARDS) may occur and probably is due to increased membrane permeability (see p. 400).

IMMUNOCOMPROMISE Bacteraemia and endotoxaemia are common because of decreases in reticuloendothelial clearance, leucocyte function, and complement activity. Spontaneous bacterial peritonitis can occur in patients with ascites.

JAUNDICE Jaundice often develops late.

INVESTIGATIONS

THE DIAGNOSIS IS CLINICAL – based mainly on encephalopathy. Investigations are necessary to find the cause of the fulminant hepatic failure, to determine prognosis, and to chart the course of the disease and its complications:

• Serology
• Hepatitis B: hepatitis B surface antigen (may be negative in patients with fulminant hepatitis); IgM and anti-HBc (antibody to he-

patitis B core antigen) rapidly becomes positive in the fulminant form of hepatitis B.

• Hepatitis A: anti-HAV (antibody to hepatitis A virus).

• Hepatitis C: anti-HCV (antibody to hepatitis C virus).

• CMV: complement-fixation test detecting IgG antibody.

• Epstein-Barr virus: 'mono-spot' or EB IgM.

• Herpes simplex virus: serum titres for herpes simplex virus.

• Paracetamol levels if drug poisoning is suspected.

• Coagulation studies: The prothrombin time is probably the most sensitive laboratory indicator of liver function in fulminant hepatic failure. It should be measured daily.

• Liver 'function tests': The functions of the liver include lipid, protein, and carbohydrate metabolism, production of bile acids, storage, and detoxification and excretion of lipid-soluble compounds. All of these functions can be tested, but few are routinely tested in clinical practice. Hepatic enzymes are crude markers of liver destruction, rather than function, and may appear 'normal' in the presence of massive liver destruction. To date, there are few clinically sensitive and specific laboratory markers of hepatic function.

• Bilirubin determinations have no value for prognosis or treatment. Serum bilirubin and bile acid levels in hepatobiliary disease are related to excretory function.

• Blood sugar levels should be measured regularly.

• Potassium should be measured as indications arise.

• Other serum electrolytes should be measured daily (sodium, calcium, magnesium, phosphate).

• Blood urea is a measure of liver (production) and renal (excretion) functions and therefore is difficult to interpret.

• Creatinine: Measure daily.

• Arterial blood gases: Measure at least twice per day.

• Chest x-ray should be obtained daily.

• EEG should be carried out on admission and regularly thereafter as an indicator of the severity of encephalopathy.

• CT scan and brain-stem evoked potentials may be helpful.

• Regular microbiological screenings should be conducted.

MONITORING

Monitoring is necessary as a guide to patient management while the liver is given an opportunity to regenerate. Because cerebral oedema, with elevated ICP, is the major cause of death among patients with fulminant hepatic failure (FHF), the cerebral perfusion pressure (CPP) and mean arterial pressure (MAP) should be continuously monitored to provide a basis for adjustments in the treatment:

CPP = MAP − ICP

Monitor

- pulse rate
- temperature
- continuous ECG
- continuous blood pressure
- central venous pressure (CVP)
- urine output
- pulse oximetry
- pulmonary artery wedge pressure (PAWP), if needed (see p. 499)
- cardiac output, if needed (see p. 502)
- oxygen consumption and delivery, if needed (see p. 376)

MANAGEMENT

Ideally, these patients should be transferred at an early stage to a specialized ICU with appropriate expertise and monitoring equipment. Early discussions with a liver transplantation unit should be undertaken.

Apart from cases of paracetamol overdose, where drug removal may be possible, the principles of treatment are meticulous monitoring and support until the liver can be given an opportunity to regenerate.

MAINTAIN CEREBRAL PERFUSION PRESSURE

Treat elevated ICP (for details, see Chapter 24).
Position the patient 30°–40° upright.
If the ICP is significantly elevated, prevent hypertensive surges to

the non-autoregulated cerebral circulation by giving small amounts of sedation before procedures. Narcotics and other sedatives depend on liver function for metabolism and should be given in only small amounts until the degree of liver damage is assessed.

Keep the patient's head straight, and avoid jugular venous compression.

Give mannitol boluses, 0.3 g/kg IV (no more than three times per day), if ICP is consistently raised [ICP > 25 mm Hg (3.3 kPa)].

Hyperventilation may be useful as a short-term measure.

Phenobarbitone, thiopentone, phenytoin, and lignocaine may also help to reduce ICP (see p. 578).

Maintain the MAP with fluids and inotropes (see p. 520).

CARDIOVASCULAR SYSTEM The cardiovascular abnormalities are very similar to those found in the presence of sepsis (see p. 184). Usually there will be high cardiac output, low MAP, and decreased peripheral vascular resistance. As in sepsis, the cardiovascular disturbances may be marked by 'delivery-dependent oxygen consumption' (see p. 376). It is crucial to avoid hypotension in patients with liver failure. Oxygen delivery to the liver should be optimized by supporting cardiac output, oxygen saturation, and haemoglobin levels. Aggressive fluid resuscitation and inotropes are often necessary. The type and dosage of inotrope are dependent on the patient's needs (see p. 520). A suggested starting regimen for hypotension, with normal filling pressures, is adrenaline or noradrenaline titrated against the response. Low-dosage dopamine (1–3 $\mu g \cdot kg^{-1} \cdot min^{-1}$) may spare the renal and mesenteric blood flow.

NUTRITION

Cease dietary protein.

Give oral lactulose (30–50 ml 8-hourly).

Avoid neomycin, as it can be absorbed and can cause renal failure.

BLOOD GLUCOSE Because the liver is a major source of glucose, hypoglycaemia can occur. Measure blood glucose hourly, and titrate against levels, with 10% or 50% dextrose intravenous infusions – large amounts may be necessary.

ELECTROLYTES Correct hypokalaemia with intravenous potassium chloride as necessary. Correct hyponatraemia with water restriction – may need to concentrate dextrose solutions and intravenous drugs in order to decrease the water intake.

FLUIDS Often, patients will require liberal amounts of fluid or blood products (see Chapter 4) because hypovolaemia and hypotension are poorly tolerated. If hypotension persists, despite adequate cardiac filling pressures, use inotropic support (see p. 520).

ACID–BASE DISTURBANCES Respiratory alkalosis does not require active treatment. For metabolic alkalosis, give acetazolamide, 500 mg IV, 8-hourly. If that fails, titrate an HCl solution (1 mol/L) intravenously (see p. 172). If there is metabolic acidosis, treat the underlying cause.

GASTRO-INTESTINAL HAEMORRHAGE H_2-receptor antagonists, although effective, will reduce blood flow to the liver, and antacids may predispose to gastric colonization (see p. 31). Sucralfate may be preferable (see p. 32).

COAGULATION ABNORMALITIES Use fresh frozen plasma, and blood and platelets where necessary, to replace coagulation factors and maintain haemoglobin levels.

RESPIRATORY FAILURE

Intubate if airway patency is in question.

Treat ARDS or acute hypoxia with an increased concentration of inspired oxygen, continuous positive airway pressure (CPAP), or ventilation with positive end-expiratory pressure (PEEP) if necessary (see p. 400).

Avoid intermittent positive-pressure ventilation (IPPV) if possible (ie use CPAP and encourage spontaneous ventilation, as increased intrathoracic pressure will decrease liver blood flow).

RENAL FAILURE

Avoid hypovolaemia and hypotension.

Low-dosage dopamine may encourage renal and mesenteric blood flow (see p. 647).

Use loop diuretics and aminoglycosides cautiously, as they can contribute to renal insufficiency.

Dialyse early if renal failure is confirmed (see p. 651).

GENERAL MEASURES Avoid sedation and analgesics unless they are being used to control ICP or to relieve pain. Use very small incremental doses in order to avoid accumulation in the absence of adequate liver detoxification.

Other forms of treatment

The following will not influence survival:

- corticosteroids
- exchange blood transfusion
- cross-circulation with humans, animals, or excised livers
- haemodialysis
- branched-chain amino acids

Charcoal perfusion with prostacyclin may improve survival rates if commenced early. Liver transplantation may play an increasing role in these patients. The results thus far indicate a survival rate higher than 50%, among selected patients, and in the absence of cerebral oedema.

Prognosis

The mortality from grade IV coma is about 80%. With early and aggressive treatment of patients with grade III encephalopathy, mortality can be reduced to about 40%.

ACUTE-ON-CHRONIC LIVER FAILURE

Acute-on-chronic liver failure and fulminant hepatic failure (FHF) are, for practical purposes, considered together. Although they have many differences, their management procedures, if not their causes, are similar. The diagnosis of acute-on-chronic liver failure is the easier of the two, because in addition to the disturbed level of consciousness, there are the obvious stigmata of chronic liver disease (jaundice, spider naevi, hepatomegaly, ascites, etc). Increasing numbers of patients with alcohol-related liver disease are being admitted to ICUs for acute deterioration (eg bleeding oesophageal varices) (see p. 692) and concurrent acute illnesses.

DIFFERENCES BETWEEN FULMINANT HEPATIC FAILURE AND ACUTE-ON-CHRONIC LIVER FAILURE

• Infection, surgery, drugs, and nitrogenous loads in the GIT can precipitate acute liver failure and hepatic encephalopathy in patients with chronic liver failure. In these patients, lactulose (30–50 ml 8-hourly orally) may be helpful. Avoid or limit sedative drugs.

• The role of cerebral oedema in acute-on-chronic liver failure has not been established.

• Short-term survival is better for acute-on-chronic failure than for FHF.

• However, among those patients with acute-on-chronic liver failure who require ventilation, mortality is about 90%.

LIVER DYSFUNCTION IN CRITICAL ILLNESS

Many patients with previously normal liver function will become jaundiced while acutely ill, especially in association with septicaemia, trauma, multiorgan failure (MOF), and shock. This is almost certainly another manifestation of the multiple splanchnic organ failure resulting from hypoperfusion. Stress ulceration and mucosal ischaemia in the GIT are other manifestations. There are two major syndromes (Table 28.1).

ISCHAEMIC HEPATITIS   Ischaemic hepatitis is characterized by acute increases in liver transaminases that occur within 24 hours of the onset of shock. Histologically there will be centrilobular necrosis, presumably as a result of an acute decrease in liver blood flow. The bilirubin will be normal or only mildly elevated. The prothrombin time usually will be prolonged.

ICU JAUNDICE   The syndrome of 'ICU jaundice' is characterized by a rising bilirubin that occurs within days of the onset of the illness that required admission to the ICU. The aetiology is multifactorial and includes

TABLE 28.1 CLINICAL FEATURES OF ISCHAEMIC HEPATITIS AND ICU JAUNDICE

Parameter	Ischaemic hepatitis	ICU jaundice
Clinical setting	Shock	Sepsis Trauma Following surgery After severe shock Multiorgan failure
Pathogenesis	Reduced liver blood flow	Reduced liver blood flow Inflammatory mediators Bilirubin load (?) Nutritional factors (?) Drugs (?)
Time of onset	Within 24 hours	Usually 1–2 weeks
Liver function tests		
Bilirubin	Normal/moderate	150–800 μmol/L
AST/ALT	>1,000 units/L	Normal/moderate
ALP/GGT	Normal/moderate	Normal/moderate
Blood glucose	Hypoglycaemia	Hyperglycaemia
Prothrombin time	Prolonged	Normal
Bile salts	Normal	Markedly elevated
Histology	Centrilobular necrosis	Intrahepatic cholestasis Steatosis Increased Kupffer cells Occasionally hepatocyte necrosis
Mortality	>50%	>50%
Clinical course	Resolves if shock is reversed Predisposes to ICU jaundice	Associated with remote organ dysfunction, immunosuppression, and abnormal inter- mediary and drug metabolism

Source: Adapted from Hawker (1991).

• decreased liver blood flow and ischaemia (artificial ventilation can, by itself, decrease liver blood flow and may potentiate liver ischaemia)

• inflammatory mediators released in response to the systemic inflammatory reaction to insults such as sepsis or trauma

- intravenous nutrition
- drugs
- blood transfusions

MANAGEMENT

Both ischaemic hepatitis and ICU jaundice will resolve spontaneously as the underlying disease resolves and the patient improves. Exclude other causes of liver dysfunction, such as hepatitis, post-anaesthetic jaundice, gallstones, and acalculous cholecystitis. Ultrasound and CT are useful investigations to exclude biliary obstruction. An iminodiacetic acid (IDA) scan can be used for diagnosing both acute and chronic cholecystitis and acute biliary obstructions and may, in fact, detect biliary-tract dilatation before it is seen on ultrasound. Avoid hypotension and hypoxia, as well as high intrathoracic pressures from artificial ventilation. Treat any underlying problem, such as sepsis, aggressively.

ASCITES

PATHOGENESIS

Portal hypertension, with increased hydrostatic pressure.
Decreases in serum albumin and colloid oncotic pressure.
Sodium retention along the entire nephron.
Impaired free-water excretion, often resulting in relatively greater water retention than sodium retention, causing hyponatraemia.
Relative hypovolaemia secondary to peripheral vasodilatation, with salt and water retention.

MANAGEMENT

BED REST AND LOW-SODIUM DIET   A low-sodium (40–50 mmol/d) diet will result in control of ascites in about 20% of patients. Sodium restriction can diminish diuretic requirements. However, many cirrhotics are anorexic and malnourished, and that can be worsened by a low-sodium diet.

DIURETIC Spironolactone (100–500 mg/d) is effective in most patients who do not have renal failure. A loop diuretic alone will produce a satisfactory response in only about 50% of cirrhotics and should be added only after failure of spironolactone.

Patients with impaired renal function do not respond well to standard doses of diuretics. Their serum concentrations of potassium and magnesium must be carefully monitored during diuretic therapy.

PERITONEOVENOUS SHUNT The LeVeen shunt consists of a perforated intra-abdominal tube connected through a one-way pressure-sensitive valve to empty into the superior vena cava. It provides short-term improvement, but is associated with a high rate of complications:

- Obstruction: 30%.
- Infection: usually with *Staphylococcus* (shunt must be removed).
- Coagulation disorders: usually mild and in the immediate postoperative period.
- Pulmonary oedema, pulmonary embolism, and endocarditis: The shunt should be reserved for patients with diuretic-resistant oedema and preserved hepatic function.

PARACENTESIS Paracentesis can predispose to hypovolaemia, hypotension, renal failure, dilutional hyponatraemia, and hepatic encephalopathy. It may be of use in combination with intravascular volume replacement.

OTHER APPROACHES
- albumin infusions: short-term benefits
- portacaval shunt: hepatic dysfunction usually so marked in cirrhotics with refractory ascites that surgery is not an option
- liver transplantation: may be considered in selected cases, especially if there is no renal impairment

PROGNOSIS Over 50% of patients with ascites from liver dysfunction are dead within 2 years. This puts ascites in the same prognostic category as many terminal malignancies.

PANCREATITIS

AETIOLOGY

Approximately 80% of cases of acute pancreatitis are associated with biliary lithiasis or chronic alcohol ingestion. Other causes include hyperlipidaemia, surgery, penetrating peptic ulcer, physical trauma, instrumentation of the pancreatic duct, hypercalcaemia, toxins, and drugs. Up to 10–20% of cases are idiopathic.

PATHOGENESIS

Acute necrotizing pancreatitis is characterized by autodigestion of the pancreas and surrounding tissues by proteolytic and lipolytic enzymes. Oedema, haemorrhage, and ischemia of the affected regions of the pancreas will eventually result in focal necrosis.

The massive initial inflammatory reaction characterizes the early toxaemic phase. Distant-organ damage and MOF can occur during this phase. These effects are attributed to release of pancreatic enzymes into the circulation and activation of the kallikrein, complement, coagulation, and fibrinolytic systems. Activated leucocytes release a variety of toxic substances, including proteases, phospholipases, lysosomal enzymes, reactive oxygen metabolites, and leukotrienes, that result in additional damage to the pancreas and distant organs. Multiorgan failure as a result of non-bacterial pancreatitis is indistinguishable from bacterial sepsis.

The initial phase can last for up to 3 days after the onset of symptoms. That is followed by the necrotic phase. Most (about 70%) patients go on to spontaneous recovery, but others can develop complications such as abscesses, haemorrhage, or pseudocyst.

DIAGNOSIS

Pancreatitis will be suspected on the basis of clinical features, supported by the finding of an elevated serum amylase. Pancreatitis must be differentiated from other acute abdominal emergencies such as ischaemia, obstruction, cholecystitis, perforation, and abdominal aneurysm. A definitive diagnosis can be made only at laparotomy. Imaging with ultrasound or CT scan can support the diagnosis. Some form of imaging should be performed early in the course of the disease in order to establish a baseline impression of the extent of the disease, in preparation for following its course and detecting complications.

CLINICAL FEATURES

• Pain is reported by more than 90% of patients – usually near the hypochondrium, but sometimes lower abdominal or flank pain. The pain usually is gradual in onset, steady, and boring, and it can be relieved by sitting up.

• Nausea and vomiting.

• The abdomen often is slightly distended, with diffuse tenderness. Sometimes there is pronounced guarding, and at other times there will be no signs at all, despite severe pain. Cullen's sign (umbilical discolouration) and Grey-Turner sign (flank discolouration) are rare and late signs, usually indicating severe necrotizing pancreatitis.

• Systemic signs and symptoms include tachycardia, tachypnoea, low-grade fever, hypotension, shock, decreased level of consciousness, and coma.

PROGNOSTIC EVALUATION

There are three main ways to evaluate the severity of acute pancreatitis: the Imrie system, Ranson scoring, and APACHE II (see p. 45). Of these, the APACHE II score is probably the most accurate.

There is no single marker that can be used to predict the severity of pancreatitis. Serial CT scanning is the most accurate technique for evaluating the extent of necrosis and the occurrence of complications.

LABORATORY ABNORMALITIES

SERUM AMYLASE

• The serum amylase concentration begins to rise 2–12 hours after onset of the attack, reaches its peak at 12–24 hours, and returns to normal within 2–5 days. Peak levels can therefore be missed, and so normal levels do not exclude the disease.

• An elevated serum amylase concentration is not specific for acute pancreatitis.

• An elevated serum amylase concentration in the absence of pancreatitis is common in the ICU.

• If the serum amylase remains elevated, suspect a pancreatic pseudocyst.

• There is no correlation between severity of disease and the serum amylase level.

OTHER TESTS There are many other non-specific abnormalities that can occur in acute pancreatitis:

• Serum lipase: The test for serum lipase is difficult to perform and is not specific for acute pancreatitis, but the lipase concentration is elevated in about 75% of cases.

• The specific serum lipase A_2 concentration is shown to correlate well with the severity of pancreatitis. However, the assay is difficult to perform and time-consuming and at present is of little clinical value.

• C-reactive protein is an acute-phase protein whose concentration correlates well with the severity of acute pancreatitis. However, the assay is non-specific.

• Serum trypsin: Protease is found exclusively in the pancreas and is increased in all cases of pancreatitis.

• Methaemalbuminaemia is no longer of clinical importance in the diagnosis of pancreatitis.

• Elevated concentrations of glucose, urea, lactic dehydrogenase, and bilirubin are all non-specific, as is leucocytosis.

• Low calcium, albumin, and magnesium concentrations are sometimes found.

• A plain abdominal x-ray may show localized ileus, pancreatic calcification, or gallstones, but x-rays are insensitive and non-specific. Its diagnostic value is mainly for exclusion of other possible causes of abdominal pain.

• Chest x-ray: In all but minor cases of pancreatitis there will be radiologically observable changes such as basal atelectasis, decreased lung volume, pleural effusions, and pulmonary infiltration.

• Ultrasound: Findings are normal in about one-third of patients with mild pancreatitis. Its greatest value is as a tool for detecting pseudo-cysts and assessing gallstones and underlying biliary disease. An inflamed pancreas often will be hidden behind dilated loops of bowel, making visualization difficult.

• CT can be valuable as a baseline investigation on admission. Its most important role is to assist in diagnosing, defining, and following the complications of pancreatitis. Being unaffected by surrounding gas, it is probably superior to ultrasound. The limitations of CT scanning include difficulty in using it to distinguish between solid necrosis and fluid collections and to predict which lesions will require surgery and which will resolve spontaneously. The changes seen with contrast-enhanced CT correlate well with the severity of the disease.

• Magnetic-resonance imaging: Its place is yet to be defined in regard to pancreatitis, and its images can be difficult to interpret because of artifacts associated with respiratory movement and bowel peristalsis.

MANAGEMENT (Table 28.2)

Supportive treatment

In 85–95% of patients, recovery occurs, without complications, within 1 week. However, among the complicated cases, 20–60% of patients die.

THE MAINSTAYS OF TREATMENT IN THESE PATIENTS ARE METICULOUS SUPPORTIVE CARE IN AN INTENSIVE CARE ENVIRONMENT, AGGRESSIVE FLUID REPLACEMENT, AND EARLY OPERATION FOR PATIENTS WITH INTRA-ABDOMINAL COMPLICATIONS.

FASTING AND NASOGASTRIC SUCTION The concept of 'resting' the pancreas has traditionally been employed, without any evidence that it affects outcome. Though fasting still is often employed, nasogastric suction is less commonly used.

STRESS ULCERATION It seems advisable to use some form of prophylaxis against stress ulceration (see p. 686). Sucralfate may be the drug of choice (see p. 32).

TABLE 28.2 MANAGEMENT OF ACUTE PANCREATITIS

Give nothing orally.

Parental maintenance fluids.

Fluid resuscitation of the intravascular space and blood if required.

Low-dosage dopamine.

Stress ulceration prophylaxis.

Pain relief.

Insulin infusion to control hyperglycaemia.

Treat hypoxia with
    increased F_{IO_2}
    maintenance of normal serum albumin levels
    restriction of crystalloid fluid
    CPAP
    IPPV and PEEP

Investigate suspected local complications or suspected site of sepsis with ultrasound or CT scan.

Carry out aggressive and repeated debridement of local collections.

Peritoneal lavage may be useful.

PARENTERAL NUTRITION It is not essential to use parenteral nutrition if acute pancreatitis resolves early (see p. 89). A feeding jejunostomy may be an effective way of providing enteral nutrition.

PAIN RELIEF Pain relief is very important during the acute stage. Continuous intravenous infusion of an opiate is a cheap and effective technique for titrating analgesia to the patient's requirements. Continuous epidural block (see p. 120) with either a local anaesthetic or a narcotic, or a combination of both, is an alternative if there are no contraindications, such as coagulopathy, thrombocytopenia, or hypotension.

There are theoretical reasons for avoiding the use of morphine in patients with pancreatitis, such as stimulation of the sphincter of Oddi. However, there does not appear to be any clinical problem with its use.

FLUID REPLACEMENT Hypovolaemia and hypotension are common with acute pancreatitis and may predispose to renal failure and MOF (see p. 137). Fluid losses can be extremely high, and large amounts of replacement fluid may be necessary. Fluid treatment should be carefully titrated against intravascular measurements such as urine output, arterial blood pressure, CVP, and, if necessary, PAWP (see p. 55).

Maintenance fluid should be hypotonic saline solution (1,000–3,000 ml/d).

METABOLIC CONSIDERATIONS Correct magnesium, phosphate, and calcium concentrations as necessary – daily measurements are required. An insulin infusion may be necessary to control hyperglycaemia. A suitable technique is to use 50 units of short-acting insulin (eg Actrapid) in 50 ml of fluid and titrate against blood glucose measured hourly.

RENAL INSUFFICIENCY In addition to aggressive fluid replacement, an intravenous infusion of 'renal'-dosage or low-dosage dopamine ($1–3$ $\mu g \cdot kg^{-1} \cdot min^{-1}$) may help to encourage renal blood flow and prevent renal failure.

RESPIRATORY COMPLICATIONS Patients often are hypoxic because of basal atelectasis and reduced lung volume, as a result of increased intra-abdominal pressure and bilaterally raised diaphragms. Hypoxia can also occur as a result of ARDS (see p. 400). Measures to alleviate hypoxia include

• increasing the FIO_2
• sitting the patient upright
• physiotherapy
• maintaining normal serum albumin and colloid osmotic pressure
• limiting sodium-containing clear fluid (crystalloids) in order to avoid interstitial oedema

If those measures fail, consider the following:

• CPAP via a mask (see p. 367). This has the advantage of improving oxygenation and increasing lung volume without necessitating intubation of the patient.

• CPAP via an endotracheal tube will be needed if the airway is compromised or if the patient is unable to tolerate the mask.
• Intermittent mandatory ventilation (IMV) with PEEP may be necessary if the patient is hypoventilating and also is hypoxic. Rarely, mandatory ventilation with IPPV is required.

The general approach to respiratory failure is covered elsewhere (see Chapter 17).

Be alert for local complications (Table 28.3)

The main local complications that will need active management are local erosion, pancreatic abscesses, pseudocysts, and infected extrapancreatic necrotic masses. Local infection can cause MOF (see p. 137) – a clinical picture the same as that for septicaemia (see p. 183). Management is aimed at supporting the patient, while aggressively diagnosing and removing the source of sepsis. Bacterial contamination or necrosis will occur in up to 40% of patients. The incidence of local infection is maximal during the third week of the disease process. However, the systemic effects of the necrotic material and infected material usually are the same. Immediate, aggressive surgery is indicated for both.

MANAGEMENT   Simple drainage sometimes can be accomplished with the aid of imaging. However, in many cases it is essential to perform wide, aggressive debridement, as well as adequate drainage. Antibiotics alone never cure abscesses and may simply select out other organisms, such as fungi. Often, multiple operations for further debridement are necessary.

Definitive treatment

There is no universal agreement on definitive treatment for acute pancreatitis. However, the following have been advocated:

PERITONEAL LAVAGE   The role of lavage is controversial. It is believed that lavage may help to remove toxic substances released from the pancreas and reverse some of the systemic effects of the early phase mediated by circulating toxins. Lavage is more successful in reducing early systemic complications than later local complications.

TABLE 28.3 COMPLICATIONS OF ACUTE PANCREATITIS

Local
Phlegmon
Abscess
Pseudocyst
Fat necrosis
Obstructive jaundice
Ascites
Local necrosis of surrounding structures (eg vessels, bowel)
Systemic
Respiratory
   Pleural effusions
   ARDS
   Atelectasis
Cardiovascular
   Hypovolaemia and shock
   Pericardial effusions
Haematological
   Disseminated intravascular coagulation
   Coagulopathies
Gastro-intestinal
   Acute stress ulceration
   Ileus
Central nervous system
   Decreased level of consciousness and coma
   Renal insufficiency or failure
Metabolic
   Hyperglycaemia
   Hypertriglyceridaemia
   Hypoalbuminaemia
   Hypocalcaemia
   Hypomagnesaemia

As yet, the subgroups of patients who would benefit from lavage have not been precisely defined. They may include patients with severe pancreatitis or early shock and marked clinical deterioration. If it is to work, it should be instituted early (ie within the first 48 hours).

The response to peritoneal lavage usually is immediate and dramatic. If there is no response, one should consider an error in diagnosis or the presence of associated biliary or systemic sepsis.

Continuous percutaneous peritoneal dialysis with an isotonic solution such as warm Ringer's lactate can be used. The catheter should be inserted in the midline just below the umbilicus. The technique is similar to peritoneal dialysis (see p. 653). Heparin should be added to each bag of fluid (500 units/L). One-litre cycles (20 minutes to run in, 20 minutes of dwell time, 20 minutes to run out) allow for adequate lavage without causing excessive abdominal distension and diaphragmatic elevation. If renal failure supervenes, the isotonic solution can be replaced by dialysate fluid (see p. 654). Lavage should be performed for 2–5 days or until the systemic effects of pancreatitis are reversed.

ENDOSCOPIC PAPILLOTOMY Endoscopic retrograde cholangiopancreatography and papillotomy, if impacted stones are present, are suggested for severe acute pancreatitis related to gallstones.

SURGERY Although pancreatectomy is used extensively in some centres, the operation involves mortality of 30–50% and does not prevent septic complications. If the pancreatitis is related to bile-duct obstruction, it is common practice to perform definitive biliary surgery during the initial hospitalization, waiting 5–7 days for the acute inflammatory process to subside.

DRUGS Aprotinin, glucagon, and prophylactic antibiotics have not been shown to influence the course or outcome of acute pancreatitis. The place of somatostatin is currently being investigated, and it appears promising in preliminary investigations.

ACUTE STRESS ULCERATION

Acute stress ulceration is defined as acute upper-GIT bleeding associated with mucosal abnormalities of the oesophagus, stomach, or duodenum. It is usually found in the critically ill. The mucosal abnormalities range from hyperaemia and small petechial haemorrhages to deeper ulceration and, rarely, perforation.

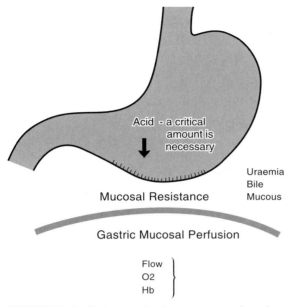

FIGURE 28.1   Pathogenesis of acute stress ulceration.

PATHOGENESIS (Figure 28.1)

DECREASED GASTRIC BLOOD FLOW AND TISSUE ANOXIA   These are most important factors, though many other factors can contribute to cellular ischaemia and hypoxia:

- hypotension
- hypoxia
- sepsis
- anaemia
- increased intrathoracic pressure
- shock
- drugs

DECREASED MUCOSAL BARRIER   This can be secondary to

- bile sales
- non-steroidal anti-inflammatory agents

- uraemia
- alcohol

INCREASED ACID AND PEPSIN   This can occur particularly in patients with burns or as a result of neurogenic causes.

Clinical features and diagnosis

Microscopic quantities of blood are found in up to 40% of patients. Macroscopic bleeding usually occurs 4–10 days after the initial insult. Only 5% of patients have clinically important bleeding.

Endoscopy is indicated for all patients with significant bleeding, to exclude other causes, such as a bleeding ulcer or oesophageal varices, which will require a different approach to management.

Management

PREVENTION (FIGURE 28.2)

• Begin aggressive management of the underlying disease (eg sepsis, liver failure, multitrauma).

• Begin rapid reversal of physiological abnormalities accompanying the critical illness that can decrease gastric blood flow and oxygen delivery to the GIT mucosa (eg hypotension, hypoxia).

• Institute enteral feeding if possible. This is as effective as neutralizing gastric acidity with drugs.

• Sucralfate (1 g every 4 hours suspended in 20 ml of water), to protect against stress ulceration without increasing gastric pH, may be as effective as H_2-receptor antagonists and antacids, without increasing gastric colonization (see p. 31).

• H_2-receptor antagonists and antacids are still used to prevent stress ulceration. They work by increasing the gastric pH to levels above 4. For effective prevention, the gastric pH should be regularly measured, with drug titrated against it. Because of the risks of bacterial colonization in an alkaline environment, H_2-receptor antagonists and antacids probably should be reserved for patients who have a history of peptic ulceration or who are suspected of active bleeding from stress ulceration.

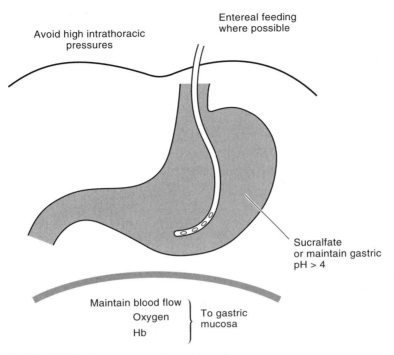

FIGURE 28.2   Prevention of stress ulceration.

DEFINITIVE MEASURES FOR ACTIVE BLEEDING   Resuscitation:

- Replenish the circulating volume (see p. 61).
- Ensure adequate haemoglobin.
- Ensure adequate oxygenation.

Aggressively treat precipitating factors such as sepsis (see p. 182).

Use endoscopy or angiography to exclude surgically treatable causes of bleeding.

Measure gastric pH hourly, and get it above 7 using antacid or H_2-receptor antagonist or both.

Manoeuvres such as selective embolization or angiographic injection with vasopressin, and intravenous vasopressin infusions have been used with varying degrees of success, but not in a controlled fashion.

Somatostatin (continuous IV infusion at 250 μg/h for 72 hours) may
  be of some benefit.
Surgery should be a last resort for diffuse bleeding, as it is associated
  with high mortality.

UPPER-GASTRO-INTESTINAL-TRACT BLEEDING

Apart from stress ulceration, other causes of upper-GIT bleeding include

- peptic ulcers
- Mallory-Weiss tears
- oesophagitis

- neoplasms
- vascular malformations
- oesophageal varices (see p. 692)

Multiple lesions are found in 15–30% of these patients.

Clinical presentation

Upper-GIT bleeding usually presents as haematemesis, melaena, or
sudden cardiovascular collapse.

Aetiology and clinical course

• Among patients with upper-GIT bleeding, 75% will stop bleeding
shortly after admission and will never rebleed.

• Of the remaining 25% with continuing or recurrent bleeding, more
than 30% will require immediate surgery or other advanced therapeutic manoeuvres. More than 30% will die.

• Severe episodes of bleeding are almost always due to ulcer disease
(40–50%), oesophageal varices (4–8%), or diffuse gastritis (10–15%).

• Elderly patients (>65 years) and those with severe underlying disease have poor prognoses.

MANAGEMENT

RESUSCITATION   The circulating volume must be restored immediately (see p. 61). Transfuse blood, after cross-matching, according to
the degree of hypovolaemia and haemoglobin levels. Urine output
should always be closely monitored and maintained.

DIAGNOSIS Once the patient is stable, and while resuscitation continues, the cause of bleeding should be sought. Diagnostic evaluation is not an urgent matter for patients in whom the bleeding stops within 1 hour of admission and who are at low risk for recurrent bleeding.

Endoscopy Endoscopy will reveal the site and nature of bleeding in approximately 80–95% of patients, even in the presence of brisk bleeding. It is the examination of choice for patients with persistent or recurrent bleeding and for those at high risk for recurrent haemorrhage. It should be performed within the first 24 hours.

Angiography Mesenteric angiography may be useful if endoscopy fails to reveal the site of bleeding. For it to be successful, the rate of bleeding usually must exceed 1.0 ml/min and be from a discrete site.

Barium A barium radiograph is not satisfactory as an early investigation for acute bleeding.

Radionuclide imaging Like angiography, this examination requires that there be active bleeding.

CONTROLLING BLOOD LOSS There are many anecdotal reports and unproven techniques in this area. One of the difficulties with proving the effectiveness of any technique is that many patients will stop bleeding spontaneously.

• H_2-receptor antagonists and antacids are often used for active bleeding from gastric and duodenal ulcers. However, there is no conclusive evidence that they influence active bleeding.

• Vasopressin (antidiuretic hormone) (10–20 units/hr, IV infusion) may be effective in patients with oesophageal varices, but intravenous vasopressin does not influence bleeding in patients with other causes of upper-GIT bleeding. Selective arterial vasopressin infusion may be more effective. As the action of vasopressin is generalized vasoconstriction, beware of ischaemia in vital organs – especially in the presence of ischaemic heart disease.

• Somatostatin (continuous IV infusion, 250 μg/h for 72 hours) may decrease bleeding by decreasing splanchnic blood flow and gastric acid secretion.

• Endoscopic coagulation, with laser photocoagulation, bipolar diathermy, or heated probes, may be successful in selected cases. Endoscopic injection at the bleeding site is also successful.

• Embolization during angiography may be effective in cases of significant bleeding from a discrete point.

• Surgery: The indications for surgery are still controversial. It should be seriously considered early for patients with severe haemorrhage (more than 2 litres in 24 hours) and for patients with active arterial bleeding from chronic ulcers, especially elderly patients. Compulsive monitoring and replenishment of intravascular volume and steps to maintain renal function are critical in these patients.

BLEEDING VARICES

It is important to suspect this as a cause of upper-GIT bleeding and to confirm it with endoscopy, because the approach to its management is different from the approach to other causes of upper-GIT bleeding. Moreover, such a patient usually will have associated liver dysfunction, often alcoholic in origin. Other causes of upper-GIT bleeding are common in the presence of oesophageal varices. Immediate endoscopy is essential to exclude those causes and to determine the site of the varices – oesophageal or gastric.

More than two-thirds of patients with oesophageal varices are dead within 1 year. The overall prognosis is related more closely to the underlying liver disease, rather than the actual bleeding varices, and has not changed in spite of more sophisticated ways of controlling bleeding in the short term.

Supportive treatment

Replenishment of the intravascular volume is most efficiently achieved with colloid or blood (see Chapter 4). There must be compulsive monitoring of the intravascular volume (see p. 55).

Reduce the potential nitrogen load from the bleeding varices by active nasogastric suction and oral lactulose (20–30 g, three or four times per day) if encephalopathy is suspected. Because neomycin is absorbed and contributes to renal failure, it should no longer be used in this setting.

Nutrition: Supplements such as vitamin K, folic acid, and thiamine should be given early if nutritional depletion or alcoholism is suspected.

Clotting factors must be monitored and replaced as necessary (see p. 712).

Control of bleeding

There are many unanswered questions concerning the best ways to control variceal bleeding. Firstly, should it be treated at all? Among those patients with severe impairments of liver function (eg with encephalopathy and coagulopathy), the immediate mortality is greater than 70%. More than half of all patients with variceal bleeding will stop bleeding, no matter what measures are used. Outcome must be looked at in the light of control of the acute bleeding, prevention of further bleeding, and long-term prognosis. Interpretation of the data from clinical trials is difficult. There are problems with entry of patients, limited numbers, lack of randomization, and whether outcome was measured in the short term or long term.

The usual approach after resuscitation is sclerotherapy, with or without prior balloon tamponade. If that fails, a vasoactive drug (eg vasopressin) can be tried, or a surgical procedure such as oesophageal transection, devascularization, or an emergency shunt procedure. All of these techniques and the combinations thereof have their proponents.

The issue of clear guidelines for long-term management to prevent further bleeding is clouded by the same problems encountered in interpreting the trial data on acute variceal bleeding.

ENDOSCOPIC VARICEAL SCLEROTHERAPY   Sclerotherapy with ethanolamine oleate or sodium tetradecyl sulphate can be used alone or in combination with tamponade to control acute bleeding. Retrosternal discomfort and fever sometimes accompany sclerosis. The decision to undertake sclerotherapy at the time of initial endoscopy depends on the rate of bleeding and the expertise of the endoscopist. Sometimes balloon tamponade is initially needed to control bleeding, and that is followed by sclerotherapy. Sclerotherapy can control bleeding for the short term in up to 90% of patients, but overall survival is not increased.

Endoscopic banding of oesophageal varices is also possible and may be technically easier.

BALLOON TAMPONADE A modified Sengstaken-Blakemore tube or Minnesota tube with a fourth channel for oesophageal aspiration is probably ideal. These are now available in disposable plastic form.

Insertion technique

Ensure the patient's airway. INTUBATION IS ALMOST ALWAYS RE-QUIRED IN THESE PATIENTS.

Check the balloon before insertion.

A pre-lubricated stiffening wire will aid insertion.

To check placement, insert 50 ml of air into the gastric balloon, and take an x-ray. If the balloon is in the stomach, insert 300 ml of air into the gastric balloon; 20 ml of 25% Hypaque can improve radiological visualization of the gastric balloon.

Draw the gastric balloon toward the cardia by gentle traction.

The tube can be taped to the face or placed on gentle traction.

The oesophageal balloon usually is not inflated, because bleeding often is controlled by the traction of the gastric balloon alone. Up to 120 ml of air, to produce a pressure of 30–50 mm Hg (4.5–6.65 kPa) in the oesophageal balloon, may sometimes be needed to control the bleeding. With both balloons clamped, their positions should be checked radiologically.

Continuous gastric and oesophageal low-pressure suction should be applied.

The pressure in the oesophageal and gastric balloons should be regularly monitored.

Complications such as aspiration pneumonia are common, and patients should be monitored in the ICU.

The tamponade should be applied for 12–24 hours, then reassessed by deflating the balloon in situ and observing for further blood loss. If the oesophageal balloon has been inflated, it should be deflated first, followed approximately 2 hours later by the gastric balloon. Balloon tamponade is only a holding procedure, and rebleeding occurs in almost half of these patients. Longer-term measures such as sclerotherapy should be considered as soon as the bleeding has been controlled with balloon tamponade.

VASOPRESSIN INFUSION Vasopressin has been largely superseded by sclerotherapy and tamponade. However, an intravenous infusion of 10–20 units per hour can control bleeding in over half of these cases. Its disadvantages include ischaemia of the heart, skin, and intestine. Rebleeding is common.

SOMATOSTATIN Somatostatin may be as efficacious as balloon tamponade and can be used alone or in conjunction with balloon tamponade (continuous IV infusion, 250 μg/h for 72 hours).

EMBOLIZATION Embolization at angiography can achieve haemostasis in many cases. However, rebleeding is common.

SURGERY Surgery should be considered after these less radical approaches have failed. Transoesophageal ligation and portacaval shunting are the most common procedures. Varices in the cardia of the stomach, as opposed to oesophageal varices, often require shunt procedures. Liver transplantation should be considered in some patients. Mortality for this type of surgery is high.

LOWER-GASTRO-INTESTINAL-TRACT BLEEDING

Clinical presentation

• Colon: usually bright rectal bleeding.
• Caecum and small intestine: maroon melaena (eg diverticular disease, polyps, angiodysplasia, trauma)

Management

RESUSCITATION Rapid replacement of intravascular volume (see p. 61) and clotting factors (see p. 712) is essential. Investigation of the site of intestinal bleeding is limited by several factors:

• Bleeding is notoriously intermittent.
• Blood travels in an antegrade and retrograde direction from the site of bleeding.
• Blood can travel long distances from the site of bleeding.

DIAGNOSIS
• Sigmoidoscopy can be used to exclude lower-colon lesions.
• Fibre-optic colonoscopy can exclude lesions up to the caecum.

• Enema and intestinal lavage may be necessary to improve observations.
• Isotope scanning with ^{99m}Tc-labelled red cells can detect bleeding rates as low as 0.1 ml/min. A specific compound, ^{99m}Tc-pertechnetate, is necessary to detect Meckel's diverticulum.
• Angiography can detect bleeding rates as low as 0.5 ml/min in over half of these patients.
• Barium enema and small-bowel series should be considered **AFTER** the bleeding has ceased and where the diagnosis is uncertain.

TREATMENT Definitive measures for stopping the bleeding depend on the site and nature of the lesion. The available methods include

• coagulation via endoscopy
• vasopressin infusion
• embolization
• early surgery for massive uncontrolled bleeding

ACUTE ABDOMINAL DISORDERS IN THE CRITICALLY ILL

It is important that the abdomen be given careful attention as part of the normal daily examination of each patient in the ICU (see p. 18). Because these patients often are unconscious, sedated, or paralysed, there may be few symptoms, and blunted signs. Nevertheless, the abdomen plays a key role in many seriously ill patients.

Many GIT manifestations of MOF, such as non-occlusive small-bowel ischaemia, ischaemic colitis, stress ulceration, and hepatocellular dysfunction, can be mediated by ischaemia related to activation of the renin-angiotensin axis.

SPECIFIC ABDOMINAL DISORDERS IN THE CRITICALLY ILL

Intestinal pseudo-obstruction

The GIT is often hypoactive in seriously ill patients. There may be decreased bowel sounds, abdominal distension, and increased nasogastric aspirate. This can simulate acute obstruction of the bowel. The cause may be related to opiate or other sedative use or electrolyte disturbances, and the condition often accompanies MOF.

Pseudo-obstruction is not a contraindication to enteral feeding, but it may have to be facilitated by nasojejunal or nasoduodenal tube in order to prevent aspiration of gastric contents.

Drugs to increase motility and enemas do not appear to have much effect on GIT stasis, and the ileus invariably resolves as the patient's underlying condition improves.

Acute acalculous cholecystitis

Acute acalculous cholecystitis can occur spontaneously in the critically ill. It can be associated with intravenous nutrition (IVN), IPPV, hypoperfusion of the gall-bladder, or increased biliary stasis.

Acalculous cholecystitis manifests as a site of intra-abdominal infection and/or occult sepsis, with all of the attending features and complications (see p. 183). Often there is a tender mass in the right upper quadrant. Ultrasound or CT may show enlargement of the gall-bladder, a thickened gall-bladder wall, or a pericholecystic collection. Laparotomy is the only way to definitively diagnose acalculous cholecystitis.

It can present as peritonitis in association with peritoneal dialysis (see p. 653) or with ascites (eg in patients with cirrhosis or nephrotic syndrome).

Although antibiotics should be commenced, surgery is the only definitive treatment – cholecystectomy and/or a drainage procedure.

Enteral feeding rather than IVN may decrease the incidence of alcalculous cholecystitis.

Mesenteric ischaemia

ASSOCIATED FACTORS Hypotension, elevated intra-abdominal pressure, post-operative surgical complications, sepsis, and vasoconstrictive drugs (eg adrenaline) can all cause mesenteric ischaemia. Despite these factors being relatively common in the critically ill, the incidence of clinically significant splanchnic ischaemia is low. Perhaps subclinical episodes are common, and overt complications such as bloody stools, abdominal distension, perforations, and peritonitis occur, leading to circulatory shock and metabolic acidosis. The diagnosis in a sedated, ventilated patient is very difficult. The creatine phosphokinase (CK) levels are often elevated.

LOCAL FACTORS Local arteriosclerosis, colonic distension, emboli, bowel strangulation, and venous occlusion can predispose to mesenteric ischaemia. Aggressive surgery is indicated in all cases of nonviable gut. The mortality remains very high.

Coincidental abdominal disorders in the critically ill

Remember that patients in an ICU can coincidentally develop acute abdominal disorders such as

- appendicitis
- cholecystitis
- tooth abscess and sinusitis
- pancreatitis
- perforation of a viscus
- volvulus

DIAGNOSIS Careful examination of the abdomen at least once each day is mandatory in all seriously ill patients as the symptoms often are non-existent, and the signs blunted. Hypotension, shock, and the signs of sepsis can accompany any acute abdominal disorder. Girth measurements are not reliable indicators of increasing intra-abdominal contents.

Intravesical pressure should be measured (see p. 699) in all patients suspected of having high intra-abdominal pressures. An upright chest x-ray should be obtained to exclude pneumoperitoneum and to elicit other signs, such as a pleural effusion, that may be secondary to the pathological abdominal condition.

Abdominal x-rays are difficult to obtain and interpret in the ICU because of the limitations of portable equipment.

Contrast studies: Apart from simple tests to exclude perforation or to identify a fistula, contrast studies have little place in the management of the acutely ill.

Ultrasound is a rapid technique involving portable equipment, but it is limited by the experience of the user and the difficulty of obtaining good images in the presence of excessive gas and in patients who have recently had surgery.

CT is useful for detecting abdominal sepsis and trauma.

Diagnostic laparotomy should be considered earlier, rather than later, for patients in whom serious intra-abdominal abnormalities are suspected and for whom other tests have not been helpful.

ABDOMINAL TAMPONADE

Abdominal tamponade due to any cause (eg intra-abdominal bleeding, ascites, pneumoperitoneum, ileus) will produce ischaemia of intra-abdominal organs. This is related in part to a decrease in cardiac output secondary to decreased venous return, as well as a direct pressure effect on the intra-abdominal organs.

The ischaemia will be marked and will affect all intra-abdominal organs. The degree of ischaemia will be proportional to the severity of the intra-abdominal pressure. One of the earliest manifestations of decreased organ blood flow is oliguria, and eventually anuria, related to decreased renal blood flow.

ASSESSMENT OF INTRA-ABDOMINAL PRESSURE

Because of inherent inaccuracies, abdominal girth measurements are of no use for assessing the degree of intra-abdominal pressure and should be discarded from our clinical practice. If there is concern about a tense abdomen, the intra-abdominal pressure should be assessed by directly measuring the intravesical pressure. One needs only a low index of suspicion to consider this measurement, as it is simple to perform and provides valuable information.

There are several techniques for measuring intravesical pressure. One of the simplest involves inserting a T-piece connector with a three-way tap at the end of the urinary catheter: Urine is allowed to drain normally until a measurement is required. Then 50 ml of isotonic saline is instilled into the bladder. The distal drainage from the urinary catheter is clamped, and the three-way tap is turned to connect to a water-manometer device for measuring CVP. The height of the column taken from the pubic symphysis represents the intravesical pressure. The bladder acts as a passive container at volumes of

50–100 ml, and intravesical pressure closely correlates with intra-abdominal pressure over the range 0–70 mm Hg (0–9.3 kPa).

Decreased renal blood flow and oliguria will begin to occur at pressures above 25 mm Hg (3.3 kPa) and will progressively become worse as the pressure increases. Consideration should be given to surgically decompressing abdominal tamponade. This can be achieved either by laparotomy, leaving the wound packed and open, or by closing the wound with material such as a Marlex graft. Surgery in these circumstances can be a challenge, especially if the tamponade is related to intra-abdominal bleeding. The bleeding may become uncontrollable if the tamponade is relieved. On the other hand, intra-abdominal organs become more ischaemic as the intra-abdominal pressure increases. Non-invasive techniques such as embolization should be considered, for example, if the source of the bleeding is from the pelvis. The intravesical pressure should be monitored regularly in all patients suspected of having elevated intra-abdominal pressure [>20 mm Hg (2.6 kPa)].

DIARRHOEA

Diarrhoea can be a problem in up to 40% of patients in an ICU. It is usually related to the underlying disease or treatment, rather than to a specific cause such as pelvic abscess. The presence of diarrhoea represents a large work load for nurses, adds to the risks of cross-infection, and, when infective, can cause systemic signs and fluid loss.

Non-infective diarrhoea

Diarrhoea is a common and non-specific precursor of generalized sepsis or infection. Non-infective diarrhoea is the most common form of diarrhoea in an ICU, and it is mainly related to enteral feeding (see p. 88). The diarrhoea is as a result of hypersecretion from the gut and can result in significant protein loss. Diarrhoea is then exacerbated by hypoalbuminaemia. It can be decreased by using iso-osmolar enteral feeds by commencing feeding at low rates, by using lactose-free feeds, or possibly by adding liquid bulking agents. However, enteral feeding should be continued in the presence of diarrhoea. Agents that will encourage bacterial action, which in turn will enhance salt and water absorption, with 'drying' of the stool, are useful for reducing the incidence of diarrhoea. Imodium (4 mg initially, and 2 mg p.r.n. up to 20 mg daily) and octreotide (dose is dependent on effect) can sometimes decrease intractable diarrhoea.

Diarrhoea can be a non-specific manifestation of MOF (see p. 135).

Antibiotic-associated diarrhoea

Antibiotic-associated diarrhoea should always be suspected in the critically ill.

Pseudomembranous colitis Most antibiotics, especially clindamycin, can predispose to pseudomembranous colitis, caused by the toxin produced by the *Clostridium difficile* bacteria. The treatment of choice is vancomycin.

Methicillin-resistant *staphylococcus aureas* enterocolitis This also occurs in association with broad-spectrum antibiotics, particularly in critically ill patients or immunocompromised hosts. It can cause systemic septicaemia and MOF.

Infective diarrhoea Other pathogens such as *Salmonella* spp., *Shigella* spp., *Campylobacter* spp., and *Escherichia coli* are only rarely the causes of diarrhoea in the ICU.

Management

Diarrhoea is a relatively common accompaniment of MOF and infection.

Always perform a rectal examination to exclude abnormalities such as impaction and spurious diarrhoea.

Adjust the enteral feeding regimen:

- Use iso-osmolar solutions.
- Avoid lactose-containing solutions.
- Add faecal bulking agents.

Replace water and electrolyte losses.

Culture stools, especially for

- *Clostridium difficile* and its cytotoxin.
- *S. aureus* (Gram stain and culture).
- Treat both pseudomembranous colitis and *S. aureus*–related diar-

rhoea with oral vancomycin, 250–500 mg, 6-hourly, for 10 days. Relapses can occur in both cases.

Employ barrier nursing if the diarrhoea is infective in origin.

FURTHER READING

General

Hillman, K. (1988). Aspects of the gastrointestinal tract in intensive care. In *Update in Intensive Care and Emergency Medicine,* ed. J.-L. Vincent, pp. 727–32.

Torsoli, G. H. (ed.) (1981). Gastrointestinal emergencies. *Clinics in Gastroenterology,* pp. 1–260 (symposium issue).

Fulminant Hepatic Failure

McIntyre, N. (1991). Hepatobiliary disease: medical emergencies. *Bailliere's Clinical Gastroenterology* 5:709–36.

Manns, M. P. (1991). New therapeutic aspects in fulminant hepatic failure. *Chest* 100:193S–6S.

Payne, J. A. (1986). Fulminant liver failure. *Medical Clinics of North America* 70:1067–79.

Acute-on-Chronic Liver Failure

Epstein, M. (1992). The hepatorenal syndrome – newer perspectives. *New England Journal of Medicine* 327:1810–11.

Murray, W. R., & MacSween, R. N. M. (1983). Hepatobiliary disturbances. In *Recent Advances in Critical Care Medicine*, 2nd ed, ed. I. M. Ledingham & C. D. Hanning, pp. 143–59. Edinburgh: Churchill Livingstone.

Zaloga, G. P., & Prough, D. S. (1988). Monitoring hepatic function. *Critical Care Clinics* 4:591–603.

Liver Dysfunction In Critical Illness

Hawker, F. (1991). Liver dysfunction in critical illness. *Anaesthesia and Intensive Care* 19:165–81.

Ascites

Arrogo, V., Gines, P., & Planas, R. (1992). Treatment of ascites in cirrhosis. *Gastroenterology Clinics of North America* 21:237–55.

Pancreatitis

Gunther, H. J., & Trede, M. (1991). Acute pancreatitis – the role of early surgery. *Gastroenterology* 5:773–86.

Potts, J. R. (1988). Acute pancreatitis. *Surgical Clinics of North America* 68:281–99.

Rattner, D. W., & Warshaw, A. L. (1988). Surgical intervention in acute pancreatitis. *Critical Care Medicine* 16:89–95.

Steinberg, W., & Tenner, S. (1994). Acute pancreatitis. *New England Journal of Medicine* 330:1198–209.

Thomas, P. D. (1985). Acute pancreatitis. *Anaesthesia and Intensive Care* 13:249–57.

Acute Gastro-Intestinal-Tract Bleeding

Dworken, H. J. (1984). Gastrointestinal hemorrhage. In *Textbook of Critical Care,* ed. W. C. Shoemaker, W. L. Thompson, & P. R. Holbrook, pp. 591–7.

Editor. (1984). Bleeding ulcers – scope for improvement? *Lancet* 1:715–17.

Laine, L., & Peterson, W. L. (1994). Medical progress: bleeding peptic ulcer. *New England Journal of Medicine* 331:717–27.

Schaffner, J. (1986). Acute gastrointestinal bleeding. *Medical Clinics of North America* 70:1055–66.

Acute Stress Ulceration

Bailey, R. W., Bolkley, G. B., Hamilton, S. R., Morris, J. B., Haglund, V. H., & Meilahn J. E. (1987). The fundamental hemodynamic mechanism underlying 'stress ulceration' in cardiogenic shock. *Annals of Surgery* 205:597–612.

Hillman, K. M. (1985). Acute stress ulceration. *Anaesthesia and Intensive Care* 13:230–40.

Oesophageal Varices

Dandson, B., Carratta, R., & Raccione Habib, N. (1991). Surgical emergencies in liver disease. *Bailliere's Clinics in Gastroenterology* 5:737–58.

Gillespie, I. E. (1986). Bleeding oesophageal varices. *British Medical Journal* 292:1479–80.

Terblanche, J., Burroughs, A. K., & Hobbs, K. E. F. (1989). Controversies in the management of bleeding oesophageal varices. *New England Journal of Medicine* 320:1393–7, 1469–75.

Westaby, D. (1988). The management of active variceal bleeding. *Intensive Care Medicine* 14:100–5.

Acute Abdominal Disorders in the Critically Ill

Golladay, S., & Byrne, W. J. (1981). Intestinal pseudo-obstruction. *Surgery, Gynecology and Obstetrics* 153:257–73.

Johnson, L. B. (1987). The importance of early diagnosis of acute acalculous cholecystitis. *Surgery, Gynecology and Obstetrics* 164:197–203.

Saclarides, T., Hopkins, W., & Doolas, A. (1986). Abdominal emergencies. *Medical Clinics of North America* 70:1093–110.

Worthy, L. I. G. (1985). Acute abdominal disorders in the paralysed patients. *Anaesthesia and Intensive Care* 13:263–71.

Abdominal Tamponade

Caldwell, C. B., & Ricotta, J. J. (1987). Changes in visceral blood flow with elevated intraabdominal pressure. *Journal of Surgical Research* 43:14–20.

Finlayson, D. F., & Muirhead, A. G. (1983). Is measurement of girth of value in assessing intraperitoneal bleeding after trauma? *British Medical Journal* 287:728.

Iberti, T. J., Lieber, C. E., & Benjamin, E. (1989). Determination of intraabdominal pressure using a transurethral bladder catheter: validation of the technique. *Anesthesiology* 70:47–50.

Platell, C., Hall, J., & Dobb, G. (1990). Impaired renal function due to raised intraabdominal pressure. *Intensive Care Medicine* 16:328–9.

Richards, W. O., Scovill, W., Shin, B., & Reed, W. (1983). Acute renal failure associated with increased intraabdominal pressure. *Annals of Surgery* 197:183–7.

Sugrue, M., Buist, M. D., Lee, A., Sanchez, D. G., & Hillman, K. M. (1994). Intraabdominal pressure measurement using a modified nasogastric tube: description and validation of a new technique. *Intensive Care Medicine* 20:558–90.

Diarrhoea

Dobb, G. J. (1986). Diarrhoea in the critically ill. *Intensive Care Medicine* 12:113–15.

Kelly, W. J., Patrick, M. R., & Hillman, K. M. (1983). Study of diarrhoea in critically ill patients. *Critical Care Medicine* 11:7–9.

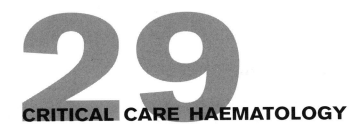

CRITICAL CARE HAEMATOLOGY

BLOOD TRANSFUSION

INDICATIONS FOR BLOOD TRANSFUSION

Fresh whole blood remains the ideal fluid for resuscitation following acute haemorrhage. However, it is rarely available today. Whole blood usually is fractionated into red-cell concentrates, plasma protein solutions, and platelet concentrates.

Blood is given to restore oxygen-carrying capacity and intravascular volume. The haemoglobin level is an important contributor to the oxygen-carrying capacity: 1.34 ml of oxygen combines with each gram of haemoglobin (Hb).

$$\text{oxygen-carrying capacity} = \text{Hb concentration} \times 1.34 \text{ ml } O_2/\text{g}$$
$$\times \text{ oxygen saturation of Hb}$$
$$\times \text{ cardiac output}$$

Critically ill patients require optimal oxygen delivery (DO_2). The ideal haemoglobin level is uncertain. It is probably greater than 10 g/dl and closer to physiological normal levels. Viscosity is rarely a clinically significant factor in blood flow, even with higher levels of haemoglobin. The balance is between increased DO_2 for each extra haemoglobin molecule and the increased viscosity caused by that extra haemoglobin molecule, which can decrease blood flow and DO_2.

Critically ill patients often require transfusion secondary to frequent blood tests, haemodilution, and extracorporeal blood losses (eg during haemofiltration).

Guidelines for transfusion are given in Table 29.1.

TABLE 29.1   BLOOD TRANSFUSION GUIDELINES

> If the patient is haemodynamically stable and the bleeding has stopped, consider supplemental iron, vitamin B_{12}, folate, and erythropoietin, rather than blood.
>
> If the patient is haemodynamically stable, but symptomatic (eg dyspnoea, palpitations, malaise), use packed red cells to restore oxygen-carrying capacity.
>
> If the patient is haemodynamically unstable, but the bleeding is controllable, use packed red cells and fluid volume replacement.
>
> If the patient is haemodynamically unstable and bleeding rapidly, use the freshest blood available, as well as
>
> • FFP
>
> • platelets
>
> and liaise with the haematology services.

CROSS-MATCHING
Serological safety of blood

	Probability of compatibility
ABO compatibility	99.4%
ABO and Rh compatibility	99.8%
ABO and Rh compatibility, with negative antibody screen	99.94%
Complete pretransfusion compatibility testing	99.95%
Autologous	100%

It is important to institute blood replacement rapidly in cases of significant haemorrhage. From the foregoing information it can be seen that un-cross-matched blood that is ABO-compatible can, if necessary, be administered in an emergency. However, a saline cross-match can be performed by most blood banks within 10 minutes. Thus, it is rarely necessary to give group O un-cross-matched blood, as resuscitation with colloid usually is satisfactory until group and saline cross-matches are performed.

BLOOD PRODUCTS

The term 'ultrafresh blood' implies collection within 4 hours without refrigeration. If it is practicable, there is an argument for using ultrafresh blood when more than the patient's own blood volume has been lost, as additional blood components will not be needed.

Fresh blood is blood that has been stored for less than 7 days. If it is not possible to use ultrafresh blood, then fresh blood is preferred for massive blood transfusion.

Stored blood is blood that has been stored for more than 7 days, and it is associated with a gradual decrease in the concentration of 2,3-diphosphoglycerate (2,3-DPG) that interferes with the oxygen-delivering capacity of haemoglobin. Platelet and granulocyte functions also deteriorate.

Microaggregates of platelets and white cells gradually accumulate with time and can cause obstruction of the pulmonary microcirculation. There has been no evidence that these microaggregates are clinically significant, and microfilters probably are not required.

Red-cell concentrate (packed cells)

- Haematocrit, 70–80%
- Volume, 200–300 ml (red cells 150–200 ml)
- Citrate phosphate dextrose (CPD): packed cells with a maximum storage time at 4°C of 21 days
- CPD with adenosine (CPD-A): can be stored at 4°C for 21 days

STORAGE CHANGES IN RED-CELL CONCENTRATE (CPD-A)

	0 days	35 days
pH	7.6	6.98
hydrogen-ion concentration (nmol/L)	25.1	106.1
sodium (mmol/L)	169	155
potassium (mmol/L)	4.0	30.0
adenosine triphosphate (ATP) (%)	100	55
plasma haemoglobin (% lysis)	0.05	0.1
2,3-DPG (%)	100	0

COMPLICATIONS OF BLOOD TRANSFUSION

Pyrexia

Pyrexia is relatively common and usually has an immunological basis.

Serological incompatibility

Most of these problems are now due to errors in identification of the patient to receive the transfusion. Initial symptoms and signs of a haemolytic transfusion reaction include rigors, nausea, vomiting, flushing, pain, and circulatory collapse. Other features include haemostatic failure, oliguria, renal failure, anaemia, and jaundice. Minor incompatibility usually occurs as a result of reaction to white cells, platelets, or plasma proteins and often results in only fever, rash, and urticaria.

Blood-borne infections associated with transfusion

BACTERIA   Bacterial infections are very rare after blood transfusion in developed countries. Contaminants that have on rare occasions been reported as causing bacteraemia include *Pseudomonas* spp., coliforms, and *Staphylococcus* spp. More recently, the possibility of infection with *Borrelia burgdorferi*, causing Lyme disease, has become a concern.

FUNGI AND PARASITES   These also are very rare in developed countries. Transfusion-transmitted malaria can pose a problem, because there is no simple and sensitive screening test.

VIRUSES   Hepatitis viruses, including hepatitis A, B, C, and D, can be transmitted by blood transfusion. Currently, screening tests exist for hepatitis A, B, and C viruses.

Cytomegalovirus (CMV), Epstein-Barr virus (EBV), and human herpes virus 6 (HHV-6) can contaminate blood. They are often associated with a syndrome that includes severe pyrexia, with or without atypical mononucleosis, 7–10 days post transfusion. This can be confused with an occult source of sepsis. It usually settles spontaneously over 2–3 weeks.

RETROVIRUSES   Human immunodeficiency virus, types 1 and 2 (HIV-1, HIV-2), and human T-cell lymphotropic virus, types I and II (HTLV-I, HTLV-II), were of great concern in the early 1980s. Screening is now routinely carried out for anti-HIV-1 and -2, as well as anti-HTLV-I and -II.

OTHER VIRUSES   Other viruses, including Colorado tick fever virus, Lassa fever virus, Rift Valley fever virus, and Ebola virus, are only very rarely found as contaminants.

IMMUNOSUPPRESSION   There is some evidence that blood transfusion can decrease graft tolerance, increase susceptibility to infection, and predispose to recurrence of cancer.

MASSIVE BLOOD TRANSFUSION

This is usually defined as replacement of more than the patient's circulating blood volume within a 24-hour period. In this situation, the circulating volume and red blood cells should be replaced rapidly with either whole blood or red blood cells and plasma solution. The blood should be as fresh as possible. **BLOOD SHOULD BE USED EARLIER, RATHER THAN LATER, IN ORDER TO PREVENT A DECREASE IN THE OXYGEN-CARRYING CAPACITY AND TO ALLOW TIME FOR THE RED BLOOD CELLS TO REGENERATE 2,3-DPG**. Avoid inflexible rules for replacement of platelets, potassium, calcium, and coagulation factors during massive blood transfusion. It is better to regularly measure the end points of transfusion and adjust treatment as necessary:

• Give haemoglobin in the form of blood-cell transfusion, as necessary.
• Platelets: Give 8–10 units when the platelet count drops below $30 \times 10^9/L$ and/or there is an indication for their use on clinical grounds.
• Coagulation profile: The need for fresh frozen plasma (FFP) (Table 29.2) or cryoprecipitate is gauged by screening tests such as the activated partial thromboplastin time (APPT), prothrombin time (PT), and thrombin time (TT). Because of delays in screening tests, FFP can be given on a qualitative basis (eg 2 FFP units for each 6 units of blood).

Complications of massive blood transfusion

IMPAIRED OXYGEN TRANSPORT   Impairment of oxygen transport during transfusion can be related to

• defective red-cell function
• impaired haemoglobin function

TABLE 29.2 ABBREVIATIONS

WBCT	whole-blood clotting time
TCT	thrombin clotting time
PT	prothrombin time
APTT	activated partial thromboplastin time
PTT	partial thromboplastin time
FDPs	fibrinogen degradation products
TT	thrombin time
DIC	disseminated intravascular coagulation
FFP	fresh frozen plasma
SPPS	stable plasma protein solution
PPF	purified protein fraction

• microaggregates
• fluid overload or hypovolaemia
• decreased lung function and adult respiratory distress syndrome (ARDS)

HAEMOSTATIC FAILURE   Haemostatic failure can be related to

• dilution and/or depletion of platelets and clotting factors
• disseminated intravascular coagulation (DIC)
• hypocalcaemia

ELECTROLYTE AND METABOLIC DISTURBANCES

Hyperkalaemia   Although stored blood has a high level of potassium, hyperkalaemia usually is not a problem, even with rapid transfusion. Potassium moves intracellularly in the higher pH environment of the body.

Hypokalaemia   Delayed hypokalaemia is more common than hyperkalaemia.

Citrate toxicity   Despite theoretical considerations, this is rarely a problem.

Hypocalcaemia   Hypocalcaemia is also a rare problem, and it is now suggested that calcium be given according to clinical signs,

ECG evidence, or concentration of ionized calcium, rather than as a routine.

Hypernatraemia   Infusion of multiple units of blood can result in hypernatraemia.

HYPOTHERMIA   Efficient blood warmers should be used to keep the temperature of infused blood above 32°C. Even mild hypothermia will have a marked effect on clotting.

JAUNDICE   Up to 30% of transfused red blood cells may not survive. This presents a large bilirubin load. In combination with liver hypoperfusion as a result of blood loss, the normally unconjugated bilirubin may be conjugated, giving a cholestatic picture. Haematoma may also contribute to the jaundice.

PLATELETS

• Volume of 1 unit: 20–50 ml (70×10^9 platelets)

• Duration of activity: 2–7 days at 20°C (optimum storage duration, 2 days)

If transfusion is indicated, an adult usually receives 300×10^9 platelets (about 4–5 units), or approximately 1 unit/10 kg. The platelet count should rise by $5–10 \times 10^9$/L for each unit transfused. Platelets should be transfused through a standard blood filter, **NOT A MICROAGGREGATE FILTER.** Ideally, platelets that are group-compatible and compatible with the patient's leucocyte antigens (HLA) should be used. Rhesus-negative (Rh-negative) platelets should be used for Rh-negative patients, as platelet concentrates are often contaminated by red blood cells.

The best measure of platelet function is bleeding time, but the platelet count at 1 hour post infusion reflects viability and correlates with bleeding time.

INDICATIONS FOR PLATELET TRANSFUSION IN INTENSIVE CARE

• Platelet count $< 10–20 \times 10^9$/L

• Low ($20–50 \times 10^9$/L) platelet count, with clinically significant bleeding

- Qualitatively defective platelets and spontaneous bleeding (eg drug-induced)

GRANULOCYTES

- Volume: 300–500 ml (2–4×10^{10} granulocytes).
- Viable for up to 12 hours.
- HLA-compatible granulocytes should be used.

INDICATIONS FOR GRANULOCYTE TRANSFUSION IN INTENSIVE CARE
There has been a reduction in the use of granulocyte transfusions in clinical practice. The safety, efficiency, and cost effectiveness of transfused granulocytes are being questioned. They are sometimes still employed on a short-term basis for neutropenic patients, either prophylactically or for established bacteraemia.

Granulocyte colony-stimulating factor elevates neutrophil numbers and is used mainly for neutropenia following chemotherapy. Its role in the critically ill is, as yet, unclear.

FRESH FROZEN PLASMA

- Volume of 1 unit: 200–300 ml.
- One unit contains approximately 10% of an adult's total clotting factors.
- Maximum storage duration is 6 months when kept below $-30°C$. It should be used within 6–24 hours after thawing.
- Contains all the coagulation factors.
- FFP also contains approximately

  sodium, 172 mmol/L
  potassium, 3.5 mmol/L
  protein, 5.5 g/dl
- FFP should be ABO-compatible.
- Commence with 10 ml/kg.

CRYOPRECIPITATE

- Volume: 15 ml.
- Stored below $-30°C$, will remain stable for about 6 months.

- Contains

  factor VIII
  fibrinogen
  von Willebrand's factor
  fibronectin

BLOOD SUBSTITUTES AND COLLOIDS

COLLOIDS   Colloids are fluids that because of their oncotic pressure are confined mainly to the intravascular space. Colloids derived from blood exert their oncotic pressure via protein particles (eg plasma and albumin solutions), whereas artificial colloids contain other particles (eg dextrans and gelatin solutions).

PLASMA EXPANDERS   Plasma expanders are colloids that contain higher concentrations of colloid particles than does plasma, and therefore they cause fluid to move from the interstitial space to expand the intravascular space (eg concentrated albumin, high-molecular-weight dextrans).

BLOOD DERIVATIVES

Human plasma protein solution

- stable plasma protein solutions (SPPS)
- purified protein fraction (PPF)
- human serum albumin (HSA)

The latter is available as fractionated and pasteurized iso-oncotic (5%) or hyperoncotic (20% or 25%) solutions. The iso-oncotic solution has protein and electrolyte concentrations approximately the same as those of circulating plasma. Other characteristics of human plasma protein solutions include the following:

- half-life for circulating protein, about 5–10 days
- long shelf life
- free from transmittable diseases
- allergic reactions very rare

ARTIFICIAL COLLOIDS

Dextrans

The dextran solutions contain polysaccharide molecules. These are classified according to their molecular weight (MW):

• Dextran 70 (MW 70,000) – intravascular half-life approximately 6 hours
• Dextran 40 (MW 40,000) – intravascular half-life approximately 3 hours

Both solutions are isotonic using either saline or dextrose.

Other characteristics include a small but significant incidence of serious anaphylactoid reactions. Dextran 40 particles are excreted in the kidneys and can block small renal tubules. There is no interference with blood cross-matching techniques using currently available dextrans. The total maximum dosage is limited to less than $1.5 \text{ g} \cdot \text{kg}^{-1} \cdot \text{d}^{-1}$, or less than a total of 1,500 ml. This limits the usefulness of these solutions for plasma volume replacement.

Modified gelatins

These are solutions containing modified gelatin and isotonic saline, with potassium and calcium. They are eliminated mainly by the kidneys, as well as via the gastro-intestinal tract and by catabolism. The intravascular half-life is approximately 4 hours. The solutions do not interfere with cross-matching, haemostasis, or renal function. They cause a very low incidence of anaphylactoid reactions.

Hydroxyethyl starch

This is a macromolecular polymer from hydrolysed corn in a solution similar to isotonic saline. It is eliminated by catabolism and excretion in urine and faeces. It has a very low incidence of anaphylactoid reactions. It does not affect renal function, but can interfere with haemostasis.

Artificial blood

Either stroma-free haemoglobin or perfluorochemicals can act as a colloid, but also have the potential to carry oxygen. They are commercially available in some countries, but their place in clinical practice awaits evaluation.

DISORDERS OF WHITE CELLS

NEUTROPHILIA

Neutrophilia is commonly seen in critically ill patients. An acute increase may indicate a new source of infection – bacterial, viral, or fungal. However, neutrophilia is also a non-specific accompaniment of many non-infectious factors, such as steroids, surgery, stress, inflammation, and acute myocardial infarction.

NEUTROPENIA

Neutropenia can be an ominous sign, especially when associated with severe sepsis. It is probably due to a combination of bone-marrow suppression and increased adherence and utilization of white cells at the site of infection.

There is a long list of drugs that can cause neutropenia. They include captopril, hydralazine, procainamide, and quinidine. Primary bone-marrow disorders, such as leukaemia, also can result in decreased white-cell production. It can be very difficult in the critical care setting to determine the exact cause of the neutropenia.

DISORDERS OF HAEMOSTASIS

DIAGNOSIS

Normal clot formation requires

- an intact vascular wall
- a normal clotting cascade
- normal platelet numbers and function

Abnormalities of haemostasis in critically ill patients commonly involve

- a hole in a vessel (ie surgical bleeding)
- an abnormality of the clotting cascade
- decreased platelet numbers

or a combination of these. One scheme for approaching the disorders of haemostasis is as follows.

Approach to bleeding

SURGICAL BLEEDING   Rule out the possibility of surgical bleeding.

HISTORY   Does the patient have renal failure, liver failure, or sepsis? Was there a recent operation? Is the patient being given drugs that can predispose to bleeding?

INITIAL COAGULATION TESTS   Check PT, APTT, TT, platelet count, and bleeding time (see Table 29.2 for abbreviations).

COAGULATION-CASCADE ABNORMALITIES

1. Prolonged PT only:
  - test the extrinsic pathway
  - factor VII abnormality (the only factor in that pathway)
  Causes include:
  - vitamin K deficiency
  - warfarin treatment
  - mild liver disease
2. Prolonged APTT only:
  - intrinsic pathway
  - factor VIII the most important factor
  Causes include:
  - haemophilia A or B
  - von Willebrand's disease
  - heparin

- blocking inhibitor (eg lupus anticoagulant, acquired anti-factor-VIII antibody)

3. Prolonged PT and APTT:

- mainly due to diseases affecting the common pathway

Causes include:

- liver disease
- DIC
- warfarin
- primary fibrinolysis
- renal disease

PLATELET ABNORMALITIES A decrease in platelet number is a more common cause of coagulation disorders in the ICU than is decreased function. The possible causes of decreased platelet numbers include

- failure of production
- increased destruction (eg DIC, loss in extracorporeal circuits)
- dilution via massive transfusion

A prolonged bleeding time will show a defect in platelet function.

This scheme should help with the diagnosis. Each of the three components of clotting will now be looked at in detail.

VASCULAR DISORDERS

Apart from a hole in a vessel, major bleeding secondary to a vascular disorder is rare. Vascular endothelial damage can be associated with infections, drug reactions, and hypersensitivity reactions (eg hereditary haemorrhagic telangiectasia).

THROMBOCYTOPENIA

The causes of thrombocytopenia can include

- a decrease in production (eg aplastic anaemia, acute leukaemia)
- an increase in destruction [eg idiopathic thrombocytopenic purpura (ITP), DIC, the use of extracorporeal circuits, such as continuous diafiltration] (see p. 657)

- dilution (eg after massive blood transfusion)
- splenic pooling or trapping in association with hypersplenism

The management of thrombocytopenia depends on the cause, the manifestations of bleeding, and platelet function and number.

GUIDELINES FOR PLATELET TRANSFUSION

1. active bleeding in conjunction with platelet count $< 50,000/\text{mm}^3$ or abnormality of platelet function (bleeding time more than twice upper limit of normal)

2. prophylaxis:
- platelet count $< 20,000/\text{mm}^3$
  OR
- preoperative platelet count $< 50,000/\text{mm}^3$
  OR
- abnormality of platelet function

3. massive transfusion: platelet count $< 50,000/\text{mm}^3$ and abnormal bleeding

DRUG-INDUCED THROMBOCYTOPENIA   Many drugs potentially can interfere with platelet function and production. Aspirin and nonsteroidal anti-inflammatory drugs interfere with platelet aggregation and can cause clinical oozing for days after a small dose. Important drugs that can cause thrombocytopenia include chloramphenicol, high-dosage penicillin, thiazide diuretics, quinine, antituberculous drugs, and antiepileptic drugs.

HEPARIN-INDUCED THROMBOCYTOPENIC SYNDROME   Thrombocytopenia is a common complication of heparin treatment, occurring in 1–30% of patients 6–12 days after commencement of treatment. As heparin is a commonly used drug in the ICU, both as a therapeutic agent and as a flushing agent in order to maintain patency of vascular catheter, a high index of suspicion is needed for the diagnosis of heparin-induced thrombocytopenic syndrome (HITS). There are two types of HITS:

Type I
  Early onset.
  Mild thrombocytopenia.

Probably due to the platelet pro-aggregating effect of heparin.
Treatment may involve
  continuing the heparin and watching the platelet count
  changing to warfarin.
Type II
  Late onset.
  Severe thrombocytopenia.
  Thrombotic complications can cause severe ischaemia.
  Caused by an immune mechanism: heparin-antibody complexes
    bind to platelets, resulting in reduced survival, thrombocytopenia, and, in some cases, thrombosis.
  Heparin should be stopped immediately. If anticoagulation is required, consider
    warfarin
    aspirin
    dextrans
    thrombolytic agents.

Usually the diagnosis is made on a clinical basis, but a heparin-dependent antibody test, using either platelet aggregometry or the ^{14}C-serotonin-release method as end point, can be used in patients suspected of having type II HITS.

Low-MW heparin (eg Fragmin) and heparinoids are being considered for use as anticoagulants in case of HITS. They may be associated with a lower incidence of HITS, as they are less reactive with platelets. However, the true incidence with these newer drugs is yet to be determined.

RENAL DISEASE Uraemia causes both platelet dysfunction and factor VIII abnormalities. Dialysis, desmopressin (DDAVP), and cryoprecipitate will help correct the defect.

COAGULATION DISORDERS

Except for factor VIII, all coagulation factors are produced in the liver. The coagulation cascade has been classified into the intrinsic and extrinsic systems. The two systems are not mutually exclusive, however, as several activated factors can react in both systems. The classic model of the two pathways is also changing (Figure 29.1). For exam-

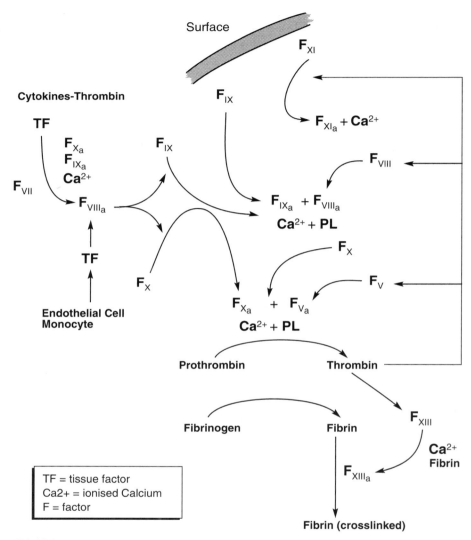

FIGURE 29.1 Coagulation cascade. This diagram represents a revised version of the traditional coagulation cascade. There is more interaction and overlap between the so-called intrinsic and extrinsic pathways.

ple, factors VIII, IX, and XI, formerly part of the intrinsic pathway, should be considered also as amplification factors of the extrinsic pathway.

Hypothermia strongly inhibits the enzymatic reactions of the co-agulation cascade and causes significant pro-coagulation of PT and APTT. This can be overlooked when interpreting coagulation profiles, especially when tested at 37°C.

Congenital disorders

HAEMOPHILIA A Haemophilia A is caused by factor VIII deficiency. If there is less than 5% of the normal factor VIII, there will be spontaneous bleeding. If there is less than 50% of the normal factor VIII, then factor VIII transfusion will be needed after surgery or trauma. The circulation half-life of factor VIII is 10–14 hours. Factor VIII is available from FFP or cryoprecipitate or as a specific concentrate.

HAEMOPHILIA B Haemophilia B, or Christmas disease, is caused by factor IX deficiency. The circulation half-life of factor IX is 24 hours. Factor IX is available as FFP or as factor IX concentrate.

VON WILLEBRAND'S DISEASE This is the commonest congenital co-agulation defect, caused by a deficiency in factor VIII quality and/or function, plus a qualitative platelet defect. Both deficits can be corrected with FFP or cryoprecipitate. Desmopressin (DDAVP) may be used for mild cases.

Vitamin K deficiency

Vitamin K is required by the liver for synthesis of factors II, VII, IX, and X. Vitamin K deficiency is seen in long-term dietary disturbances (eg poor oral intake) and is exacerbated by antimicrobial gut steril-ization. Inhibition of vitamin K is seen with the use of oral anticoag-ulants, coumarin, or indandione derivatives (see p. 727).

Vitamin K_1, 10 mg, twice weekly, subcutaneously, should be given to long-term patients in the ICU. Some preparations of vitamin K_1 are based in cremophor, which can cause anaphylaxis, especially when given intravenously. Vitamin K_1 takes 6 hours before coagulation-factor synthesis begins. Thus, FFP will have to be used initially for bleeding related to vitamin K deficiency.

Liver disease

Clotting-factor synthesis is one of the most accurate indicators of liver function. The vitamin-K-related factors decrease first. All of the factors produced in the liver have short circulating half-lives and will eventually decrease. The liver's ability to degrade activated clotting factors can be compromised, causing DIC.

Massive blood transfusion (see p. 709)

Cardiopulmonary bypass

Cardiopulmonary bypass surgery causes damage to red cells, decreases platelet number and function, and activates factor XII.

DISSEMINATED INTRAVASCULAR COAGULATION

Disseminated intravascular coagulation is not so much a separate disease as an exaggeration of the normal haemostatic processes in response to a wide variety of insults. The usual clinical manifestation of DIC is bleeding. Widespread intravenous activation of clotting and deposition of fibrin lead to consumption of platelets and clotting factors. Microvascular obstruction and varying degrees of end-organ damage can result. Secondary fibrinolysis then occurs, which accentuates the bleeding.

SOME CONDITIONS ASSOCIATED WITH DIC

• tissue damage (eg burns, heatstroke, dissecting aortic aneurysm, drowning, head injury, crush injury)
• severe infections (bacterial, viraemia, parasites)
• immunological (allograft rejection, immune-complex disorders, incompatible blood transfusion)
• obstetric (abruptio placentae, amniotic fluid embolism, retained foetal products, eclampsia, hypertonic saline abortion)
• metabolic (diabetic ketoacidosis)

- neoplastic (mucin-secreting adenocarcinoma, promyelocytic leukaemia)
- miscellaneous (evenomation, fat embolism, venous thrombosis)

DIAGNOSIS The diagnosis is based on (1) clinical evidence of bleeding from many sites and (2) laboratory tests:

Screening tests
- prolonged PT
- prolonged APTT: more sensitive than PT
- hypofibrinogenaemia (<1 g/L): poor sensitivity
- thrombocytopenia (<100 $\times$ 10^9/L): poor specificity

Rarely will all four of these tests show normal findings in the presence of DIC. More specific tests are needed for confirmation.

Confirmatory tests These tests are to show the following:
- A clot has been formed.
- The fibrinolytic system is activated (formation of plasmin) and has lysed the clot (formation of fibrin products)
- Fibrin monomer: Detection of fibrin monomer indicates that plasmin has been formed.
- Fibrin degradation products (FDPs): Their presence also indicates that plasmin has been formed, but does not distinguish between primary and secondary fibrinolysis. In some patients with severe DIC there may be no elevation in FDPs, because of inhibition of the fibrinolytic response.
- Fragment E and d-dimer: These distinguish secondary fibrinolysis – that a clot has been formed and then lysed. Although the d-dimer assay is more SPECIFIC than the FDP assay, it is less SENSITIVE:

	Sensitivity	Specificity
FDP	100%	56%
d-dimer	85%	97%
Combined	100%	97%

Abnormalities in three or more of the screening tests constitute presumptive evidence for DIC. Fibrin degradation products and d-dimer assays provide confirmatory evidence in the proper clinical setting. Other laboratory studies do not improve the diagnostic accuracy.

DISSEMINATED INTRAVASCULAR COAGULATION IN THE ICU   Many patients in intensive care have thrombocytopenia, abnormal coagulation, and equivocally raised FDPs, especially in association with multiorgan failure and sepsis. It is debatable that this condition deserves the label DIC. These patients rarely require any specific treatment, and the 'DIC' resolves as the precipitating disease process resolves.

Management of disseminated intravascular coagulation

1. REMOVE THE PRECIPITATING CAUSE OF THE DIC. THIS IS BY FAR THE MOST IMPORTANT PRINCIPLE (eg urgent delivery of the foetus in case of abruptio placentae or eclampsia, drainage and/or antibiotics for infection). Because DIC is not a specific disorder, but rather a pathophysiological process caused by a variety of underlying diseases, treatment must be tailored toward the underlying condition.

2. Maintain
   • circulation – important to correct hypovolaemia (see p. 61)
   • oxygenation (see p. 363)

3. Fluid replacement: Despite objections about 'fueling the fires', most clinicians will replace platelets, blood, and clotting factors as necessary until the underlying disease process is controlled. Moreover, there are sufficient inhibitors present in the replacement fluids to prevent amplification of the system. Apart from FFP, cryoprecipitate may also be necessary to replace factor VIII and fibrinogen. Regular laboratory measurements must be used to guide replacement.

   Guidelines for platelet transfusion:
   • For surgery or brain injury, maintain the platelet count higher than 100,000/ml.
   • For mild bleeding into the gastro-intestinal tract, maintain the platelet count higher than 50,000/ml.

4. Heparin: Despite theoretical attractions, heparin is rarely used for DIC. A possible exception may be acute promyelocytic leukaemia. Start with an intravenous bolus of 500–1,000 units, followed by 500 units per hour, and increase the dosage, depending on laboratory and clinical data. Other possible indications include purpura fulminans and retained dead foetus. Low-molecular-weight heparin (LMWH) may prove more useful.

5. Future directions may involve specific inhibition of the extrinsic pathway and neutralization of the triggering factors, such as tissue factor and factor VIIa.

Primary fibrinolysis

This is a rare disorder, of which the major component is fibrinogenolysis (ie lysis before a stable clot is formed). Burns, certain types of surgery (neurosurgery, prostatic surgery), and malignancy can release inappropriately large quantities of plasminogen activator, which is converted to circulating plasmin. This attacks fibrinogen and factor VIII. It can present as sudden catastrophic haemorrhage.

DIAGNOSIS Excessive fibrinolysis is recognized on the basis of

- prolonged TT
- decreased serum fibrinogen
- increased FDPs
- decreased euglobin clot lysis time

MANAGEMENT Treat the precipitating factors. Antifibrinolytic agents such as ϵ-aminocaproic acid (EACA) and tranexamic acid may prove effective in these circumstances.

Lupus anticoagulant

Despite giving a prolongation of the APTT, the lupus anticoagulant is rarely associated with bleeding, mainly thrombosis. Also, despite its name, it is rarely associated with systemic lupus! The lupus anticoagulant is an antiphospholipid antibody that interferes with the clotting cascade at sites where phospholipid is required.

Anti-factor-VIII antibody

This is autoantibody against the patient's own factor VIII molecule.

ANTICOAGULANTS

HEPARIN

Actions:

• Heparin binds to and potentiates antithrombin III, which is the main physiological inhibitor of the coagulation cascade.
• Heparin enhances platelet aggregation.

Uses:

• For deep vein thrombosis (DVT) prophylaxis, give heparin, 5,000 units SC, 8–12-hourly. No monitoring required.
• For systemic anticoagulation:
  loading dose, 5,000 units IV
  continuous infusion, 20,000–40,000 units/24 h

Monitoring:

• No single test is an accurate measure of heparin activity:
  APPT or TT will be two to four times normal
  heparin levels (0.2–0.6 units/ml)

Reversal:

• Protamine sulphate, 1 mg/100 units heparin, or 50 mg empirically and assess effect.
• Protamine itself can cause coagulation problems and anaphylactoid reactions. Give slowly intravenously.

Low-molecular-weight heparin

Compared with heparin, low-molecular-weight heparin has these features:

• lower MW!
• longer half-life
• smaller dose for the same antithrombotic effect
• less severe platelet effects
• can be partially reversed by protamine (1 mg/100 units Fragmin)
• unknown incidence of HITS

Uses:

• DVT prophylaxis (Fragmin, 2,500 units, once daily). No monitoring required.
• Systemic anticoagulation, 100 units $\cdot$ kg^{-1} $\cdot$ h^{-1}, either subcutaneously by 12-hourly or continuous intravenous infusion.

Monitoring:

• Anti-Xa levels: for a continuous infusion of Fragmin anti-Xa levels, 0.5–1.0 unit/ml.

WARFARIN

Actions:

• Warfarin is a vitamin K antagonist that prevents the vitamin-K-dependent clotting factors II, VIII, IX, and X from becoming active.
• The rate of the anticoagulant action is determined by the half-lives of the clotting factors, from factor VII (5 hours) up to factor II (60 hours).
• Larger doses will not hasten the onset of anticoagulation.

Uses:

• Can be given when heparin starts. Takes approximately 1 week to achieve stability.

Monitoring:

• Initially PT will become abnormal (factor VII).
• Full anticoagulation is not achieved until APPT is abnormal.
• Usually monitored with PT (two times normal).

Reversal:

• FFP will replace clotting factors in an emergency.
• Vitamin K, 10 mg, will take approximately 6 hours to work.

Special points:

• Drugs that are highly protein-bound will displace warfarin and may exacerbate bleeding.

• Patients may become hypercoagulable initially because of decreased protein C levels.

THROMBOLYTIC AGENTS

All thrombolytic agents act directly or indirectly as plasminogen activators. They can be given systemically or locally to lyse arterial or venous thrombi. The commonly used agents and their properties are listed in Table 29.3.

Optimal dosing regimens are known for patients with myocardial infarction, but they have not yet been determined for those with pulmonary emboli, strokes, and peripheral venous and arterial thrombi.

Common complications include bleeding, haemorrhagic stroke, and allergic reactions (streptokinase and APSAC).

Contraindications to the use of thrombolytics:

Absolute
• active haemorrhage
• recent central nervous system (CNS) infarction, haemorrhage, surgery, trauma, malignancy (<3 months)

Relative
• recent surgery (within 10 days)
• recent trauma
• recent gastro-intestinal haemorrhage
• recent external cardiac massage
• coagulation disorders
• pregnancy, or 10 days post partum
• severe hypertension (diastolic > 130 mm Hg)
• conditions with a potential for CNS embolism (eg bacterial endocarditis)

As yet there is no reliable monitor to assess the thrombolytic effect or the risk of bleeding. Fibrinogen levels and FDPs have poor sensitivity and specificity.

Other drugs

APROTININ   Aprotinin is used mainly with cardiopulmonary bypass to decrease peri-operative bleeding. The mechanism of action is un-

TABLE 29.3 PROPERTIES OF THROMBOLYTIC AGENTS

Property	Streptokinase	Urokinase	Tissue plasminogen activator	APSAC[a]
Source	Streptococcal culture	Heterologous mammalian tissue culture	Heterologous mammalian tissue culture; recombinant bacterial product	Streptococcal culture
Molecular mass (daltons)	47,000	37,000	68,000	131,000
Type of agent	Bacterial pro-activator	Tissue plasminogen activator	Bacterial pro-activator	Tissue plasminogen activator
Plasma half-life (min)	23–29	15–18	6	90
Fibrinolytic activation	Systemic	Systemic	Systemic	Systemic
Fibrin specificity	Minimal	Minimal	Moderate	Minimal
Antigenicity	Yes	No	No	Yes
Allergic reactions	Yes	No	No	Yes
Cost	Cheapest	More expensive	Most expensive	More expensive

[a]APSAC, anisoylated plasminogen streptokinase activator complex.

certain (probably inhibits the increased fibrinolysis secondary to the use of extracorporeal circuits).

DESMOPRESSIN (DDAVP) Desmopressin is used clinically for haemophilia, von Willebrand's disease, and uraemia and to reduce blood loss during surgery. It increases the circulating levels of factor VIII coagulant activity and von Willebrand factor and will shorten bleeding times.

FURTHER READING

Bell, W. R., & Streiff, M. B. (1993). Thrombolytic therapy. A comprehensive review of its use in clinical medicine. *Journal of Intensive Care Medicine* 8:56–72, 115–29.

Burnum, J. F. (1986). Medical vampires. *New England Journal of Medicine* 314:1250–1.

Cate, H., Brandjes, D. P. M., Wolters, H. J., & von Deventer, S. J. H. (1993). Disseminated intravascular coagulation: pathophysiology, diagnosis and treatment. *New Horizons* 1:312–23.

Chong, B. H. (1992). Heparin induced thrombocytopenia. *Australian and New Zealand Journal of Medicine* 22:145–52.

Fischback, D. P., & Fogdall, R. P. (1981). *Coagulation. The Essentials*. Baltimore: Williams & Wilkins.

Gould, S. A., Lakshman, R. S., Hansa, L. S., et al. (1992). Artificial blood, current status of haemoglobin solutions. *Critical Care Clinics* 8:293–310.

Gregory, S. A., McKenna, R., Sassetti, R. J., & Knospe, W. H. (1986). Hematological emergencies. *Medical Clinics of North America* 70:1149.

Higgins, M. J., & Klein, H. G. (1989). Massive transfusion in the intensive care unit. *Journal of Intensive Care Medicine* 4:221–33.

Irving, G. A. (1992). Perioperative blood and blood component therapy. *Canadian Journal of Anaesthesia* 39:1105–15.

Isbister, J. D. (1986). *Clinical Haematology – A Problem Orientated Approach*. Baltimore: Williams & Wilkins.

Mollison, P. L. (1983). *Blood Transfusion in Clinical Medicine*, 7th ed. Oxford: Blackwell.

Schaier, A. H. (1991). Disseminated intravascular coagulation: pathogenesis and management. *Journal of Intensive Care Medicine* 6:209–28.

Thijs, L. G., de Boer, J. P., de Groot, M. C. M., & Hack, C. E. (1993). Coagulation disorders in septic shock. *Intensive Care Medicine* 19:S8–S15.

Ulstad, D. R., Godfrey, P. M., Robbins, R., & Camilli, A. E. (1990). Red cell transfusion in a critical care unit. *Journal of Intensive Care Medicine* 5:204–8.

30

CRITICAL CARE ENDOCRINOLOGY

SEVERE UNCONTROLLED DIABETES

PATHOPHYSIOLOGY

Most diabetic emergencies arise as a result of insulin deficiency, either absolute or relative, that causes decreased uptake of glucose into the cells and increased hepatic glycogenolysis and gluconeogenesis (Figure 30.1).

Increased amounts of regulatory hormones, such as glucagon, catecholamines, and cortisol, are released in response to the stress of hypoglycaemia. These hormones, along with the decreased insulin concentration, stimulate lipolysis and generation of fatty acids, and oxidation of these fatty acids in the liver results in ketone-body formation and metabolic acidosis. Hyperosmolar hypoglycaemic non-ketotic coma (HHNKC) occurs as a result of relative insulin deficiency or resistance, but with minimal counter-regulatory hormonal activation.

An increased serum glucose concentration will lead to osmotic diuresis, with extensive water losses, equally from all of the body's fluid compartments. Poor tissue perfusion will eventually lead to lactate formation, which in turn will exacerbate the metabolic acidosis. The metabolic acidosis will also lead to decreased total-body levels of potassium and magnesium, as these ions not only are exchanged for extracellular hydrogen ions but also are lost in the urine as a result of the osmotic diuresis, along with sodium, water, phosphate, and glucose.

CLINICAL FEATURES

A wide spectrum of biochemical and clinical abnormalities can occur in acute uncontrolled diabetes (Table 30.1), extending from pure hyperglycaemia without ketosis or HHNKC to pure ketosis without hy-

731

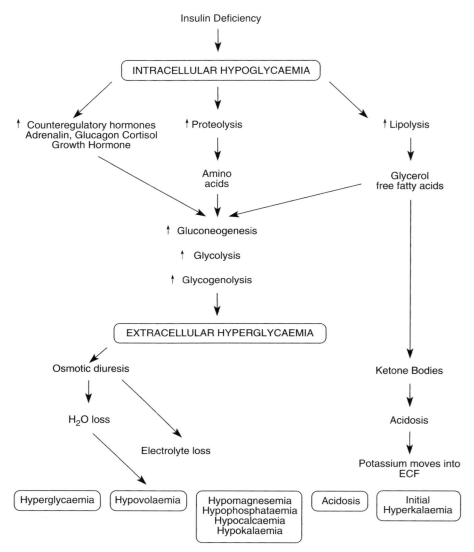

FIGURE 30.1 Pathophysiology of diabetic emergencies.

perglycaemia (euglycaemic ketoacidosis). Between the ends of this spectrum of presentation there is a mixture of ketosis and hyperglycaemia that is the classic diabetic ketoacidosis, accounting for about 70% of admissions for diabetes.

TABLE 30.1 FEATURES OF DIABETIC EMERGENCIES

Parameter	Euglycaemic ketoacidosis	Diabetic ketoacidosis	Hyperosmolar non-ketotic coma
Age	Usually young	Any age	Usually old
Previous history	Insulin-dependent	Known or new diabetic	Insulin-dependent or on oral hypo-glycaemics
Prodromal period	Hours	Days	Days to weeks
Acidosis	+++	+++	0/+
Fluid loss	0/+	++	+++
Change in level of consciousness	0	++	+++
Blood sugar	0/+	++	+++

The clinical features can include

• Fatigue, thirst, nausea, and abdominal pain.

• Decreased level of consciousness, irritability, and confusion.

• Hyperventilation (Kussmaul respirations) as a response to the metabolic acidosis.

• Clinical dehydration as a result of large water and electrolyte losses. Signs such as dry mucous membranes, sunken eyes, and loss of tissue turgor may be seen.

• Varying degrees of hypovolaemia occur in all patients, with hypovolaemic shock occurring in the more severe cases. Because of the osmotic diuresis induced by glucosuria, urine output may be maintained in spite of decreased renal blood flow.

• Ketones can be smelt on the breath of ketotic patients.

PRECIPITATING FACTORS Although there may be no obvious reason for a sudden deterioration in an otherwise stable diabetic, there are some possible precipitating factors:

• infection

• poor patient compliance due to inadequate instruction

• acute illness (eg surgery, myocardial infarction)

INVESTIGATION AND MONITORING

• Intravascular fluid replacement must be monitored in terms of blood pressure, pulse rate, peripheral perfusion, central venous pressure (CVP), and, if necessary, pulmonary artery wedge pressure (PAWP) and cardiac output. Urine output is an unreliable indicator, as it is affected by the osmotic diuresis.

• Take hourly Dextrostix readings, confirmed by regular blood sugar measurements. Dextrostix are not accurate when the blood sugar levels are over 20 mmol/L, in which case formal determinations of blood sugar should be made.

• Determine the serum potassium concentration hourly, until stable.

• Make initial and then daily serum sodium, magnesium, calcium, and phosphate determinations.

• Make daily determinations of serum osmolality, urea, creatinine, haemoglobin, and white cells, and obtain a chest x-ray.

• Carry out blood culture, urine microscopy and culture, sputum culture, and 12-lead ECG on admission and then as indicated.

• Use plasma Ketostix, and determine the serum lactate if necessary, to exclude a source of acid other than ketosis.

• Urinary electrolyte concentrations may help in the selection of a replacement fluid.

MANAGEMENT

Mortality from severe diabetic ketoacidosis remains around 5%, and from hyperosmolar coma, around 50% – treatment must be aggressive and meticulous (Table 30.2).

The principles of treatment to be outlined next apply to classic diabetic ketoacidosis. Hyperosmolar hypoglycaemic non-ketotic coma and euglycaemic ketoacidosis are discussed separately.

Fluid resuscitation

1. Correct hypovolaemia and reverse shock   Initially, 2 litres or more may have to be infused rapidly, then 50–300 ml/h, with boluses of 200 ml as necessary, until the circulating volume is restored.

TABLE 30.2 SUMMARY OF MANAGEMENT IN
DIABETIC EMERGENCIES

1. Aggressive control of airway – endotracheal tube if necessary.
2. Aggressive resuscitation from hypovolaemia and shock. Colloid is more efficient than crystalloids for this purpose. Avoid rigid regimens, and use measurements of the intravascular space (eg blood pressure, pulse rate, CVP, peripheral perfusion) as guidelines for resuscitation.
3. Replace total body water losses with 5% dextrose or hypotonic solutions, 100–300 ml/h, depending on degree of dehydration.
4. Replace fluid losses with half-normal saline or other suitable dextrose/saline solution if there is no evidence of hypovolaemia.
5. Replace potassium, magnesium, and phosphate according to measured levels.
6. Commence intravenous infusion of short-acting insulin at 1 unit per hour for diabetic ketoacidosis and 0.5 unit per hour from HHNKC, and adjust the infusion according to regularly measured blood glucose concentrations.
7. Correct acidosis with bicarbonate, 1 mmol/kg, only if arterial pH < 6.9 or is persistently less than 7.2.
8. Concurrently treat the underlying cause of the diabetic emergency.
9. Give low-dosage prophylactic heparin.

Many recommendations for fluid treatment are based on inflexible recipes that may be irrelevant to a patient's individual needs. The approach to fluid loss in a patient with glycosuria is the same as for a patient with hypovolaemia or shock. It would be equally illogical to recommend an inflexible fluid regimen for shock as a result of a ruptured spleen. Each patient's fluid needs must be assessed individually, and then continually reassessed (Figure 30.2). Body water follows glucose into the cells when insulin administration is commenced, and this can exacerbate any underlying hypovolaemia. Fluid should be titrated against regularly measured end points reflective of circulating volume, such as blood pressure, pulse rate, CVP, and peripheral perfusion. Colloid probably is more efficient than isotonic saline for correcting hypovolaemia, but isotonic saline is still widely used and is recommended as the first-line fluid for resuscitation (see p. 67).

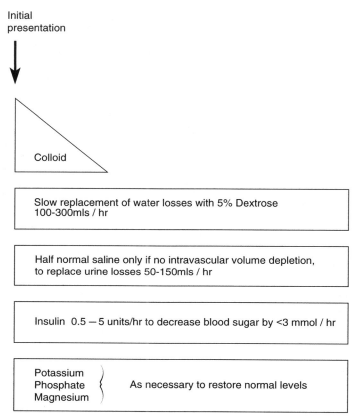

Initial presentation

Colloid

Slow replacement of water losses with 5% Dextrose 100-300mls / hr

Half normal saline only if no intravascular volume depletion, to replace urine losses 50-150mls / hr

Insulin 0.5 – 5 units/hr to decrease blood sugar by <3 mmol / hr

Potassium
Phosphate } As necessary to restore normal levels
Magnesium

FIGURE 30.2 Management of acute diabetic emergencies. Colloid is initially used to re-suscitate the circulating volume. Simultaneously, 5% dextrose is used to replace water losses. If there is no intravascular volume depletion, half-normal saline can be used to offset polyuria. Insulin is commenced at a low rate and increased as necessary. Electrolytes are replaced according to frequently measured levels.

The disadvantage of isotonic saline is that it is ultimately distributed mainly to the interstitial space, which does not need urgent resuscitation and is not responsible for hypovolaemia or shock. Moreover, isotonic saline as a first-line fluid for resuscitation is inefficient in correcting hypovolaemia and inappropriate for correcting the water loss. The average urinary sodium losses as a result of the osmotic diuresis are approximately 50–70 mmol/L and will be adequately replaced by the sodium in the colloid needed for initial resuscitation.

2. Correct water losses   If there has been minimal fluid loss and there is no hypovolaemia, one can use a solution approximating the sodium concentration in the fluid lost as a result of the polyuria. This will be approximately equivalent to half-normal saline.

Although the first priority is to correct hypovolaemia, the total losses of body water should be concurrently and slowly corrected with 5% dextrose or a hypotonic dextrose/saline solution. The extra sugar added in the form of the dextrose-containing solutions is only a small amount and is easily controlled by adjusting the insulin infusion. The amount of fluid given will depend on the degree of dehydration. As a guideline, 2–6 litres (100–300 ml/h) should be given in the first 24 hours, with infusion continuing until the patient is tolerating oral fluids. WATER LOSSES FROM THE INTERSTITIAL AND INTRACELLULAR SPACES ARE NOT IMMEDIATELY LIFE-THREATENING, BUT RAPID CORRECTION CAN BE. IT IS IMPORTANT THAT THE WATER LOSSES BE CORRECTED SLOWLY (OVER 24–72 HOURS), TO ALLOW FOR GRADUAL OSMOTIC EQUILIBRATION BETWEEN THE BODY FLUID SPACES.

If a patient is severely hypovolaemic, the urine output may be low, despite glycosuria. Once the intravascular space has been restored, the urine output will rise, driven by glycosuria. It is important that the total fluid infused be greater than the urine output.

Electrolytes

POTASSIUM   The serum potassium concentration should be measured on admission and hourly until it stabilizes, and then 2–4-hourly for the first 12 hours. Almost half of all diabetic patients are hyperkalaemic on admission. Some diabetic patients will have compromised renal function and difficulty in excreting potassium.

After checking the initial serum potassium concentration, commence giving potassium at 5–40 mmol/h for the first 2 hours, and adjust the rate according to subsequent serum potassium concentrations measured every hour until stable.

Average requirements:

- 20 mmol/h for 6 hours
- 10 mmol/h for the next 12 hours

PHOSPHATE   Initial and daily measurements of phosphate are necessary during the acute stage. Hypophosphataemia can have many complications, including respiratory failure (see p. 83).

If the concentration is low on admission, commence phosphate replacement at a rate of 5 mmol/h until corrected. Because phosphate solutions also contain potassium, the rate of potassium replacement may have to be adjusted.

MAGNESIUM   Depending on the initial and daily measurements, magnesium may also have to be given.

Guideline: 20 mmol of magnesium intravenously over 1 hour, and repeat as necessary.

SODIUM   Sodium losses are usually corrected by the initial fluid used for resuscitation. Measurement of serum sodium will be affected by the blood glucose and will appear lower.

$$\text{real Na} = \text{measured Na} + \frac{\text{blood glucose (mmol/L)}}{4}$$

Hyperglycaemia

INSULIN   Use short-acting insulin (Figure 30.3). The use of human insulin is recommended. Use a continuous intravenous insulin infusion system for better control of glucose. Hourly Dextrostix measurements and routine checks against blood sugar determinations are essential.

Insulin causes potassium, magnesium, and phosphate, as well as water, to move intracellularly. IT IS ESSENTIAL NOT TO REDUCE THE BLOOD GLUCOSE RAPIDLY, AS THESE OSMOLAR FLUID AND ELECTROLYTE SHIFTS CAN CAUSE SEVERE COMPLICATIONS. Some patients are very sensitive to insulin. An initial loading dose of insulin is unnecessary; it could exacerbate hypovolaemia and cause cell swelling and hypokalaemia.

Guidelines

Commence insulin at 1–2 units/h until the rate of decrease in glucose can be estimated.

Blood glucose should be allowed to decrease by no more than 3 mmol/h, to allow osmotic gradients time to equilibrate gradually.

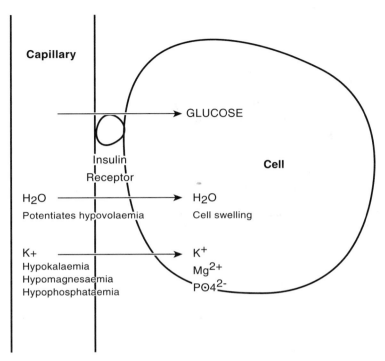

Capillary

GLUCOSE

Insulin
Receptor

Cell

H_2O ⟶ H_2O
Potentiates hypovolaemia   Cell swelling

K+ ⟶ K^+
Hypokalaemia Mg^{2+}
Hypomagnesaemia
Hypophosphataemia PO_4^{2-}

FIGURE 30.3 Effects of insulin in diabetic emergencies.

If higher infusion rates are needed, double the infusion rate, and keep on doubling the rate periodically until control is achieved.

A rate of 0.5–3 units/h usually will maintain the blood glucose concentration when it has dropped to below 10 mmol/L.

Insulin adsorption on plastic syringes and giving sets is not a clinical problem, as infusion rates are titrated against regularly measured blood sugar levels. Special carrier solutions usually are not necessary.

Poor responses to insulin often are related to uncorrected hypovolaemia and inadequate resuscitation. Also check the insulin delivery mechanism.

Intramuscular regimens are less reliable because of diminished absorption, but sometimes they are necessary because of lack of equipment and under-staffing. Their guidelines are as follows:

• hourly Dextrostix measurement

- 20 units initial dose
- 6 units/h

ACIDOSIS The acidosis usually will correct itself if the foregoing management principles are followed.

Consider giving HCO_3 at 1 mmol/kg if the initial arterial pH is less than 6.9, and repeat the pH measurement in 30 minutes. Otherwise, consider giving HCO_3 at 1 mmol/kg if the pH is persistently less than 7.2. Check the adequacy of intravascular volume replacement and the insulin delivery mechanism.

Over-correction of acidosis with HCO_3 is associated with

- sodium overload and exacerbation of hyperosmolality
- paradoxical increase in intracellular acidosis
- exacerbation of hypokalaemia

TREAT THE UNDERLYING CAUSE
- Concurrently, infection should be excluded by Gram stain and cultures.
- Exclude myocardial infarction.
- Better patient education and ready access to medical advice and outpatient and hospital facilities have proved to be significant advances in the management of diabetes mellitus, and when applied effectively, they have largely prevented acute diabetic emergencies.

HYPEROSMOLAR HYPOGLYCAEMIC NON-KETOTIC COMA

The same basic principles as for diabetic ketoacidosis should be used for HHNKC, with the following differences:

- Coma and decreased level of consciousness are more common in HHNKC. Aggressive airway control with an endotracheal tube is often necessary.

- Because of larger fluid losses, it is even more important to avoid isotonic saline in patients with HHNKC. Use colloid initially for resuscitation, and concurrently commence 5% dextrose solution. These patients can be very sensitive to under-treated hypovolaemia and shock, because of their greater age and increased incidences of associated conditions such as ischaemic heart disease.

• Because the fluid losses are usually higher, more colloid may be needed for initial resuscitation, followed by more 5% dextrose to replace the gross water deficit. WHILE RAPIDLY REVERSING SHOCK WITH COLLOID, AIM TO CORRECT WATER LOSSES OVER 24–72 HOURS (average infusion rate, 100–300 ml/h). The rate is empirical and will depend on clinical assessment of fluid depletion and the time since onset. The longer since the onset, and the more severe the dehydration, the more severe the osmotic and metabolic disturbances. In order to enable these complex derangement to adjust, correction of water deficits should occur slowly in these patients.

• Resuscitation of the intravascular space should occur rapidly.

• These patients are older and require careful monitoring of fluid replacement (see Chapter 4).

• Insulin requirements in these patients usually are lower than those for patients with diabetic ketoacidosis. A SLOW INFUSION IS ESSENTIAL, TO ALLOW OSMOTIC EQUILIBRATION AND TO PREVENT RAPID FLUID AND ION SHIFTS: AIM TO SLOWLY REDUCE BLOOD GLUCOSE OVER AT LEAST 24–72 HOURS. The rate of reduction of blood glucose will depend on the onset of hyperglycaemia – the slower the onset, the more carefully the blood sugar should be reduced.

• Potassium requirements are usually higher. Phosphate and magnesium losses may also be high.

• Drowsiness, disorientation, and coma often are prolonged and can occur up to 6 days after the commencement of treatment. If there is no specific intracerebral lesion, total recovery can be expected.

• Prophylactic heparin should be given – the incidence of venous thrombosis is high among patients with HHNKC.

EUGLYCAEMIC KETOACIDOSIS

The same principles of management as for classic diabetic ketoacidosis apply, with the following differences:

• Minimal fluid loss – may need only 5% dextrose, not colloid.

• Insulin infusion is the mainstay of management.

• Acidosis usually will correct itself.

• Because of the lack of dehydration and the presence of normal blood sugars, the diagnosis often can be overlooked. Beware of the confused unco-operative young diabetic with relatively normal blood sugar.

ALCOHOLIC KETOACIDOSIS

Alcoholic ketoacidosis is not related to a lack of insulin. Indeed, these patients are very sensitive to insulin. It is typified by hypoglycaemia and ketoacidosis.

THYROID GLAND DISORDERS

'SICK-EUTHYROID' SYNDROME

Up to 70% of critically ill patients will have altered thyroid function and yet will be clinically euthyroid. The sick-euthyroid state is a response that prevents hypermetabolism when the body is stressed. It is important to differentiate this syndrome from true hypothyroidism. It requires no treatment.

1. Low-T_3 syndrome is very common in the seriously ill:

• low serum concentration of T_3 caused by decreased peripheral conversion of T_4 to T_3 and reduced protein binding

• serum thyroid-stimulating hormone (TSH) low or normal, with thyroid-releasing hormone (TRH) stimulation producing a normal or blunted TSH response

2. High-T_4 syndromes are less common:

• elevated T_4, usually as a result of increased concentration of thyroid-binding globulin (TBG)

• free T_3 is low and rT_3 high

3. Low-T_4 and -T_3 syndrome is a variant of low-T_3 syndrome, but is less common.

• hyposecretin of T_4 from the thyroid gland, and decreased protein binding of T_4

• TSH usually decreased, TSH response to TRH stimulation blunted

Thyroid function tests can be difficult to interpret in the seriously ill. Provided the patient is not receiving glucocorticoids, dopamine, or T_4 replacement, a normal TSH assay is a reliable predictor of euthyroidism.

HYPOTHYROIDISM

Clinical features of myxoedematous coma

- coma or decreased level of consciousness
- cardiovascular collapse (bradycardia, hypotension, hypovolaemia, pericardial effusion)
- hypothermia and reduced metabolic rate
- hypotonia and delayed relaxation of tendon reflexes
- respiratory failure (may be due to collapse, atelectasis, aspiration, pleural effusion, hypercarbia, hypoventilation)
- features of other endocrine disturbances (eg hypopituitarism, hypoparathyroidism)
- external features of coarse hair, a large tongue, loss of external one-third of eyebrows, yellow coarse skin, hoarse voice, non-pitting oedema, and possibly signs of thyroid enlargement or atrophy, depending on the cause

Many non-thyroid serious diseases mimic hypothyroidism, especially in the intensive care setting. The extreme of hypothyroidism, usually known as myxoedematous coma, is the profound physiological expression of lack of thyroid hormone.

Diagnosis

The diagnosis of true hypothyroidism depends on

- an accurate history of previous thyroid abnormalities or symptoms associated with hypothyroidism, such as cold intolerance, hoarse voice, lethargy, constipation, alopecia, weight gain despite appetite loss, and amenorrhoea.
- physical findings such as bradycardia, a neck scar, dry skin, hypothermia, respiratory failure, and those clinical features mentioned under myxoedematous coma.

Laboratory findings

- low T_3 and T_4 concentrations
- high TSH if hypothyroidism is primary, or low TSH if it is secondary to pituitary disturbance
- elevated serum cholesterol
- anaemia
- ECG: may show low-amplitude QRS complex and/or features of ischaemia
- Chest x-ray: may show pericardial or pleural effusion
- Metabolic findings: hyponatraemia, respiratory acidosis, and hypoglycaemia

Further investigations may include a thyroid scan, CT scan, and investigation of pituitary and parathyroid functions.

Hypothyroidism can be differentiated from sick-euthyroid states on the basis of the presence of low concentrations of free T_3 and rT_3, as well as an exaggerated response of TSH to TRH. Treatment should be commenced on clinical grounds.

Management

- Secure the airway
- Use oxygenation and ventilation (see p. 363) if necessary.
- Fluid replacement and circulatory support with inotropes are often necessary (see p. 520), as for other seriously ill patients.
- Excessive water replacement should be avoided, as these patients usually experience water retention.
- Slowly and passively rewarm.
- Correct other metabolic disorders such as hyponatraemia.
- Treat hypoglycaemia with 50% dextrose intravenously.
- Treat pericardial and pleural effusions as necessary.
- Exclude complications such as skin necrosis, compartment syndrome (see p. 297), rhabdomyolysis (see p. 642), and renal failure (see p. 640) as a result of coma.

MONITORING These patients need careful monitoring of their cardiorespiratory status, especially after commencement of hormone replacement, as there can be

- a rapid increase in oxygen consumption
- an increase in cardiac output
- myocardial ischaemia

DRUG TREATMENT Initially, only very small doses (eg 2.0-μg increments) of T_3 should be administered orally, except in the presence of paralytic ileus, where it should be given in even smaller doses intravenously and monitored carefully (intravenous infusion of 20 μg/d). T_3 theoretically is preferable to T_4, because it crosses more rapidly from the serum to the cerebrospinal fluid, does not depend on a converting enzyme, and has a shorter half-life than T_4.

Hydrocortisone, 100 mg IV, 6-hourly, is often given as well.

THYROID STORM

Thyroid storm is a life-threatening clinical extreme of hyperthyroidism. It is very rare nowadays because of better long-term control. It usually occurs in a patient known to have hyperthyroidism who has an intercurrent acute illness, such as a severe infection, myocardial infarction, or diabetic ketoacidosis, or undergoes surgery or childbirth.

Clinical features

- Hyperthermia (can be extreme).
- Cardiovascular collapse (related to arrhythmias, cardiomyopathy, and fluid loss). Initially there is hyperdynamic circulation.
- Restlessness, confusion, tremor, and coma are common.
- Hyperventilation.
- Nausea, vomiting, diarrhoea, epigastric pain, cachexia, and liver dysfunction are often found.
- Hypokalaemia and hyponatraemia.
- Hypercalcaemia and hyperglycaemia.

Diagnosis

Treatment should be initiated on clinical grounds. The hormone levels cannot be determined rapidly and will be no different from levels found in uncomplicated hyperthyroidism. Ultrasound examination of the thyroid gland and TSH assays may help with the diagnosis.

Management

GENERAL SUPPORTIVE MEASURES

- Treat any precipitating factor.
- Secure the airway.
- Correct hypovolaemia and other fluid losses (see p. 61).
- Correct metabolic abnormalities.
- Support the circulation (see p. 518).
- Ventilate and oxygenate if necessary (see p. 363).
- Cool with tepid sponging and fanning.

DRUGS Drug treatment aims to

- inhibit the effects of circulating hormones (β-blockers are usually used for this purpose)
- inhibit the release of thyroid hormone (iodine)
- block synthesis of and inhibit peripheral conversion of T_4 to T_3 (propylthiouracil).

1. β-adrenergic blockade should be administered cautiously to suppress the signs and symptoms of thyrotoxicosis. Give propranolol, 40 mg orally, 8-hourly, or 1 mg intravenously, as required. However, β-blockers by themselves are not effective for thyroid storm.

2. Give propylthiouracil, 1 g orally, stat, then 150 mg orally, 6-hourly. This drug blocks the synthesis of and inhibits the peripheral iodination of T_4 to T_3.

3. Give potassium iodide, 500 mg orally, 8-hourly, or 200 mg in 500 ml of isotonic saline intravenously over 2 hours, given twice daily, 1 hour AFTER PROPYLTHIOURACIL. Iodine inhibits the release of thyroid hormone.

4. Plasmapheresis, dialysis, and resin haemoperfusion have been used successfully in cases that were refractory to the foregoing measures.

5. Dexamethasone, 2 mg IV, 6-hourly, is sometimes used.

ADRENAL GLAND DISORDERS

ADRENAL INSUFFICIENCY

In the intensive care setting, adrenal insufficiency occurs most commonly in patients treated with glucocorticoids. Less often it can occur where adrenal tissue has been destroyed by autoimmune disease, tuberculosis, meningococcal or other infection (eg AIDS), haemorrhage, or infiltration by malignancy. Addisonian crisis usually occurs as a result of bilateral destruction of the adrenal cortices and usually is precipitated by an intercurrent catastrophe such as severe infection or surgery.

Clinical features

• Weakness, malaise, abdominal discomfort, fasting hypoglycaemia, skin pigmentation (if long-term).

• Dehydration, weight loss, hypotension, and tachycardia may occur simultaneously with high cardiac output and low systemic vascular resistance.

• Hyponatraemia, hyperkalaemia, and metabolic acidosis.

• Hypoglycaemia.

Diagnosis

• Low plasma cortisol concentration, with a high concentration of adrenocorticotrophic hormone (ACTH).

• In the seriously ill, a single plasma cortisol determination can be helpful. Increased levels are expected in acutely ill patients with normal adrenal function; a low cortisol level is a good indication of hypofunction.

• Abdominal CT may demonstrate the cause of the adrenal abnormality.

Treatment

• Isotonic saline (approximately 6–8 litres in 24 hours) to correct the hyponatraemia and fluid loss.
• Hydrocortisone, 100 mg IV, 6-hourly.
• Aldosterone, 0.5 mg IM. This is unnecessary when large amounts of hydrocortisone are used.
• Treat the precipitating cause.

STEROID WITHDRAWAL

Corticosteroids are widely used in medicine, and their withdrawal can cause an Addisonian-type picture within 24 hours:

• general malaise, anorexia, abdominal discomfort
• postural hypotension, pyrexia, and Addisonian crisis

  Treatment:

• hydrocortisone, 100 mg IV, 6 hourly
• isotonic saline

Adrenal suppression is increasingly likely after long-term use (2–10 years). Therefore, withdrawal of steroids must be gradual. After steroid treatment for more than 8 years, adrenal cortical suppression may be permanent.

If there is doubt about adrenal suppression, an ACTH stimulation test (Synacthen test) can be performed. This can reveal a lack of adrenocortical reserve, as opposed to total absence of activity. Administration of ACTH to these patients should result in diminished cortisol responses:

• Give tetracosactrin [synthetic 1–24-ACTH (Synacthen)], 250 μg IM.
• Take blood samples at 30 and 60 minutes post injection, and measure for cortisol.

PHAEOCHROMOCYTOMA

Phaeochromocytoma is a rare catecholamine-secreting tumour originating from the chromaffin cells of the sympathetic nervous system:

- 90% develop in the adrenal medulla
- 10% are malignant

Clinical presentation

The symptoms range from mild to severe and can be sustained or paroxysmal. They include

- sweating attacks
- tachycardia
- headaches
- hypertension
- autonomic dysfunction
- possibly arrhythmias, angina, and pulmonary oedema

Diagnosis

Determination of urinary metanephrine is a good screening test.
Determination of urinary vanillylmandelic acid is a less sensitive screening test.
Determination of urinary catecholamines is also a good screening test.
Plasma catecholamine measurement is technically difficult to perform.
Localization:

- CT scan of the abdomen
- [131I]metaiodobenzylguanidine scintigraphy.

Management

Surgical removal is the only definitive treatment. Careful pre-operative preparation is essential and must include

- α-blockers (usually phenoxybenzamine) commenced 2–3 weeks before operation
- β-blockers only after α blockade has been commenced
- Fluid replacement usually is necessary as the circulation vasodilates.
- Potassium replacement.

FURTHER READING

Arieff, A. I., Carroll, H. J. (1972). Nonketotic hyperosmolar coma with hyperglycaemia: clinical features, pathophysiology, renal function, acid–base balance, plasma–cerebrospinal fluid equilibria and the effects of therapy in 37 cases. *Medicine* 51:73–94.

Bagdade, J. D. (1986). Endocrine emergencies. *Medical Clinics of North America* 70:1111–28.

Breslow, M. J., & Ligier, B. (1991). Hyperadrenergic states. *Critical Care Medicine* 19:1566–78.

Chernow, B. (1982). Hormonal and metabolic considerations in critical care medicine. In *Critical Care: State of the Art*, vol. 3, ed. W. C. Shoemaker & W. L. Thompson, pp. J1–52. Fullerton, CA: Society of Critical Care Medicine.

Daggett, P. (1982). Endocrine emergencies. In *Care of the Critically Ill Patient*, ed. J. Tinker & M. Rapin, pp. 593–608. Berlin: Springer-Verlag.

Felicetta, J. V., & Sowers, J. R. (1987). Endocrine changes with critical illness. *Critical Care Clinics* 5:855–69.

Griffith, D. N. W., & Yuakin, J. S. (1986). Diabetic ketoacidosis. *British Journal of Hospital Medicine* 8:82–7.

Hawker, F. (1988). Endocrine changes in the critically ill. *British Journal of Hospital Medicine* 39:278–88.

Hillman, K. M. (1991). The management of acute diabetic emergencies. *Clinical Intensive Care* 2:154–62.

Johnston, D. G., & Alberti, K. G. M. M. (1980). Diabetic emergencies: practical aspects of the management of diabetic ketoacidosis and diabetes during surgery. *Bailliere's Clinical Endocrinology and Metabolism* 9:437–60.

Knowlton, A. I. (1989). Adrenal insufficiency in the intensive care setting. *Journal of Intensive Care Medicine* 4:35–45.

Smallbridge, R. C. (1992). Metabolic and anatomic thyroid emergencies. A review. *Critical Care Medicine* 20:276–91.

Teich, S., Sharpe, S., & Chernow, B. (1985). Endocrine function in the critically ill. *Clinics in Anaesthesiology* 3:999–1026.

31

CRITICAL CARE PAEDIATRICS

CARDIORESPIRATORY ARREST

Cardiac arrest in children is usually due to hypoxia. Unless the cause of the hypoxia can be rapidly reversed (eg relief of upper-airway obstruction), these patients have little chance of survival: Hypoxia that is severe enough to cause cardiac arrest in a healthy child almost certainly will have resulted in irreversible brain damage. Asystole, preceded by bradycardia as a result of overwhelming hypoxia, is the usual mechanism of cardiorespiratory arrest in children. Primary tachyarrhythmias are rare in children, with the exception of those patients with congenital heart disease.

Prevention of hypoxia and early recognition of the signs of hypoxia, with immediate oxygenation, are the key elements to successful paediatric resuscitation. BEWARE THE QUIET, UNRESPONSIVE YET IRRITABLE INFANT. Other signs of hypoxia include inability to feed, signs of respiratory distress, and cool and cyanosed peripheries. Sinus bradycardia in this setting is often a pre-arrest rhythm. Hypoxia can be rapidly confirmed by oxygen-saturation monitoring with pulse oximetry.

MANAGEMENT

1. CLEAR THE AIRWAY. Suction the posterior pharynx after adequate visualization with a laryngoscope. In the out-of-hospital setting, a 'finger sweep' of the mouth and posterior pharynx will suffice.

2. SECURE THE AIRWAY. Intubate with an endotracheal tube (ETT) the same size as the child's fifth finger or the same diameter as the external nares (Table 31.1). Remember that an infant's larynx is more superior and anterior than an adult larynx. The epiglottis is larger and floppier, often requiring a straight-blade laryngoscope for elevation and visualization of the vocal cords. If rapid intubation cannot

TABLE 31.1 DIMENSIONS OF ENDOTRACHEAL AND NASOTRACHEAL TUBES FOR CHILDREN

Age	Endotracheal tube diameter (mm)	Nasotracheal tube minimal length (cm)
Newborn (<1 kg)	2.5	7–11
Newborn (1–3.5 kg)	3.0	12–13
3 months	3.5	13–15
6 months	4.0	15
12 months	4.0	16
18–24 months	4.5	17
4 years	5.0	18
6 years	5.5	20
8 years	6.0	22
10 years	7.0	23
12 years	7.0	24
14 years	8.0	27

be achieved, then an appropriately sized Guedel airway should be inserted, and bag-and-mask ventilation commenced. Remember that a child has a large tongue in a small mouth, and the Guedel airway can push the tongue into the posterior pharynx and cause obstruction (Table 31.2).

3. VENTILATION. Restoration of oxygenation and ventilation is paramount. Intubation often can be performed in more controlled circumstances if ventilation is commenced with a bag and mask. Observe the chest for adequate ventilation. Common causes of inadequate ventilation are as follows:

When bagging
• occlusion of the airway by hyperextension of the neck
• over-vigorous submandibular pressure
• inappropriate Guedel airway

When intubated
• displaced tube in oesophagus or pharynx or down the right mainstem bronchus

TABLE 31.2 HOW CHILDREN DIFFER FROM ADULTS REGARDING THE AIRWAY

Children:
Big floppy head
Short neck
Small mouth
Large tongue
Anterior larynx
Large floppy epiglottis
Smallest part of the airway is the cricoid ring
Short trachea
Endotracheal tubes:
Uncuffed until the age of 10 years
Should have a leak around the ETT at 25 cm H_2O airway pressure

Barotrauma from too vigorous ventilation, especially when an adult bag is being used, can occur. Ventilation should be at a rate appropriate to the child's age.

4. CARDIAC MASSAGE. Check for a pulse in the femoral, brachial, or axillary area. An infant's short neck and large head make palpation of the carotid pulse difficult. A physician's hands may be able to encircle the chest of a baby, allowing both thumbs to compress the chest. Otherwise, two fingers can be used to depress the sternum, with the baby placed on a firm surface. Adequate cardiac output can be assessed by palpation of a femoral pulse. Inadequate depth of chest compression and inappropriate cardiac compression can result in inadequate cardiac output (Table 31.3).

5. SECURE VASCULAR ACCESS. Often it is impossible to gain venous access during cardiac arrest because of the difficulties associated with peripheral shutdown and increased subcutaneous fat. It may be advisable to insert an intraosseous needle, rather than waste time attempting to cannulate small peripheral veins. Alternatively, an experienced operator may be able to blindly cannulate the long saphenous vein. The intraosseous needle should be inserted on the flat medial aspect of the tibia just below the tibial tuberosity. It is best to make a small skin incision first before commencing the vig-

TABLE 31.3 CARDIOPULMONARY RESUSCITATION IN CHILDREN

Age	Hand position	Compression depth (cm)	Compression rate (cycles/ min)	Respiratory rate (breaths/ min)
<1 year	Two fingers or encircling hands at one finger width below nipple line on the sternum	2–3	100–120	20
1–7 years	One hand at two finger widths up from xiphisternum	2–3	80–100	15–20
>8 years	Two hands – as for adults	4–5	80	15

orous rotating movements required to pass the needle through the bone cortex. Keep the needle at 90° to the bone surface. There will be a sudden 'give' as the needle enters the medulla of the tibia. Drugs and fluids can be administered via this route in the same dosages and volumes as for intravenous access. Once the circulation has been restored, venous access can be gained in more controlled circumstances.

An ETT can be used to administer drugs. However, this is a poor substitute for vascular access. Up to 10 times the normal intravenous dose should be used, with dilution of the drug in isotonic saline (1 ml for infants, 3 ml for pre-schoolers, and 5 ml for older children). Adrenaline, lignocaine, and atropine can be safely given via this route, but bicarbonate and calcium can cause lung damage.

6. RESTORATION OF THE CIRCULATION. As most cardiac arrests in children are due to asystole, adrenaline doses of 0.1 mg/kg can be used repeatedly in an attempt to restore cardiac rhythm. Repeated doses of bicarbonate (1 mmol/kg) may be more useful in children than in adults who have suffered cardiac arrest, because of the profound metabolic acidosis that often is present after prolonged hypoxia in metabolically active children. Ventricular fibrillation must be treated with immediate cardioversion (2–5 J/kg). Adult paddles can be used as long as they do not connect with each other during defibrillation. Hypovolaemia is also common, and repeated boluses of colloid or blood at 20 ml/kg should be administered until the circulation is restored.

7. TERMINATION OF RESUSCITATION. Survival is unlikely after 15 minutes of normothermic asystolic arrest. The use of inotropes for out-of-hospital asystolic cardiac arrest has led to poor outcomes. The decision to terminate resuscitation efforts should be made after appropriate details of the arrest are known – in particular, the duration and adequacy of out-of-hospital resuscitation efforts. Priorities then must change to supporting the grieving parents and family.

RESUSCITATION OF THE NEWBORN

Assessment: APGAR scoring system

The APGAR scoring system was developed as a tool to assess a baby's condition at birth. Five physical signs are examined and scored at birth and 5 minutes after birth.

	Score		
Sign	0	1	2
Heart rate	Absent	<100/min	>100/min
Respiratory rate	Absent	Slow, irregular	Good, crying
Colour	Blue, pale	Body pink, extremities blue	Pink
Reflex irritability (response to nasal-catheter insertion)	Absent	Grimace	Cough/sneeze
Muscle tone	Limp	Some flexion of extremities	Active motion

Major causes of asphyxia

• Primary fetal abnormalities (eg prematurity and multiple births)

• Primary placental abnormalities (eg eclampsia or ante-partum haemorrhage)

• Conditions of labour and delivery (eg breech presentation, prolapsed cord, or analgesics given to mother)

• Postnatal problems (eg respiratory distress)

Management

AIRWAY Use airway suctioning and intubation if necessary.

VENTILATION Use bag-and-mask ventilation initially, then intubation and intermittent positive-pressure ventilation (IPPV) with 100% oxygen initially. It is important to remove meconium from the pharynx and trachea before instituting IPPV.

CIRCULATION Venous access should be rapidly established using umbilical or peripheral veins. Initially administer bicarbonate, 1 mmol/kg (8.4% solution). Determine acid–base status, and deliver more bicarbonate accordingly. Because asphyxiated infants are commonly hypovolaemic, transfuse colloidal solution 10 ml/kg, rapidly, and repeat as necessary.

Cardiac massage: Use two fingers or thumbs applied to midsternum, at a rate of 100–120/min to a depth of approximately 2.0 cm.

DRUGS These are the recommended dosages when the following drugs are indicated:

• adrenaline, 1 ml of 1:10,000 solution stat (ie 0.1 mg), repeated as necessary

• lignocaine, 1 mg/kg, repeated every 5 minutes, up to 3 mg/kg

• atropine, 0.02 mg/kg IV

• calcium chloride, 0.1 mg/kg IV

• sodium bicarbonate, 1 mmol/kg stat, repeated according to acid–base status.

CORRECT ANY CORRECTABLES

• hypoglycaemia (50% dextrose solution, 0.5–1.0 ml/kg IV)

• seizures (diazepam, 0.3 mg/kg IV, over 5 minutes)

• perfusion pressure (maintain its adequacy)

• anaemia

• ventricular fibrillation (although extremely rare) (external 2–5 J/kg)

• hypothermia (keep warm)

ACUTE UPPER-AIRWAY OBSTRUCTION

Treatment and diagnosis must go hand in hand in this medical emergency. The airway must be secured while the cause of the obstruction is being sought. Children with such obstructions usually are otherwise fit and healthy, and although the episode is immediately life-threatening, the cause of the obstruction usually will be completely reversible. There are few moments in medicine in which so much depends on rapid implementation of the attending physician's skills and experience.

AETIOLOGY

The most common causes are

- acute laryngotracheitis (viral croup) (**MOST COMMON**)
- acute epiglottitis (**MOST COMMON**)
- foreign body (usually heralded by an attack of coughing)
- staphylococcal tracheolaryngobronchitis (pseudomembranous croup)
- angioneurotic oedema (evidence of swelling elsewhere)

DIFFERENTIATING BETWEEN LARYNGOTRACHEITIS AND EPIGLOTTITIS REQUIRES VISUALIZATION OF THE EPIGLOTTITUS UNDER ANAESTHESIA.

ACUTE LARYNGOTRACHEITIS (VIRAL CROUP)

- usually occurs at 6 months to 3 months of age
- afebrile, or a mild fever
- stridor, especially when upset
- hoarse cough
- upper-respiratory-tract infection for 2–3 days
- far more common than epiglottitis

EPIGLOTTITIS

- usually occurs at 2–6 years of age, but can occur at any age
- toxic appearance
- sitting upright, mouth open, drooling secretions

- history less than 24 hours
- no cough

CLINICAL PRESENTATION

- **STRIDOR.**
- Tachypnoea.
- Exhaustion supervenes, with bradypnoea, cyanosis, and brady-cardia.

Radiographic examination of the upper airways and chest can provide information about a foreign body or the patency of the upper airways. However, there is little place for x-rays in patients with viral croup and epiglottitis. If such x-rays are taken, the child must be continuously monitored during the entire period.

MANAGEMENT

SECURE THE AIRWAY WITHOUT DELAY. All but minor cases of epiglottitis will need intubation, whereas only approximately 5% of patients with viral croup will need intubation. However, it can be difficult to distinguish between the two diseases in the presence of severe stridor or where the clinical diagnosis is uncertain. **IN THESE CIRCUM-STANCES, LARYNGOSCOPY AND/OR INTUBATION ARE INDICATED WITHOUT DELAY.**

Anaesthesia for Laryngoscopy or intubation

A skilled team of experienced personnel is needed:

- anaesthetist
- ear, nose, and throat (ENT) surgeon or someone capable of performing an emergency tracheostomy
- assistants

Leave the child in a sitting position on the parent's lap. No attempt should be made to lay the child down prior to induction of anaesthesia.

Inhalation technique: Use oxygen and an agent such as halothane, administered after pre-oxygenation with 100% oxygen.

Intravenous access should be secured only AFTER the child is anaesthetized.

Make sure the child is deeply anaesthetized before laryngoscopy is attempted.

Topical lignocaine (2 mg/kg) may be applied, and the larynx examined under deep anaesthesia.

Insert an uncuffed orotracheal tube. Assess the size by the presence of a leak at 25 cm H_2O airway pressure. A tube of the correct size can then be inserted through the nose, and the orotracheal tube removed (Table 31.3). The tube should be firmly secured, and splints should be applied to both arms to prevent extubation. Sedation is rarely needed, as these tubes usually are well tolerated. The tip of the tube should be above the carina at approximately the second thoracic vertebra.

Adequate humidification is essential.

Regular bagging and instillation of warm saline (0.5–1.0 ml), followed by tracheal suction, are required in order to prevent lung collapse.

Some units are experienced in the use of intravenous induction agents and muscle relaxants for induction. However, those are not recommended techniques for most clinicians.

Specific treatment

EPIGLOTTITIS The diagnosis of epiglottitis is made via laryngoscopy, where an enlarged cherry-like epiglottis can be visualized, with surrounding supraglottic enlargement. Blood cultures should be examined before antibiotics are commenced:

- ampicillin, 25–50 mg/kg, 6-hourly
  AND
  ceftriaxone, 50 mg/kg IV, 12-hourly, or cefotaxime, 50 mg/kg IV, 6–8 hourly should be given until sensitivities are known, as some strains of *Haemophilus influenzae* are resistant to ampicillin.

Steroids have not been shown to influence the course of the disease, and cold-mist treatment is contraindicated.

Non-cardiogenic pulmonary oedema following relief of the airway obstruction has been reported. It should be managed according to standard principles (see p. 353).

To avoid inadvertent extubation, it is important to use restraining devices on the child, such as a combination of elbow splints and 'boxing-glove' bandages on the hands.

The responses to treatment usually are rapid, with extubation possible within 24 hours. Laryngoscopy usually is not necessary before extubation.

ACUTE LARYNGOTRACHEITIS OR CROUP Avoid upsetting the child. Encourage intake of oral fluids, and avoid intravenous cannulation until the patient is intubated.

There is anecdotal evidence that a warm, humid environment may be helpful. Cold mists, however, can worsen matters.

Use continuous nebulised adrenaline, 2–5 ml of a 1:1000 solution, nebulized over 10 minutes, and repeat every 1–2 hours as necessary. Continuous ECG monitoring is essential. This often will result in dramatic improvement and preclude the need for intubation in serious cases. Alternatively, give 0.5 ml of 2.25% racemic adrenaline solution diluted to 4 ml with water or saline, nebulised 1–2-hourly, as necessary. Racemic adrenaline has been said to have less severe cardiovascular side effects than adrenaline, and it is widely used in North America. However, there is no pharmacological basis nor clinical evidence to support that contention.

Antistaphylococcal antibiotics are indicated only if bacterial tracheitis is suspected.

Steroids may beneficially influence the natural course of laryngotracheitis.

Fewer than 5% of patients with croup will need intubation. The indications for intubation derive from clinical grounds: when the child is not improving, but is showing signs of exhaustion. The procedure for intubation has already been outlined.

FOREIGN BODY Inhalation of a foreign body is especially common in children from 6 months to 2 years of age, often heralded by coughing and accompanied by stridor, continuing coughing, wheezing, and aphonia. Many foreign bodies can be visualized radiographically, and gas trapping distal to the foreign body may be obvious. Removal should be by laryngoscopy or bronchoscopy under anaesthesia.

SEVERE PAEDIATRIC INFECTIONS

FEATURES

The presenting signs and symptoms associated with severe paediatric infections can be more subtle than those seen in adults, especially in the early stages. These include irritability, lethargy, poor feeding, vomiting, and irregular or rapid breathing. Unfortunately, these can be the prodromal features of a mild viral infection as well as a severe bacterial infection. The Glasgow coma scale for children is shown in Table 31.4

Fever is usually a feature of severe bacterial infection, but some patients can be hypothermic. A fever of more than 40°C in an infant younger than 3 months often is associated with serious infections, such as sepsis, meningitis, and pneumonia.

EXAMINATION

The child should be thoroughly examined, looking for features of the underlying cause, such as localized infection, rash, signs of meningoencephalitis (eg bulging fontanelle, seizures, exaggerated irritability when moved, and, less commonly, a stiff neck), or signs of pneumonia (eg tachypnoea, bronchial breath sounds).

The effects of the underlying disease process can include fever, hypotension, dehydration, lethargy, mental confusion, and restlessness, prior to increasing coma and cardiovascular collapse. Features of hypoxia in young infants include pallor, apnoea, bradycardia, hypotension, and expiratory grunting. In older infants, hypoxia causes features similar to those in adults (eg cyanosis, tachypnoea, tachycardia, and hypertension).

INVESTIGATIONS

• Blood cultures must be performed.

• Cultures from suspected sites of infection (eg lumbar puncture, suprapubic bladder aspiration, thoracentesis, tympanocentesis, paracentesis, percutaneous lung aspiration, aspiration of infected fluid from soft-tissue sites).

• Gram staining of specimens and/or antigenic identification of organisms.

TABLE 31.4 GLASGOW COMA SCALE FOR CHILDREN

	<1 years	>1 year
Eye opening	4 Spontaneously	4 Spontaneously
	3 To shout	3 To verbal commands
	2 To pain	2 To pain
	1 No response	1 No response
Best motor response	4 Localizes pain	4 Localizes pain
	3 Flexion to pain	3 Flexion to pain
	2 Extension to pain	2 Extension to pain
	1 No response	1 No response

	0–2 years	2–5 years	5 years
Best verbal response	5 Smiles/coos, cries appropriately	5 Appropriate words and phrases	5 Oriented and converses
	4 Cries appropriately	4 Inappropriate words	4 Disoriented and converses
	3 Inappropriate crying and/or screams	3 Cries and/or screams	3 Inappropriate words
	2 Grunts	2 Grunts	2 Incomprehensible sounds
	1 No response	1 No response	1 No response

Note: Add the scores from eye opening, best motor response, and best verbal response. The total is expressed out of a possible score of 13. Note that this is different from the adult GCS, which is out of 15.

• Lumbar puncture: microbiological investigation as well as protein and glucose determinations.
• White-cell count: A high neutrophil count supports a diagnosis of severe bacterial infection, but a normal count does not exclude it.
• Arterial blood gases and pH.
• Blood glucose determination.
• Serum electrolytes and liver function tests.
• Coagulation studies.
• Chest x-ray.

MANAGEMENT

The management principles for septicaemia and severe infections in children are the same as those for adults and are discussed in detail elsewhere (see Chapter 13). They include:

• fluid resuscitation (see Chapter 4)
• cardiovascular support (see Chapter 22)
• respiratory support (see Chapter 20)
• central nervous system support (see Chapter 24)

Initial antibiotic treatment

The range of possible bacterial infections in children is different from that in adults. In the immunologically normal child, the following may be encountered:

SEPTICAEMIA Among newborns, the causative organisms usually are Gram-negative bacteria or group B streptococci. In the older group, septicaemia is often caused by *Neisseria meningitidis*.

Less than 1 month of age
• ampicillin, 50–100 mg · kg^{-1} · d^{-1} IV (6-hourly intervals)
  +
  gentamicin, 7.5 mg · kg^{-1} · d^{-1} IV (8-hourly intervals)
          5 mg · kg^{-1} · d^{-1} IV (12-hourly intervals) for neonates
  levels reached: peak, 0.5–10 mg/L
                trough, <2 mg/L

OR

- cefotaxime, 150–200 mg · kg^{-1} · d^{-1} (6–8-hourly intervals)

More than 1 month of age
- penicillin, 60 mg/kg IV, 4-hourly
  +

  cefotaxime, 50 mg/kg IV, 4-hourly
  OR
- chloramphenicol, 25 mg/kg IV (8-hourly intervals) (to cover *H. influenzae, Streptococcus pneumoniae, N. meningitidis*]
  ±

  ampicillin, 200–300 mg/kg IV (6-hourly intervals)

PNEUMONIA

Newborns Pneumonia in newborns is usually caused by organisms derived from the mother's genital tract (eg group B streptococci and coliform bacteria). Treat with

- ampicillin, 50–100 mg · kg^{-1} · d^{-1} IV (6-hourly intervals)
  +

  gentamicin 7.5 mg · kg^{-1} · d^{-1} (8-hourly intervals)
  levels reached: peak, 0.5–10 mg/L
            trough, <2 mg/L

Infants under 1 month Gram-negative organisms and group B streptococci are the important pathogens. Treat with antibiotics (same as for septicaemia in the same age group).

Children 1 month–4 years Most pneumonia in this group is viral, and the respiratory syncytial virus (RSV) is the commonest cause. The pneumococcus and *H. influenzae* are the commonest bacterial pathogens. Treat with

- ampicillin, 200–300 mg · kg^{-1} · d^{-1} IV (6-hourly intervals)
  ±

  flucloxacillin or gentamicin if severely ill.

Children past 4 years *Mycoplasma pneumoniae* is the most frequently identified organism. Treat with

- erythromycin, 15–20 mg · kg^{-1} · d^{-1} IV (6-hourly intervals)

MENINGITIS

Neonatal meningitis The most common organisms in this group are Gram-negative organisms or group B streptococci. Initial antimicrobial treatment:

- ampicillin, 50–100 mg · kg^{-1} · d^{-1} IV (6-hourly intervals)
  +
  gentamicin, 5 mg · kg^{-1} · d^{-1} IV (8-hourly intervals)
  OR
- cefotaxime, 150–200 mg · kg^{-1} · d^{-1} IV (4-hourly intervals)

Over the age of 1 month *H. influenzae, S. pneumoniae,* and *N. meningitidis* are the most common organisms. Treat with antibiotics:

- penicillin, 60 mg/kg IV, 4-hourly
  +
  cefotaxime, 50 mg/kg IV, 4-hourly
  OR
- chloramphenicol, 75–100 mg · kg^{-1} · d^{-1} IV (6-hourly intervals)
  ±
  ampicillin, 200–300 mg · kg^{-1} · d^{-1} IV (6-hourly intervals)

All who come into close contact with the patient should receive prophylaxis in the form of rifampicin, 20 mg · kg^{-1} · d^{-1} (maximum 600 mg) for 4 days.

All of the antibiotics suggested here must be reviewed and changed if necessary, pending the microbiological results and sensitivity determinations.

Dexamethasone (0.15 mg/kg IV), given 15–20 minutes before initiation of antibiotic treatment, may improve outcomes from childhood meningitis.

FLUIDS AND ELECTROLYTES

MAINTENANCE SOLUTIONS: INTRAVENOUS

The figures that follow are only guidelines that must be modified according to careful and continuous monitoring of hydration (eg skin turgor) and circulating volume [eg urine output, blood pressure, central venous pressure (CVP), and occasionally pulmonary artery wedge pressure (PAWP)], as well as urine osmolality. Serum sodium is the best guide to the total body water.

Factors that can modify 'maintenance' fluid requirements include fever, hypothermia, ambient temperature, humidification of inspired gases, and whether the patient is active or paralysed:

INFANTS
- 1 day old   5% or 10% dextrose, 2 ml · kg^{-1} · h^{-1} (+ KCl, 20 mmol/L, and NaCl, 40 mmol/L)
- 2 days old   5% or 10% dextrose, 3 ml · kg^{-1} · h^{-1} (+ KCL, 20 mmol/L, and NaCl, 40 mmol/L)
- 3 days–1 year   5% or 10% dextrose, 4 ml · kg^{-1} · h^{-1} (+ KCl, 20 mmol/L, and NaCl, 40 mmol/L)

CHILDREN
- For the first 10 kg, give 5% or 10% dextrose, 4 ml · kg^{-1} · h^{-1} (+ NaCl, 40 mmol/L, and KCl, 20 mmol/L)
- Plus, for the next 10 kg, give 5% or 10% dextrose, 2 ml · kg^{-1} · h^{-1} (+ NaCl, 40 mmol/L, and KCl, 20 mmol/L)
- Plus, for every 1 kg above 20 kg, give 5% or 10% dextrose, 1 ml · kg^{-1} · h^{-1} (+ NaCl, 40 mmol/L, and KCl, 20 mmol/L)

ELECTROLYTES

Serum concentrations of potassium, sodium, magnesium, calcium, and phosphate must be measured regularly and replenished as needed. Daily maintenance electrolyte guidelines:

sodium	2–3 mmol · kg^{-1} · d^{-1}
potassium	2–3 mmol · kg^{-1} · d^{-1}
calcium	1 mmol · kg^{-1} · d^{-1}
magnesium	0.2 mmol · kg^{-1} · d^{-1}
phosphate	0.5 mmol · kg^{-1} · d^{-1}
zinc	0.5 µmol · kg^{-1} · d^{-1}

Assessment of dehydration

5%   thirst, oliguria, slightly sunken eyes and fontanelle, dry skin and mucous membranes

10%   oliguria, markedly sunken eyes, loss of skin turgor, soft eye-
        balls, hypovolaemia (tachycardia, thready pulse, mottled
        skin, hypotension)
15%   shock

Replacement fluids

Shock is a medical emergency that must be corrected as soon as possible. The intravascular fluid must be rapidly replenished: appropriate fluid at 20 ml/kg, and then repeated boluses of the same amount
until the circulating volume is normal. Blood should be given for
haemorrhage, and otherwise either a colloid (eg protein-containing
solution, modified gelatin solution) (see p. 61) or isotonic saline. Other
fluid deficits usually can be corrected by increasing the amount of
maintenance fluid according to the degree of dehydration. The sodium
concentration of the replacement fluid may have to be adjusted according to the serum sodium concentration. Severe hyponatraemia
and hypernatraemia should be corrected slowly after the circulating
volume has been corrected.

NUTRITIONAL SUPPORT

Whenever possible, enteral feeding should be encouraged. However,
sometimes that is not possible, and in those cases, because the nutritional reserves of children are much lower than those of adults,
parenteral nutrition must be considered early in the disease process.
Whenever possible, parenteral nutrition for children, especially small
ones, should be supervised by an experienced paediatric team.

PARENTERAL NUTRITION REGIMEN

Commence at the lower end of the recommended ranges for fluid and
parenteral nutrition (Table 31.5), and gradually increase to maximum
levels as tolerated over approximately 6 days.

Counselling of the patient and relatives is essential, explaining the
purpose and possible complications fully.

The central venous lines should be used exclusively for parenteral
nutrition, not for blood sampling, intravenous injections, blood administration, or administration of other fluids.

TABLE 31.5 PARENTERAL NUTRITION REQUIREMENTS

Item	Infants (<1 month or <10 kg)	Children
Energy – non-nitrogen $(kJ \cdot kg^{-1} \cdot d^{-1})$	170–360	210–300
Fluid $(ml \cdot kg^{-1} \cdot d^{-1})$	100–150	60–150
Amino acids $(g \cdot kg^{-1} \cdot d^{-1})$	1.0–2.5	1–3
Glucose $(g \cdot kg^{-1} \cdot d^{-1})$	10–14	5–15
Fat $(g \cdot kg^{-1} \cdot d^{-1})$	1–3	2–4
Vitamins and trace elements[a]		
folic acid (mg/d)	0.5	1
vitamin K (mg/d)	0.5	1

[a]Other vitamins and trace elements should be given empirically, as required, usually in the form of a commercial preparation.

Strict guidelines and protocols must be established and enforced regarding insertion and maintenance of central venous lines, as well as infusion of parenteral nutrition.

Monitoring of patients receiving parenteral nutrition

Daily	*Three times per week*	*Weekly*
Weight	Electrolytes	Arterial blood gases
Fluid balance	Urea	Serum zinc
Regular measurement of vital signs	Serum calcium and phosphorus	Liver function tests
		Bilirubin
Dextrostix (12-hourly for first week)	Lipid profile	Serum copper
Serum (for lipaemia)		
		Haemoglobin, white-cell count differential
Examination of IV site		Platelet count
Urinalysis and specific gravity		Iron, transferrin
Urea and electrolytes for 1 week		

Complications

If infection is suspected, take the following steps:

- Inspect the catheter site (change if it looks suspicious).
- Exclude all other possible causes of infection.
- Examine appropriate cultures [eg blood, urine, cerebrospinal fluid (CSF), pharyngeal secretions].
- Take haemoglobin and full blood counts and chest x-ray.
- Inspect the infusing solution for cloudiness (undetectable unless organisms $> 10^9$/L).
- If systemically septic, cease parenteral nutrition, and commence appropriate antimicrobials. If sepsis is not controlled within 24 hours, remove the intravenous line, even if it does not appear to be infected. Send the intradermal portion or tip for culture.

Consider fungal infection if there is no response to antimicrobials after 48–72 hours.

Other complications

Hyperlipidaemia
Hypoglycaemia
Hyperglycaemia
Pancreatic and gastro-intestinal-tract atrophy
Complications associated with intravenous-line insertion
Liver dysfunction
Acidosis
Hyperosmolar dehydration
Deficiencies of essential fatty acids
Trace-element deficiencies
Hyperammonaemia
Acidosis
Hypoproteinaemia

DRUGS COMMONLY USED IN PAEDIATRIC PRACTICE

| Adrenaline | Stat dose, 0.1 mg/kg IV (1:10,000 solution = 0.1 mg/ml) |

	0.2–0.5 mg/kg via ETT
	Infusion: start at 0.05 $\mu \cdot kg^{-1} \cdot min^{-1}$
Aminophylline	Loading dose, 8 mg/kg over 20 minutes
	Infusion, 1.2 mg $\cdot kg^{-1} \cdot h^{-1}$ (25–31 $\mu g \cdot kg^{-1} \cdot min^{-1}$)
	Therapeutic range, 55–110 $\mu mol/L$ theophylline
	Aminophylline = 80–85% theophylline
Ampicillin	For children <1 month, 50–100 mg $\cdot kg^{-1} \cdot d^{-1}$ (6-hourly intervals)
	For children >1 month, 200–300 mg $\cdot kg^{-1} \cdot d^{-1}$ (6-hourly intervals)
Atropine	0.01–0.02 mg/kg
Calcium	Maintenance, 1 mmol $\cdot kg^{-1} \cdot d^{-1}$
	$CaCl_2$ 10% solution: 0.7 mmol Ca per 1 ml
	Ca gluconate 10% solution: 0.23 mmol Ca per 1 ml
Charcoal (activated)	2 g/kg stat 0.25 g $\cdot kg^{-1} \cdot h^{-1}$, via nasogastric tube
Chloramphenicol	Neonates 25 mg $\cdot kg^{-1} \cdot d^{-1}$ IV (12-hourly intervals)
	Older infants and children, 50–100 mg $\cdot kg^{-1} \cdot d^{-1}$ IV (6-hourly intervals)
	Levels reached: peak, 15–25 mg/L
	trough, 7.15–15 mg/L
Clindamycin	20–40 mg $\cdot kg^{-1} \cdot d^{-1}$ IV (6-hourly intervals)
Dexamethasone	Loading dose, 0.2 mg/kg (maximum 10 mg)
	Maintenance, 0.3 mg $\cdot kg^{-1} \cdot d^{-1}$
Digoxin	Loading dose, 15 $\mu g/kg$ stat
Dopamine	Infusion: start at 1.0 $\mu g \cdot kg^{-1} \cdot min^{-1}$
Dobutamine	Infusion: start at 1.0 $\mu g \cdot kg^{-1} \cdot min^{-1}$
Erythromycin	15–20 mg $\cdot kg^{-1} \cdot d^{-1}$ IV (6-hourly intervals)
Frusemide	0.5–1.0 mg/kg IV (6–12-hourly)
Gentamicin	Neonates, 5 mg $\cdot kg^{-1} \cdot d^{-1}$ IV (12-hourly intervals)
	Others, 7.5 mg $\cdot kg^{-1} \cdot d^{-1}$ IV (8-hourly intervals)
	Levels reached: peak, 0.5–10 mg/L
	trough, <2 mg/L
Glucose	For hypoglycaemia, 50% dextrose solution, 0.5–1.0 ml/kg IV

	For hyperkalaemia, 0.5–1 g/kg, and insulin, 0.1 unit/kg IV
Heparin	Loading dose, 50–100 units/kg
	Maintenance, 20–30 units $\cdot$ kg^{-1} $\cdot$ h^{-1}
Hydralazine	Stat dose, 0.2 mg/kg IV
	Maintenance, 1.5–3.0 mg $\cdot$ kg^{-1} $\cdot$ d^{-1}
Insulin	For diabetic ketoacidosis, 0.05–0.1 unit $\cdot$ kg^{-1} $\cdot$ h^{-1}, and titrate against regularly measured blood sugars
Isoprenaline	0.025 μg $\cdot$ kg^{-1} $\cdot$ min^{-1} IV (maximum 1.0 mg)
	Infusion: start at 0.1–1.0 μg $\cdot$ kg^{-1} $\cdot$ min^{-1}
Lignocaine	Stat dose, 1.0 mg/kg IV
	Infusion, 10–50 μg $\cdot$ kg^{-1} $\cdot$ min^{-1}
Magnesium	Maintenance, 0.2 mmol $\cdot$ kg^{-1} $\cdot$ d^{-1} IV
Mannitol	0.2–0.5 g/kg IV (8-hourly intervals)
Morphine	Stat dose, 0.1–0.2 mg/kg
	Infusion, 10–20 μg $\cdot$ kg^{-1} $\cdot$ h^{-1} titrated against effect
Naloxone	0.005 mg/kg IV, can be repeated in 5–10 minutes
Neostigmine	0.07 mg/kg IV
Nitroglycerin	Infusion: start at 0.1 μg $\cdot$ kg^{-1} $\cdot$ min^{-1}
Nitroprusside	Infusion: start at 0.5–0.8 μg $\cdot$ kg^{-1} $\cdot$ min^{-1}
Noradrenaline	Infusion: start at 0.1–1.0 μg $\cdot$ kg^{-1} $\cdot$ min^{-1}
Pancuronium	Stat dose, 0.15 mg/kg, then 0.1 mg/kg (1–2-hourly intervals)
Paraldehyde	0.1–0.15 ml/kg IM or orally
	Infusion: 2–4 ml $\cdot$ kg^{-1} $\cdot$ h^{-1}, using 5% solution (dilute 2.5 ml in 50 ml of 5% dextrose)
Penicillin	50,000–100,000 units $\cdot$ kg^{-1} $\cdot$ d^{-1} 6 hourly intervals
Phenobarbitone	Seizures: loading dose, 20 mg/kg IV, slowly maintenance, 3–5 mg $\cdot$ kg^{-1} $\cdot$ d^{-1} IV (12-hourly intervals)
Phenoxybenzamine	Loading dose, 1 mg/kg IV, over 1 hour
	Maintenance, 0.5–2.0 mg $\cdot$ kg^{-1} $\cdot$ d^{-1} (6-hourly intervals)
Phentolamine	Loading dose, 0.02–0.1 mg/kg
	Maintenance, 5–50 μg $\cdot$ kg^{-1} $\cdot$ min^{-1}
Phenytoin	Loading dose, 20 mg/kg IV, over 1 hour

	Maintenance, 4–8 mg/kg IV, 12-hourly
	Levels: 40–80 μmol/L
Phosphate	0.5 mmol · kg⁻¹ · d⁻¹

Maintenance, 4–8 mg/kg IV, 12-hourly
Levels: 40–80 μmol/L

Phosphate 0.5 mmol $\cdot$ kg^{-1} $\cdot$ d^{-1}

Potassium 2 mmol $\cdot$ kg^{-1} $\cdot$ d^{-1}

Propranolol Stat dose, 0.01–0.05 mg $\cdot$ kg^{-1} $\cdot$ d^{-1} IV, slowly, up to 0.2 mg/kg

Maintenance, 1–2 mg $\cdot$ kg^{-1} $\cdot$ d^{-1} orally (6-hourly intervals)

Prostaglandin E Infusion, 0.05–0.1 μg $\cdot$ kg^{-1} $\cdot$ min^{-1}

Rifampicin Prophylaxis: meningococcal infection, 20 mg $\cdot$ kg^{-1} $\cdot$ d^{-1} orally (12-hourly intervals for 48 hours) (maximum 600 mg per dose)

H. influenzae infection, 20 mg $\cdot$ kg^{-1} $\cdot$ d^{-1} orally (12-hourly intervals for 96 hours)

Salbutamol Inhalation of 0.5% solution, 0.3 ml/kg

Infusion: loading dose, 5 μg/kg

maintenance, 0.2–10.0 μg $\cdot$ kg^{-1} $\cdot$ min^{-1} (increase by 1 μg $\cdot$ kg^{-1} $\cdot$ min^{-1} every 10 minutes)

Suxamethonium 1.0–2.0 mg/kg

Thiopentone Stat dose, 3–5 mg/kg IV

Infusion, 2–4 mg $\cdot$ kg^{-1} $\cdot$ h^{-1}

Vasopressin 0.01–0.02 unit $\cdot$ kg^{-1} $\cdot$ h^{-1}

FURTHER READING

Baines, D. B., Wark, H., & Overton, J. H. (1985). Acute epiglottis in children. *Anaesthesia and Intensive Care* 13:25–8.

Behrman, R. E. (1991). *Nelson Textbook of Pediatrics,* 14th ed. Philadelphia: Saunders.

Dashefsky, B. (1991). Life threatening infections. *Paediatric Emergency Care* 7:244–53.

Editor (1988). Pneumonia in childhood. *Lancet* 1:741–3.

Holbrook, P. R. (ed.) (1988). Issues in pediatric critical care. *Critical Care Clinics* 4:645–885.

Holbrook, P. R. (1988). Issues in airway management. *Critical Care Clinics* 4:787–802.

Khilnani, P. (1992). Electrolyte abnormalities in children. *Critical Care Medicine* 20:241–50.

Lloyd-Thomas, A. R. (1990). Paediatric trauma. *British Medical Journal* 301:336–8, 380–2.

Mackway-Jones, K., Molyneux, E., Phillips, B., & Wieteska, S. (eds.) (1993). *Advanced Paediatric Life Support*. London: BMJ Group.

Pfenninger, J. (1993). Neurological intensive care in children. *Intensive Care Medicine* 19:243–50.

Rogers, M. C. (1989). *Handbook of Pediatric Intensive Care*. Baltimore: Williams & Wilkins.

32

OBSTETRIC EMERGENCIES

> • Obstetric emergencies involve young patients who are at the limits of normal physiological adaptation, because of late pregnancy, and who can develop catastrophic multisystem disease.
> • One must understand the normal physiology of both patients and be aware of how these two patients interact with each other and with the underlying disease.
> • The obstetrician, neonatologist, and intensivist must work closely together in managing these patients.

Physicians dealing with critically ill obstetric patients are encouraged to familiarize themselves with the normal physiology (Table 32.1, Figure 32.1) and pathophysiology of pregnancy by reading text-books such as *The Critically Ill Obstetric Patient,* by Baldwin and Hanson, or collections such as *Obstetric Emergencies,* edited by Clark, as cited at the end of this chapter. Many rare and spectacular presentations of critical illness, such as post-partum capillary-leak syndrome, fulminant hepatic failure of pregnancy, and post-partum cardiomyopathy, can be encountered in obstetric practice. Many other, more common complications, such as massive bleeding, will also be encountered. Only pre-eclampsia, eclampsia, post-partum haemorrhage, abruptio placentae, and amniotic fluid embolism will be discussed here.

Often there is doubt about the most suitable place to manage these emergencies – in an obstetric environment or an intensive care environment. All hospitals should develop their own policies, depending on their respective experiences and the severity of the illness. If there is any doubt, the patient should be managed in an intensive care environment until the threat to the patient's life abates. Intensivists quite understandably can become very nervous when consulting with obstetricians. Severely ill obstetric patients are amongst the most challenging in intensive care.

TABLE 32.1 SOME PHYSIOLOGICAL CHANGES
DURING PREGNANCY

Increased pulse rate (to 85–90 beats/min)
Decreased blood pressure in second trimester (by 5–15 mm Hg)
Cardiac output increases (by 1–1.5 L/min)
Reduction in peripheral resistance
Maternal blood volume increases by 25–50% by late pregnancy
Uterine blood flow increases from 50 to 500 ml/min at term (10% of cardiac output)
Renal blood flow and glomerular filtration rate increases
Tidal volume increase by 40%
Respiratory rate unchanged
Respiratory alkalosis
Delayed gastric emptying
Hypercoagulability

ECLAMPSIA AND PRE-ECLAMPSIA: PREGNANCY-INDUCED HYPERTENSION

Definition

Eclampsia and pre-eclampsia are parts of the spectrum of pregnancy-induced hypertension. Hypertension during pregnancy is defined as a systolic blood pressure ≥ 140 mm Hg and/or a diastolic blood pressure ≥ 90 mm Hg, or, alternatively, a rise in systolic blood pressure of more than 25 mm Hg or a rise in diastolic blood pressure of more than 15 mm Hg from the pressure recorded before conception or during the first trimester. Pregnancy-induced hypertension affects approximately 15% of primigravidas.

Hypertension during pregnancy is usually classified as follows:

Pre-eclampsia
   mild
   severe
Chronic hypertension
   essential
   secondary
Pre-eclampsia superimposed on chronic hypertension

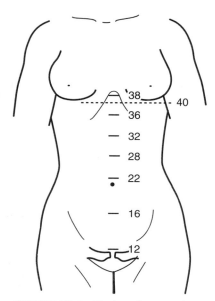

FIGURE 32.1 Uterine size at various stages of pregnancy (in weeks).

The definitions of eclampsia and pre-eclampsia remain controversial. Moreover, the components of the classic triad of hypertension, proteinuria, and oedema do not always occur simultaneously, can occur alone in other disease states, and can even be present during normal pregnancy.

PRE-ECLAMPSIA   Pre-eclampsia is also known as pregnancy-induced hypertension (PIH). It is associated with proteinuria, oedema, and high blood pressure occurring after the 20th week of gestation, and usually abating within 24–48 hours of delivery in the absence of a history of hypertension or renal disease in a patient who had normal blood pressure before pregnancy. It is usually a disease of primigravidas. Oedema is of uncertain significance in the definition. The more severe the proteinuria, the more severe the pre-eclampsia.

ECLAMPSIA   Eclampsia is PIH with superimposed convulsions. It can occur in patients with mild or severe forms of pre-eclampsia.

PATHOPHYSIOLOGY

The pathophysiology of PIH is uncertain, though theories abound. The result, whatever the cause, is widespread maternal vasospasm and intravascular volume contraction leading to organ hypoperfusion. Dysfunctions occur primarily in renal, hepatic, haematological, neurological, and uteroplacental vascular beds secondary to thrombosis and vasospasm.

MONITORING AND INVESTIGATION

Exclude other possible causes of hypertension, such as essential, primary renal abnormalities, phaeochromocytoma, and coarctation of the aorta.

The initial assessment of patients with severe PIH (Table 32.2) must include neurological assessment, cardiorespiratory evaluation, and laboratory determinations of haematological, renal, and hepatic functions.

ROUTINE MONITORING   The following are only guidelines. The extent and frequency of repeated monitoring will depend on the severity of the illness, the gestational age of the fetus, and the timing of the delivery:

- blood pressure   4-hourly
- pulse rate   4-hourly
- midstream urine specimen for urinalysis   daily
  and microscopy
- full blood count   daily
- clotting studies and platelet count   daily
- liver function tests and serum uric acid   daily
- renal function tests   daily
- plasma protein, creatinine, urea, and urine output   daily
- continual ECG monitoring, regular determinations of arterial blood gases, central venous pressure (CVP), and pulmonary artery wedge pressure (PAWP) in severe cases
- fetal growth and well-being: fetal movements, and serial ultrasound of fetal size

TABLE 32.2 DIAGNOSTIC CRITERIA FOR SEVERE
PREGNANCY-INDUCED HYPERTENSION

Cardiac
Diastolic BP $\geq$ 110 mm Hg
Pulmonary oedema
Neurological
Visual disturbances
Convulsions
Hyperreflexia with clonus
Renal
Serum creatinine $>$ 100 μmol/L
Proteinuria $>$ 2+ on dipstick testing
Oliguria
Serum uric acid $>$ 0.40 mmol/L
Hepatic
Epigastric pain
Elevated plasma bilirubin
Elevated aspartate transaminase
Haematological
Thrombocytopenia
Haemolysis
Fetal
Growth retardation
Abnormal cardiotocograph

Source: From Brown (1989), with permission.

• more intensive fetal monitoring in severe PIH, such as cardiotocography (CTG), biophysical profile, Doppler velocimetry, and amniocentesis to determine maturation of fetal lungs

MANAGEMENT

Prevention

Whereas diuretics and salt restriction will not influence the incidence of pre-eclampsia, supplemental calcium and low-dosage aspirin may prove to have some beneficial effects.

Sedation

Where possible, sedation should be avoided, because the drugs can cross into the fetal circulation and have prolonged effects. Prophylactic anticonvulsants are commonly given (see p. 782).

Fluid balance

The paradox of pre-eclampsia is the simultaneous presence of peripheral oedema and hypovolaemia. The average plasma volume deficit is 400–600 ml. To address this problem, give minimal amounts of crystalloids and hypotonic solutions in order to reduce excessive salt and water retention. Excessive fluid can cause not only peripheral oedema but also pulmonary oedema. Simultaneously, give intravenous colloids or blood as necessary in order to maintain the intravascular volume (see p. 61). Colloid solutions may be preferable to crystalloid solutions, as they will maintain the intravascular volume without exacerbating oedema and at the same time will increase rather than decrease the colloid oncotic pressure. It is particularly important to give fluid when antihypertensives are used, as the underlying hypovolaemia will be exacerbated by the vasodilation. Maintain the colloid osmotic pressure with a protein solution if necessary. Avoid diuretics, as they would exacerbate the relative hypovolaemia.

Control of hypertension

Hypertension can result in complications such as cerebral haemorrhage and placental abruption. Medical intervention is necessary when the systolic or diastolic pressure exceeds 170 or 110 mm Hg, respectively. Attempt to maintain the diastolic blood pressure between 90 and 110 mm Hg.

AVOID RAPID DECREASES IN BLOOD PRESSURE, WHICH COULD COMPROMISE PLACENTAL PERFUSION. PLACENTAL BLOOD FLOW IS NOT AUTOREGULATED AND IS TOTALLY DEPENDENT ON MATERNAL BLOOD PRESSURE.

TO AVOID HYPOVOLAEMIA, INTRAVENOUS FLUID IS ALMOST ALWAYS NECESSARY, ESPECIALLY WHEN VASODILATION OCCURS AS A RESULT OF ANTIHYPERTENSIVE AGENTS (see Chapter 23).

BLOOD PRESSURE SHOULD BE CONTINUOUSLY MONITORED DURING ANTIHYPERTENSIVE TREATMENT, EITHER INVASIVELY OR NON-INVASIVELY.

DRUG TREATMENT

Hydralazine   Give hydralazine, 5–10 mg IV, over 15 minutes, with frequent measurements of blood pressure. Alternatively, a continuous intravenous infusion can be used: 5–20 mg/h, titrated against response. The mechanism of action is through direct relaxation of arteriolar smooth muscle. This is the most common first-line drug.

Labetalol   Give labetalol by intravenous infusion, 5–500 μg/min.

Nifedipine   Give nifedipine, 5 mg sublingually initially, with repeated doses of 5–10 mg no more frequently than every 30 minutes.

Sodium nitroprusside   Give sodium nitroprusside as a continuous infusion (50 mg/50 ml), commencing at 5 μg/min, up to a maximum of 500 μg/min, SLOWLY and SMOOTHLY, to prevent precipitous falls in blood pressure. Measure plasma cyanide levels when using prolonged high-dosage infusions.

Diazoxide   Diazoxide has been used extensively for severe hypertension in patients with pre-eclampsia (15–30 mg every 10–15 minutes). However, it can cause rapid drops in blood pressure that can be dangerous for maternal and fetal perfusions.

Avoid diuretics and angiotensin-converting enzyme (ACE) inhibitors, as the circulating volume is low, and precipitous falls in blood pressure can result. ACE inhibitors have also been associated with fetal retardation. Non-steroidal anti-inflammatory drugs (NSAIDs) should also be avoided, as they can precipitate a hypertensive crisis and renal failure.

Epidural analgesia

For many years, the fear of systemic hypotension and fetal distress as a result of sympathetic blockade and peripheral vasodilation resulted in avoidance of epidural anaesthesia. However, with careful fluid administration to prevent hypovolaemia, it is now becoming the technique of choice for labour and Caesarean section.

Epidural analgesia helps to control maternal blood pressure and increase placental perfusion. The intravascular volume must be main-

TABLE 32.3 GUIDELINES FOR DELIVERY IN PRE-ECLAMPSIA

Maternal
Inability to control blood pressure
Deteriorating liver function
Deteriorating renal function
Progressive thrombocytopenia
Neurological complications
Fetal
Non-reactive, positive spontaneous- or induced-contraction stress test with deceleration
Intrauterine growth retardation

tained, and only small doses should be given to achieve a satisfactory block, while monitoring the blood pressure. Epidurals are contraindicated in the presence of coagulopathy and local infection.

Coagulopathy

A full blood count, platelet count, and coagulation profile should be performed at least daily for all severely ill patients with pre-eclampsia.

The basis of treatment consists in correction of the underlying disorder and replacement of coagulation factors as necessary (see p. 712).

Timing of delivery

After the patient has been resuscitated and stabilized, delivery should be considered in severe cases (Table 32.3), no matter what the gestational age of the fetus, as this is the only definitive way of arresting pre-eclampsia. The indications for delivery are outlined in Table 32.3. Each case must be considered individually, and the indications viewed as guidelines only.

In the meantime, nurse the mother in the left lateral position, when possible, in order to decrease caval compression and maintain uterine blood flow.

Most cases of severe pre-eclampsia require Caesarean section. Adequate analgesia is important both during and after delivery. Oxytocin, not ergometrine, should be used, in order to avoid excessive hypertension.

Close monitoring must be maintained for at least 48 hours post partum.

Epidural analgesia will provide pain relief and help to control the blood pressure. If it is not possible to use an epidural, a continuous intravenous infusion of narcotic can be used after delivery (see p. 116).

Prevention of convulsions

This is a controversial area. Magnesium treatment is commonly used in North America as seizure prophylaxis, whereas in Europe and Australasia, phenytoin (15 mg/kg as a loading dose, and then according to levels) (see p. 617) and other, more standard anticonvulsants such as benzodiazepines and barbiturates, are used (see p. 617). As yet, controlled comparative trials have not demonstrated which, if any, of the drugs are most efficacious in preventing seizures.

MAGNESIUM TREATMENT Magnesium has been used with success in patients with severe pre-eclampsia in order to prevent convulsions. Unlike other antiepileptic drugs, it has the advantage of not being detrimental to fetal function in therapeutic doses.

Before commencing treatment, assess renal function, and determine the plasma magnesium concentration. The use of magnesium in the presence of renal insufficiency is hazardous.

Use a continuous intravenous infusion of magnesium, preferably via a central vein using a multilumen catheter, with one lumen dedicated to the infusion in order to prevent inadvertent bolus injections. The infusions should be continued for 24–72 hours post partum:

- magnesium sulphate:
Loading dose, 4 g, over 20 minutes (20 ml of 20% magnesium, or approximately 16 mmol magnesium)
Infusion, 1 g/h (4 mmol magnesium per hour)
   OR
- magnesium chloride:
Loading dose, 2 g, over 20 minutes (20.8 mmol magnesium)
Infusion, 0.5 g/h (5.2 mmol magnesium per hour)

These are only guidelines to achieve plasma levels of magnesium within the therapeutic range of 2.0–3.5 mmol/L. Clinically, the rate should be titrated in order to avoid effects such as decreased reflexes and muscle weakness. Beware of the prolonged actions of neuromuscular blocking agents, even when magnesium is in the therapeutic range.

EFFECTS OF INCREASING PLASMA MAGNESIUM LEVELS

	Plasma magnesium (mmol/L)
Normal	0.8–1.1
Therapeutic range	2.0–3.5
ECG changes (increased PR interval and widening QRS complex)	>3.0
Drowsiness	>4.0
Absence of deep-tendon reflexes	>4.0
Respiratory arrest	>5.0
Heart block	>7.5
Cardiac arrest	>10.0

Determine magnesium levels hourly, until stable levels are achieved. The myocardial- and skeletal-muscle effects of magnesium can be partially reversed by intravenous calcium.

ECLAMPSIA

The exact causes of seizures in patients with pre-eclampsia are unknown, but hypertensive encephalopathy, vasospasm, ischaemia, haemorrhage, and cerebral oedema may be responsible. The standard treatment is rapid control of the seizures, control of the airway, if necessary, and delivery of the fetus.

CONVULSIONS MUST BE RAPIDLY CONTROLLED, AS THEY CAN BE LIFE-THREATENING (see p. 613):

- diazepam, 2–5 mg increments intravenously
- phenytoin, 20 mg/kg IV, over 20 minutes (<50 mg/min), as a loading dose, then 5 mg/kg IV daily, as a single dose, over 1 hour
- thiopentone, 25–50 mg increments intravenously – may potentiate hypotension, which should be rapidly corrected with fluid replacement

Control and clear the airway.

Administer oxygen.

Prevent aortocaval compression and pulmonary aspiration.

Endotracheal intubation and ventilation may be necessary.

Continually assess the fetal state. An emergency Caesarean section may be necessary.

Exclude other possible causes of seizures (eg cerebral oedema or intracerebral bleed) if they are not being controlled.

HELLP SYNDROME

The term 'HELLP syndrome' is derived from the combination 'Haemolysis, Elevated Liver enzymes, and Low Platelet count'. The term is being used less frequently and probably should be discarded, as it is only a manifestation of severe pre-eclampsia. It can even occur without overt hypertension. Haemolysis and thrombocytopenia are the results of peripheral cellular destruction. The elevated liver enzymes are another manifestation of this multisystem disease. Hepatic infarction, haemorrhage, and even rupture can occur with severe pre-eclampsia and the HELLP syndrome.

Its management is similar to that for pre-eclampsia and ultimately depends on delivery of the fetus. Complete recovery may be delayed in some cases, even after delivery. Plasmapheresis may sometimes be indicated.

POST-PARTUM HAEMORRHAGE

Post-partum haemorrhage (PPH) is empirically defined as loss of more than 500–1,000 ml of blood following delivery. PPH remains a significant cause of maternal morbidity and mortality.

AETIOLOGY

Early causes (<24 hours)

• Uterine atony continues to be the most common cause of PPH.

• Lower-genital-tract tears are also common causes, associated with interventions or prolonged and precipitous delivery.

• Uterine rupture is a rare cause and is associated with previous uterine surgery, operative vaginal delivery, and high parity.

• Uterine inversion is rare and usually obvious.

• Retained placental products can be associated with early or delayed PPH.

• Coagulopathies can directly cause PPH or exacerbate existing PPH (eg in association with sepsis, amniotic-fluid embolism, PIH).

Delayed causes (>24 hours)

• Infection.

• Retained products of conception.

MANAGEMENT

Prevention

Predisposing factors, such as multiple gestation, high parity, previous Caesarean section, polyhydramnios, previous history of PPH, PIH, and uterine polyps, should be identified early.

• Avoid premature administration of agents, such as Pitocin, that are used to facilitate placental delivery.

• Carefully inspect the placenta for intact delivery.

• Manual removal of placenta may be appropriate if it has not been delivered within 10 minutes of birth.

• Oxytocin infusion is commonly employed in order to optimize uterine tone after placental delivery.

Active management

1. Determine the cause and treat it at the same time as the patient is being resuscitated.

2. Early recognition and aggressive treatment of blood loss are essential.

3. Establish intravenous access, and begin replenishment of the intravascular volume early (see p. 61). Give high-flow oxygen via mask.

4. Monitoring:

   (a) Vital signs

- blood pressure
- pulse rate
- respiratory rate
- urine output

   (b) Estimation of blood loss

   (c) More complex monitoring, such as ECG, pulse oximetry, CVP, and pulmonary artery catheterization, may be necessary in severe cases.

5. Rapidly perform

   (a) Blood cross-match

   (b) Complete blood count

May also need

   (a) Coagulation screen

- prothrombin time
- partial thromboplastin time
- fibrinogen level
- fibrin split products

   (b) Arterial blood gases

6. Rapidly replace lost blood with fluid, according to vital signs (see p. 61). Blood losses tend to be under-estimated. It is very difficult to over-transfuse patients with PPH. Fresh frozen plasma and other components may also be needed (see p. 712).

7. Specific causes:

   (a) Uterine atony

- fundal compression
- oxytocin infusion (10–40 units in 100 ml of isotonic saline)
- other measures (eg prostaglandin $F_{2\alpha}$ by intrauterine or intramuscular injection)

   (b) Other

- Examine the perineum, vagina, and cervix for tears and for material in the cervix.
- Manual examination and removal of these products should be conducted if necessary.

8. If bleeding persists, consider
- curettage of the uterus
- ligation of pelvic arterial vessels
- angiographic embolization
- hysterectomy

ABRUPTIO PLACENTAE

Abruptio placentae is characterized by complete or partial separation of the placenta prior to birth. It is usually as a result of bleeding into the decidua basalis.

Causes

- There is no unifying theory.
- Associated with a high incidence of maternal hypertension.
- As many as 10% of patients with severe PIH have abruption.
- Other causes can include blunt trauma (see p. 305).

DIAGNOSIS

Abruptio placentae is divided into three grades:

Grade I
- about 40% of cases
- slight vaginal bleeding
- normal maternal blood pressure, and no coagulopathy
- no fetal distress

Grade II
- about 45% of cases
- greater amount of vaginal bleeding
- maternal hypofibrinogenaemia
- fetal distress

Grade III
- about 15% of cases
- heavy vaginal bleeding

- uterine tenderness
- maternal coagulopathy and thrombocytopenia
- fetal death usually occurs

COMMON SIGNS AND SYMPTOMS

- Vaginal bleeding in the third trimester. Haemorrhage is overt in 80% of cases and is concealed in the remainder.
- Pain in about 50% of cases.
- Uterine tenderness and contractions in about 20% of cases.
- Signs of maternal blood loss.
- Perinatal ultrasound may assist in the diagnosis.
- Fetal distress and death.

The differential diagnosis must include uterine rupture, placenta praevia, and polyhydramnios.

INVESTIGATIONS AND MONITORING

There should be regular monitoring of maternal vital signs:

- blood pressure
- pulse rate
- urine output
- respiratory rate

More complex monitoring may be needed if blood loss is severe (see p. 499). The following investigations and determinations are necessary:

- full blood count and cross-match
- coagulation tests (see p. 716)
- arterial blood gases
- urea, creatinine, and electrolytes

Fetal monitoring must include the following:

- Fetal heart rate.
- Determine gestational age, fetal weight and viability, and placental location with ultrasound examination.

MANAGEMENT

• The major problems are maternal blood loss, coagulopathy, and fetal distress or death. Assessment and resuscitation should be carried out simultaneously. Fluid resuscitation is much the same as for PPH (see p. 785). Establish an intravenous line, and replenish the intravascular volume with colloid or crystalloid solution and blood if necessary. Blood losses often are under-estimated.

• Disseminated intravascular coagulopathy is seen in about 10% of cases (see p. 722). It usually occurs only after massive blood loss or when the fetus is dead. It should be clinically suspected when bleeding is excessive or when oozing is seen from venous puncture sites. Coagulation factors and platelets may also be needed (see p. 711).

• The definitive treatment is delivery of the fetus and placenta. This will depend on maternal and fetal condition, as well as gestational age.

AMNIOTIC-FLUID EMBOLISM

Amniotic-fluid embolism is a rare complication of pregnancy, labour, and the post-partum period. It is characterized by hypotension, hypoxia, and coagulopathy and is associated with mortality as high as 80%. Half of all patients die within 1 hour.

It occurs more frequently in elderly multiparous patients.

The amniotic fluid probably enters the circulation through a tear in the membranes. It can occur during abortion in the first or second trimester, or as a result of abdominal trauma, amniocentesis, or hysterotomy, or even in the post-partum period. However, most episodes occur during labour.

PATHOGENESIS

The pathogenesis of this condition still is not completely understood. It is a biphasic process apparently triggered by embolization of amniotic fluid or debris of fetal origin into the maternal venous circulation. The initial phase is acute cardiorespiratory collapse, followed by a consumptive coagulopathy. Either of the phases can predominate.

Amniotic fluid in the pulmonary circulation causes

- pulmonary vascular obstruction, with sudden decreases in left atrial pressure and cardiac output associated with hypotension and cardiac arrest
- acute cor pulmonale
- gross ventilation/perfusion inequality and severe hypoxia

CLINICAL FEATURES

- respiratory distress and pulmonary oedema
- cyanosis
- cardiovascular collapse
- convulsions and coma
- bleeding diathesis and haemorrhage

DIAGNOSIS

- The diagnosis is usually made on clinical grounds.
- Elements of amniotic fluid and fetal cells occasionally are found in the maternal circulation, but their exact clinical significance is unknown.
- At post-mortem examination, amniotic-fluid material is often found in lung, coronary arteries, kidney, and brain.
- The differential diagnosis should include septic shock, aspiration pneumonitis, acute myocardial infarction, pulmonary embolism, placental abruption, and an accidental high spinal block during epidural analgesia.

MANAGEMENT

Treatment is aimed at resuscitation and support.

Cardiovascular support

- Intravenous fluids to restore circulatory balance (see p. 61).
- Monitor left- and right-side pressures via pulmonary artery catheter in severe cases.
- Inotropic support may also be necessary (see p. 520).

• Careful pulmonary vascular dilation with drugs such as prostacyclin or sodium nitroprusside, with appropriate pressure monitoring, may be indicated.

Respiratory support

Increases in the inspired oxygen, positive end-expiratory pressure, continuous positive airway pressure, intermittent positive-pressure ventilation, and other general measures may be needed to correct hypoxia.

Haematological support

There are few guidelines for management of the severe coagulopathies that accompany amniotic-fluid embolism. Some authors recommend correction of coagulation-factor deficiencies, including the hypofibrinogenaemia, and others suggest heparin. Although there is confusion, the advice of a clinical haematologist should be sought, and each coagulation abnormality must be treated on its merits.

Fetal management

The fetus will also suffer from the effects of anoxia and hypotension and should be closely monitored and delivered rapidly, with full resuscitation facilities.

FURTHER READING

Australasian Society for the Study of Hypertension in Pregnancy (1993). Consensus statement: management of hypertension in pregnancy, executive summary. *Medical Journal of Australia* 158:700–3.

Brown, M. A. (1989). Pregnancy induced hypertension. *Current Concepts* 17:185–97.

Clark, S. L. (ed.) (1991). Obstetric emergencies. *Critical Care Clinics* 7:763–929 (symposium issue).

Cotton, D. B., & Clark, S. L. (eds.) (1986). Critical care in obstetrics. *Clinics in Perinatology* 13:695–885 (symposium issue).

Cunningham, F. G., & Lindheimer, M. D. (1992). Hypertension in pregnancy. *New England Journal of Medicine* 326:927–32.

Morgan, M. (1979). Amniotic fluid embolism. *Anaesthesia* 34:20–34.

Nolan, T. E., Wakefield, M. L., & Devoe, L. D. (1992). Invasive hemodynamic monitoring in obstetrics. A critical review of its indications, benefits, complications and alternatives. *Chest* 101:1429–33.

Peterson, E. P., & Taylor, H. B. (1970). Amniotic fluid embolism: an analysis of 40 cases. *Obstetrics and Gynecology* 35:787–93.

SI UNITS

BASIC AND DERIVED UNITS

metre	m	unit of length (L)
kilogramme	kg	unit of mass (M)
second	s	unit of time (T)
kelvin	K	unit of temperature
candela	cd	unit of luminous intensity
bel	b	unit of sound intensity, 1 decibel = 0.1 bel
ampere	A	unit of electrical current, $1\ A = 2 \times 10^{-7}\ \text{N/m}$
hertz	Hz	unit of frequency (one cycle per second)
mole	mol	unit of amount of substance in grams
newton	N	unit of force that will give 1 kilogramme of mass an acceleration of 1 metre per second ($1\ \text{N} = 1\ \text{kg} \cdot \text{m} \cdot \text{s}^{-2}$)
pascal	Pa	unit of pressure expressed as force per unit area ($1\ \text{Pa} = 1\ \text{N/m}^2$)
joule	J	unit of energy or work (force through a distance) ($1\ \text{J} = 1\ \text{N} \cdot \text{m}$)
watt	W	unit of power (energy per second) ($1\ \text{W} = 1\ \text{N} \cdot \text{m} \cdot \text{s}^{-1} = 1\ \text{J} \cdot \text{s}^{-1}$)
coulomb	C	unit of electric charge ($1\ \text{C} = 1\ \text{A} \cdot \text{s}$)
volt	V	unit of electrical potential difference ($1\ \text{V} = 1\ \text{W} \cdot \text{A}^{-1} = 1\ \text{J} \cdot \text{A}^{-1} \cdot \text{s}^{-1}$)
ohm	Ω	unit of electrical resistance ($1\ \Omega = 1\ \text{V} \cdot \text{A}^{-1}$)

Prefixes to SI units to indicate fractions or multiples

10^{12}	tera	T	10^{-15}	femto	f
10^{9}	giga	G	10^{-12}	pico	p
10^{6}	mega	M	10^{-9}	nano	n
10^{3}	kilo	k (K)	10^{-6}	micro	μ
10	deca	da (D)	10^{-3}	milli	m
			10^{-1}	deci	d

2 NORMAL BIOCHEMICAL VALUES

'Normal' values will vary between laboratories. The figures are representative of normal values, but should be checked with your own laboratory.

Blood specimen tube:

C	Clotted sample
L	Lithium heparin tube
H	Heparinized whole blood
*	Seek lab advice
EDTA	Sequestrone tube

Name	Values in old units		Values in SI units		Blood specimen required and comments
Adrenaline	0.01	μg/%	0.546	nmol/L	*
Alanine-aminotrans-ferase (ALT)			5–35	U/L	C
Ammonium	20–50	μg/%	12–31	μmol/L	L (to lab without delay)
Amylase	0–180	Somogyi U/%	70–300	U/L	L
Aspartate-aminotrans-ferase (AST)			5–35	U/L	C
Bicarbonate					
actual	24–30	mEq/L	24–30	mmol/L	L
standard	21–25	mEq/L	21–25	mmol/L	L
Bilirubin					
total	0.2–1.0	mg/%	3–17	μmol/L	C
conjugated	<0.4	mg/%	<7.0	μmol/L	C

Caeruloplasmin	30–60	mg/dl	300–600	mg/L	C
Calcium					
total	8.5–10.6	mg/%	2.25–2.65	mmol/L	C
ionized	4–5	mg/%	1.0–1.25	mmol/L	C
Catechola-mines	1	μg/%	<54.6	nmol/L	*
Chloride	95–105	mEq/L	95–105	mmol/L	L
Cholesterol	150–300	mg/%	3.9–7.5	mmol/L	L
Cholinesterase					
acetyl	—		9–25	μmol · ml^{-1} · mm^{-1}	C
plasma	40–100	U/%	—		
Complement					
C3			0.7–1.8	g/L	*
C4	0.16–0.45	g/L			
Copper	76–165	μg/%	12–26	nmol/L	EDTA
Cortisol					
0900 h	10–25.3	μg/%	280–700	nmol/L	L
2400 h	<5–10	μg/%	<140–280	nmol/L	L
Creatinine	0.7–1.7	mg/%	70–150	μmol/L	L
Creatine phospho-kinase (CK)					
male	100	U/L	25–195	U/L	C
female	60	U/L	25–170	U/L	C
Creatinine clearance	120	ml/min	—		*
Fibrinogen	200–500	mg/%	2.0–5.0	g/L	* (citrate bottle)
Folate	3–20	ng/ml	3–20	μg/L	C
Glucose					
fasting	72–108	mg/%	4.0–6.0	mmol/L	fluoride bottle
postprandial	<180	mg/%	<10	mmol/L	
Gamma glutamyl transferase	7–25	U/L	10–55	U/L	
Growth hormone					
male			<6	mU/L	*
female			<16	mU/L	*

Insulin (fasting)			<20	mU/L	
Iodine, total	3.5–8.0	μg/%	273–624	nmol/L	C
Iodine, protein-bound	4.0–7.5	μg/%	300–600	nmol/L	C
Iodine 131 uptake	20–50% of dose in 24 h				C
Iron	80–160	μg/%	14–30	μmol/L	C
Total iron-binding capacity (TIBC)	302–420	μg/%	54–75	μmol/L	C
Isocitric dehydrogenase (ICH)	2–4	U/L	20–140	U/L	C
Ketones	0.8–2.4	mg/%	80–140	μmol/L	L
Lactate	3.5–15	mg/%	0.4–1.6	mmol/L	*
Lactate dehydrogenase	100–300	units/L	30–90	U/L	C
Lead	10–40	μg/%	0.5–2.0	μmol/L	EDTA
Lipids, total	400–1,000	mg/%	4.0–10.0	g/L	C
S particles	0–550	mg/%	0–5.5	g/L	C
M particles	0–240	mg/%	0–2.4	g/L	C
L particles	0–28	mg/%	0–0.28	g/L	C
Magnesium	1.4–2.8	mEq/L	0.7–1.00	mmol/L	C
Manganese	2.2	μg/L	40.0	nmol/L	*
Methaemoglobin	0.01–0.5	g/%	0.1–5	g/L	EDTA
Mercury	0–5	μg/dl	0–0.25	μmol/L	*
Nitrogen (non-protein)	18–30	mg/%	12.8–21.5	mmol/L	C
Noradrenaline	0.05	μg/%	<2.95	nmol/L	*
Osmolality	280–300	mOsm/kg	280–300	mOsm/kg	L
Phosphate (inorganic)	2.0–4.5	mg/%	0.8–1.4	mmol/L	C
Phosphatase					
acid	1–5	KA units	1–7	U/L	C
alkaline	3–13	KA units	30–100	U/L	C

Phospholipids	5–10	mg/%	1.6–3.2	mmol/L	C
Potassium	3.5–5.0	mEq/L	3.5–5.0	mmol/L	L
Protein, total	6.0–8.0	g/%	60–80	g/L	C
albumin	3.5–5.0	g/%	35–50	g/L	C
globulin	2.4–3.7	g/%	24–37	g/L	C
IgA	80–500	mg/%	0.8–5.0	g/L	C
IgG	700–1,900	mg/%	7–19	g/L	C
IgM	50–200	mg/%	0.5–2.0	g/L	C
Pyruvate	0.4–0.7	mg/%	45–80	μmol/L	*
Sodium	135–145	mEq/L	135–145	mmol/L	L
Sulphate	1–1.8	mg/%	0.31–0.56	mmol/L	C
Thyroid-stimulating hormone (TSH)	—		1–11	munits/L	*
T_3	—		1.3–2.9	nmol/L		*
T_4	5.0–12.0	μg/%	69–150	nmol/L	C
Triglycerides	30–150	mg/%	0.34–1.7	mmol/L	C
Transferrin	120–200	mg/%	1.2–2.0	g/L	C
T_3 uptake	95–115	%	95–115	%	C
Urate	2–7	mg/%	0.1–0.4	mmol/L	C
Urea	15–40	mg/%	2.5–6.5	mmol/L	L
Urea nitrogen	10–20	mg/%	1.6–3.3	mmol/L	L
Uric acid					
male	3.5–8.0	mg/%	0.21–0.48	mmol/L	C
female	2.5–6.5	mg/%	0.15–0.39	mmol/L	C
Zinc	1–2	mEq/L	0.5–1	mmol/L	C

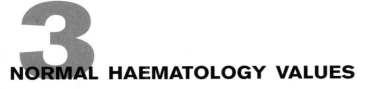

NORMAL HAEMATOLOGY VALUES

Haemoglobin (Hb)	
male	13.0–18.0 g/dl
female	11.5–16.5 g/dl
Red-blood-cell count (RBC)	
male	$4.5–6.5 \times 10^{12}$/L
female	$3.5–5.0 \times 10^{12}$/L
White-blood-cell count (WBC)	$4.0–11.0 \times 10^{9}$/L
Neutrophils (40–75%)	$2.5–7.5 \times 10^{9}$/L
Lymphocytes (20–45%)	$1.5–3.5 \times 10^{9}$/L
Monocytes (2–10%)	$0.2–0.8 \times 10^{9}$/L
Eosinophils (1–6%)	$0.04–0.44 \times 10^{9}$/L
Basophils (0–1%)	$0–0.1 \times 10^{9}$/L
Platelet count	$150–400 \times 10^{9}$/L
Reticulocyte count	0–2% of RBCs
Sedimentation rate (ESR)	
male	0–5 mm/h
female	0–7 mm/h
Haematocrit (HCT)	
male	0.40–0.54
female	0.37–0.47
Mean corpuscular volume (MCV)	76–96 fl (femtolitre)
Mean corpuscular haemoglobin concentration (MCHC)	32–36 g/dl
Mean corpuscular haemoglobin (MCH)	27–32 pg (picogram)

Routine clotting screen

Activated partial thromboplastin time (APTT)	21–36 seconds
Bleeding time	<9 minutes
d-dimers	<0.25 mg/L
Fibrin degradation products (FDP)	<10 μg/ml
Fibrinogen	1.5–4.0 g/dl

International normalized ratio used to control warfarin treatment (INR)	2–2.5 as prophylaxis for deep venous thrombosis (DVT)
	2–3 as treatment for DVT and pulmonary embolism
	3–4.5 for recurrent DVT and pulmonary embolism, arterial disease and grafts, cardiac prosthetic valves
Platelet count	$150–400 \times 10^9$/L
Prothrombin index (PI)	80–100%
Prothrombin time (PT)	10–14 seconds
Prothrombin ratio (PT/control) (PTR)	1.0–1.3

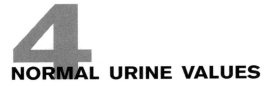

NORMAL URINE VALUES

Name	Values	
Adrenaline	<100	nmol/24 h
Aldosterone	<50.0	μmol/24 h
Ammonium	18–60	mmol/24 h
Amylase	100–1,000	units/24 h
Calcium	2.5–7.5	mmol/24 h
Catecholamines		
Hydroxymethoxymandelic acid (HMMA) or vanillylmandelic acid (VMA)	15–75	μmol/24 h
Noradrenaline	30–592	nmol/24 h
Chloride	100–300	mmol/24 h
Cortisol	0.2–1.0	μmol/24 h
Creatinine	10–20	mmol/24 h
Creatinine clearance	120	ml/min
Copper	0.2–1.0	μmol/24 h
Coproporphyrin	150–300	nmol/24 h
Folic acid	3.5–23.5	μg/24 h
Glomerular filtration rate	105–140	ml/min
Glucose	0–11	$mmol \cdot L^{-1} \cdot d^{-1}$
Hydroxyproline	0.08–0.25	mmol/24 h
5-Hydroxyindoleacetic acid (5-HIAA)	15–75	μmol/24 h
17-keto steroids	34–100	μmol/24 h
Lead	<0.40	μmol/24 h
Magnesium	3.3–5.0	mmol/24 h
Oestriol (after 30-week pregnancy)	30–140	μmol/24 h
Oestrogens		
pregnant	14–86.7	μmol/24 h
non-pregnant	14–347	μmol/24 h
Osmolality	300–1,000	mOsm/24 h
Oxalate	<300	μmol/24 h
Phosphate	15–50	mmol/24 h
Potassium	40–120	mmol/24 h
Protein (albumin)	0.02–0.1	g/24 h
pH (hydrogen ion)	10–30,000	nmol/24 h

		(pH 4.5–8.0)
Phosphatase, acid		
male	164	KA units/24 h
female	217	KA units/24 h
Porphobilinogen	1–10	μmol/24 h
Renal plasma flow	500–800	ml/min
Sodium	50–250	mmol/24 h
Specific gravity	1,003–1,030	
Urea	50–500	mmol/24 h
Urea clearance	60–95	ml/min
Urate	2–6	mmol/24 h
Urobilinogen	0–6.7	μmol/24 h
Uroporphyrin I and II	0–30	nmol/24 h

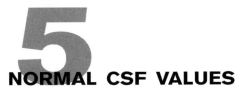

NORMAL CSF VALUES

Parameter	Values in SI units
Pressure	7.0–15.0 cm H_2O (0.93–2.0 kPa)
Volume	120–140 ml
Hydrogen ion	50–54 mmol/L (pH 7.30–7.35)
Specific gravity	1,007
Osmolality	306 mOsm/kg
Calcium	1–1.5 mmol/L
Chloride	120–130 mmol/L
Glucose	2.7–4.5 mmol/L (1.0 mmol/L less than blood sugar)
Lactate	<2.8 mmol/L
Magnesium	0.36–3.2 mmol/L
Sodium	140 mmol/L
Phosphate	0.13–0.23 mmol/L
Potassium	3–4 mmol/L
Lymphocytes	$0–5 \times 10^6$/L
Protein	0.15–0.45 g/L
globulin	0–20 mg/L
IgG	<0.05 g/L
IgG : total-protein ratio	5–15%

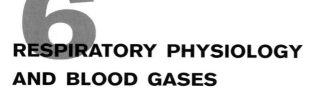

RESPIRATORY PHYSIOLOGY AND BLOOD GASES

BLOOD GASES

Arterial

H^+ concentration (pH)	36–44 nmol/L (7.35–7.44)
Pao_2	11.3–13.3 kPa (85–100 mm Hg)
$Paco_2$	4.8–5.9 kPa (36–44 mm Hg)
O_2 content	8.9–9.4 nmol/L (20–21 volumes/dl)
CO_2 content	21.5–22.5 nmol/L (48–50 volumes/dl)

Venous

H^+ concentration (pH)	38–46 nmol/L (7.34–7.42)
$P\bar{v}o_2$	5–5.6 kPa (37–42 mm Hg)
$P\bar{v}co_2$	5.6–6.7 kPa (42–50 mm Hg)
O_2 content	6.7–7.2 nmol/L (15–16 volumes/dl)
CO_2 content	23.5–24.0 nmol/L (52–54 volumes/dl)

pH CONVERSION TO NANOMOLES

pH units	H^+ concentration (nmol/L)
6.0	1,000.0
6.1	794.2
6.2	630.9
6.3	501.2
6.4	398.1
6.5	316.3
6.6	251.2
6.7	199.5
6.8	158.5
6.9	125.9
7.0	100.0
7.1	79.4
7.2	63.1

7.3	50.1
7.4	39.8
7.5	31.6
7.6	25.1
7.7	19.9
7.8	15.8
7.9	12.6
8.0	10.0

PRESSURE CONVERSION

1 kPa = 7.5 mm Hg
1 mm Hg = 0.133 kPa
1 mm Hg = 1.36 cm H_2O

VENTILATORY ABBREVIATIONS

Primary symbols

C	concentration of gas in the blood
D	diffusing capacity
F	fractional concentration of a dry gas
f	frequency of respiratory (breaths/minute)
P	gas pressure or partial pressure
Q	volume of blood
$\dot{Q}$	volume of blood per unit time
R	respiratory exchange ratio
S	saturation of haemoglobin with oxygen or carbon dioxide
$\overset{\cdot}{V}$	gas volume
$\dot{V}$	volume of gas per unit time

Secondary symbols

A	alveolar gas
a	arterial gas
B	barometric
c	pulmonary capillary blood
c′	pulmonary end-capillary blood
cj	conjunctival
D	dead-space gas
d	difference
E	expired gas

I	inspired gas
i	ideal
jv	jugular vein
L	lung
tc	transcutaneous
T	tidal gas
$\bar{v}$	mixed venous blood

RESPIRATORY MEASUREMENTS

These are only approximate figures for adults, and they are subject to age and weight variations.

Airway resistance	$0.5\text{–}3.4$ cm $H_2O \cdot L^{-1} \cdot s^{-1}$
Alveolar ventilation ($\dot{V}A$)	4.2 L/min ($2\text{–}2.5$ L $\cdot$ min$^{-1} \cdot$ m^{-2})
Alveolar air equation	13.3 kPa (100 mm Hg), approximately
Alveolar–arterial oxygen difference	
breathing air	$5\text{–}20$ mm Hg ($0.7\text{–}2.7$ kPa)
breathing 100% oxygen	$10\text{–}60$ mm Hg ($1.3\text{–}8.0$ kPa)
Compliance	
chest wall	200 ml/cm H_2O
lung	200 ml/cm H_2O
lung & chest wall	100 ml/cm H_2O
Dead space (vD)	150 ml (2.2 ml/kg)
Diffusing capacity of carbon monoxide (Dco)	$17\text{–}20$ ml CO $\cdot$ min$^{-1} \cdot$ (mm Hg)$^{-1}$
Forced expiratory volume in 1 second (FEV$_1$)	$70\text{–}80\%$ of VC
Maximum ventilatory volume (MVV)	120 L/min ($35 \times$ FEV$_1$)
Minute volume (VE)	$5{,}000\text{–}6{,}000$ ml/min (100 ml/kg)
Peak expiratory flow rate (PEFR)	$300\text{–}700$ L/min
Peak inspiratory flow rate (PIFR)	$200\text{–}700$ L/min
Pulmonary capillary blood flow ($\dot{Q}c$)	$5{,}400$ ml/min
Pulmonary capillary blood volume (Qc)	60 ml
Respiratory quotient	0.8 (on normal diet)
Respiratory rate	$12\text{–}14$ bpm
Venous admixture	$5\text{–}10\%$ of cardiac output
Work of breathing	
maximum	98 J/min
quiet	4.9 J/min

Oxygen consumption	115–165 ml $\cdot$ min^{-1} $\cdot$ m^{-2}
Oxygen delivery	900–$1,000$ ml $\cdot$ min^{-1} $\cdot$ m^{-2}

LUNG VOLUMES

Tidal volume (V$_T$)	400–600 ml (7–10 ml/kg)
Total lung capacity (TLC)	5,000–6,500 ml
Vital capacity (VC)	4,200–4,800 ml (52 ml/kg)
Inspiratory capacity (IC)	3,600–4,300 ml
Inspiratory reserve volume (IRV)	3,100–3,750 ml
Expiratory reserve volume (ERV)	950–1,300 ml
Functional residual capacity (FRC)	2,300–2,800 ml
Residual volume (RV)	1,200–1,700 ml

NORMAL PARTIAL PRESSURE OF GASES

A bar above a symbol indicates a mean value.
A dot above a symbol indicates a value per unit time.

Inspired air

P$_{IO_2}$	158 mm Hg (21.06 kPa)
P$_{ICO_2}$	0.3 mm Hg (0.04 kPa)
P$_{IN_2}$	596 mm Hg (79.46 kPa)
P$_{IH_2O}$	5 mm Hg (0.67 kPa)

Expired air

P$_{EO_2}$	116 mm Hg (15.47 kPa)
P$_{ECO_2}$	28 mm Hg (3.73 kPa)
P$_{EN_2}$	568 mm Hg (75.73 kPa)
P$_{EH_2O}$	47 mm Hg (6.27 kPa)

Arterial blood gases

Pa$_{O_2}$	90–110 mm Hg (12.0–14.67 kPa)
Pa$_{CO_2}$	34–46 mm Hg (4.53–6.13 kPa)
Pa$_{N_2}$	573 mm Hg (76.39 kPa)
C$_{H^+}$	44–36 nmol/L (7.35–7.44)

Mixed venous blood gases

P$\bar{v}_{O_2}$	37–42 mm Hg (4.93–5.60 kPa)
P$\bar{v}_{CO_2}$	40–52 mm Hg (5.53–6.93 kPa)
P$\bar{v}_{N_2}$	573 mm Hg (76.39 kPa)
C$_{H^+}$	38–46 nmol/L (7.34–7.42)

Alveolar gas

P$_{AO_2}$	103 mm Hg (13.73 kPa)
P$_{ACO_2}$	40 mm Hg (5.33 kPa)
P$_{AN_2}$	570 mm Hg (75.99 kPa)
P$_{AH_2O}$	47 mm Hg (6.27 kPa)

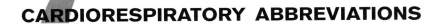

CARDIORESPIRATORY ABBREVIATIONS

$(A\text{-}\overline{v})DO_2$	arterial–mixed-venous oxygen content difference
BSA	body surface area
BP	blood pressure
CI	cardiac index
CO	cardiac output
HR	heart rate
LVSW	left ventricular stroke work
LVSWI	left ventricular stroke-work index
MAP	mean arterial pressure
$\overline{PAP}$	pulmonary artery pressure
PAP	mean pulmonary artery pressure
PAWP	pulmonary artery wedge pressure
$\overline{PAWP}$	mean pulmonary artery wedge pressure
PEO_2	partial pressure of O_2 in expired gas
$PECO_2$	partial pressure of CO_2 in expired gas
PVR	pulmonary vascular resistance
RAP	right atrial pressure
RQ	respiratory quotient
SI	stroke index
SV	stroke volume
SVR	systemic vascular resistance
$\dot{Q}_S/\dot{Q}_T$	venous admixture or pulmonary shunt
$\dot{V}O_2$	oxygen consumption
DO_2	oxygen delivery

CARDIORESPIRATORY EQUATIONS

Body surface area (BSA)	$BSA = (\text{weight})^{0.425} \times (\text{height})^{0.725} \times 71.84 \times 10^{-4}\ m^2$
Cardiac output (CO)	$CO = \text{heart rate (HR)} \times \text{stroke volume (SV)}$
Cardiac index (CI)	$CI = \dfrac{CO}{BSA}\ ml \cdot min^{-1} \cdot m^{-2}$
Stroke volume index (SVI)	$SVI = \dfrac{SV}{BSA}\ ml \cdot beat^{-1} \cdot m^{-2}$

Left ventricular stroke-work index (LVSWI)

$$LVSWI = (MAP - PAWP)(SVI) \times (0.0136) \; g \cdot m \cdot m^{-2}$$

Right ventricular stroke-work index (RVSWI)

$$RVSWI = (PAP - RAP)(SVI) \times (0.0136) \; g \cdot m \cdot m^{-2}$$

Systemic vascular resistance (SVR)

$$SVR = \frac{MAP - RAP}{CO} \times 80 \; dyn \cdot s \cdot cm^{-5}$$

Pulmonary vascular resistance (PVR)

$$PVR = \frac{PAP - PAWP}{CO} \times 80 \; dyn \cdot s \cdot cm^{-5}$$

Respiratory quotient (RQ)

$$RQ = \frac{CO_2 \; produced}{O_2 \; consumed}$$

Alveolar air equation

$$P_{AO_2} = P_{IO_2} - \frac{Pa_{CO_2}}{RQ}$$

OR

$$P_{AO_2} = P_{IO_2} - Pa_{CO_2} \frac{P_{IO_2} - P_{EO_2}}{P_{ECO_2}}$$

Alveolar–arterial difference in partial pressure of oxygen

$$P_{AO_2} - Pa_{O_2}$$

Physiological dead space (Bohr's equation)

$$\frac{V_D}{V_T} = \frac{Pa_{CO_2} - P_{ECO_2}}{Pa_{CO_2}} \quad or \quad \frac{V_D}{V_T} = \frac{Pa_{CO_2} - P_{ECO_2}}{Pa_{CO_2}}$$

Venous admixture

$$\frac{\dot{Q}_S}{\dot{Q}_T} = \frac{Cc'_{O_2} - Ca_{O_2}}{Cc'_{O_2} - C\bar{v}_{O_2}}$$

Oxygen consumption ($\dot{V}_{O_2}$)

$$\dot{V}_{O_2} = (CI)(Ca_{O_2} - C\bar{v}_{O_2}) \; ml \cdot min^{-1} \cdot m^{-2}$$

Oxygen delivery (D_{O_2})

$$D_{O_2} = (CI)(Ca_{O_2}) \; ml \cdot min^{-1} \cdot m^{-2}$$

CARDIOVASCULAR MEASUREMENTS

Cardiac output	4–7 L/min
Cardiac index	3.5–4 L/min
Stroke volume	42–52 ml/beat
Stroke index	36–48 ml/m²
Ejection fraction	0.55–0.75
End-diastolic volume	60–95 ml/m²
End-systolic volume	18–32 ml/m²
Right atrial pressure	1–8 mm Hg (0.13–1.06 kPa)
Pulmonary artery wedge pressure	5–15 mm Hg (0.67–2.0 kPa)
Right ventricular systolic pressure	15–25 mm Hg (2.0–3.3 kPa)
Right ventricular diastolic pressure	0–8 mm Hg (0–1.06 kPa)
Pulmonary artery systolic pressure	15–25 mm Hg (2.0–3.3 kPa)
Pulmonary artery diastolic pressure	8–15 mm Hg (1.06–2.0 kPa)

Pulmonary artery mean pressure	10–20 mm Hg (1.3–2.7 kPa)
Left ventricular stroke-work index	44–55 $g \cdot m \cdot m^{-2}$
Right ventricular stroke-work index	7–10 $g \cdot m \cdot m^{-2}$
Systemic vascular resistance	1,500–3,000 $dyn \cdot s \cdot cm^{-5}$
Pulmonary vascular resistance	100–250 $dyn \cdot s \cdot cm^{-5}$

8

TOXICOLOGY

These data are only approximations. Allowances must be made for individual responses. If in any doubt, contact your local Poison Centre.

Drug	Normal or therapeutic range	Toxic levels
Amitriptyline	0.05–0.2 mg/L	>0.40 mg/L
Aminophylline (theophylline)	10–20 mg/L	>20 mg/L
Amphetamine	0.1–3.0 mg/L	>3 mg/L
Arsenic (blood)	<30 μg/L	>1.0 mg/L
Barbiturates		
Amylobarbitone	2–4 mg/L	>8 mg/L
Barbitone	5–15 mg/L	>20 mg/L
Butobarbitone	2–4 mg/L	>8 mg/L
Cyclobarbitone	2–4 mg/L	>8 mg/L
Heptabarbitone	2–4 mg/L	>8 mg/L
Hexabarbitone	2–4 mg/L	>8 mg/L
Pentobarbitone	2–4 mg/L	>8 mg/L
Phenobarbitone	5–20 mg/L	>25 mg/L
Bromide	50 mg/L	>500 mg/L
Cadmium (blood and urine)	<10 μg/L	>50 μg/L
Carbamazepine	3–13 mg/L	>15 mg/L
Carbon monoxide	1% saturation	>15% saturation of Hb
Chloral hydrate	10–50 mg/L	>50 mg/L
Chloramphenicol	2–6 mg/L	>10 mg/L
Chlordiazepoxide	3–7 mg/L	8 mg/L
Chlormethiazole	0.5–2.0 mg/L	>6 mg/L
Chlorpromazine (free drug)	0.2–0.5 mg/L	>0.8 mg/L
Copper (serum)	0.8–1.5 mg/L	>5.0 mg/L
Cyanide	0.15 mg/L	>2 mg/L

DDT	10 μg/L	>50 μg/L
Desipramine	0.5–1.4 mg/L	>5 mg/L
Dextropropoxyphene	0.2–0.8 mg/L	>1.0 mg/L
Diazepam	0.5–2.5 mg/L	>5 mg/L
Digitoxin	20–35 μg/L	>50 μg/L
Digoxin	1–2 μg/L	>2.5 μg/L
Diphenhydramine	0.5 mg/L	>1.0 mg/L
Ethambutol	3–5 mg/L	>6 mg/L
Ethanol	0.05 g/L (legal Australian driving limit)	0.3 g/L (clinically drunk)
Ethchlorvynol	10–20 mg/L	>20 mg/L
Ethosuximide	40–80 mg/L	100 mg/L
Ethylene glycol	—	>1.5 g/L
Fenfluramine	0.1–0.15 mg/L	>0.2 mg/L
Fluoride	0.5 mg/L	>2 mg/L
Gentamicin	8–12 mg/L	>15 mg/L
Glutethimide	2–4 mg/L	>8 mg/L
Imipramine	0.1–0.3 mg/L	>0.5 mg/L
Indomethacin	0.7–1.3 mg/L	—
Iron	500 mg/L (erythrocytes)	6 mg/L (serum)
Lead	0.05–1.0 mg/L	>1.5 mg/L
Lignocaine	2–5 mg/L	>5.0 mg/L
Lithium	0.8–1.2 mmol/L	>1.5 mmol/L
Meprobamate	5–20 mg/L	>25 mg/L
Mercury (blood)	—	>40 μg/L
Methadone	0.05–1.0 mg/L	>1.0 mg/L
Methaqualone	2–4 mg/L	>5 mg/L
Methsuximide	10–40 mg/L	>40 mg/L
Methanol	—	>100 mg/L
Morphine	0.1–0.5 mg/L	>1.0 mg/L
Nortriptyline	0.05–0.15 mg/L	>0.25 mg/L
Oxazepam	1–2 mg/L	>2 mg/L
Paracetamol	5–25 mg/L	>30 mg/L (see p. 340)
Pethidine	0.2–0.8 mg/L	>2.0 mg/L
Phenacetin	5–25 mg/L	>30 mg/L
Phenylbutazone	50–100 mg/L	>100 mg/L
Phenytoin	10–20 mg/L	>20 mg/L
Procainamide	3–8 mg/L	>10 mg/L
Propranolol	0.025–0.2 mg/L	>8 mg/L
Quinidine	3–5 mg/L	>6 mg/L

Salicylate	150–250 mg/L	>300 mg/L
Sodium valproate	50–100 mg/L	>100 mg/L
Strychnine	—	>2 mg/L
Tobramycin	5–8 mg/L	10–12 mg/L
Tricyclics	50–200 μg/L	>400 μg/L
Warfarin	1–10 mg/L	>10 mg/L

INDEX